Phlebology, Vein Surgery and Ultrasonography

Eric Mowatt-Larssen • Sapan S. Desai
Anahita Dua • Cynthia E.K. Shortell
Editors

Phlebology, Vein Surgery and Ultrasonography

Diagnosis and Management of Venous Disease

Springer

Editors
Eric Mowatt-Larssen
Vein Specialists of Monterey
Monterey, CA
USA

Sapan S. Desai
Department of Surgery
Duke University Medical Center
Durham, NC
USA

Department of Cardiothoracic and Vascular Surgery
University of Texas at Houston Medical School
Houston, TX
USA

Anahita Dua
MSB 5.030
University of Texas-Houston
Houston, TX
USA

Cynthia E.K. Shortell
Department of Vascular Surgery
Duke University Medical Center
Durham, NC
USA

ISBN 978-3-319-01811-9 ISBN 978-3-319-01812-6 (eBook)
DOI 10.1007/978-3-319-01812-6
Springer Cham Heidelberg New York Dordrecht London

Library of Congress Control Number: 2013956742

Printed on acid-free paper

Springer is part of Springer Science+Business Media (www.springer.com)

Foreword

The latter half of the twentieth century saw very little advancement or innovation in the diagnosis and treatment modalities of venous disease. The standard diagnostic testing for deep venous disease, whether for acute or chronic thrombosis or for insufficiency, consisted primarily of venography, with treatment options limited to compression, leg elevation, anticoagulation, and occasionally open surgical intervention. For superficial venous disease, diagnostic testing at that time was limited even more to physical examination, with treatment being standard surgical high ligation and stripping with avulsion phlebectomy and perforator ligation.

Venous disease diagnostics were dramatically improved late in the twentieth century by advances in imaging modalities. The first and most important among these was duplex ultrasound, followed by computerized tomography (CT) and magnetic resonance imaging (MRI). More recently, diagnostic vascular enhancement techniques have made CT and MRI even more useful. We have also been reaping further diagnostic benefits from advancements in ultrasound testing, using intravascular ultrasound (IVUS), for example, to diagnose deep venous disease. While not perfect, duplex ultrasound has become the gold standard for at least the initial diagnostic maneuver for most venous disorders, even including those related to lymphedema and vascular malformations.

These diagnostic advancements have allowed scientific investigators worldwide to gain a clearer understanding of venous disorders and have resulted in truly dramatic changes in the therapeutic realm. We are moving rapidly toward evermore minimally invasive treatments for both deep and superficial venous disorders. An international explosion of interest in venous disease is bringing a wide spectrum of expertise to bear upon our understanding of venous pathophysiology. This has allowed the field to move from one mostly dominated by art and anecdotal science to one based on rigorous investigation and scientific principles. Hugo Partsch describes this as a transition from "eminence-based medicine" to "evidence-based medicine." Such advancements must be very gratifying to the venous practitioners working in the field for the past half century. They certainly are stimulating to those entering the field from other disciplines.

Phlebology, Vein Surgery and Ultrasonography is an excellent description of current thinking regarding venous disorders, but I think of this text as simply a progress report on the journey to greater understanding of venous disorders. By reading this book, you will, I hope, be stimulated to add to this fund of knowledge with scientific investigations of your own or in support of others, with the goal of producing high-quality reports to help us care for the vast number of patients with venous disorders.

Nick Morrison

Preface

Phlebology is in the midst of a revolution brought on by technological advancements. Duplex ultrasound is used before treatments to map reflux and see clots and obstructions in diagnosis, during many procedures to ensure accurate treatments, and used afterward to check technical success and avoidance of complications. Furthermore, because it allows noninvasive monitoring of venous pathology, it has acted much like the invention of the telescope and allowed paradigm-challenging observations about the natural history of reflux. It turns out the understandings of Rima and Trendelenburg from the nineteenth century are incorrect, and reflux often spreads proximally up the great saphenous vein over time. We have not figured out the implications of these findings.

Meanwhile, endovascular techniques have become dominant, even as surgical techniques have continued to improve and advance. Laser ablation, radiofrequency ablation, and chemical ablation (sclerotherapy) compete with high ligation with or without stripping, ambulatory phlebectomy, powered phlebectomy, and subfascial endoscopic perforator surgery. Three-dimensional venography and intravascular ultrasound allow us to diagnose and treat proximal venous problems at ilio-caval and pelvic veins few physicians even considered only 10 years ago.

All this intellectual fervor has led to two new certifications. Physicians who are diplomates of the American Board of Phlebology specialize in venous disease management. Physicians and ultrasonographers can attain certification as a registered phlebology sonographer.

I hope the reader will sense some of the excitement of the birth of this new specialty in this book. The authors come from a wide range of specialties, consistent with the history of phlebology, which has always smartly embraced the diverse perspectives of multiple different medical fields. The faculty is also international, an overt acknowledgement that the work of our international colleagues has been instrumental in moving our understanding of venous disease forward. Finally, ultrasound is integrated into this text, because it is my belief that good ultrasound is essential in providing excellent care for our patients.

Although phlebology is young, venous diseases are common, and the shoulders we stand on are ancient. The high risk of reflux in our species may well be primarily the result of bipedalism, which magnifies the impact of gravity when venous valves fail. Compression is seen in cave paintings from our hunter-gatherer origins from over 5000 years ago. All the ancient cultures who left written records described vein symptoms and treatments. Recent rapid developments in our understanding were only possible through the work of several organizations, such as the International Union of Phlebology, American College of Phlebology, and American and European Venous Forums. Important textbooks were written and edited by giants in the field, such as Craig Feied, Robert Weiss, Helane Fronek, Mitchell Goldman, John Bergan, JJ Guex, and Peter Gloviczki.

This volume would have been impossible without the amazing technical skills of Dr. Sapan Desai. He has already impacted the arena of medical education in profound ways and you will see the fruits of his abilities in the pages which follow. I owe many thanks also to Dr. Cynthia Shortell. Besides her contributions to the editing for this book, she has taught me a tremendous amount over our years of collaboration.

To the reader: please read, challenge, enjoy, and savor!

Monterey, CA, USA Eric Mowatt-Larssen

Contents

Contributors

Ali Azizzadeh, MD Department of Cardiothoracic and Vascular Surgery, University of Texas at Houston Medical School, Houston, TX, USA

Naga Ramesh Chinapuvvula, MD Department of Radiology, University of Texas-Houston, Memorial Hermann Hospital, Houston, TX, USA

Mitchell Cox, MD Department of Surgery, Duke University Medical Center, Durham, NC, USA

Stephanie M. Dentoni, MD, FSVM California Vein and Vascular Institute, Stockton, CA, USA

Sapan S. Desai, MD, PhD, MBA Department of Surgery, Duke University Medical Center, Durham, NC, USA

Department of Cardiothoracic and Vascular Surgery, University of Texas at Houston Medical School, Houston, TX, USA

Craig F. Feied, MD, FACEP, FAAEM, FACPh Department of Emergency Medicine, Georgetown University School of Medicine, Washington, DC, USA

Daniel F. Geersen, MPAP, PA-C Division of Vascular Surgery, Duke University Medical Center, Durham, NC, USA

Sergio Gianesini, MD Vascular Disease Center, University of Ferrara, Ferrara, Italy

David L. Gillespie, MD, RVT, FACS Division of Vascular Surgery, Heart and Vascular Center, Southcoast Health System, Charlton Hospital, Fall River, MA, USA

Department of Surgery, Uniformed Services University of the Health Sciences, F. Edward Hebert School of Medicine, Bethesda, MD, USA

Carlos J. Guevara, MD Division of Vascular and Interventional Radiology, Department of Radiology, Duke University Medical Center, Durham, NC, USA

Jennifer Heller, MD Department of Surgery, Johns Hopkins Vein Centers, Johns Hopkins University, Baltimore, MD, USA

Mark N. Isaacs, MD, FACPh, FAAFP, RPhS Vein Specialists of Northern California, Walnut Creek, CA, USA

Joyce Jackson, RN, MSN, ANP, BC Belmont Aesthetic and Reconstructive Surgery, Chevy Chase, MD, USA

Berman Skin Institute, Palo Alto, CA, USA

Sean Johnston, MD Department of Radiology, University of Texas-Houston, Memorial Hermann Hospital, Houston, TX, USA

David O. Joseph, MD, MS Department of Anesthesia, University of Texas at Houston Medical School, Houston, TX, USA

Darcy M. Kessler, RVT Division of Vascular Surgery, Straub Clinic and Hospital, John A. Burns School of Medicine, Honolulu, HI, USA

Charles Y. Kim, MD Division of Vascular and Interventional Radiology, Duke University Medical Center, Durham, NC, USA

Brian S. Knipp, MD, MC, USN Division of Vascular Surgery, School of Medicine and Dentistry, University of Rochester, Rochester, NY, USA

SreyRam Kuy, MD, MHS Division of Vascular Surgery, Medical College of Wisconsin, Milwaukee, WI, USA

James Laredo, MD, PhD, FACS, RVT, RPVI Department of Surgery, Division of Vascular Surgery, George Washington University Medical Center, Washington, DC, USA

Byung Boong Lee, MD, PhD, FACS George Washington University Medical Center, Washington, DC, USA

Jovan N. Markovic, MD Department of Surgery, Duke University Medical Center, Durham, NC, USA

Elna M. Masuda, MD Division of Vascular Surgery, Straub Clinic and Hospital, John A. Burns School of Medicine, Honolulu, HI, USA

Robert B. McLafferty, MD, FACS, RVT Division of Vascular Surgery, Department of Surgery, Southern Illinois University, School of Medicine, Springfield, IL, USA

Jason McMaster, MD Obstetrics and Gynecology, Medical College of Wisconsin, Milwaukee, WI, USA

Frank R. Miele, MSEE Pegasus Lectures, Inc., Forney, TX, USA

Eugene W. Moretti, MD, MHSc. Department of Anesthesiology, Duke University Medical Center, Durham, NC, USA

Nick Morrison, MD, FACPh, FACS, RPhS Morrison Vein Institute, Scottsdale, AZ, USA

Eric Mowatt-Larssen, MD, FACPh, RPhS Vein Specialists of Monterey, Monterey, CA, USA

Cary Munschauer, BA Department of Surgery, The Venous Institute of Buffalo, Buffalo, NY, USA

Jessica L. Myers, MD Department of Anesthesiology, Duke University Medical Center, Durham, NC, USA

Diana L. Neuhardt, RVT, RPhS CompuDiagnostics, Inc., Phoenix, AZ, USA

Thomas L. Ortel, MD, PhD Departments of Medicine and Pathology, Duke University Medical Center, Durham, NC, USA

Marc A. Passman, MD Section of Vascular Surgery and Endovascular Therapy, University of Alabama at Birmingham, Birmingham, AL, USA

Elaheh Rahbar, PhD Department of Surgery, Center for Translational Injury Research, University of Texas Medical School at Houston, Houston, TX, USA

Mohammad Hossein Rahbar, PhD Department of Epidemology and Biostatistics, Human Genetic and Environmental Sciences, University of Texas School of Public Health at Houston, Houston, TX, USA

Marlin W. Schul, MD, MBA, RVT, FACPh Venous and Lymphatic Medicine, Lafayette Regional Vein and Laser Center, A division of Unity Healthcare, LLC, Lafayette, IN, USA

Cynthia K. Shortell, MD, FACS Department of Vascular Surgery, Duke University Medical Center, Durham, NC, USA

Julianne Stoughton, MD, FACS Department of Vascular Surgery, Massachusetts General Hospital, Boston, MA, USA

Michael A. Vasquez, MD, FACS, RVT SUNY Buffalo Department of Surgery, The Venous Institute of Buffalo, Buffalo, NY, USA

Paolo Zamboni, MD Vascular Disease Center, University of Ferrara, Ferrara, Italy

Joseph A. Zygmunt Jr., RVT, RPhS Covidien Vascular Therapies, Global Clinical Education, San Jose, CA, USA

Part I

Basic Sciences

Anatomy

1

Brian S. Knipp and David L. Gillespie

Contents

Abstract

Embryology and Development of the Venous System

This chapter focuses on the key embryology, anatomy, and histology of the venous system. The embryology and development of the venous system are intimately related. In normal embryologic development of the central venous system, venous channels arise within the fourth week with completion by the seventh to eighth week of development. The extremity venous system begins with primitive vascular channels developing in the limb during the third week of gestation. The veins of the foot along with the great and small saphenous system, auxiliary superficial venous systems, deep venous system, and perforators constitute the anatomic makeup of the lower limb.

B.S. Knipp, MD, MC, USN
Division of Vascular Surgery,
School of Medicine and Dentistry,
University of Rochester, Rochester, NY, USA
e-mail: brian_knipp@urmc.rochester.edu

D.L. Gillespie, MD, RVT, FACS (✉)
Division of Vascular Surgery,
Heart and Vascular Center,
Southcoast Health System,
Charlton Hospital, Fall River, MA 02720, USA

Department of Surgery, Uniformed Services
University of the Health Sciences,
F. Edward Hebert School of Medicine,
Bethesda, MD 20854, USA
e-mail: david_gillespie@urmc.rochester.edu

1.1 The Central Venous System

In normal embryologic development, venous channels arise within the fourth week. At this point, paired vascular channels run along the dorsum of the developing embryo and are joined in the middle forming a rough "H" shape.

The superior-most vessels, known as the anterior cardinal veins, are the precursors of the superior vena caval system. The cranial aspects of these vessels persist as the internal jugular veins. Venous buds from the upper extremities develop

E. Mowatt-Larssen et al. (eds.), *Phlebology, Vein Surgery and Ultrasonography*,
DOI 10.1007/978-3-319-01812-6_1, © Springer International Publishing Switzerland 2014

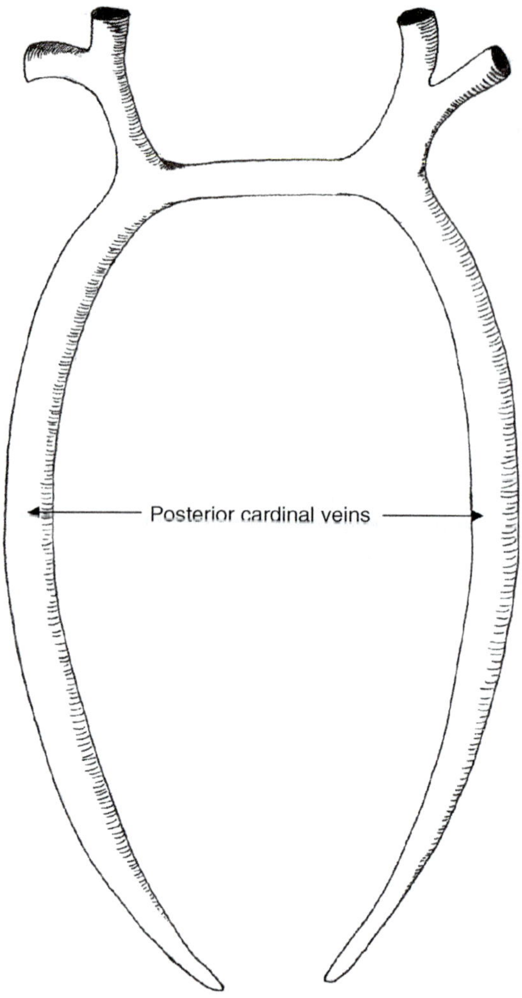

Fig. 1.1 In the fourth week of embryologic development, paired vascular channels, known as the anterior and posterior cardinal veins, arise and join in the midline at the sinus venosus, the site of development of the cardiac system

anastomoses to the anterior cardinal system and give rise to the subclavian and brachiocephalic veins. The inferior vessels are known as the posterior cardinal veins and serve as the precursors to the inferior vena cava (IVC) and iliac venous system. At the midpoint of the channels, there is a lateral connection known as the sinus venosus, which represents the developing cardiac system. The anterior cardinal veins, cranial to the sinus venosus, are the precursors of the superior vena cava (SVC) and the venous system draining the head and upper extremities (Fig. 1.1).

Starting in the sixth week of development, the posterior cardinal veins begin to regress in the middle, whereas the distal posterior cardinal veins develop a weblike anastomosis. At the cranial extent of the posterior cardinal veins, just inferior to the sinus venosus, a new pair of venous channels arises, known as the subcardinal veins, lying anteromedial to the posterior cardinal veins. These vessels join near the mesonephric to form a midline anastomosis, known as the preaortic intersubcardinal anastomosis. In addition, at this point, the primitive hepatic venous system begins to develop as the vitelline veins, which drain the yolk sac, coalesce into the portal venous system. Near the connection with the right subcardinal vein, this system is interrupted by hepatic sinusoids, the site of the developing liver parenchyma. These sinusoids are in turn drained by the efferent venae revehentes, which combine to form the left and right hepatic veins, which drain into the right atrium. Downward extension of the venae revehentes anastomoses with the developing inferior vena cava (Fig. 1.2).

In the seventh week of embryologic development, the posterior cardinal veins have nearly completely regressed with the exception of the cranial and caudal extent, the latter of which has joined to form the iliac venous bifurcation. The mesonephric anastomosis of the subcardinal veins develops into the aortic collar; the usual developmental pattern is regression of the retroaortic component, leaving a preaortic left renal vein. The failure of the retroaortic segment to regress leads to a circumaortic or retroaortic left renal vein, depending on the persistence or regression of the preaortic segment. The subcardinal vein regresses at this point in all areas except for the suprarenal IVC. A new pair of venous channels arises at this time: the supracardinal veins. The right supracardinal vein anastomoses with the right subcardinal vein to become the renal segment of the vena cava and persists caudally as the postrenal segment until it anastomoses with the posterior cardinal vein remnant at the iliac venous bifurcation (Fig. 1.3).

Finally, the cranial components of the supracardinal veins persist as the azygous and hemiazygous

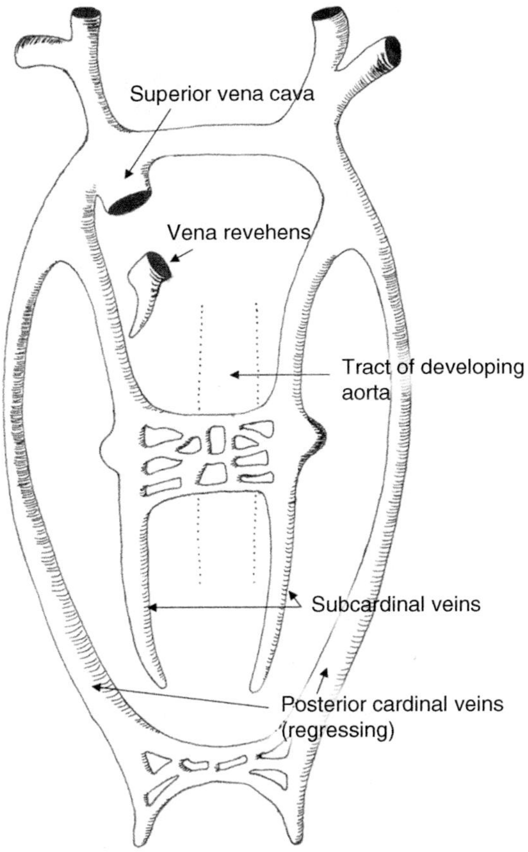

Fig. 1.2 In the sixth week of embryologic development, the posterior cardinal veins begin to regress in their midpoint and join distally to form the future iliac venous bifurcation. The subcardinal veins develop and anastomose in the perinephric region. The venae revehentes develop as an outflow tract for the portal venous circulation and hepatic sinusoids, draining into the right atrium and forming an inferior anastomosis with the developing inferior vena cava

systems. The completed development of the central venous system is shown in Fig. 1.4.

1.2 The Extremity Venous System

Primitive vascular channels occur in the limb during the third week of gestation. Initially, only a capillary network is present. This coalesces into larger plexuses and eventually, by the end of the third week, into large channels with the appearance of veins, arteries, and lymphatics [1].

One of the fundamental principles of extremity vascular development is that the vasculature tends to parallel major neural structures as the axons and Schwann cells secrete vascular endothelial growth factor, attracting vascular growth and encouraging differentiation [2]. In the leg, the sciatic nerve induces development of the deep venous plexus and, below the knee, the small saphenous vein (SSV). The femoral nerve guides the development of the great saphenous vein (GSV). Alterations in the dominance and reabsorption of primitive venous channels can lead to venous anomalies such as an axiofemoral trunk (predominance of the profunda femoris vein in the thigh and distal anastomosis to the proximal popliteal vein; the femoral vein is a small collateral channel) or bifidity of the femoral vein [3].

1.3 Histology of the Vein Wall

There are three layers to the vein wall, just as in the arterial system, namely, intima, media, and adventitia. However, there is a variance in proportion in the venous system. The intima is generally a single layer of cells lying on a thin connective tissue skeleton. In the GSV, there is a relatively thick media which resists dilatation. However, tributary vessels tend to be quite fragile with minimal media. Deep veins tend to have fewer smooth muscle cells and a greater proportion of connective tissue.

1.4 Anatomy of the Lower Extremity Venous System

1.4.1 Veins of the Foot

In the original *Terminologia Anatomica* description, all the venous structures of the foot were classified as superficial. However, in the latest interdisciplinary consensus conference on nomenclature, while the dorsal venous drainage of the foot is primarily superficial in its named structures, the plantar venous drainage is considered a deep venous system [4].

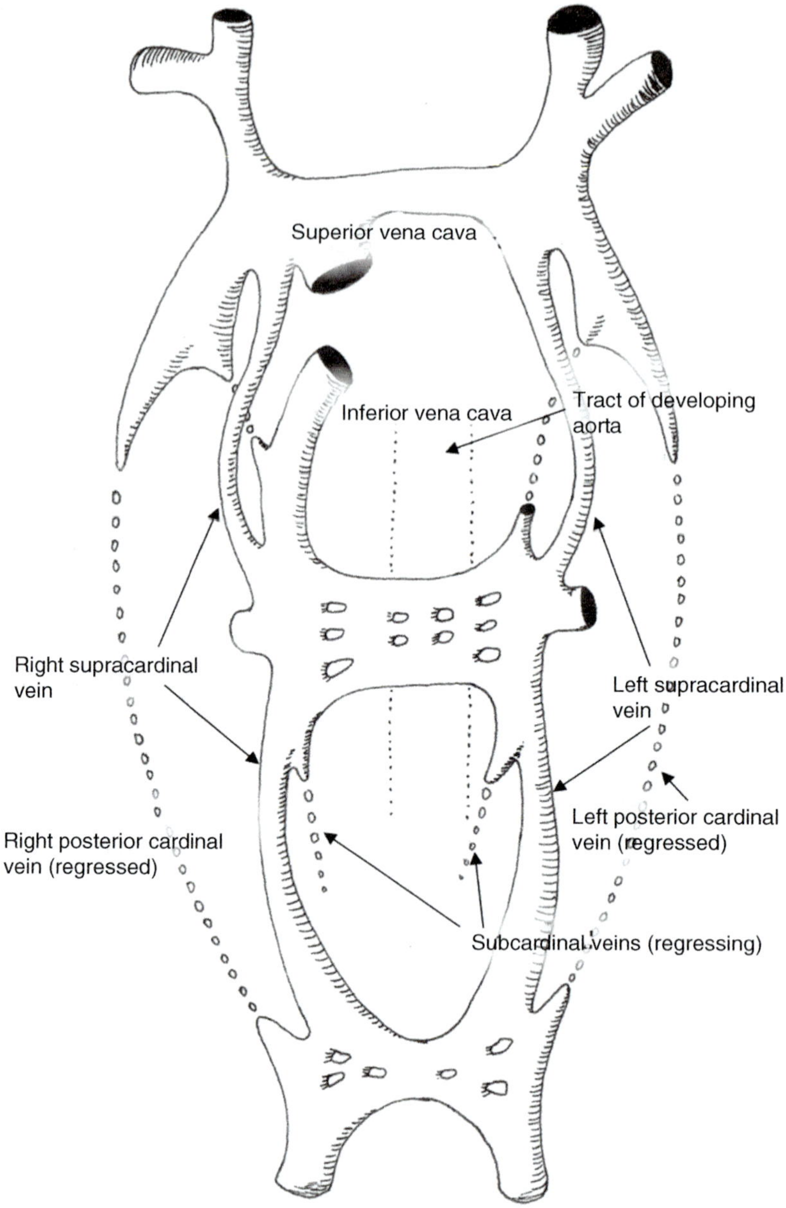

Fig. 1.3 In the seventh week of embryologic development, the posterior cardinal veins have regressed completely aside from the caudal extent forming the iliac bifurcation. The mesonephric anastomosis of the subcardinal veins develops into the renal segment of the IVC and the left and right renal vein; the cranial extent of the right subcardinal vein persists as the suprarenal IVC. The supracardinal veins develop and form the infrarenal segment of the IVC as well as contribute to the renal segment

The venous drainage of the dorsal surface of the foot can be divided into a well-defined superficial system and an ill-defined deep system. The superficial system is comprised of a discrete dorsal venous arch which gives rise to the medial and lateral marginal veins, which drain into the great saphenous vein and the small saphenous vein, respectively. The dorsal deep venous system of the foot consists of the venae comitantes of the dorsalis pedis artery, which join to form the pedal vein, continuing as the anterior tibial veins. The anterior tibial veins enter the anterior compartment of the leg and run cephalad along the course of the anterior tibial artery. Perforating veins connect these two systems [4, 5] (Fig. 1.5).

On the plantar surface, the anatomy is deep system dominant due to the weight-bearing nature of the foot. The superficial veins tend to be ill-defined. The plantar venous network consists of the deep plantar arch which connects the

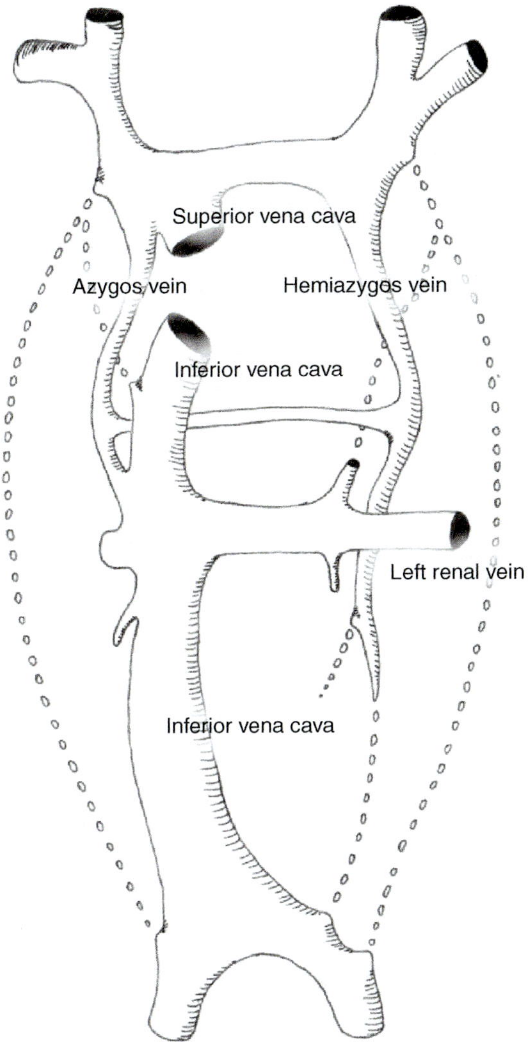

Fig. 1.4 In the completed central venous system, the anterior cardinal veins have developed into the SVC and brachiocephalic venous system. The subcardinal system has developed into the suprarenal and renal segment of the IVC as well as the left and right renal vein. The supracardinal system has developed into the infrarenal IVC as well as the azygous and hemiazygous systems. And the vitelline veins have coalesced to form the portal venous system which drains through the developing liver into the hepatic veins which arise from the venae revehentes

medial and lateral plantar veins. These veins join to form the posterior tibial veins which then pass posterior to the medial malleolus and track in a cephalad direction along the posterior tibial artery. Perforators exist along the medial and lateral foot, but not appreciably in the plantar surface. Small accessory veins may drain the surface of the forefoot and flow directly into the peroneal or posterior tibial veins [4, 5] (Fig. 1.6).

1.4.2 Great Saphenous System

The great saphenous vein (GSV) system begins in the dorsal venous arch of the foot, which drains medially through the medial marginal vein to enter the caudal GSV. This then ascends anterior to the medial malleolus of the ankle, crosses the tibia, and continues to ascend the medial calf. In the distal two-thirds of the calf, this vein is intimately associated with the saphenous nerve, which supplies cutaneous innervation to the medial calf. The GSV then crosses the medial surface of the knee and continues cranially along the medial thigh to enter the deep system at the saphenofemoral junction, passing through the fossa ovalis located 3 cm inferior and 3 cm lateral to the pubic tubercle (Fig. 1.7).

In their study of 1,400 venous studies, Kupinski et al. documented the following size ranges for the superficial venous system: 2.2–10.0 mm in the proximal thigh, 1.5–8.8 mm in the distal thigh, 1.2–7.3 mm in the proximal calf, and 1.0–5.5 mm in the distal calf [6].

Several tributaries can enter the vein along its length. In the calf, both the anterior and posterior accessory GSV of the calf may be present, draining the lateral and posteromedial calf, respectively. Above the knee, the anterior accessory GSV of the thigh, if present, drains the lateral thigh and may provide a communication between the lateral superficial venous plexus and the GSV system. The posterior accessory GSV of the thigh drains the medial thigh and runs posterior to the GSV. There may also be an anterior and/or a posterior thigh circumflex vein draining the lateral and medial thigh, respectively, inferior to the accessory saphenous veins. The key differentiation between the actual GSV and accessory or tributary vessels is the saphenous fascial envelope, which runs along the entire length of the GSV. This separate saphenous compartment is bounded superficially by

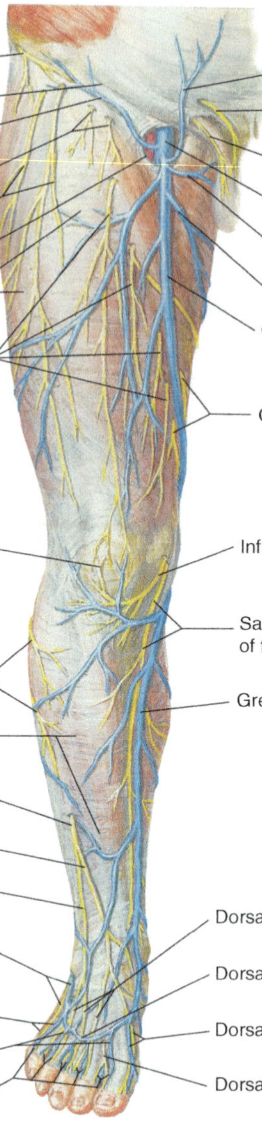

Fig. 1.5 The superficial venous drainage of the dorsal foot. The primary drainage is through the dorsal venous arch, which connects to the great saphenous vein via the medial marginal vein and to the small saphenous vein via the lateral marginal vein. Perforators in the dorsal, medial, and lateral positions connect this system to the dorsal deep venous system (Copyright Elsevier. Used with permission)

hyperechoic saphenous fascia and deeply by the muscular fascia and contains the saphenous veins, nerves, and small arteries. Saphenous tributaries and accessory, collateral, and communicating veins lie external to this compartment [4, 7] (Fig. 1.8). This fascial compartment has been described as an "Egyptian eye" on ultrasonographic examination, providing a reproducible sign useful for identification [8].

The GSV has a great degree of variability. Kupinski et al. reviewed over 1,400 evaluations in 1,060 patients with duplex ultrasonography. The indication for the study was infrainguinal bypass in 86 % and coronary artery bypass in 14 % [6]. The standard arrangement most commonly described in anatomy textbooks is a single medial-dominant vein, and a single anterior-dominant vein in the calf occurs in 38–55 % of

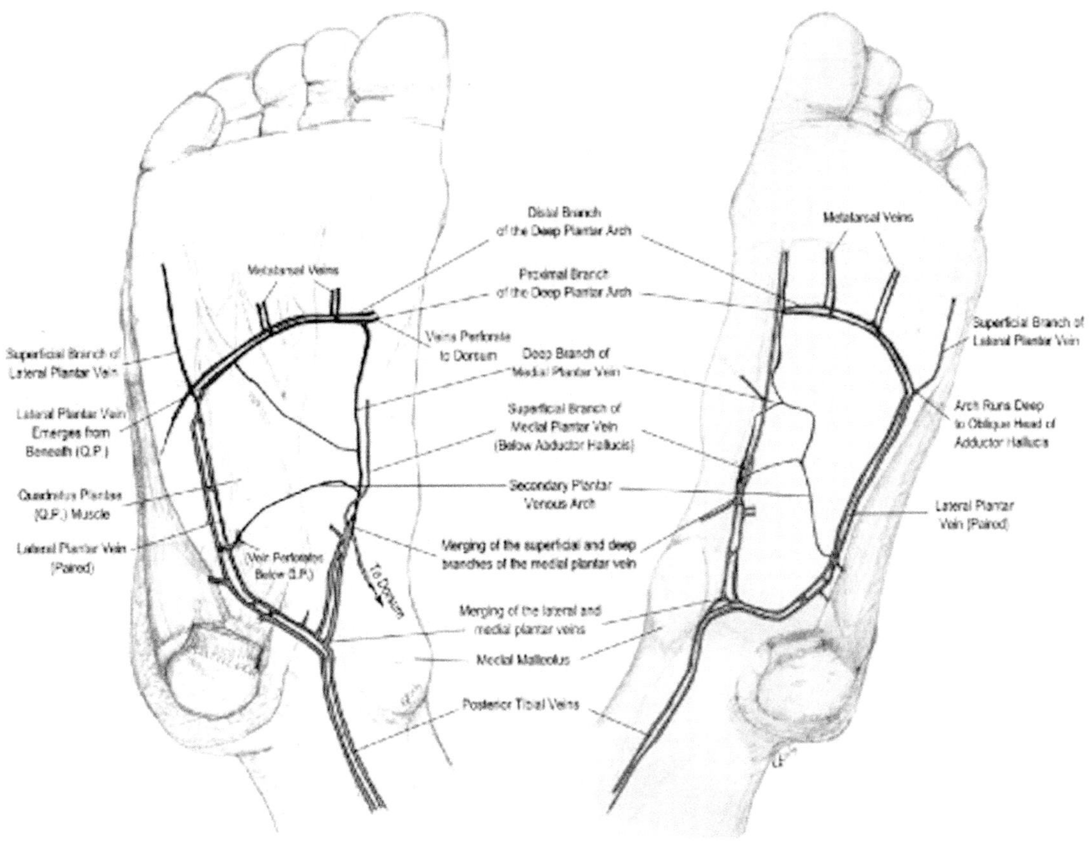

Fig. 1.6 The deep plantar venous system consists of the deep plantar arch, which drains the metatarsal veins and carries blood proximally via the medial and lateral plantar veins. These veins then join at the posterior medial malleolus to form the posterior tibial veins. Perforating veins enter at the medial and lateral plantar veins

limbs studied [6, 9]. Variations in this system occur in both the thigh and the calf. In the thigh, there are five primary arrangements described by Kupinski: a single medial-dominant system (59 %), a branching double system (18 %), a complete double system (8 %), a single system with a closed loop (7 %), and a single lateral-dominant system (8 %). In less than 1 %, a more complex arrangement was found. In the calf, there were four major arrangements: single vessel anterior-dominant (58 %), double vessel anterior-dominant (27 %), double vessel posterior-dominant (8 %), and single vessel posterior-dominant (7 %). Rare cases of triple systems or complex systems below the knee were seen in less than 1 % of cases. Awareness of these variations is important when attempting to identify the great saphenous vein, as incorrect identification can lead to ineffective surgical treatment of venous disease or harvest of insufficient conduit for arterial bypass [6].

The saphenofemoral junction (SFJ), also known as the confluence, or "crosse" in a historical sense, is the entry point of the GSV to the deep system by way of the fossa ovalis. There is a terminal valve located within 1–2 mm of the anastomosis of the GSV with the common femoral vein. Approximately 80 % of individuals will also have another valve approximately 2 cm distal to this anastomosis. Between these valves, the GSV receives inflow from the anterior and posterior accessory GSVs, which are considered the "distal" veins, as their drainage pattern is distal to the SFJ. By similar logic, the "proximal" veins draining the anterior superficial abdominal wall, which include the superficial circumflex iliac vein, the superficial epigastric vein, and the external pudendal vein, also drain into the SFJ [8].

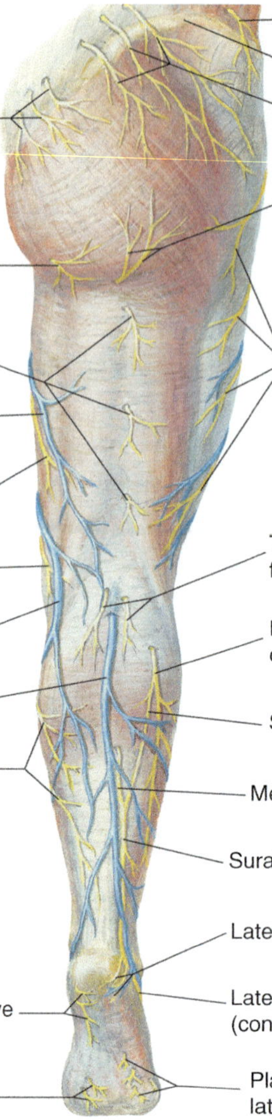

Fig. 1.7 The great saphenous vein arises from the medial marginal vein as it passes anterior to the medial malleolus at the ankle. It rises in the calf region just medial to the tibial edge, in most cases. As it approaches the knee, it generally receives contributions from a posterior and/or anterior accessory saphenous vein. It then crosses the medial surface of the knee and runs along the medial thigh. As it nears the groin, it often is joined by accessory anterior and/or posterior saphenous veins. At the level of the saphenofemoral junction, additional tributaries such as the superficial epigastric, superficial circumflex iliac, and the external pudendal veins join as it then enters the common femoral vein (Copyright Elsevier. Used with permission)

1.4.3 Small Saphenous System

The course of the small saphenous vein (SSV) is quite consistent, running along the posterior aspect of the calf. The SSV originates via the lateral marginal branch of the dorsal venous arch and passes anterior to the lateral malleolus. It runs in a dorsal midline subcutaneous plane along the posterior calf and enters the fascia between the heads of the gastrocnemius muscle. In most cases the SSV enters the deep system approximately 5 cm cephalad to the knee crease by draining into the popliteal vein. In 22 % of cases, however, the SSV continues above the

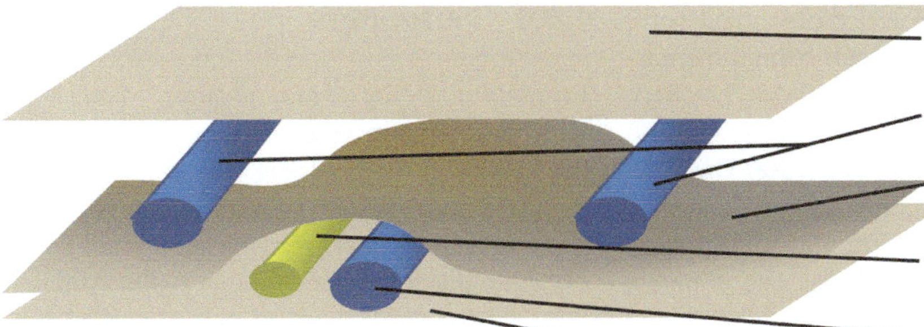

Fig. 1.8 The saphenous compartment is bound superficially by the saphenous fascia and deeply by the muscular fascia. Contained within are the saphenous veins and saphenous nerve. The saphenous tributary vein is outside this compartment

knee, terminating in the SFV. The mean diameter of the SSV is 3.0±0.17 mm proximally and 2.7±0.11 mm distally [6].

In the caudal two-thirds of the SSV, the sural nerve is in close approximation to the vein, a clinically relevant issue in cases of SSV ablations where the thermal energy used to ablate the vein can lead to nerve damage and disabling neuropathic pain in some patients.

1.4.4 Auxiliary Superficial Venous Systems

The lateral thigh and leg superficial venous network forms a plexus known as the lateral venous system. There is a great deal of variability in this system. It tends to drain into the GSV and SSV systems through communicating veins or into the deep venous network through perforating veins.

In many patients, a branch of the SSV system, known as the cranial extension of the SSV, continues cephalad to the anastomosis with the popliteal vein, penetrating the fascia back into the superficial system. Frequently, this vein will then drain via the intersaphenous vein (also known as the vein of Giacomini) via a posteromedial route into the GSV system. Alternatively, this cranial extension of the SSV may terminate in a superficial venous communicating vein or a perforating vein or veins; this arrangement is not the classically described vein of Giacomini.

1.4.5 Deep Venous System

As the deep venous system leaves the foot, the medial and lateral plantar veins coalesce into the paired posterior tibial veins which run along the course of the posterior tibial artery. These veins pass behind the medial malleolus and enter the posterior deep space, passing between the flexor digitorum longus and the tibialis posterior muscles and run under the deep posterior space fascia to provide the primary venous drainage of this compartment. At their cephalad extent, they pass through the soleus muscle close to its bony origin to continue as the popliteal vein. Some of the most clinically important perforator veins in the leg, the medial calf perforators, drain into the posterior tibial veins, draining the superficial posterior compartment. The peroneal veins, also paired structures intimately associated with the peroneal artery, originate in the distal third of the calf and ascend, also, in the deep posterior space deep to the flexor hallucis longus muscle. These veins receive peroneal perforator veins, as well as several large veins from the soleus. The anterior tibial paired veins originate from the venae comitantes of the dorsalis pedis artery via the pedal vein and enter the anterior compartment of the leg, running behind the tibialis anterior and the extensor hallucis longus muscles on top of the interosseous membrane along the course of the anterior tibial artery.

The anterior tibial, posterior tibial, and peroneal veins join in the upper calf behind the gastrocnemius to form the popliteal vein. The SSV enters the popliteal vein in most cases approximately 5 cm above the popliteal crease. The other major tributaries of the popliteal system are the gastrocnemius veins which form a major portion of the calf muscle pump system. The popliteal vein is often duplicated in segments of its length and forms a network around the popliteal artery. As the popliteal vein rises in the leg and passes through the adductor ("Hunter's") hiatus, it becomes known as the femoral vein. This vein was previously labeled the "superficial femoral" vein, but due to confusion by some practitioners about its nature as a part of the deep system and the need to anticoagulate patients with thrombosis of this segment, the recent consensus committee on nomenclature has changed the name of the structure. This vessel starts out lateral to the femoral artery at the caudal extent of the adductor canal and then passes medial to the artery as it courses cranially. It is joined by the profunda femoris vein to form the common femoral vein approximately 9 cm below the inguinal ligament. The profunda femoris vein drains the thigh by providing deep femoral communicating veins which run along the perforating arteries of the profunda femoris artery (PFA). These are *not* perforators in the venous sense as they do not connect the deep and superficial systems; they are venae comitantes of the arterial perforating branches of the PFA. In 84 % of cases, the distal profunda femoris vein forms an anastomosis with the femoral or popliteal vein which forms a collateral pathway for drainage in case of proximal thrombosis. The common femoral vein receives the GSV system tributaries (including the accessory saphenous veins, the superficial epigastric vein, and the external pudendal vein) via the saphenofemoral junction (Fig. 1.9). It also receives the medial and lateral circumflex femoral veins. These vessels often form important collateral routes in cases of iliofemoral thrombotic obstruction by anastomosing proximally to the iliac veins. At the inguinal ligament, the common femoral vein becomes the external iliac vein.

1.4.6 Perforators

In addition to the communication of the GSV with the common femoral vein at the SFJ and the SSV with the popliteal vein at the saphenopopliteal junction (SPJ), there are numerous perforating veins which provide additional routes of communication from the superficial system to the deep system. These vessels generally have unidirectional valves and are generally thought to contribute to chronic venous insufficiency in cases of incompetence of the valve, although this has never been scientifically established [10–12]. There are two primary subclassifications of perforators: direct perforators which connect superficial veins directly to the deep system (e.g., the GSV to the posterior tibial veins) and indirect perforators which connect superficial veins to intramuscular venous sinuses.

There are a large number of perforator veins in the lower extremity, over 150 in most limbs. There has been a shift in nomenclature from eponymous terminology (e.g., Cockett perforators, the Sherman perforator) to a topographic classification (Fig. 1.10). In the foot, there are perforators in the dorsal, lateral, medial, and plantar surfaces. At the ankle level, there are medial, lateral, and anterior perforators.

In the calf, the medial perforators are felt by many investigators to be particularly significant in that reflux in these vessels is often associated with significant venous ulceration. The medial calf perforators are subdivided into two groups: the paratibial perforators connect the GSV to the posterior tibial veins, whereas the posterior tibial perforators connect the posterior accessory saphenous vein of the calf to the posterior tibial veins (the well-described Cockett perforators). In a study of 40 cadaver limbs, an average of 13.8 perforators were identified in the medial calf. Fifty-two percent of these vessels were direct, 41 % were indirect, and 7 % were undetermined. Two primary groups were identified in the distal leg, located 7–9 and 10–12 cm, respectively, from the inferior edge of the medial malleolus. These

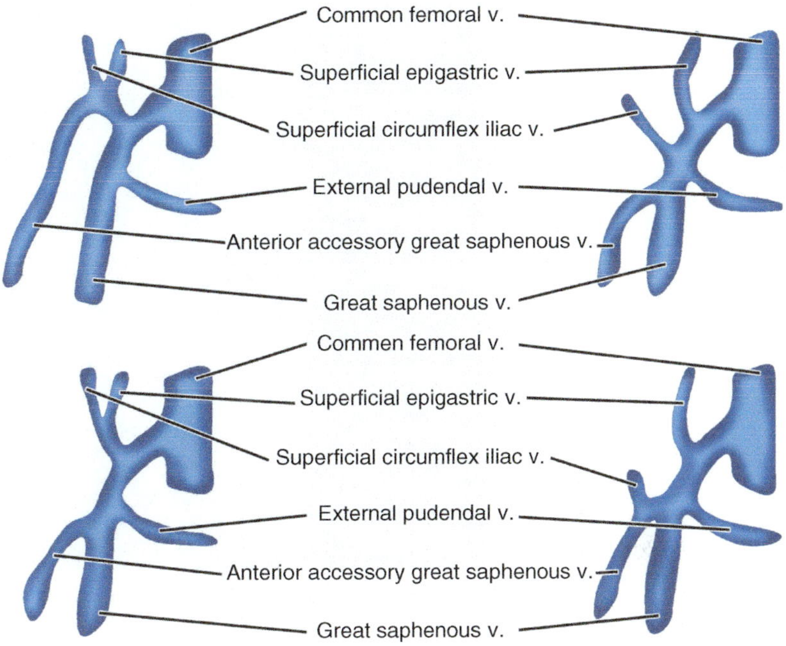

Fig. 1.9 Variation in anatomy of the sapheno-femoral junction (Copyright Surgisphere Corporation. Used with permission)

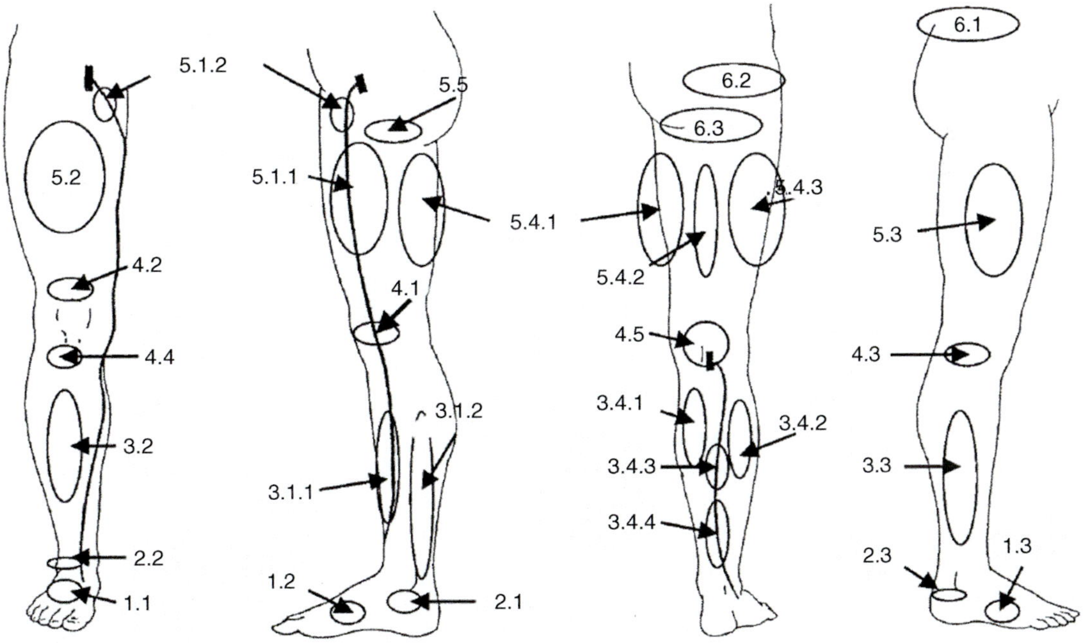

Fig. 1.10 Schematic representation of the topography of the main groups of perforating veins (PVs). Foot PVs: *1.1* dorsal foot PV, *1.2* medial foot PV, *1.3* lateral foot PV. Ankle PVs: *2.1* medial ankle PV, *2.2* anterior ankle PV, *2.3* lateral ankle PV. Leg PVs: *3.1.1* paratibial PV, *3.1.2* posterior tibial PV, *3.2* anterior leg PV, *3.3* lateral leg PIT, *3.4.1* medial gastrocnemius PV, *3.4.2* lateral gastrocnemius PV, *3.4.3* intergemellar PV, *3.4.4* para-achillean PV. Knee PVs: *4.1* medial knee PV, *4.2* suprapatellar PV, *4.3* lateral knee PV, *4.4* infrapatellar PV, *4.5* popliteal fossa PV. Thigh PVs: *5.1.1* PV of the femoral canal, *5.1.2* inguinal PV, *5.2* anterior thigh PV, *5.3* lateral thigh PV, *5.4.1* posteromedial thigh PV: *5.4.2* sciatic PV, *5.4.3* posterolateral thigh PV, *5.5* pudendal PV. Gluteal PVs: *6.1* superior gluteal PV, *6.2* midgluteal PV, *6.3* lower gluteal PV (Reproduced from Caggiati et al. [4] with permission)

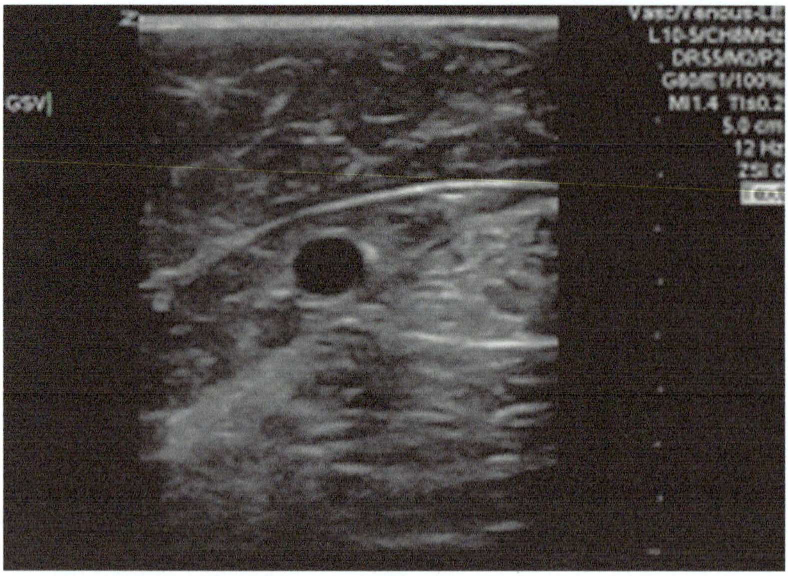

Fig. 1.11 An example of the fascial sheath of the GSV

perforators generally lie within what has been described as the "venous triangle," the space defined by the subcutaneous tibial border anteriorly, the anterior border of the soleus posteriorly, and the flexor retinaculum inferiorly [10]. Proximally, the paratibial perforators were identified in three groups located within 1 cm of the lateral tibial edge: 18–22, 23–27, and 28–32 cm from the lower edge of the medial malleolus [11].

Lateral calf perforators were discretely studied by de Rijcke et al. in a series of 16 limbs in 12 cadavers. They found an average of 22 perforating veins in the lateral calf. Over half of these veins (54 %) were less than 1 mm in diameter, 35 % were 1–2 mm in diameter, and 11 % were greater than 2 mm in diameter. Most of the perforating veins (69 %) were unrelated to the SSV; those that had an association with the SSV tended to be greater than 2 mm in diameter. Perforators unrelated to the SSV tend to lie along the intermuscular septum between the anterior and lateral or the lateral and superficial posterior compartments [12].

Other leg perforators are the anterior leg perforators and the posterior leg perforators, which are subdivided into the medial gastrocnemius, lateral gastrocnemius, intergemellar, and the para-Achillean perforators. Perforators in the knee region are divided into medial, lateral, suprapatellar, infrapatellar, and popliteal fossa perforators. In the thigh, the perforators are divided into perforating veins of the femoral canal, inguinal, anterior thigh, lateral thigh, posteromedial thigh, sciatic, posterolateral thigh, and pudendal perforators. Finally, gluteal perforators are divided into superior, midgluteal, and lower gluteal perforators.

1.4.7 Fascial Compartments

There are four discrete levels of fascial compartments in the lower extremity. The most superficial has been termed the epifascial layer. This layer, which consists of the subcutaneous tissues to the depth of the perimuscular fascia, contains all of the superficial venous vessels with the exception of the saphenous veins. A separate saphenous sheath, comprised superficially of the saphenous fascia and deep by the perimuscular fascia, surrounds the saphenous system and aids in the differentiation of this vein from the rest of the superficial system (Fig. 1.11).

The other two compartments exist below the fascia. The large vessels of the deep venous system run in the intermuscular regions, along the named arterial vessels. The other major compartment is the intramuscular veins of the calf muscle pump, such as the gastrocnemius and soleal veins.

1.4.8 Calf Muscle Venous Anatomy

The venous drainage of the gastrocnemius and the soleus together constitute the calf muscle pump, a physiologic structure thought to augment venous outflow from the leg. Blood initially flows into the muscle from superficial veins through indirect perforators. These vessels join with blood flow from the muscle's postcapillary network to empty into high-capacitance venous sinuses, thin-walled channels deep within the muscle bellies. These sinuses then coalesce into primary outflow channels, the gastrocnemius and soleal veins. Whereas the sinuses have no valves, there are multiple valves in the gastrocnemius and soleal veins. As the calf muscles contract, blood is compressed from the venous sinuses into the trunk veins and into the deep veins; the soleal veins drain into the posterior tibial and peroneal veins, and the gastrocnemius veins drain primarily into the popliteal vein, although they occasionally drain to the posterior tibial, peroneal, or tibioperoneal truncal veins. Aragao et al. presented an anatomic study of 40 cadaver limbs. They identified a mean of 4.6 veins per gastrocnemius muscle head and 1.2 main trunks per muscle head. In their series, 87 % of the main trunks emptied into the popliteal vein. They classified four anatomic arrangements for the gastrocnemius complex. The most common arrangement was characterized by veins emerging from each gastrocnemius head and draining into an axial venous trunk which then became the main trunk, emptying into the popliteal vein. A second type of venous drainage included greater ramifications, again coalescing into main trunks prior to entry into the popliteal vein. The third type was characterized by multiple veins joining as axial trunks which then entered the deep system directly. Finally, veins emerging directly from the muscle and entering the deep system without converting to trunks were the final described type [13] (Fig. 1.12).

1.4.9 Valves

Valves of the lower extremity venous system were described in detail by Calotă et al. They define five components to the valvular segment: the valvular insertion ring, the entrance orifice, the valvular opening, the exit orifice, and the valvular sinus [14]. Valves are bicuspid structures ensuring unidirectional flow of blood out of the leg.

The location and number of valves in the lower extremity venous system vary significantly, but there do tend to be several patterns. In terms of the superficial system, the SSV has numerous valves, between 4 and 13 in most cases. The GSV ranges from 14 to 25 valves. They function to secure unidirectional flow of blood toward the heart. Tributaries to the superficial system will often also have valves, which orient blood flow from the SSV system toward the GSV system.

In the deep venous system, valves are also frequent and predominate in the distal aspects of the extremity. In the foot and tibial veins, valves tend to occur every 2 cm. They become much less frequent starting at the popliteal vein; only one to two valves occur on average in the popliteal and distal femoral vein. The proximal femoral vein generally has three or more valves, with one usually being distal to the profunda femoris vein takeoff. The common femoral has one valve in most patients and a second valve above the confluence with the GSV in two-thirds of patients. The iliocaval system is valveless [15].

Disclaimer The views expressed in this chapter are those of the author and do not necessarily reflect the official policy or position of the Department of the Navy, Department of Defense, nor the US Government.

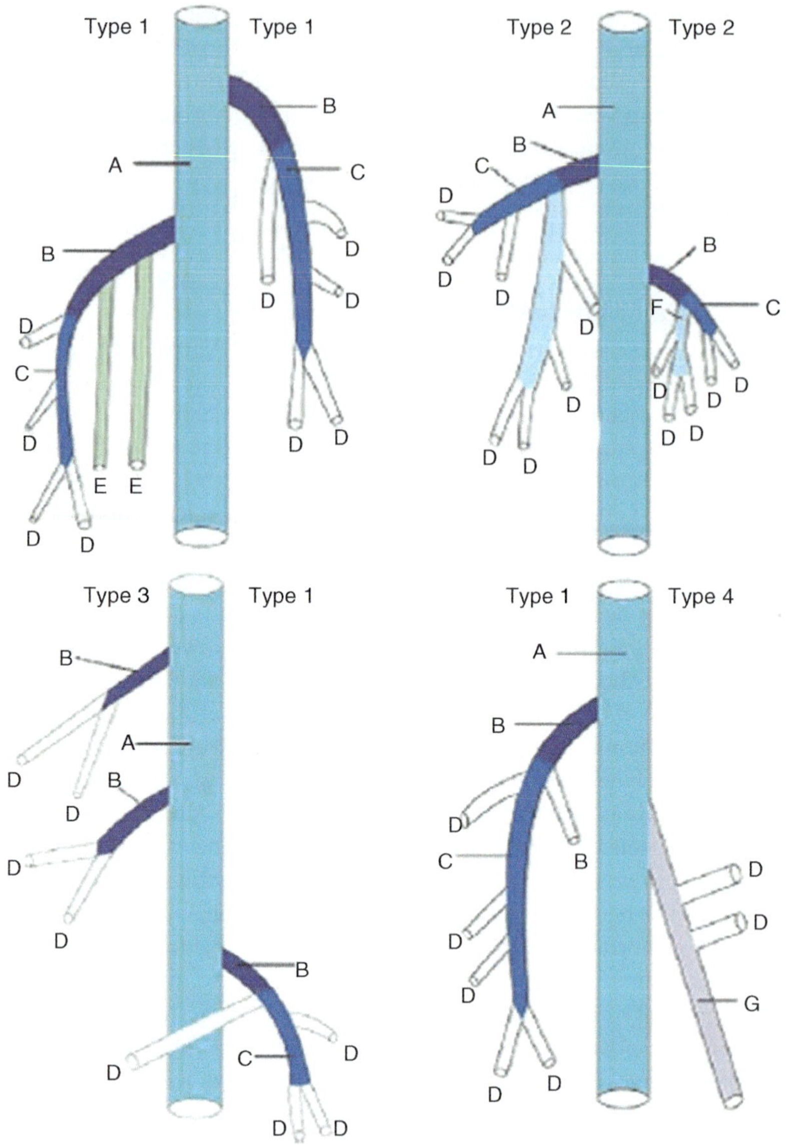

Fig. 1.12 Diagram showing the distribution of gastrocnemius encilia network types 1, 2, 3 and 4. *A* popliteal vein, *B* mairt gashocnernius venous trunk, *C* axial gastroimemilis venous trunk, *D* gastroirnemiusveins, *E* soleal veins, *F* small aphennus vein,, *G* collaleral gastmenemius venous trunk (Reproduced from Aragão et al. [13], with permission)

References

1. Belov S. Anatomopathological classification of congenital vascular defects. Semin Vasc Surg. 1993;6(4): 219–24.
2. Risau W. Mechanisms of angiogenesi. Nature. 1997;386(6626):671–4. doi:10.1038/386671a0.
3. Uhl JF, Gillot C, Chahim M. Anatomical variations of the femoral vein. J Vasc Surg. 2010;52(3):714–9. doi:10.1016/j.jvs.2010.04.014. Elsevier Inc.
4. Caggiati A, Bergan JJ, Gloviczki P, Jantet G, Wendell-Smith CP, Partsch H, International Interdisciplinary Consensus Committee on Venous Anatomical Terminology. Nomenclature of the veins of the lower limbs: an international interdisciplinary consensus statement. J Vasc Surg. 2002;36:416–22. Presented at the Journal of Vascular Surgery: Official Publication, the Society for Vascular Surgery [and] International Society for Cardiovascular Surgery, North American Chapter.
5. Mozes G. New discoveries in anatomy and new terminology of leg veins: clinical implications. Vasc Endovascular Surg. 2004;38(4):367–74. doi:10.1177/153857440403800410.
6. Kupinski AM, Evans SM, Khan AM, Zorn TJ, Darling RC, Chang BB, Leather RP, et al. Ultrasonic characterization of the saphenous vein. Cardiovasc Surg. 1993;1(5):513–7.

7. Caggiati A. Fascial relationships of the long saphenous vein. Circulation. 1999;100(25):2547–9.
8. Cavezzi A, Labropoulos N, Partsch H, Ricci S, Caggiati A, Myers K, Nicolaides A, et al. Duplex ultrasound investigation of the veins in chronic venous disease of the lower limbs—UIP consensus document. Part II. Anatomy. Eur J Vasc Endovasc Surg. 2006;31(3):288–99. doi:10.1016/j.ejvs.2005.07.020.
9. Shah DM, Chang BB, Leopold PW, Corson JD, Leather RP, Karmody AM. The anatomy of the greater saphenous venous system. J Vasc Surg. 1986;3(2):273–83.
10. Thomson H. The surgical anatomy of the superficial and perforating veins of the lower limb. Ann R Coll Surg Engl. 1979;61(3):198–205.
11. Mozes G, Gloviczki P, Menawat SS, Fisher DR, Carmichael SW, Kadar A. Surgical anatomy for endoscopic subfascial division of perforating veins. J Vasc Surg. 1996;24(5):800–8.
12. de Rijcke PAR, Schenk T, van Gent WB, Kleinrensink G-J, Wittens CHA. Surgical anatomy for subfascial endoscopic perforating vein surgery of laterally located perforating veins. J Vasc Surg. 2003;38(6):1349–52. doi:10.1016/S0741-5214(03)01045-0.
13. Aragão JA, Reis FP, Pitta GBB, Miranda Jr F, Poli de Figueiredo LF. Anatomical study of the gastrocnemius venous network and proposal for a classification of the veins. Eur J Vasc Endovasc Surg. 2006;31(4):439–42. doi:10.1016/j.ejvs.2005.10.022.
14. Calotă F, Mogoantă SS, Vasilescu M-M, Vasile I, Paşalega M, Stoicea MC, Camen D, et al. The valvular segment of the lower limbs venous system: anatomical, physiological and physiopathological aspects. Rom J Morphol Embryol. 2010;51(1):157–61.
15. Delis KT. Leg perforator vein incompetence: functional anatomy. Radiology. 2005;235(1):327–34. doi:10.1148/radiol.2351031598.

Pathophysiology of Reflux

2

Sergio Gianesini and Paolo Zamboni

Contents

Abstract

Physiological Venous Hemodynamics Physics Laws Governing Flow

A review of the physical laws governing fluid motion is required to understand reflux pathophysiology. Venous blood flows not just because of a pressure gradient, as is commonly believed, but because of an energy gradient, in which pressure is only a single determinant. In accordance with the thermodynamics zero principle, there will be no energy exchange between systems presenting with the same energy values: no venous flow will occur. In accordance with the thermodynamics second principle, energy exchange will occur from a system presenting higher energy values to one at a lower energy state: venous flow will occur. Considering that reflux, like every physiological flow, needs an energy gradient to be generated, a simple but highly selective and reasoned therapeutic action against the escape, and in favor of the reentry, points will lead to a conservative but effective venous drainage restoration.

2.1 Physics Laws Governing Flow

In order to understand reflux pathophysiology deeply, a review of the physical laws governing fluid motion is required. The venous system presents several energy determinants making its physiology at least as intriguing as the arterial

S. Gianesini, MD (✉) • P. Zamboni, MD
Vascular Disease Center,
University of Ferrara, Ferrara, Italy
e-mail: sergiogianesini@hotmail.com; zambo@unife.it

E. Mowatt-Larssen et al. (eds.), *Phlebology, Vein Surgery and Ultrasonography*,
DOI 10.1007/978-3-319-01812-6_2, © Springer International Publishing Switzerland 2014

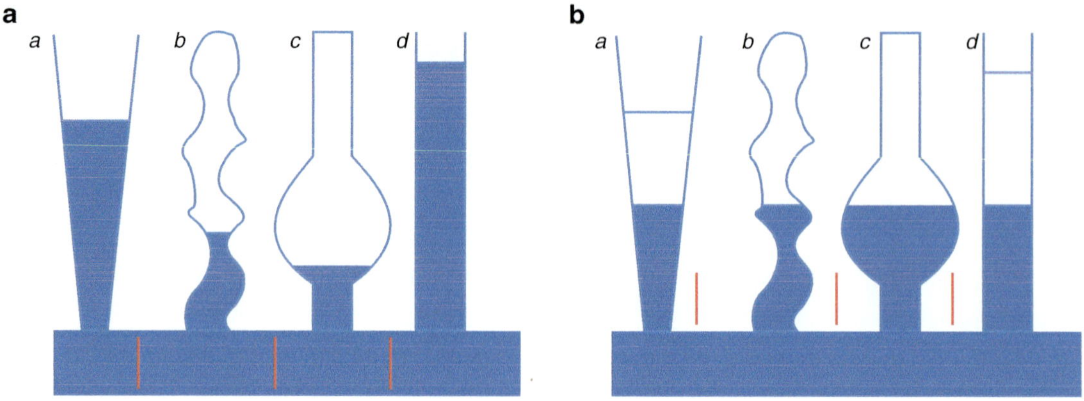

Fig. 2.1 The communicating vessel principle. (**a**) Noncommunicating hydrostatic columns presenting different heights, which lead to different energy states (column *d* presents the highest energy value). (**b**) Communicating columns in which flow moves from the higher to the lower energy state systems, until a common energy balance is reached

one. Venous blood flows not just because of a pressure gradient, as is commonly believed, but because of an energy gradient, in which pressure is only a single determinant [1–4].

In accordance with the thermodynamics zero principle, there will be no energy exchange between systems presenting with the same energy values: no venous flow will occur. In accordance with the thermodynamics second principle, energy exchange will occur from a system presenting higher energy values to one at a lower energy state: venous flow will occur. The communicating vessel principle (Fig. 2.1) describes the result of these two phenomena: regardless of the vessel shape and volume, the fluid will flow from the system presenting a higher energy state to the one at lower energy value, until an energy balance is achieved [4].

If there is no communication between vessels (Fig. 2.1a), the columns present different energy states, which vary just according to the same column height. In fact, in this static situation, the only energy level determinant is the potential gravitational energy value, which is expressed by the following formula:

$$\text{Potential gravitational energy} = \rho g h$$

(ρ represents the fluid density, g the gravity constant, h the height above the surface)

Whenever the different systems are in communication (Fig. 2.1b), fluid flows from the higher to the lower column, thus settling into a balanced common energy state, in which all the column heights are equal [5].

The venous system works both in stasis and in dynamics, so it is the Bernoulli's law which better describes the involved determinants. In ideal conditions, it states that the energy factors governing the venous hemodynamic are the kinetic energy ($\rho v^2/2$; ρ represents the fluid density, v the fluid velocity) together with the potential energy. The potential energy is constituted by the lateral pressure (p), linked to the vessel wall elastic properties, and gravitational pressure, produced by the blood column weight.

The sum of them ($\rho v^2/2 + p + \rho g h$) is constant at any point:

$$\text{Bernoulli s principle}: \rho v^2 / 2 + p + \rho g h = \text{constant}$$

This means that in the stasis condition, the potential energy will be at its maximum, while it will decrease proportionally to the flow velocity increase. The obvious but determinant consequence is that the lateral pressure, exerted on the venous wall, will decrease proportionally to the velocity reached by the fluid (Fig. 2.2).

According to Bernoulli's principle, in two communicating vessels, the one presenting a higher flow velocity will display a lower lateral pressure: a gradient will be created and the blood will flow from the slower to the faster vessel. The aspiration effect performed by the higher velocity vessel is universally known as the Venturi's principle. Venturi's principle is strictly linked to the

Castelli's law (Fig. 2.3) which states that flow velocity (v) is inversely proportional to the vessel cross-sectional area (A):

$$\text{Castelli s law}: A_1 v_1 = A_2 v_2 = \text{Flow}(Q)$$

The implication is that, whenever the vessel divides into several branches, if the sum of the areas of the branches is smaller than the original vessel, an increased flow velocity will be expected. The opposite will be realized if the total area of the branches increases.

2.2 Transmural Pressure and Venous Compliance

Transmural pressure (TMP) is a key factor in understanding venous hemodynamics. It is the difference between the internal venous pressure (IVP), acting on the internal vessel side to expand it, and the external venous pressure (EVP), acting on the external parietal wall to collapse it (Fig. 2.4). TMP and vessel permeability represent the determinants of intravascular-extravascular exchanges (Starling's law).

Together with an energy gradient, another necessary element in producing a flow is the vessel capacity to receive a certain amount of fluid. As a collapsed, elliptical vein begins to fill, it can receive a large volume of fluid with little increase in pressure, a property conferring the blood reservoir function to the venous system. Much more pressure is required to stretch the vessel with additional fluid volume once it has become circular.

The physical property of a vessel to increase its volume with increasing TMP is known as compliance (C) and is expressed by the change in volume (ΔV) divided by the change in pressure (ΔP):

$$\text{Compliance} = \Delta V / \Delta P$$

Compliance is strictly linked not only to the filling degree but also to the geometric vessel properties (length and radius), together with its wall elasticity.

A pressure-diameter curve (Fig. 2.5) highlights the nonlinear relationship in the initial filling phase, which is due to the great increase in vessel caliber following tiny pressure augmentations. On the contrary, in a distension phase, starting from pressure values around 20 mmHg, a volume/pressure linearity has been demonstrated.

Up to this point, all of our physics law applications have been made considering the vessel and the blood as an ideal conduit and liquid,

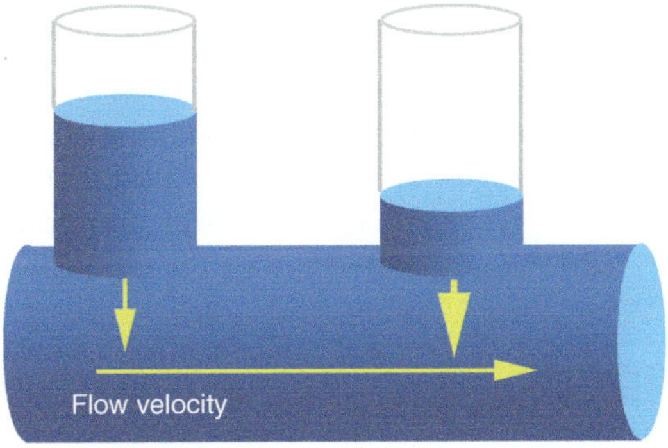

Fig. 2.2 Bernoulli's principle related lateral pressure (LP) drop. Decreasing lateral pressure values, according to flow velocity increase

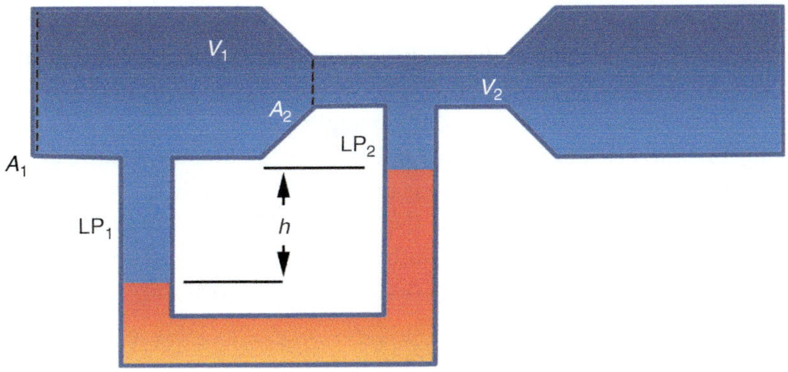

Fig. 2.3 Castelli's law andVenturi's effect. Flow velocity (v) inverse proportionality to vessel cross-sectional area (A) (Castelli's law) and consequent LP variation ($LP_1 > LP_2$) leading to the fluid aspiration determined by the Venturi's effect

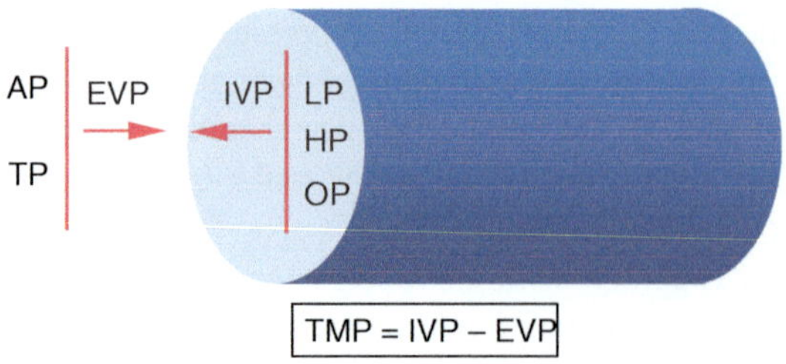

Fig. 2.4 Transmural pressure. *AP* atmospheric pressure, *TP* tissue pressure, *EVP* external venous pressure, *IVP* internal venous pressure, *LP* lateral pressure, *HP* hydrostatic pressure, *OP* oncotic pressure. TMP is the crucial parameter in tissue drainage and venous caliber regulation

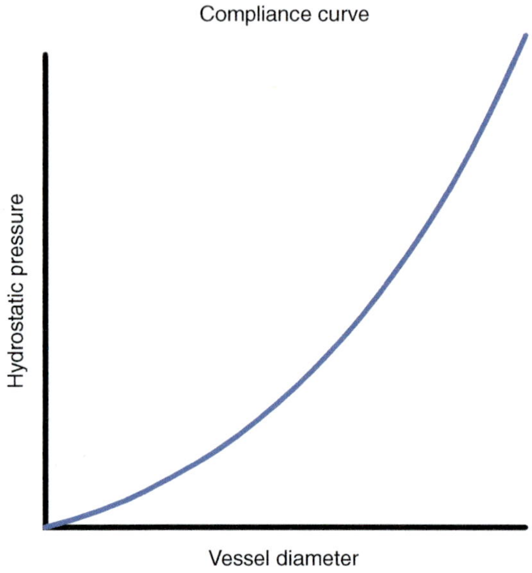

Fig. 2.5 Compliance curve. The pressure-diameter curve highlights an exponential pressure increase over a little volume amount in an initial filling phase. After the achievement of a certain distension phase, the volume–pressure ratio (compliance) shows a linear relationship: in the saphenous system, this happens around the pressure value of 20 mmHg

respectively. The human body, however, produces friction through blood contact. An extension of the thermodynamics second principle, the entropy law, states that in case of nonideal conduits or liquids, part of the energy is dissipated as heat generation, thus increasing the amount of unavailable energy (entropy). The human body solution to counteract this energy dissipation has been the creation of the several pump mechanisms placed in series all along the cardiovascular system.

2.3 Anatomical and Physiological Pathways of Venous Drainage

The venous drainage occurs from the superficial to the deep tissues and from the distal areas to the heart. The only two exceptions are represented by the foot sole venous system, where the blood is directed toward the dorsal network through marginal veins and the saphenofemoral junction tributaries, some of which drain reversely from the abdomen toward the groin.

Three anatomical compartments are identifiable in the venous system:

Anatomical compartment 1 (AC1) is located underneath the deep fascia and contains the deep venous system (femoral, popliteal, tibial, peroneal, gastrocnemius, and soleal veins).

Anatomical compartment 2 (AC2) is located between the superficial and the deep fascia and contains the saphenous system (great, accessory, small saphenous, and intersaphenous veins).

Anatomical compartment 3 (AC3) is located above the superficial fascia and contains the tributary veins.

One of the most important vein features is their being endowed with bicuspid unidirectional valves. These are thin but extremely strong structures lying at the base of a vein segment which is expanded into a sinus. This anatomical peculiarity allows the valve to open without completely touching the parietal wall, thus resulting in a fast closure with blood flow reversal [6].

Valve density is significant in determining drainage pathways. The density of AC2 valves is lower at the leg than at the thigh (Fig. 2.6), and it always remains lower than that belonging to the AC1. This anatomical arrangement puts into practice the communicating vessel principle

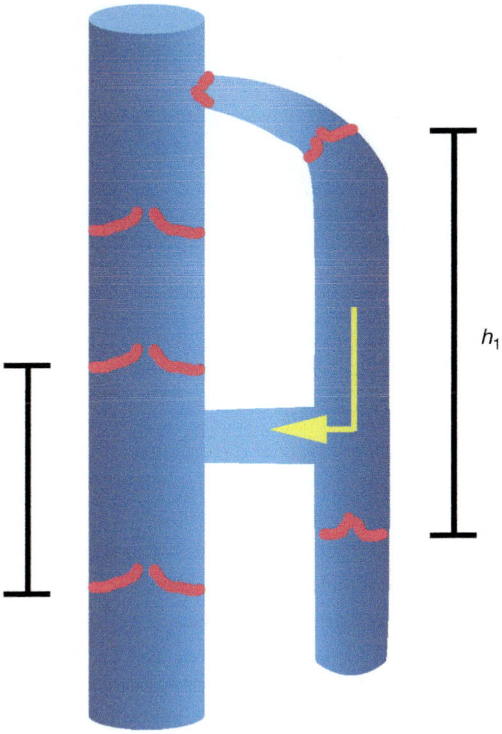

Fig. 2.6 Valve density in the deep and saphenous compartments. The valvular density of the saphenous compartment is lower than that of the deep venous system. This anatomical organization creates higher hydrostatic columns in the saphenous system. Following the communicating vessel principle, blood will flow from the superficial to the deep compartments, through the perforating veins

(Fig. 2.1), thus representing the first determinant in the hierarchical emptying order from the superficial to the deep venous system [7].

The different anatomical compartment locations confer the second determinant of the physiological lower limb drainage. In fact, the muscle pump, which is mainly developed in the calf, assumes the main antagonist role against the force of gravity. The soleal and gastrocnemial contractions exert an EVP between 40 and 200 mmHg, thus reducing the TMP and displacing the blood toward the heart. The generated pressure wave will be transmitted to the surrounding veins proportionally to their own proximity to the muscular fascia investments.

In AC1, all the veins are in direct contact with the muscle mass and are surrounded by the rigid counterforce provided by the deep fasciae. At this level, the calf muscle pump is able to exert its maximum activity in opposing the force of gravity. The saphenous system, being above the muscular compartment and banded between the superficial and the deep fasciae, receives from the calf systole a higher energetic amount than that of its tributaries but also a significantly smaller one than that received by AC1. The decreasing muscular pump effect from AC1 to AC3 is shown by the decrease of concomitant flow velocities: 20–40 cm/s in AC1, 10–20 cm/s in AC2, and 0.05 cm/s in capillary plexuses (Fig. 2.7). The above-described deceleration creates a Venturi's effect. This in turn governs the so-called physiological venous hierarchical order of emptying from the superficial to the deep compartments (from AC3 to AC2 to AC1) of the leg (Fig. 2.8).

Two others "pumps" have to be considered among venous flow determinants: the cardiac and thoracoabdominal. The heart is the main blood propeller providing volume, pressure, and flow to the system in the supine position when the hydrostatic pressure is null (in the standing position, the cardiac-created energy gradient needs to be integrated with the muscular pump because of the hydrostatic pressure increase).

Moreover, the right heart greatly influences venous hemodynamics, increasing the central venous pressure during its systole and the venous flow during its diastole. The close link between heart pump and venous circulation is shown by the evident cardiac pulsations in lower limb venous tracings and by the venous edema seen in congestive heart failure patients.

The thoracoabdominal pump influences the venous return by means of the diaphragm movements, which in the end determines the intra-abdominal pressure. During inspiration, intra-abdominal pressure increases, thus compressing the inferior vena cava and reducing the venous blood flow; usually the venous outflow from the lower limbs can temporarily cease. During expiration, the intra-abdominal pressure falls again, the inferior vena cava expands, and the

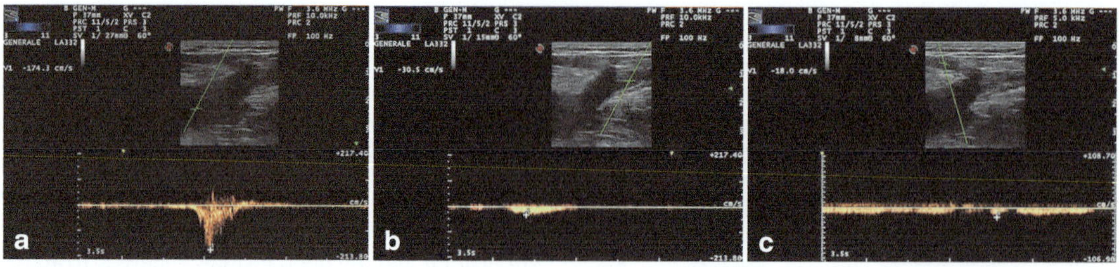

Fig. 2.7 Decreasing flow velocities from the deep to the superficial venous compartment. The phenomenon is mainly due to a muscular pump minor energy transfer to the superficial veins. The Doppler sample was placed in the common femoral vein just above the saphenous confluence (**a**), in the great saphenous vein underneath the preterminal valve (**b**), in the superficial epigastric vein just before its saphenous confluence (**c**)

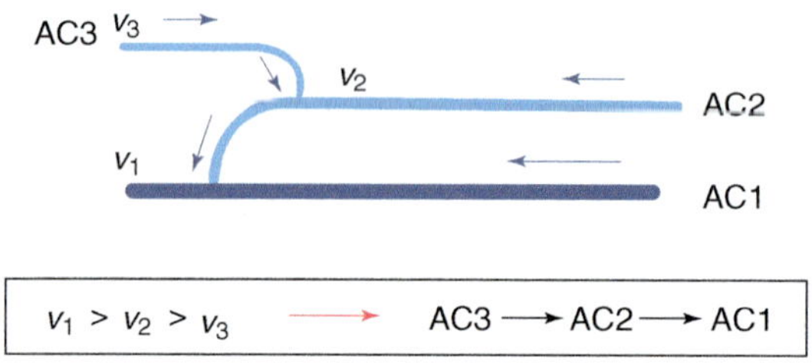

Fig. 2.8 The hierarchy of venous compartment emptying. The physiological venous emptying from the superficial to the deep tissues is made possible by the blood aspiration exerted by the Venturi's effect application

venous blood from the lower limbs can flow to the heart. In conclusion, in order to establish a flow, two factors are needed: an energy gradient (potential plus kinetic) and a system with a compliance capable of receiving a certain fluid amount [4].

2.4 Pathophysiological Venous Hemodynamics

2.4.1 Reflux Establishment and Definition

A retrograde segmental superficial and/or deep venous flow lasting less than 0.5 s (except in the femoropopliteal system, where 1.0 s is allowed) is considered physiological in the muscular diastolic phase. The communicating vessel principle predicts blood displacement from the higher hydrostatic columns to the lower ones, until an energy balance is reached.

The distance between two competent valvular planes is not long, even if greater in AC2 than in AC1. Thus, a physiological retrograde flow exhibits slow velocities, which render this blood movement undetectable by Doppler (Fig. 2.9a). On the other hand, in the case of valvular incontinence or absence, the height of the hydrostatic columns becomes progressively higher (Fig. 2.9b): if the system presents a compliance capable of receiving a blood overload, a diastolic flow at high velocity will be produced and revealed by Doppler.

A reflux is defined as a flow that is inverted with respect to the physiological direction and that lasts more than 0.5 s (except 1.0 s for the femoropopliteal system). Thus, it is a flow that displaces blood toward the distal areas of the lower limbs and from the deeper to the more superficial compartments; in this sense, reflux can be defined as a change in the hierarchical order of emptying (from AC1 to AC3).

Therefore, two main scenarios are possible in reflux characterization: it is a retrograde flow running down in the same conduit, or it is an inverted flow jumping into an anatomical compartment more superficially placed. The first situation is common in healthy but long-standing subjects, thus not strictly pathological. The second scenario is certainly a pathological one because of the loss in the hierarchical order of venous emptying. Unfortunately, the actual definition does not differentiate between the two different hemodynamic situations, thus offering an issue for a future-related consensus.

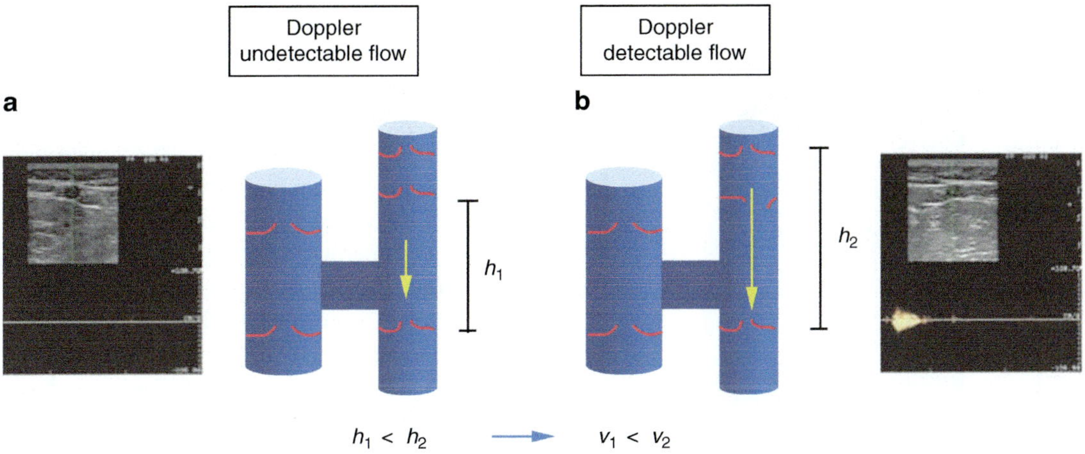

Fig. 2.9 Valvular derangement consequence on flow velocity. (**a**) In physiological conditions, the distance between two competent valves does not allow a significant retrograde flow velocity enhancement. No Doppler signal will be revealed. (**b**) In case of valvular derangement, the distance between two competent valves becomes significant. The consequent refluxing flow velocity increase will permit a Doppler signal transmission

Reflux is a flow, so to be established, it needs an energy gradient and a system compliance capable to receive it. Moreover, a reflux needs a connection between the venous segment acting as the flow source (the escape point) and the vessel destined to receive the blood overload (the reentry point).

The escape and reentry points are not to be considered just for their anatomical relevance. In fact, their first meaning is their hemodynamic significance. The energy gradient between the escape and the reentry points is the *conditio sine qua non* for the reflux creation. If the venous network receiving the refluxing blood (the reentry point) was not in a lower energy state as a consequence of its smaller hydrostatic columns created by competent valves, no flow motion would be developed. Every time a reflux is detected, a reentry point must be expected.

The pathological reflux compartment jump has two main causes: an increase in the deep pressure (following a Valsalva maneuver or a thrombotic occlusion) or a superficial pressure decrease. In the last case, the energy drop is linked to the aspiration caused by the reentry gradient, which in turn is responsible for an acceleration of the refluxing blood, thus creating a Venturi's effect which reduces the lateral pressure, thus aspirating on the reflux source itself in a closed circuit (Fig. 2.10).

The vicious cycle of the previously described circuit is defined as a "private circulation." This is a pathological blood recirculation which is established between two linked venous networks in which a certain amount of venous blood refluxes into the reentry point during diastole and then, during systole, flows back to the escape point, thus supplying the same shunt once again [8–10].

2.4.2 Reflux Pathogenesis in the Superficial Network: The Descending vs. Ascending Theories

The pathogenesis of superficial venous reflux is controversial [11, 12]. Descending and ascending theories are promoted. The descending or valvular hypothesis was first described by Trendelenburg in the nineteenth century. He proposed that reflux begins because of an incompetent terminal saphenofemoral valve, which is overwhelmed by the hydrostatic column pressing on it. Reflux then progresses in a retrograde direction, progressively causing incompetence of more distal valves.

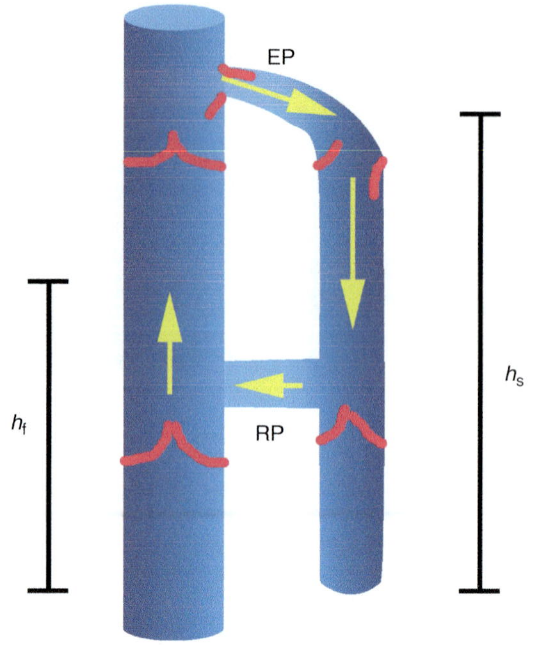

Fig. 2.10 Venturi's effect and communicating vessel principle application on the anatomical venous compartments jump. In this figure, the saphenofemoral junction represents the reflux source (escape point [*EP*]). The blood reversal takes place because of the aspiration effect exerted by the higher femoral flow velocity (v_f) through the reentry perforator (*RP*). The incompetent proximal saphenous vein valves allow a blood recirculation into the saphenous axis itself. Together with the communicating vessel principle, this causes a progressive increase in the reversed flow velocity (v_s). This leads to a reduction in the saphenofemoral confluence lateral pressure, which in turn promotes the establishment of a refluxing closed circuit (femoral hydrostatic column height [h_f], saphenous hydrostatic column height [h_s])

The ascending theory was proposed in the 1980s based on histological, biochemical, and functional investigations demonstrating how the venous wall can undergo pathological alterations in segmental localizations, irrespective of the site and functional state of the valves. In this pathophysiological explanation, reflux begins as a local alteration, possibly developing in any part of the lower limb, and valve failure progresses in an anterograde fashion [13].

Even if the location of reflux genesis is controversial, recent researchers have proposed a unifying pathogenetic theory. Primary structural changes of the venous valve or wall lead to an initial reflux. Increased metalloproteinases (MMPs) activity, following high wall tension values, has been recently demonstrated. The consequent derangement of the endothelium and smooth muscle cells causes altered venous constriction/relaxation properties, together with the leukocyte chemotaxis. A vicious circle involving valvular incompetence, venous wall alteration, vessel dilation, and increasing reflux is created. Thus, parietal damage leading to vessel dilation seems to be antecedent to the valvular incompetence instauration; a cascade of events is than executed by the activation of MMPs, with consequent progressive venous drainage impairment. The unbalanced proteolytic activity in varicose vein tissues is nowadays fully documented in the literature: MMP 1, MMP 2, MMP 9, and MMP 13 upregulation has been observed in stasis dermatitis, ratios of tissue inhibitors of MMPs to activated MMPs have been found to be higher in varicose patients, and unregulated levels of inflammation-related TGF-beta have been assessed into the dilated vein wall [1]. All these molecular events become the final executor of the pathological cascade which, in the end, leads to the macroscopic varicose derangement.

2.4.3 Reflux Pathogenesis in the Deep Network

Agenesis, malformations, and post-thrombotic damages are the most frequent causes of deep valvular incompetence linked to deep venous reflux. In past years, deep venous incompetence was considered to cause significant hemodynamic derangements. Several recent investigations have pointed out how different deep segments carry with them different hemodynamic impacts. Iliac axis incompetence is considered hemodynamically less relevant than the deep lower leg veins, whose alteration can lead to even irreversible muscle pump damage. The femoral vein is still a matter of debate. Some data suggested it is irrelevant, while other data highlight severe disturbances following its incompetence. Selective saphenous vein ablation in the case of combined saphenous

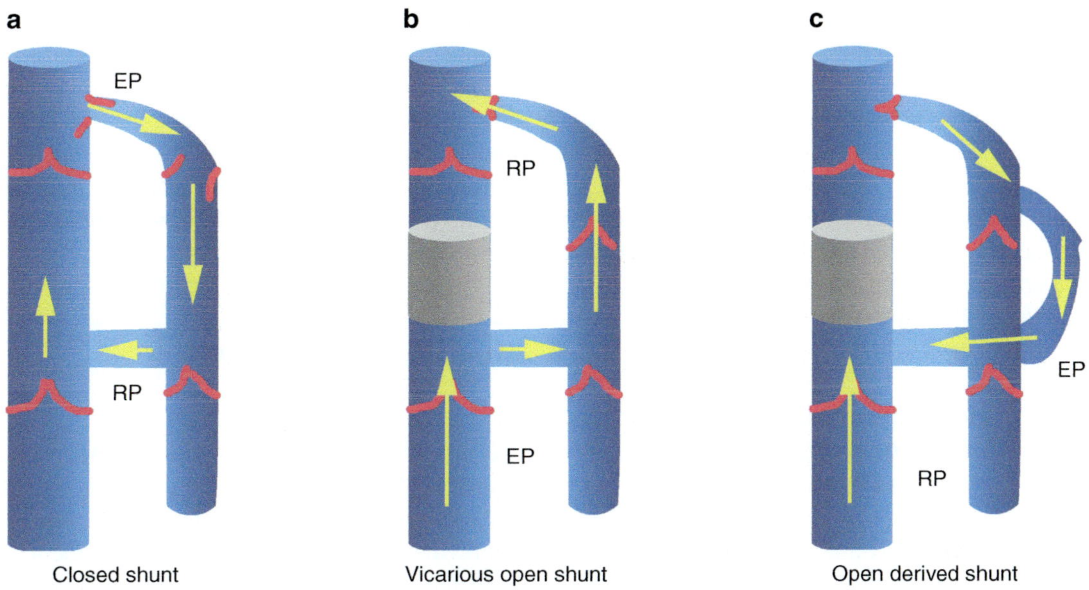

Fig. 2.11 (**a**) Closed shunt. Recirculation from an escape point (*EP*) through a reentry perforator (*RP*) during the diastole following the muscular pump activation. A private circulation is established and excluded by the remaining draining network. (**b**) Vicarious open shunt. Collateral circulations are activated in order to bypass an obstacle (e.g., thrombosis, vicarious varicose veins following non-hemodynamic therapeutic approaches). (**c**) Open derived shunt. Diastolic retrograde flow overload from a competent confluent vein because of an incompetent collateral link to a reentry perforator which directly drains into a deeper compartment. No recirculation is established because the EP and the RP belong to different networks

and femoral vein refluxes usually restores normal venous hemodynamics despite persisting femoral vein insufficiency. Femoral vein incompetence seems not to cause severe hemodynamic derangements if the lower legs are competent [14, 15].

2.4.4 Shunts and Reflux Patterns

A venous shunt is a pathway carrying two different types of flow: the physiologically draining one and the pathologically deviated blood. Anatomically and hemodynamically, it starts in a refluxing (or escaping) point and terminates in the so-called reentry point. Three main shunt networks are described: closed, vicarious open, and open derived.

In *closed shunts* (Fig. 2.11a), a vicious circle is created between the escape and the reentry points. The deviated flow recirculates at each energy gradient inversion like in a closed electrical circuit. A classic example is an incompetent saphenofemoral junction (escape point) letting the femoral blood drain along the saphenous trunk in a retrograde fashion toward a reentry perforator during muscular pump diastole. At the systolic energy gradient inversion, the femoral blood will flow back to the saphenofemoral junction and then will be deviated again along the saphenous compartment. In this way, a closed shunt will be established, and a certain amount of blood will be excluded by the systemic venous network because it is entrapped in the previously described private circulation [4].

A *bypassing open shunt* (Fig. 2.11b) is a natural bypass exploited by the venous network to go over an obstacle. The use of a collateral route to bypass what is usually a thrombotic occlusion is desirable, as it reduces the drainage resistance. In this type of shunt, there is no recirculation, and it is fed by the residual draining pressure together with the proximal cardiac and thoracoabdominal aspiration. It may be either antegrade or retrograde.

An *open derived shunt* (Fig. 2.11c) is a flow diversion into an incompetent vein caused by a reversed energy gradient usually generated during muscular pump diastole. The blood overload is directed to a reentry perforator which drains directly into a network not linked to the escape point one: no recirculation occurs. A typical example is an incompetent saphenous tributary endowed with a reentry perforator draining into the deep venous system: the blood overload will "jump" from AC2 to the saphenous tributary AC3 and then will flow down directly toward AC1 [4].

2.5 Hemodynamic Role of Perforators in Chronic Venous Disease

Perforating veins connect the superficial to the deep compartments by piercing the muscular fascia. A physiological draining direction from surface inward is guaranteed by unidirectional valves. In the past, perforator incompetence was considered a main initial reflux trigger. Several ligation or disruption methods, including subcutaneous endoscopic surgery, have been in use for many years. Nowadays, the evidence suggests that nonselective ligation or ablation of calf perforators is ineffective. When they are dilated, these veins should be analyzed and treated, taking into consideration their hemodynamic significance (escape or reentry points). Large perforating veins are not always directly responsible for trophic disorders, and, even if dynamic tests highlight a systolic outflow, the net flow direction is usually toward the deep venous system. On the other hand, a perforating vein is considered pathological whenever refluxing during the diastolic phase of a dynamic test.

Thus, a perforating vein may be treated depending on its hemodynamic role and on the shunt type it constitutes. For example, treatment of a reentry perforator belonging to a closed (Fig. 2.12a) or open derived shunt would be erroneous because that impairs the physiological blood return to the heart (Fig. 2.12b). On the contrary, elimination of a refluxing perforator feeding the closed or open derived shunt (escape point) is mandatory to perform a hemodynamic correction of the venous return (Fig. 2.12c).

Bidirectional flow can take place into the perforating system afflicted by primary chronic venous disease (CVD). Moreover, most of the time, these dilated veins are not the cause of venous hypertension but the consequence of voluminous saphenous system refluxes, flowing into the deep venous network through the perforating system [16].

2.6 Reflux Hemodynamic Implications

The first consequence of venous hypertension, linked to the refluxing blood overload, is an increase in the IVP and thus a rise in TMP values. As previously described, TMP is a key element in balancing the liquid compartments and so in ruling the tissue drainage. An excessive TMP results in an accumulation of toxic metabolites, which in turn becomes responsible for pathognomonic CVD skin changes.

The high TMP assessed in CVD patients leads to extravasation of red blood cells through the capillary sinusoids. Hemoglobin degradation in the interstitial compartment becomes the source of the iron-mediated oxidative reactions that are the final executor of this pathological tissue damage. Clinically, even with genetic and molecular individual peculiarities, the previously described hemodynamic phenomenon causes the typical edema, hyperpigmentation, lipodermatosclerosis, necrosis, and ulcer.

Another main reflux consequence is represented by the changes in flow physical characteristics. Physiologically, blood flow is laminar. It is comparable to several concentric cylinders sliding one over the other at decreasing velocities from the vessel central axis to the parietal layers. The cylinder adjacent to the vessel wall is the one most greatly involved by the parietal friction, thus the one presenting the lowest velocity.

The kinematics of fluid motion is significantly affected by blood viscosity, wall friction, geometric conduit characteristics, and flow velocities. All these factors are summarized in a dimensional parameter known as Reynolds number, which, if higher than 2,000, is predictive of

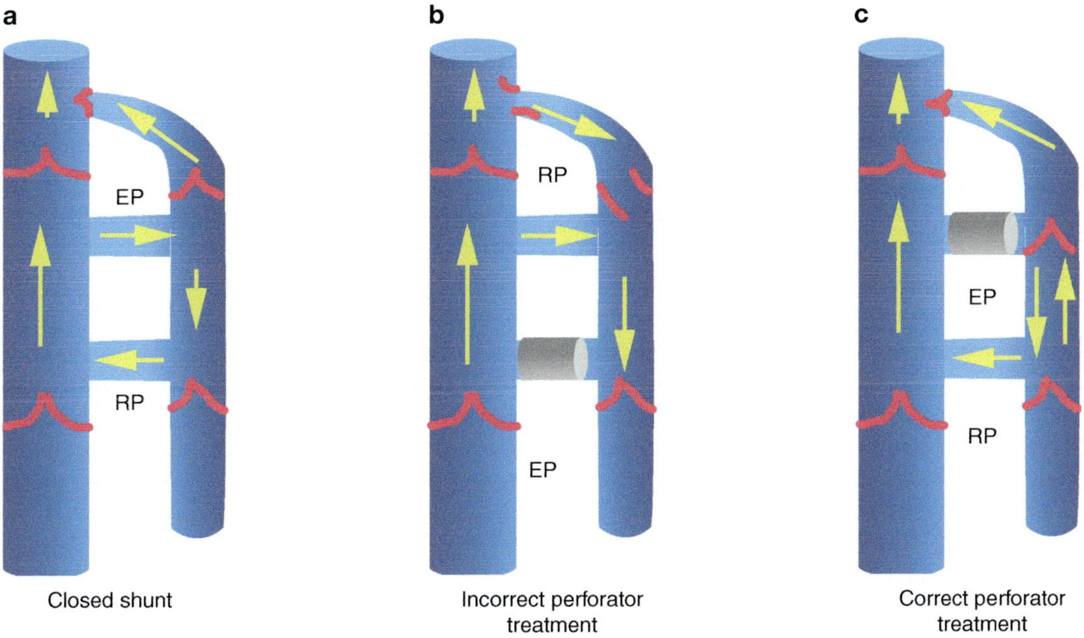

Fig. 2.12 (**a**) Closed shunt. Recirculation from an EP represented by a Hunterian perforator through a more distal RP. (**b**) Incorrect perforator treatment. Suppressing the RP energy gradient leads to a lateral pressure increase in the more superficial network which will suffer the consequent dilation progressively undergoing valves incompetence. This phenomenon will cause an increased hydrostatic overload, which will worsen the hemodynamic impairment. (**c**) Correct perforator treatment. Suppressing the EP will lead to an abolition of the shunted blood overload. The lightened superficial network will possibly decrease its diameter, assuring valvular competence and physiological drainage

turbulent flow. Turbulent refluxing flow is a flow presenting a derangement of the kinetic energy vectors, which are no longer linear but chaotically orientated in all the directions. Thus, an energy waste is produced together with a tendency toward vascular wall dilation.

Dilation is more related to the energy gradient alteration than to just a pressure increase. The importance of turbulence and not just pressure is suggested by the use of the saphenous vein for arterial bypasses. Despite the increased pressure, the graft does not develop varicosities because of the arterial laminar flow (Fig. 2.13).

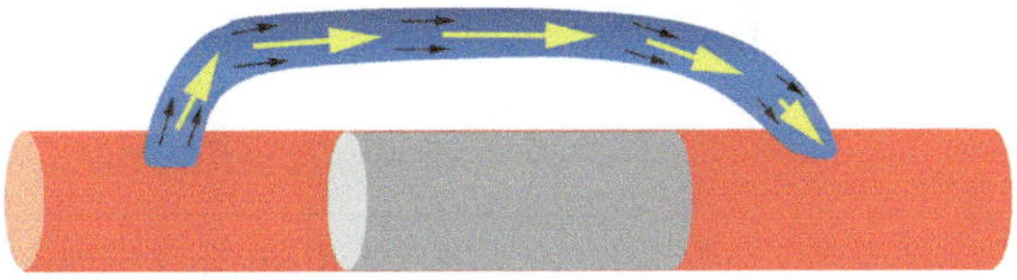

Fig. 2.13 Turbulence and vessel dilation. A vein graft in an arterial bypass does not develop varicosities despite the high-pressure values. This phenomenon is explained by the laminar flow draining into the vein and offers evidence of the importance of turbulence in the pathophysiology of varicose veins

2.7 Reflux Assessment

Understanding the pathophysiological background of the various reflux assessment techniques is mandatory for a correct interpretation of the performed investigations. A deeper description of the different diagnostic tools will follow in Sect. 2.2. Nowadays, invasive ascending and descending venography has been largely replaced by ultrasound scans [17]. The noninvasive Doppler evaluation is proved to be comparable to venography in providing deep and superficial venous reflux staging. Descending contrast venography remains important in cases of severe deep venous occlusive disease leading to venous bypasses, valve repair, or transplantation procedures.

The ideal reflux assessment tool should provide both anatomical and hemodynamic data in a dynamic evaluation. Venography, photoplethysmography, and air plethysmography assessments, although particularly useful in providing standardized data on global venous hemodynamics, are unable to detect those isolated segmental refluxes and hemodynamic changes that are related to the muscular pump and gravitational energy gradient activation.

Ultrasonography, even if operator dependent, not only allows precise reflux anatomic localization and hemodynamic quantification but also evaluates the venous system under conditions that simulate the normal venous system pump function (Valsalva, compression/relaxation, Paranà, oscillation, toe-flexion, active foot dorsiflexion, rising-on-tiptoes maneuvers). Moreover, echo and color Doppler scanning represents the ideal tool to quantify reflux characterizing parameters, such as reflux time (RT), Psathakis (PI), and dynamic reflux indexes (DRI).

The exact cutoff time for reflux definition remains an actual topic of debate. Recent consensus opinion defines reflux as abnormal flow lasting over 0.5 s for all veins except the femoropopliteal system, where the value is 1.0 s [18]. Independently by its duration, RT is a parameter not necessarily proportional to the reflux severity. The smaller the leaking valvular hole is, the longer lasting RT will be. Moreover, RT has been proved not to be proportional to the clinical severity class. It also changes according with the type of assessment maneuver utilized.

Psathakis (PI) and dynamic reflux indexes (DRI) also offer a potential means to quantify the hemodynamic impairment. PI is a parameter assessed in the deep network during compression/relaxation maneuver and is expressed by the following formula:

$$\mathrm{PI} = \frac{(\text{diastolic reflux velocity surface})}{(\text{systolic velocity flow surface})}$$

This parameter is considered pathological when greater than 0.40, but it takes into account the reflux volume without assessing the flow. The DRI expresses both the reflux volume and the flow rate, through the following formula:

$$\mathrm{DRI} = \frac{\left[(\text{diastolic reflux mean velocity})^2 \times (\text{diastolic reflux time})\right]}{\left[(\text{systolic reflux mean velocity})^2 \times (\text{diastolic flow time})\right]}$$

DRI varies according to the reflux flow rate, and it expresses the reflux severity degree more completely than PI or RT.

2.8 Hemodynamic Rationale of Reflux Suppression

As previously described, venous reflux leads to a venous hypertension related to an excessive TMP. The therapeutic aim becomes either a reduction of the IVP or an increase in EVP. When IVP is moderately high, the EVP increase caused by elastic stocking compression can counteract the hypertension caused by the reflux. The elastic compression stocking assists the muscular fasciae and induces blood acceleration. Compression is responsible for a lateral pressure drop (Bernoulli's principle), thus favoring the hierarchical order of venous drainage by means of a blood aspiration toward the deepest networks (Venturi's effect).

Following valvular incompetence and venous wall degeneration, the hydrostatic columns can significantly increase their values. In this case, the therapeutic strategy needs to be addressed by

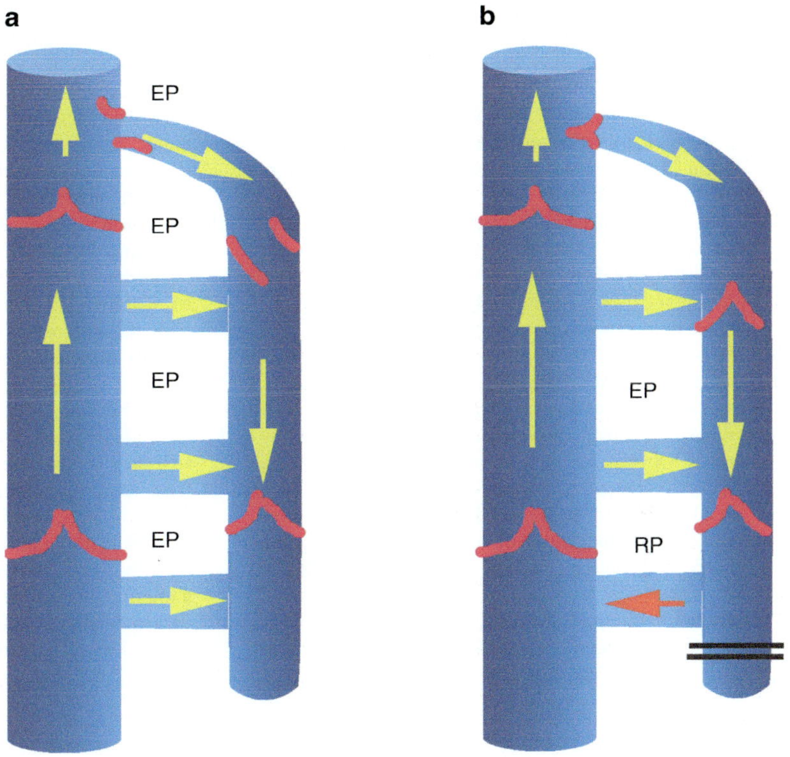

Fig. 2.14 Perforating vein terminalization. A simple ligation, or even a finger compression, below a perforating vein originally representing an EP of reflux can break off the private circulation. The consequent reflux disappearance is caused by the reduced diastolic reflux velocity, together with the private circulation compliance reduction. The result is an energy gradient inversion, which favors blood drainage toward the deep compartment. A perforator would then be transformed from an EP (**a**) to an RP (**b**)

fragmentation of such valve distances. Surgical correction can be offered by means of valve repair or permanent hydrostatic pressure fractionation through perforating veins "terminalization" [19].

Hydrostatic pressure fractionation is a conservative hemodynamic approach consisting in a ligation below a perforator belonging to a private circulation. The consequent reduction in the hydrostatic column leads to a decrease of the reflux velocity and system compliance, which in turn is associated to an increased lateral pressure. The consequence is an inversion of the refluxing gradient in favor of its aspiration into the deep circulation (Fig. 2.14).

Applying the physics laws, the strategy to conservatively achieve a reflux abolishment becomes understandable. Considering that reflux, like every physiological flow, needs an energy gradient to be generated, a simple but highly selective and reasoned therapeutic action against the escape, and in favor of the reentry points, will lead to a conservative but effective venous drainage restoration [20].

References

1. Bergan JJ, Shmid-Schonbein GW, Smith PD, Nicolaides AN, Boisseau MR, Ekloff B. Chronic venous disease. N Engl J Med. 2006;355(5):488–98.
2. Bjordal R. Simultaneous pressure and flow recordings in varicose veins of the lower extremity. Acta Chir Scand. 1970;136:309–17.
3. Chien M. Venous pathophysiology. Semin Intervent Radiol. 2005;22(3):157–61.
4. Franceschi C, Zamboni P. Principles of venous hemodynamics. Hauppauge, NY: Nova Science Publishers; 2009.
5. Rutherford RB. Vascular surgery. 6th ed. Philadelphia: Saunders; 2005.
6. Van Bemellen PS, Beach K, Bedford G, Strandness Jr DE. The mechanism of venous valve closure. Its relationship to the velocity of reverse flow. Arch Surg. 1990;125(5):617–9.
7. Sales C, Rosenthal D, Petrillo K, Jerivs HS, Matsura J, Clark MD, Pontoriero MA, Syracuse DC, Luka N. The valvular apparatus in venous insufficiency: a problem of quantity? Ann Vasc Surg. 1998;12:153–5.
8. Naoum JJ, Hunter GC, Woodside KJ, Chen C. Current advances in the pathogenesis of varicose veins. J Surg Res. 2007;141:311–6.

9. Raju S, Neglen P. High prevalence of not thrombotic iliac vein lesion in chronic venous disease: a permissive role in pathogenicity. J Vasc Surg. 2006; 44(1):136–43.
10. Venruri M, Bonavina L, Annoni F, Colombo L, Butera C, Perachia A. Biochemical assay of collagen and elastin in the normal and varicose vein wall. J Surg Res. 1996;60:245–8.
11. Tibbs JD, Fletcher EWL. Direction of flow in superficial veins as a guide to venous disorders in lower limbs. Surgery. 1983;93(6):758–67.
12. Labropoulos N, Giannoukas AD, Delis K, et al. Where does venous reflux start? J Vasc Surg. 1997;26: 736–42.
13. Bernardini E, De Rango P, Piccioli R, Bisacci C, Pagliuca V, Genovese G, Bisacci R. Development of primary superficial venous insufficiency: the ascending theory. Observation and hemodynamic data from a 9-year experience. Ann Vasc Surg. 2010;24:709–20.
14. Hu ZJ, Wang SM, Wang YH, Huang XL. Quantitative assessment of the degree of deep venous reflux of the lower extremities. Asian J Surg. 2003;26(2): 108–11.
15. Maleti O, Lugli M. Neovalve construction in postthrombotic syndrome. J Vasc Surg. 2006;43(4):794–9.
16. Delis KT, Husmann M, Kalodiki E, Wolfe JH, Nicolaides A. In situ hemodynamics of perforating veins in chronic venous insufficiency. J Vasc Surg. 2001;33:773–82.
17. Chauveau M, Gelade P, Cros F. The venous return simulator: comparison of simulated with measured ambulatory venous pressure in normal subjects and in venous valve incompetence. Vasa. 2011;40(3):205–17.
18. Gloviczki P, Comerota A, Dalsing M, Eklof B, Gillespie D, Gloviczki M, Lohr J, McLafferty R, Meissner M, Murad M, Padberg F, Pappas P, Passman M, Raffetto J, Vasquez M, Wakefield T. The care of patients with varicose veins and associated chronic venous diseases: clinical practice guidelines of the Society for Vascular Surgery and the American Venous Forum. J Vasc Surg. 2011;53:2S–48.
19. Carandina S, Mari C, De Palma M, et al. Varicose vein stripping versus hemodynamic correction (CHIVA): a long term randomised trial. Eur J Vasc Endovasc Surg. 2008;35:230–7.
20. Escribano JM, Juan J, Bofill R, Maeso J, Rodriguez-Mori A, Matas M. Durability of reflux elimination by a minimal invasive CHIVA procedure on patients with varicose veins: a 3 years prospective case study. Eur J Vasc Endovasc Surg. 2003;25:159–63.

Presentation of Chronic Venous Disease

3

Michael A. Vasquez and Cary Munschauer

Contents

Abstract

An estimated 20–25 million people in the USA have varicose veins, while up to 20 % of people worldwide have CVI. Diagnosis, treatment, and surveillance may be routine and singularly focused or may be staged and multifactorial. An area that has proven to benefit from the use of protocols and standardized surveys is surveillance. Follow-up care of patients with varying disease severity over time has been successfully performed using the Clinical-Etiology-Anatomy-Pathophysiology (CEAP) classification and the Venous Clinical Severity Score (VCSS), evaluation scales that provide reproducible results. This chapter examines assessment, epidemiology, and symptoms and physical findings in patients with CVD and CVI.

3.1 Introduction

Chronic venous disease (CVD) and chronic venous insufficiency (CVI) are widely prevalent worldwide, with causes and symptoms ranging from straightforward to complex. According to the Vascular Disease Foundation, an estimated 20–25 million people in the USA have varicose veins, while up to 20 % of people worldwide have CVI [1]. Venous disease has a significant financial effect in the USA, with missed work-days and costs related to medical care estimated to exceed $1 billion annually [2].

M.A. Vasquez, MD, FACS, RVT (✉)
SUNY Buffalo Department of Surgery,
The Venous Institute of Buffalo,
Buffalo, NY, USA
e-mail: mvasquezmd@roadrunner.com

C. Munschauer, BA
Department of Surgery,
The Venous Institute of Buffalo,
Buffalo, NY, USA
e-mail: cmunsch@earthlink.net

E. Mowatt-Larssen et al. (eds.), *Phlebology, Vein Surgery and Ultrasonography*,
DOI 10.1007/978-3-319-01812-6_3, © Springer International Publishing Switzerland 2014

Diagnosis, treatment, and surveillance may be routine and singularly focused or may be staged and multifactorial. The progress of diagnostic tools, treatment options, and surveillance methods has been rapid over the last several years, with the goal being a continuum of care and the choice of appropriate therapy for each patient. Straightforward protocol-driven diagnostic algorithms are difficult to apply in chronic venous conditions owing to the myriad of signs and symptoms present at different stages of the disease and their varying effects on patient health status and quality of life. Treatment options range from the conservative use of compression stockings to combination therapy with ablation, ligation, and sclerosing agent to address complex or recurrent disease. Chronic venous disease and insufficiency are not conditions easily addressed with a single procedure and declared cured. Rather, appropriate treatment involves an individual strategy that addresses the progression of disease and considers the effect on the patient's lifestyle. An area that has proven to benefit from the use of protocols and standardized surveys is surveillance. Follow-up care of patients with varying disease severity over time has been successfully performed using the Clinical-Etiology-Anatomy-Pathophysiology (CEAP) classification and the Venous Clinical Severity Score (VCSS), evaluation scales that provide reproducible results [3–5]. Several other evaluation instruments that consider different facets of venous disease are available for uniform surveillance [6].

The end of the twentieth century and the first decade of the twenty-first century have been a time of compilation, contemplation, and advancement in regard to venous disease and therapy. While treatments were being offered to patients for many vascular conditions, the outcomes were being only sporadically evaluated. The realization that diagnostic methods and treatment options cannot exist in isolated incarnations has focused the attention of the scientific community on analyzing this information to provide a framework of commonality in clinical practice and research.

After years of debate to identify the standard for outcome reporting, the consensus is that scoring instruments should provide uniform, accurate, reproducible measurements and should be modifiable to reflect the chosen therapy [7]. According to Dayal and Kent, they should "define essential terms and make recommendations regarding the following: clinical classification of disease; criteria for improvement, deterioration, and failure; a grading system for risk factors; categorization of operations and interventions; complications encountered with grades for severity or outcome," as well as allow results to be reported in a common language, which facilitates comparison of outcomes across studies [8]. The responsibility of the physician is to rigorously evaluate new developments through analysis of data and to share the findings with patients and other physicians [9].

The complex nature of venous disease makes ultrasonography an ideal diagnostic medium to assist the physician in evaluation and treatment planning. The ability to use venous mapping to evaluate the severity of disease and plan a treatment strategy is invaluable. Ultrasonography has an additional benefit in the ability to evaluate the patient throughout the treatment period, differentiating recurrent varices from disease progression and assisting in the long-term strategy [10].

As awareness of the morbidity and socioeconomic consequences of CVD has increased, so has the technology available for treatment. A critical need now exists for outcome assessment instruments that reflect the morbidity associated with CVD and the response to treatment. Several instruments have been developed to describe the severity of disease or to measure clinical outcomes.

3.2 CEAP Classification

One example of a useful outcome reporting method in CVD is the CEAP classification. The basic design of CEAP is to function as a universally accepted system for quantifying all degrees of CVD, leading to a common platform for clinical intervention and scientific inquiry [11]. CEAP was adopted in 1994 by an international ad hoc committee of the American Venous Forum and over time has become "the accepted standard for classifying chronic venous disorders" [12]. CEAP meets the desired criteria for an assessment in the range of systems and symptoms included, the nature of the severity measurements, and inclusion of a disability score [11].

The *clinical* component of CEAP is scored from 0 to 6 and indicates increasing disease severity, ranging from none (0 points) to active ulcers (6 points). The *etiologic* component is used to denote whether the venous disease is congenital, primary, or secondary in nature. The *anatomic* classification pinpoints the veins involved as superficial, deep, or perforating. The *pathophysiologic* classification identifies the presence or absence of reflux in the superficial, communicating, or deep systems, as well as the existence of outflow obstruction [7]. CEAP scores can be determined from the results of clinical evaluation and Doppler testing, making it an easily quantifiable instrument in the diagnosis of CVI [13].

In 2004, CEAP was revised to increase its descriptive functionality and to provide 2 levels of classification for different applications [11]. A simpler basic CEAP was introduced to clarify some of the classification elements and to make the system readily accessible in clinical practice. The highest descriptive element is used for the "C" classification, and the "E," "A," and "P" are derived from the Doppler examination and are modified with "s," "p," and "d" descriptors for *superficial*, *perforator*, and *deep*. In this way, the relevant revisions to CEAP can be used in a format that allows straightforward, easily reproducible results. The advanced CEAP classification may be most beneficial to researchers because it allows patients to be grouped and subgrouped based on relevant elements and then reevaluated throughout treatment [11].

With advanced CEAP, patients having similar manifestations of venous disease can be accurately grouped for analysis. Correlating CEAP scores with subjective symptoms and diagnostic testing (e.g., ultrasonography) can provide relevant data on the relationship between subjective complaints and objective findings in CVD [14]. The advanced CEAP classification breaks each category down into component parts to allow more detailed descriptions. Advanced CEAP is especially useful in research and in publishing applications [15].

The major drawback to CEAP is the static nature of assessment in measuring severity at a single time point. Venous disease, like many other chronic conditions, involves a continuum of symptoms and severity. Change in status following therapy is an ongoing process. This is especially true for C4 and C5 disease (Figs. 3.1, 3.2, and 3.3). The static nature of these measurements makes it difficult for a physician to track changes over time in response to therapy [16]. Some investigators have proposed combining CEAP with other outcome assessment measures to increase its specificity for longitudinal assessment [17, 18].

3.3 Venous Clinical Severity Score

The VCSS is a longitudinal measure of nine categories considered universally relevant in the diagnosis and management of CVD. It was designed to supplement CEAP and to provide an evaluative longitudinal assessment of change following treatment and disease progression [16]. It was also designed to give additional weight to more severe manifestations of CVD [18].

The VCSS is generated by the clinician during the course of patient examination and can be followed up readily. It can be used to assess the broader spectrum of CVD, as well as to compare patients with post-thrombotic syndrome and those undergoing different treatment modalities of saphenous venous ablation, stenting for venous obstruction, and pharmacomechanical thrombolysis. Although useful, the *original* VCSS had drawbacks. Ambiguity in the clinical descriptors was identified as a primary shortcoming of the instrument [19]. In response to these issues, the VCSS has recently been revised [20]. The specific language of proven quality-of-life instruments was used to better address the issues of patients at the lower end of the venous disease spectrum. The language that patients use in describing their symptoms has been considered as well. This revision is designed primarily to

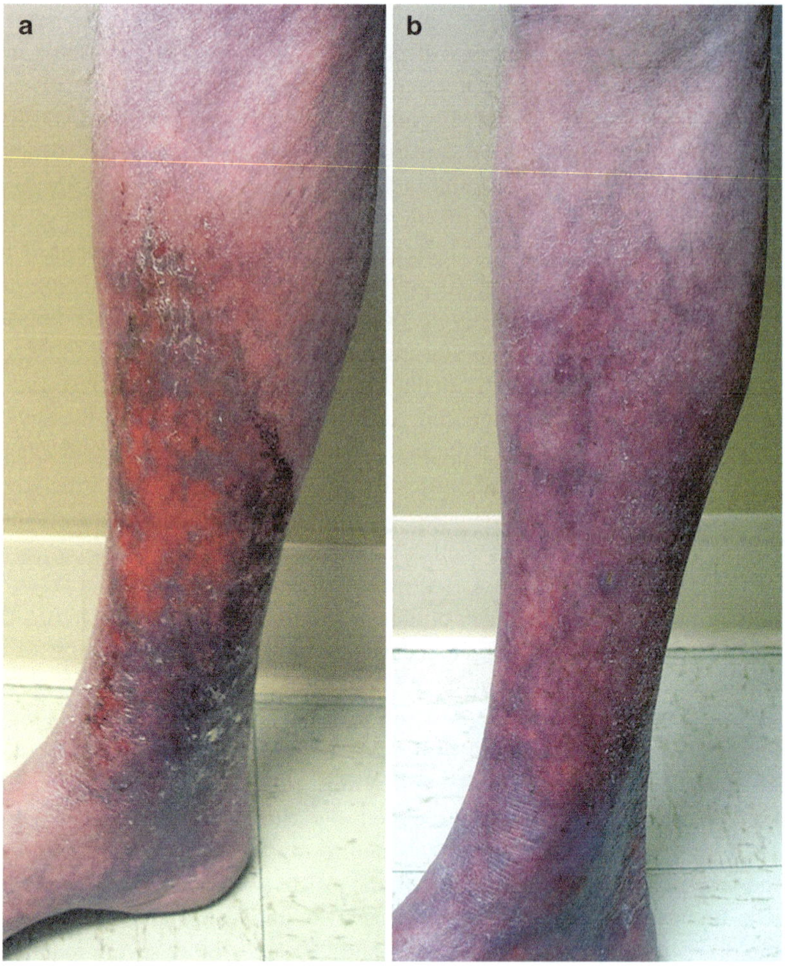

Fig. 3.1 (**a**) Before treatment Clinical C4 – VCSS 16. (**b**). Four months after treatment, patient remains Clinical C4. Now C4 – V9

clarify the clinical descriptors and make the instrument more precise (Tables 3.1 and 3.2). It has demonstrated good correlation with the results of ultrasonography, and its simplicity makes it easy to administer and score [4]. Recently, a valuable application for the VCSS has arisen in the form of its visual descriptive power. The "visual language of VCSS" is a common framework for consistent physician scoring of venous disease (Fig. 3.4). Similarity in scoring and in descriptions of venous sequelae adds to the structure of the language of CVD.

The pain component has been adapted to include patient-reported symptoms, such as ache, heaviness, fatigue, soreness, and burning. These symptoms are often found in communicating pain of venous origin. The varicose vein category has been changed to mirror the revised CEAP classification. Corona phlebectatica has been added to this category as a mild finding (Fig. 3.5). The venous edema and skin pigmentation categories (Fig. 3.6) have been changed to reflect the extent of the findings over the surface of the leg. The inflammation category was changed to include terms that indicate acute changes, namely, *erythema*, *cellulitis*, *venous eczema*, and *dermatitis* (Fig. 3.7). The induration category added the terms *chronic edema with fibrosis*, *hypodermitis*, *white atrophy*, and *lipodermatosclerosis* to indicate severity and chronicity (Fig. 3.8). Ulcer categories were refined in regard to ulcer size and duration (Fig. 3.9). The category on the use of compression therapy eliminated leg elevation and addresses only the wearing of compression garments [20].

Progression of CVD over time can be documented by the VCSS. In addition, some patients will develop recurrent disease after treatment

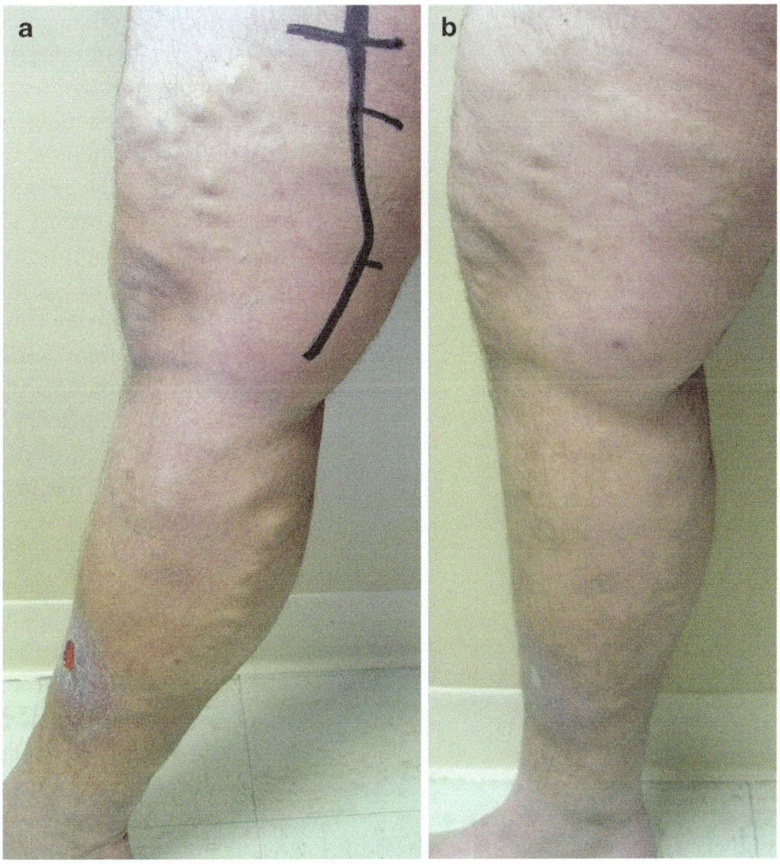

Fig. 3.2 (**a**) Prior to treatment Clinical C6 – V18. (**b**). One month after treatment Clinical C5 – V11

[21, 22]. The VCSS has a role in assessing these patients as well. The Revised VCSS coupled to clinical CEAP provides a standard clinical language to report and compare differing approaches to CVD management. For example, CEAP C6 disease can only ever improve to C5; C4 disease may remain unchanged, despite diminishing signs and symptoms; and the clinical status of patients with C2 and C3 disease varies widely. Linking the VCSS to clinical CEAP conveys a large amount of complementary information that enhances communication (Figs. 3.1, 3.2, and 3.3).

3.4 Key Definitions

The terms *chronic venous disease* and *chronic venous insufficiency*, often used interchangeably, have distinct meanings. The 2009 VEIN-TERM document gives definitions of CVD and CVI and adds a third global term, *chronic venous disorder* [21]. Chronic venous disorder "includes the full spectrum of morphological and functional abnormalities of the venous system" [21]. Chronic venous disease refers to "any morphological and functional abnormalities of the venous system of long duration manifested either by symptoms and/or signs indicating the need for investigation and/or care" [21]. *Chronic venous insufficiency* (C3–C6) is "a term reserved for advanced chronic venous disease, which is applied to functional abnormalities of the venous system producing edema, skin changes or venous ulcers" [21]. Bergan et al. in 2006 wrote that "chronic venous disease encompasses the full spectrum of signs and symptoms associated with classes C0–C6, whereas the term chronic venous insufficiency is generally restricted to disease of greater severity, (i.e., classes C4–C6)" [23].

Meissner and colleagues define CVI as "those manifestations of venous disease resulting from ambulatory venous hypertension, defined as a failure to reduce venous pressure with exercise" [13]. In the same year, Thorisson et al. wrote

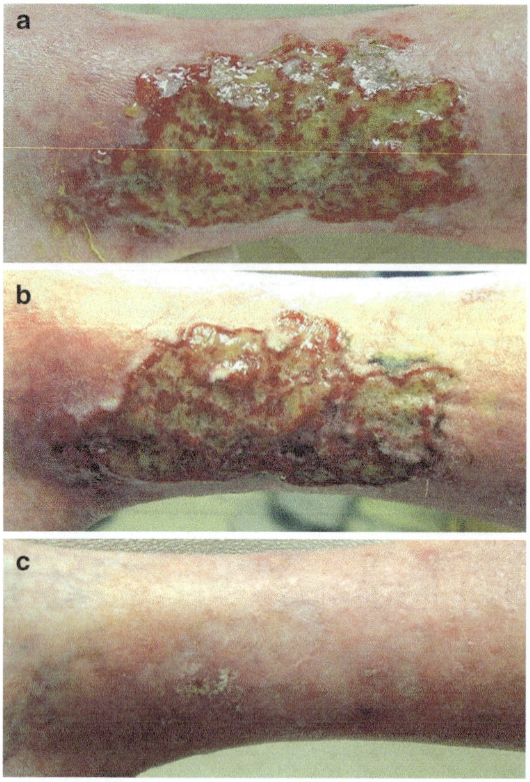

Fig. 3.3 The broadened language of uniting VCSS with CEAP in CVD. Substantial information is relayed in stating C6 – V25 to C6 – V21 and at last C5 – V7. (**a**) Pre-treatment. (**b**) One week post treatment. (**c**) Two months post treatment

that "chronic venous insufficiency (CVI) of the superficial and/or deep venous systems of the lower extremities is an extremely common condition and is estimated to occur in one of every five Americans. The most common manifestation is varicose veins…the clinical significance of CVI is not merely cosmetic because many patients experience debilitating symptoms ranging from lower extremity pain, swelling, heaviness, warmth, itching, cramping, and muscle fatigue to inflammatory dermatitis and ultimately venous stasis ulcers" [24].

3.5 Epidemiology

Standardized reporting of clinical outcomes in venous disease is expected by physician societies, hospitals, third-party payers, and government agencies. Such practices are required to compare devices and other therapeutic methods intended to improve outcomes. Despite recent increases in venous technology use and procedural volume, clinical outcome reporting is sporadic at best [6, 25]. The selection of outcome variables to study and report is crucial. Clinical outcomes measure improvement in survival, symptoms, or quality of life as a result of therapy. Surrogate outcomes include diagnostic tests, physical signs, or physiologic variables. The literature is filled with surrogate outcomes, including occlusion rates, stent patency, hemodynamic changes, and ulcer healing rates. We have an obligation to demonstrate that interventions are evidence based and to report outcomes of importance to the patient and to society, rather than isolated surrogate markers. These often provide quantifiable results in a limited follow-up period. However, it is important to note that surrogate outcomes should be held to the same standards as clinical outcomes. The change in response to treatment should still be predictive of benefit to the patient, and the relationship between the two should be clear and well defined. Surrogate outcomes should not simply be correlated with clinical outcomes but should be predictive [26].

Initial epidemiology investigations in venous disease were not standardized for data collected or results reported. Evaluation techniques varied among studies, and prevalence results for varicose veins, CVI, and specific sequelae of venous disease differed widely across geographic regions. Beginning in 2003, epidemiologic studies were published that had been performed based on the CEAP classification. The more precise definitions of the components of venous disease helped to unify the data. While there was still some variation in research methods, these studies reported results that could be compared and applied to further research [27].

The Bonn Vein Study was a population study based on CEAP [27, 28]. This German study evaluated 3,072 participants and was designed to assess the rate of occurrence and severity of CVD among the general public. Patients were enrolled from the community without prior knowledge of their venous disease status. Using standard

Table 3.1 Revised Venous Clinical Severity Score [20]

Pain Or other discomfort (i.e., aching, heaviness, fatigue, soreness, burning) Presumes venous origin	**None:** 0	**Mild:** 1 Occasional pain or other discomfort (i.e., not restricting regular daily activity)	**Moderate:** 2 Daily pain or other discomfort (i.e., interfering with but not preventing regular daily activities)	**Severe:** 3 Daily pain or discomfort (i.e., limits most regular daily activities)
Varicose veins "Varicose" veins must be ≥3 mm in diameter to qualify	**None:** 0	**Mild:** 1 Few: scattered (i.e., isolated branch varicosities or clusters) Also includes corona phlebectatica (ankle flare)	**Moderate:** 2 Confined to calf or thigh	**Severe:** 3 Involves calf and thigh
Venous edema Presumes venous origin	**None:** 0	**Mild:** 1 Limited to foot and ankle area	**Moderate:** 2 Extends above ankle but below knee	**Severe:** 3 Extends to knee and above
Skin pigmentation Presumes venous origin Does not include focal pigmentation over varicose veins or pigmentation due to other chronic diseases (i.e., vasculitis purpura)	**None:** 0 None or focal	**Mild:** 1 Limited to perimalleolar area	**Moderate:** 2 Diffuse over lower third of calf	**Severe:** 3 Wider distribution above lower third of calf
Inflammation More than just recent pigmentation (i.e., erythema, cellulitis, venous eczema, dermatitis)	**None:** 0	**Mild:** 1 Limited to perimalleolar area	**Moderate:** 2 Diffuse over lower third of calf	**Severe:** 3 Wider distribution above lower third of calf
Induration Presumes venous origin of secondary skin and subcutaneous changes (i.e., chronic edema with fibrosis, hypodermitis) Includes white atrophy and lipodermatosclerosis	**None:** 0	**Mild:** 1 Limited to perimalleolar area	**Moderate:** 2 Diffuse over lower third of calf	**Severe:** 3 Wider distribution above lower third of calf
Active ulcer number	0	1	2	≥3
Active ulcer duration (longest active)	N/A	<3 months	>3 months but <1 year	Not healed for >1 year
Active ulcer size (largest active)	N/A	Diameter <2 cm	Diameter 2–6 cm	Diameter >6 cm
Use of compression therapy	0 Not used	1 Intermittent use of stockings	2 Wears stockings most days	3 Full compliance: stockings

questionnaires, ultrasonography, and physical examination, it was possible to evaluate the rate of occurrence of CVD and its effect on several quality-of-life variables. Risk factors were determined for varicose veins (advanced age, female sex, and number of times pregnant) and for CVI (advanced age, obesity, and living in an urban setting).

The San Diego Population Study, also based on the CEAP classification, involved a large cohort evaluated specifically for telangiectases, varicose veins, skin changes, and edema [29].

Table 3.2 Instructions for using the Revised Venous Clinical Severity Score [20]

On a separate form, the clinician will be asked to: "For each leg, please check 1 box for each item (symptom and sign) that is listed below"	
Pain or other discomfort (i.e., aching, heaviness, fatigue, soreness, burning)	
The clinician describes the four categories of leg pain or discomfort that are outlined below to the patient and asks the patient to choose, separately for each leg, the category that best describes the pain or discomfort the patient experiences	
None = 0	None
Mild = 1	Occasional pain or discomfort that does not restrict regular daily
Moderate = 2	Daily pain or discomfort that interferes with, but does not prevent, regular daily activities
Severe = 3	Daily pain or discomfort that limits most regular daily activities
Varicose veins	
The clinician examines the patient's legs and, separately for each leg, chooses the category that best describes the patient's superficial veins	
Veins must be ≥3 mm in diameter to qualify as "varicose veins"	
None = 0	None
Mild = 1	Few, scattered, varicosities that are confined to branch veins or clusters. Includes "corona phlebectatica" (ankle flare), defined as >5 blue telangiectases at the inner or sometimes the outer edge of the foot
Moderate = 2	Multiple varicosities that are confined to the calf or the thigh
Severe = 3	Multiple varicosities that involve both the calf and the thigh
Venous edema	
The clinician examines the patient's legs and, separately for each leg, chooses the category that best describes the patient's pattern of leg edema. The clinician's examination may be supplemented by asking the patient about the extent of leg edema that is experienced	
None = 0	None
Mild = 1	Edema that is limited to the foot and ankle
Moderate = 2	Edema that extends above the ankle but below the knee
Severe = 3	Edema that extends to the knee or above
Skin pigmentation	
The clinician examines the patient's legs and, separately for each leg, chooses the category that best describes the patient's skin pigmentation. Pigmentation refers to color changes of venous origin and not secondary to other chronic diseases (i.e., vasculitis purpura)	
None = 0	None, or focal pigmentation that is confined to the skin over varicose veins
Mild = 1	Pigmentation that is limited to the perimalleolar area
Moderate = 2	Diffuse pigmentation that involves the lower third of the calf
Severe = 3	Diffuse pigmentation that involves more than the lower third of the calf
Inflammation	
The clinician examines the patient's legs and, separately for each leg, chooses the category that best describes the patient's skin inflammation. Inflammation refers to erythema, cellulitis, venous eczema, or dermatitis, rather than just recent pigmentation	
None = 0	None
Mild = 1	Inflammation that is limited to the perimalleolar area
Moderate = 2	Inflammation that involves the lower third of the calf
Severe = 3	Inflammation that involves more than the lower third of the calf
Induration	
The clinician examines the patient's legs and, separately for each leg, chooses the category that best describes the patient's skin induration. Induration refers to skin and subcutaneous changes such as chronic edema with fibrosis, hypodermitis, white atrophy, and lipodermatosclerosis	
None = 0	None
Mild = 1	Induration that is limited to the perimalleolar area
Moderate = 2	Induration that involves the lower third of the calf
Severe = 3	Induration that involves more than the lower third of the calf

Table 3.2 (continued)

Active ulcer number	
The clinician examines the patient's legs and, separately for each leg, chooses the category that best describes the number of active ulcers	
None=0	None
Mild=1	1 ulcer
Moderate=2	2 ulcers
Severe=3	≥3 ulcers
Active ulcer duration	
If there is at least one active ulcer, the clinician describes the four categories of ulcer duration that are outlined below to the patient and asks the patient to choose, separately for each leg, the category that best describes the duration of the longest unhealed ulcer	
None=0	No active ulcers
Mild=1	Ulceration present for <3 months
Moderate=2	Ulceration present for 3–12 months
Severe=3	Ulceration present for >12 months
Active ulcer size	
If there is at least one active ulcer, the clinician examines the patient's legs, and separately for each leg, chooses the category that best describes the size of the largest active ulcer	
None=0	No active ulcer
Mild=1	Ulcer <2 cm in diameter
Moderate=2	Ulcer 2–6 cm in diameter
Severe=3	Ulcer >6 cm in diameter
Use of compression therapy	
Choose the level of compliance with medical compression therapy	
None=0	Not used
Mild=1	Intermittent use
Moderate=2	Wears stockings most days
Severe=3	Full compliance: stockings

The study evaluated 2,211 individuals using a combination of surveys, ultrasonography, and physical examination. The results were presented as overall characteristics of venous disease, risk factors, symptoms, and quality of life. Similar to the Bonn Vein Study, risk factors found in the San Diego Population Study were advanced age and obesity, as well as family history, hormonal factors, and activity level [27, 28].

The San Diego Population Study expanded the reported results with a consideration of visual and functional ramifications of venous disease [29]. Visible hallmarks of venous disease, including telangiectases, varicose veins, and skin changes, were compared with anatomic (functional) ultrasonographic findings of superficial or deep venous reflux or obstruction. Visible disease was defined as varicose veins or skin changes, not simply telangiectases or spider veins, and functional disease was defined as the ultrasonographic presence of superficial or deep reflux or obstruction. The agreement between visible and functional disease was 92.0 %, with 17.4 % agreement for the presence of disease and 74.6 % agreement for the absence of disease. The determination was made that "visible disease did not invariably mark underlying functional disease, and functional disease was sometimes present in the absence of any visible venous disease" [29].

Venous disease, and varicosities in particular, is diagnosed with increasing frequency worldwide, with varicosities being the most frequently diagnosed vascular anomaly [16]. Chronic venous disease is a complex condition with numerous possible presentations and manifestations. Diagnosis is not always straightforward,

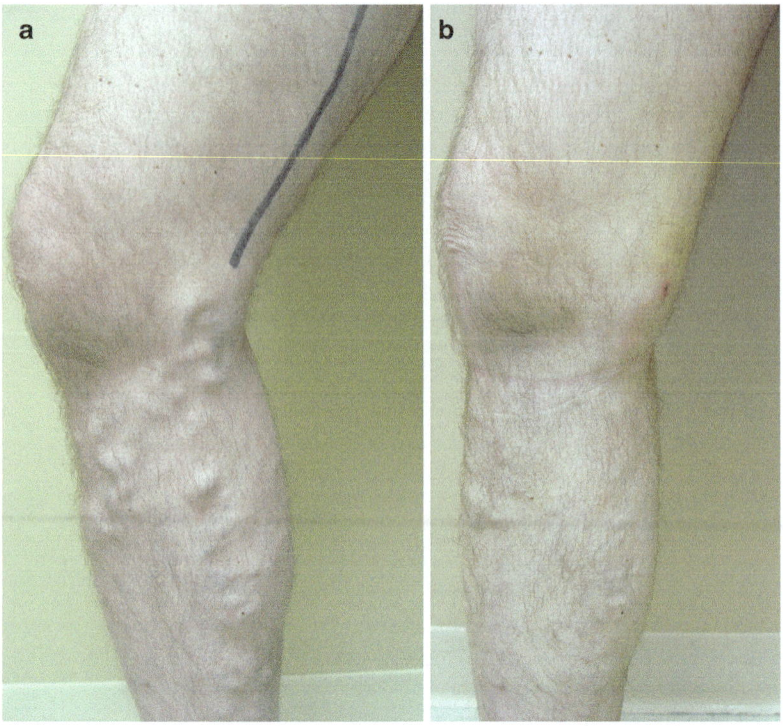

Fig. 3.4 (**a**) The "visual language" of VCSS. Consistency in physician scoring and reporting allows a common language of venous disease to emerge. Basic Clinical CEAP 3 – VCSS 7. (**b**) After treatment scoring changes to Clinical CEAP 2 – VCSS 3

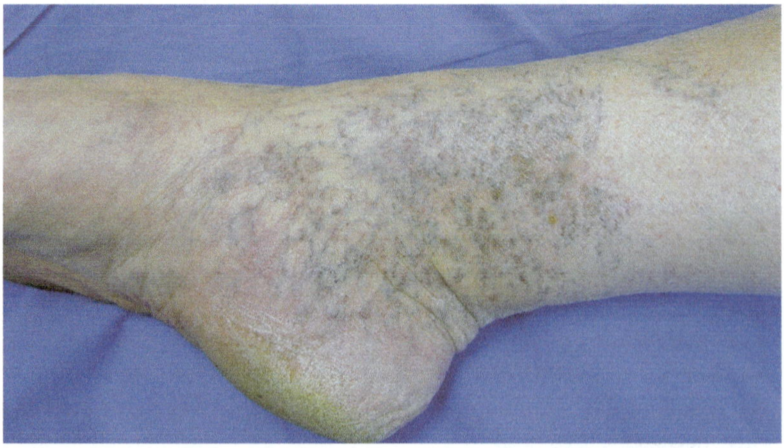

Fig. 3.5 Corona phlebectatica

generally requiring a combination of clinical experience and diagnostic testing.

Treatment for venous disease has evolved over the years, and outcome assessment has had a role in the acceptance of new procedures. Great saphenous vein stripping was generally considered the standard of care for venous disease. Removing the saphenous vein from circulation virtually ensured resolution of symptoms attributed to it. However, recurrent symptoms were seen when all levels of underlying disease were not addressed, sometimes necessitating additional invasive procedures. O'Donnell wrote in 1999: "The adoption of a surgical strategy that corrects the abnormal superficial venous system alone (saphenous veins and perforators) in the face of deep venous reflux requires that the therapeutic outcomes of such a strategy be judged with objective criteria" [30]. Implementation of results-focused analysis means that the outcome

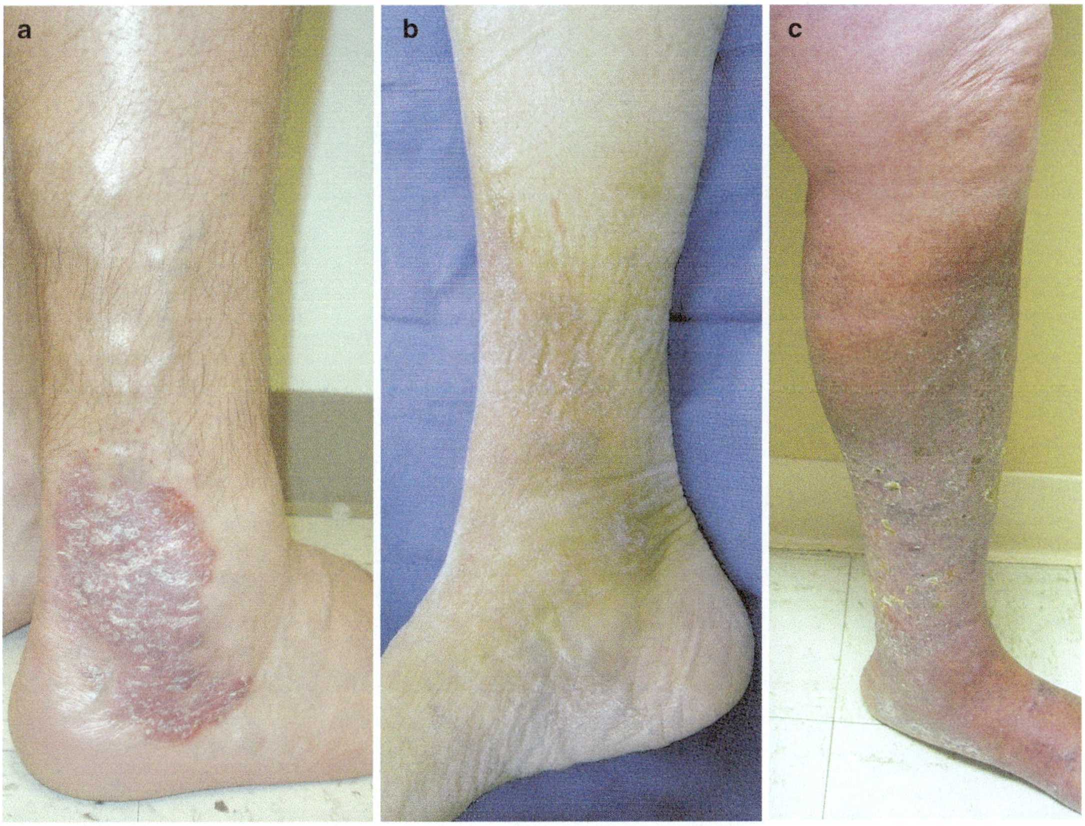

Fig. 3.6 Skin pigmentation. (**a**) Perimalleolar. (**b**) Lower third calf. (**c**) Above lower third calf

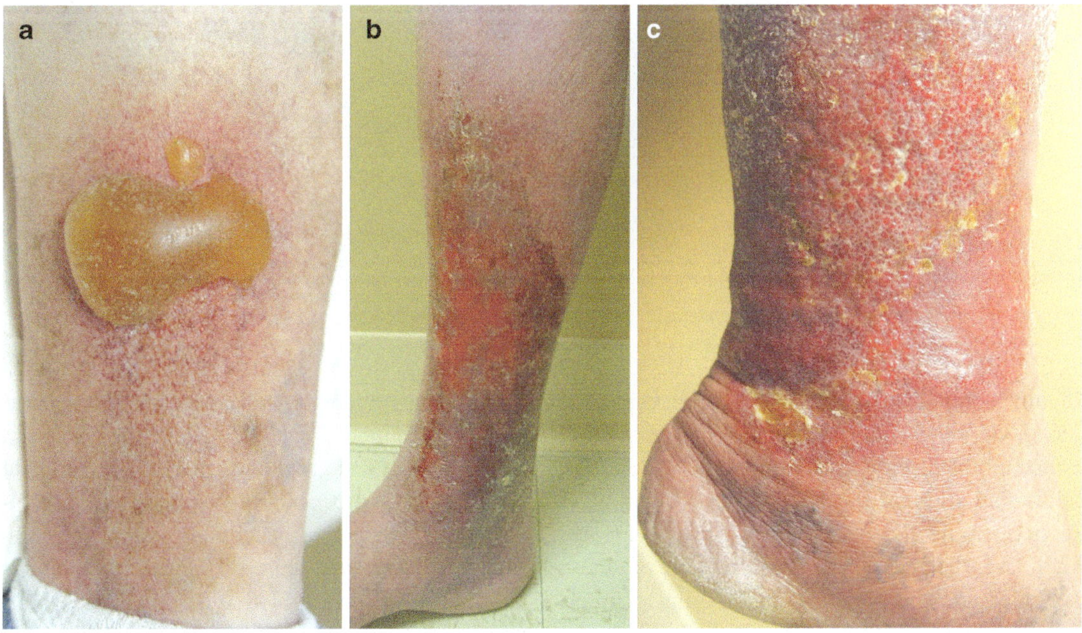

Fig. 3.7 Inflammation. (**a**) Cellulitis. (**b**) Dermatitis. (**c**) Venous eczema

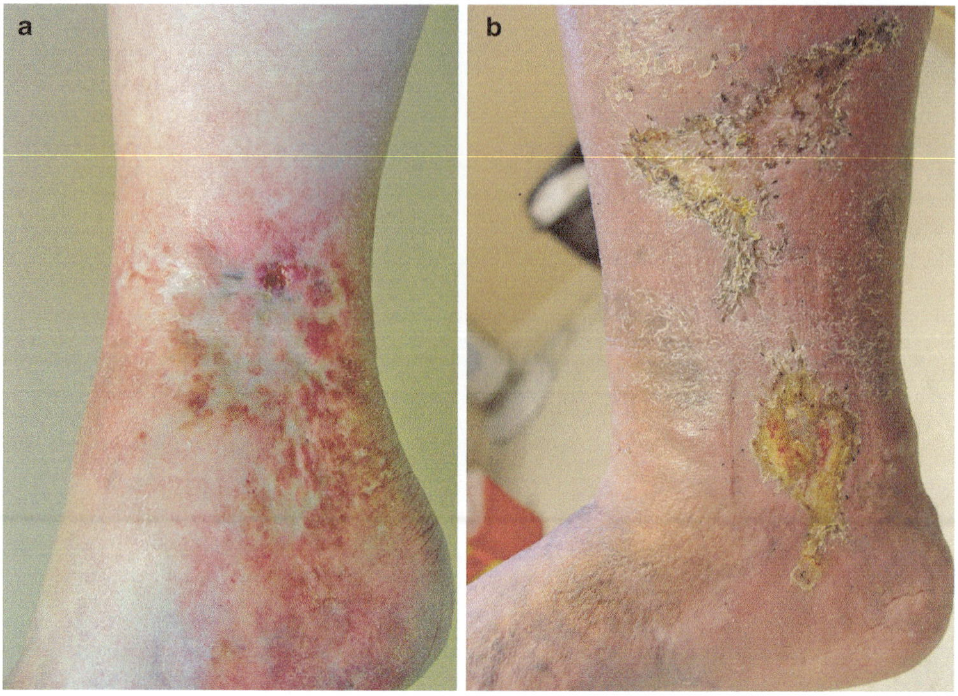

Fig. 3.8 Induration. (a) White atrophy. (b) Lipodermatosclerosis

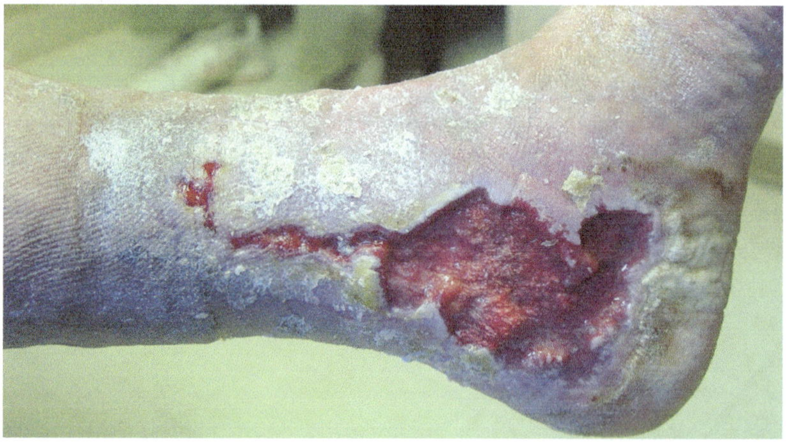

Fig. 3.9 Number of active ulcers (remains one in healing phase)

of any surgical procedure should be evaluated alongside other options, including the natural course of the disease itself, nonsurgical therapies, additional surgical interventions, or other ways of performing the intervention being evaluated [25]. Eventually, the results of this type of analysis enter into the planning and staging of interventions, with the ultimate goal of obtaining the best results with fewer invasive procedures.

The movement toward less-invasive therapeutic techniques has affected venous surgery. Modern surgical methods for CVD include superficial venous ablation, deep venous reconstruction, injection of sclerosing foam, and ligation of perforating veins. Endovascular venous ablation is proving effective as part of the strategy to address superficial veins, tributaries, and perforators. Recurrence of clinical symptoms and the emergence of new veins generally occur infrequently in patients treated with ablation, and outcome assessment of the procedure over 5 years or longer indicates that it provides a standard of care comparable to saphenous vein stripping [31].

Because of variability in the presentation of CVD, thorough outcome reporting instruments have been difficult to devise. Meissner and colleagues wrote in 2002: "The ideal clinical outcome measure for CVD would include the full spectrum of disease and be sufficiently sensitive to allow stabilization, improvement or deterioration to be precisely quantified" [5]. The goal of treating venous disease can vary widely in the opinion of the physician versus the patient. Morbidity and mortality statistics, while useful, report only the direct clinical outcome of an intervention, failing to consider other factors of potential importance to others. For an outcome to be fully evaluated, its effect on the physician, patient, and community must be considered [32].

3.6 Symptoms

Chronic venous disease encompasses many symptoms in many manifestations. Patients may experience one or all, and symptoms may improve and worsen many times throughout the course of evaluation, treatment, and follow-up care.

Initially, telangiectases and reticular and varicose veins may be asymptomatic, with patients noticing only discolored or prominent veins. As venous disease progresses, leg symptoms may develop, including achiness, heaviness, burning, throbbing, or itching, and may be accompanied by physical manifestations that include edema, eczema (Fig. 3.7), pigmentation changes (Fig. 3.6), induration (Fig. 3.8), or possibly ulceration (Fig. 3.9) [33].

Patient motivation to seek treatment for venous disease can occur at any stage of severity and is likely not triggered by any one symptom [4]. Many individuals live with severe sequelae of CVD without ever seeking treatment, some are seen only when edema or ulcers are beyond self-care, and others seek evaluation early with cosmetic concerns representing very mild venous disease.

Some patients are concerned that their symptoms may be related to peripheral artery disease. Hallmarks of peripheral artery disease include claudication, sensory or motor changes in the legs, coolness, pallor, slow hair and nail growth and shiny skin on the affected limb, weakening or loss of palpable pulse in the affected limb, or open sores that are difficult to heal [34]. It is important to rule out peripheral artery disease before initiating treatment for venous disease.

3.7 Physical Findings

When evaluating patients for CVD, several elements should be used to derive an appropriate clinical assessment and treatment plan. Eklöf et al. stratify this process into levels. Level 1 consists of the initial visit and examination, level 2 is noninvasive vascular laboratory testing, and level 3 comprises additional imaging or invasive studies [11]. A detailed clinical examination is the first step in diagnosis and should be repeated at each reevaluation. The initial visit should also include assessment of venous disease manifestations (including edema, varicose veins, telangiectases, phlebitis, pigmentation and skin-quality changes, lipodermatosclerosis, venous stasis dermatitis, and ulcers). This objective assessment should be combined with a review of the patient's history that includes weight, smoking, pregnancies, venous thromboembolic event, physical activity, and family history of venous disease, along with relevant patient-reported symptoms (including pain, aching, tingling or burning, heaviness, and fatigue) [12–14, 21, 35].

The somewhat subjective elements of clinical examination make diagnostic testing a useful objective measure [12]. Laboratory evaluations are important not only in assisting with the diagnosis of CVI but also in identifying or excluding other conditions, such as arterial disease, deep vein thrombosis, deep venous reflux, perforator disease, and venous obstruction. While primary venous disease involves reflux, a sequela of venous hypertension, secondary CVD may involve reflux and an obstructive event [36]. The obstruction may be related to venous compression or the results of a deep vein thrombosis (post-thrombotic syndrome) [36–38].

Duplex Doppler is the usual first level of laboratory evaluation, providing data on reflux (superficial or deep) and valvular incompetence, deep vein thrombosis, and obstruction, but may be insufficient to demonstrate the hemodynamic significance of obstruction or reflux [39]. Ultrasonography is beneficial in locating a duplicated femoral vein, which can be an unidentified source of deep vein thrombosis. Evidence has shown that the incidence of duplicated femoral vein is about 40 %, a significant figure because it represents possible undetected deep vein thrombosis; expanded ultrasonographic examination was recommended to rule out duplicated femoral vein in the case of leg swelling without an identifiable source [40]. Invasive diagnostic methods, including venography and intravascular ultrasonography, provide greater detail about the hemodynamic significance of venous abnormalities [39]. Although not generally used in uncomplicated venous disease, venography is indicated in complex disease, multilevel disease, and obstructive disease, including deep vein thrombosis, post-thrombotic syndrome, and non-thrombotic compressive phenomena, such as May-Thurner syndrome and non-thrombotic iliac vein lesions [38–43]. Symptoms of these lesions may mimic CVI but may also consist of severe left leg swelling and pain that may interfere with normal activity [38].

The treatment of CVI is multifactorial and depends on many variables. From conservative therapy (weight loss, leg elevation, and the use of compression stockings) to direct intervention (open surgery, endovascular therapy, or a combination of the two), the goals of therapy should be established and agreed on by the patient and the provider [44]. Regardless of the initial choice of therapy, patients need to be aware that interventions for CVI are intended to treat manifestations and slow progression of disease, not to provide a cure. Furthermore, all interventions will affect patient lifestyle, from wearing compression stockings to practicing general leg hygiene following surgery [35]. While the patient may seek treatment simply to remove unsightly and painful varicose veins, the surgeon understands that obliteration of refluxing veins may be the optimal choice for long-term relief and ultimate satisfaction [44]. In our practice, a combination of clinical examination, duplex Doppler study, and Revised VCSS is used to diagnose CVD, plan intervention, and track outcomes. Any of these elements on its own would most likely provide insufficient information to plan a treatment strategy, but by integrating all three components, a more complete picture of the clinical severity of venous disease and factors that are most important to the patient can be developed. This three-spoke strategy has proven most successful.

3.8 Basics of Recurrent Varices

The REVAS (recurrent varices after surgery) study by Perrin et al. followed up 170 patients (199 limbs) from 14 institutions seen with varicosities after venous surgery [22]. Three classifications of recurrence were identified: actual recurrent varices, residual veins with reflux, and new varicose veins due to disease progression. A classification system was developed that works in conjunction with CEAP to identify the area, cause, source, and factors leading to recurrent varices. In the combined system, the site of recurrence, source of reflux, contributing factors, and cause are classified according to REVAS, while the clinical, etiologic, anatomic, and pathophysiologic patterns are presented according to CEAP. The advanced CEAP classification was used to analyze subgroups of patients scored under REVAS. The long follow-up period (mean, 136 months) and variety of initial procedures provided insight into the nature of varicose vein presentation following initial intervention. The authors concluded that recurrence is common after venous surgery, that incompetent perforating veins not addressed at the initial procedure contribute significantly to symptoms and incidence of recurrent varices, and that a significant amount of time had elapsed for most patients between their initial procedure and the onset of recurrent varicosities. The information gained from this study provided insight for following up patients after interventions. Surveillance and future therapy can be planned within a common framework, which facilitates discussion about concomitant or staged adjunct procedures.

As endovenous ablation becomes more prevalent, questions about the timing and necessity of adjunct procedures have arisen. With endovenous ablation, there are two schools of thought: first, that adjunct procedures should be performed in the same setting to address all issues and avoid reintervention and, second, that adjunct procedures should be delayed to derive the maximum benefit from the initial ablation and obviate reintervention [45].

Min and colleagues followed up a group of 423 patients (499 limbs) after endovenous ablation to assess outcomes and complications [46]. During the 2-year follow-up period, 93.4 % of all treated veins remained occluded. Their examination of these veins by ultrasonography revealed that "...what is found on the duplex imaging early is predictive of what will be seen later, with none of the treated patients developing recanalization of successfully occluded GSVs [greater saphenous veins] at 2 or 3 years that was not seen before 9 months" [46]. According to the authors: "Although symptomatic resolution and significant improvement in the appearance of the leg is usually noted after endovenous laser treatment alone, most patients will need additional complementary procedures to fully realize the restorative benefits of treatment" [46].

Based on the results of clinical assessment, patient reporting, REVAS, CEAP, and VCSS, we now recommend that adjunct procedures be delayed at least 4 months following ablation to allow the full effect to be demonstrated. In our experience, most varices present at radiofrequency ablation diminished in size or resolved over the 4 months following the initial procedure but then leveled off in terms of change [4].

On assessment, our patients fell into several groups. First were those who had an anterolateral saphenous tributary that was recognized and treated but only over a short segment (10–15 cm). These tributary varices ran over a longer course in the leg and were more frequently treated than tributary calf varices. This has been observed by others [47]. Second, most of our greater saphenous vein ablations at the time were performed to the knee. Failure to recognize a high calf (Boyd) perforator or a non-saphenous connecting tributary resulted in below-knee greater saphenous vein reflux and reintervention. We have since adapted our preoperative mappings to look for these to preemptively treat. This also has been substantiated by others [22, 48]. Third, reflux often occurs via perforators posteriorly or laterally in the thigh or calf, with resultant varices and no connection to saphenous systems. These require direct treatment. Perforator reflux was most often noted in patients with C4–C6 disease. We occasionally saw this in patients with C3 disease, with more localized swelling, symptoms, and varices at and below the site of the perforator in the medial low calf. Endothermal ablation of perforators has mixed success; however, we now often use a combination of radiofrequency (RF) ablation and ultrasonography-guided foam ablation to treat the entire tributary bed under the diseased skin. In general, ultrasonography-guided foam ablation, instead of microphlebectomy, for tributary veins has increased in our practice, with excellent results.

We have noted certain patterns of reintervention [4]. No neovascularization was identified following radiofrequency ablation. Most patients who required intervention had residual first-order or second-order varices in the distribution of the treated saphenous segment. Residual reflux via an anterolateral saphenous, small saphenous, below-knee saphenous, or perforator vein constituted the second most common source of reintervention. Progression of disease (usually among patients with more severe disease) was the least common pattern of reintervention.

Limbs with higher initial CEAP and VCSS were significantly less likely to require further intervention than those with lower baseline CEAP and VCSS [4]. The reason for this is not entirely clear. Patients with higher initial CEAP had a greater drop in their overall VCSS. The relief obtained through ablation alone may have met these patients' expectations. It may be that patients with milder disease tend to focus on their residual varices.

The choice and timing of adjunct procedures are important to providing the best patient care and are a matter of increasing debate. Delaying adjunct procedures allows many patients to avoid potentially unnecessary procedures. Whether considering disability, pain, complications, or cost, this strategy has clear benefits. Delaying adjunct procedures allows the clinician to formulate a more directed treatment plan that can best address the individual needs of the patient as they arise. Increasing use of ultrasonography-guided foam ablation may change this paradigm.

3.9 Summary

In the realm of following outcomes in the treatment of CVD, what is the best means to report procedural outcomes as a function of clinical resolution and patient quality of life? Many advanced minimally invasive treatments for venous disease have been developed. Despite these innovations, the same question remains: How should new therapies be assessed to provide a common framework for treating patients at all levels of venous disease? We have learned over time that patients with even minor symptoms improve after superficial vein ablation, albeit not as dramatically as those with severe disease. How do we accurately assess improvement in all patients, regardless of initial disease severity? How do we appropriately stage therapy while simultaneously evaluating success from interventions and improvement in symptoms related to disease progression?

We need to establish what is medically relevant for patients with venous disease. To properly do so, we need to hear their concerns described in their own words and then infuse medical understanding into it. After treatment, we listen again and reevaluate. As providers, we need to look forward, establish goals for outcome measures, and move toward an era of commonality in reporting standards. Outcome assessment is not a new concept. Physicians, surgeons, and scientists have been engaging in discussions using the common language of outcomes for years. What has changed in recent times to bring this topic to the forefront, in America and beyond, is the need to quantify the benefit of a service in light of increasingly competitive and dwindling healthcare dollars. Outcome studies promote understanding of the diseases we treat and the results of treatment we provide. They allow us to stratify disease and therapy, as well as to compare results using a common language. The choice of a valid and reliable assessment tool is crucial. It is incumbent on us to look critically at ourselves and to objectively improve on what we do. Quality-of-life instruments and surveys are valuable indicators of patient perspective and are proven to be practical and reliable. Combining the patient-generated language of quality-of-life instruments with physician-generated surveys, such as CEAP and Revised VCSS, seems to be a good starting point for outcome assessment. The most important factor in improving treatment outcomes is the decision to examine results and to share them in a meaningful way.

References

1. Vascular Disease Foundation. Learn about vascular disease. http://www.vdf.org/. Accessed 27 Oct 2011.
2. Venous Disease Coalition. Learn about venous disease. http://www.venousdiseasecoalition.org/. Accessed 27 Oct 2011.
3. Gloviczki P, Comerota AJ, Dalsing MC, Eklöf BG, Gillespie DL, Gloviczki ML, Lohr JM, McLafferty RB, Meissner MH, Murad MH, Padberg FT, Pappas PJ, Passman MA, Raffetto JD, Vasquez MA, Wakefield TW. The care of patients with varicose veins and associated chronic venous diseases: clinical practice guidelines of the Society for Vascular Surgery and the American Venous Forum. J Vasc Surg. 2011; 53:2S–48.
4. Vasquez MA, Wang J, Mahathanaruk M, Buczkowski G, Sprehe E, Dosluoglu HH. The utility of the Venous Clinical Severity Score in 682 limbs treated by radiofrequency saphenous vein ablation. J Vasc Surg. 2007;45:1008–15.
5. Meissner MH, Natiello C, Nicholls SC. Performance characteristics of the Venous Clinical Severity Score. J Vasc Surg. 2002;36:889–95.
6. Vasquez MA, Munschauer CE. Venous Clinical Severity Score and quality-of-life assessment tools: application to vein practice. Phlebology. 2008; 23:259–75.
7. Dayal R, Kent KC. Standardized reporting practices. In: Rutherford RB, editor. Vascular surgery. 6th ed. Philadelphia: WB Saunders; 2005. p. 41–52.

8. Kundu S, Lurie F, Millward SF, Padberg F, Vedantham S, Elias S, Khilnani NM, Marston W, Cardella JF, Meissner MH, Dalsing MC, Clark TWI, Min RJ. Recommended reporting standards for endovenous ablation for the treatment of venous insufficiency: joint statement of the American Venous Forum and the Society of Interventional Radiology. J Vasc Surg. 2007;46:582–9.
9. Gloviczki P. Presidential address: venous surgery: from stepchild to equal partner. J Vasc Surg. 2003; 38:871–8.
10. Min RJ, Khilnani NM, Golia P. Duplex ultrasound evaluation of lower extremity venous insufficiency. J Vasc Interv Radiol. 2003;14:1233–41.
11. Eklöf B, Rutherford RB, Bergan JJ, Carpentier PH, Gloviczki P, Kistner RL, Meissner MH, Moneta GL, Myers K, Padberg FT, Perrin M, Ruckley CV, Smith PC, Wakefield TW, American Venous Forum International Ad Hoc Committee for Revision of the CEAP Classification. Revision of the CEAP classification for chronic venous disorders: consensus statement. J Vasc Surg. 2004;40:1248–52.
12. Meissner MH, Gloviczki P, Bergan J, Kistner RL, Morrison N, Pannier F, Pappas PJ, Rabe E, Raju S, Villavicencio JL. Primary chronic venous disorders. J Vasc Surg. 2007;46:54S–67.
13. Meissner MH, Moneta G, Burnand K, Gloviczki P, Lohr JM, Lurie F, Mattos MA, McLafferty RB, Mozes G, Rutherford RB, Padberg F, Summer DS. The hemodynamics and diagnosis of venous disease. J Vasc Surg. 2007;46:4S–24.
14. Chiesa R, Marone EM, Limoni C, Volonte M, Petrini O. Chronic venous disorders: correlation between visible signs, symptoms and presence of functional disease. J Vasc Surg. 2007;46:322–30.
15. Kistner RL, Eklöf B. Classification and etiology of chronic venous disease. In: Gloviczki P, editor. Handbook of venous disorders. 3rd ed. London: Hodder Arnold; 2009. p. 37–46.
16. Kakkos SK, Rivera MA, Matsagas MI, Lazarides MK, Robless P, Belcaro G, Geroulakos G. Validation of the new venous severity scoring system in varicose vein surgery. J Vasc Surg. 2003;38:224–8.
17. Ricci MA, Emmerich J, Callas PW, Rosendaal FR, Stanley AC, Naud S, Vossen C. Evaluating chronic venous disease with a new venous severity scoring system. J Vasc Surg. 2003;38:909–15.
18. Rutherford RB, Padberg FT, Comerota AJ, Kistner RL, Meissner MH, Moneta GL. Venous severity scoring: an adjunct to venous outcome assessment. J Vasc Surg. 2000;31:1307–12.
19. Gillett JL, Perrin MR, Allaert FA. Clinical presentation and venous severity scoring of patients with extended deep axial vein reflux. J Vasc Surg. 2006; 44:588–94.
20. Vasquez MA, Rabe E, McLafferty RB, Shortell CK, Marston WA, Gillespie D, Meissner MH, Rutherford RB. Revision of the Venous Clinical Severity Score: venous outcomes consensus statement: special communication of the American Venous Forum Ad Hoc Outcomes Working Group. J Vasc Surg. 2010;52:1387–96.
21. Eklöf B, Perrin M, Delis KT, Rutherford RB, Gloviczki P, American Venous Forum; European Venous Forum; International Union of Phlebology; American College of Phlebology; International Union of Angiology. Updated terminology of chronic venous disorders: the VEIN-TERM transatlantic interdisciplinary consensus document. J Vasc Surg. 2009;49:498–501.
22. Perrin MR, Labropoulos N, Leon Jr LR. Presentation of the patient with recurrent varices after surgery (REVAS). J Vasc Surg. 2006;43:327–34.
23. Bergan JJ, Schmid-Schönbein GW, Smith PD, Nicolaides AN, Boisseau MR, Eklöf B. Chronic venous disease. N Engl J Med. 2006;355:488–98.
24. Thorisson HM, Pollack JS, Scoutt L. The role of ultrasound in the diagnosis and treatment of chronic venous insufficiency. Ultrasound Q. 2007;23(2):137–50.
25. Rutherford RB. Presidential address: vascular surgery: comparing outcomes. J Vasc Surg. 1996;23:5–17.
26. Meissner MH. "I enjoyed your talk, but…": evidence-based medicine and the scientific foundation of the American Venous Forum. J Vasc Surg. 2009;49(1):244–8.
27. Rabe E, Pannier F. Epidemiology of chronic venous disorders. In: Gloviczki P, editor. Handbook of venous disorders. 3rd ed. London: Hodder Arnold; 2009. p. 105–10.
28. Rabe E, Pannier F. What have we learned from the Bonn Vein study? Phlebolymphology. 2006;13:188–94.
29. Criqui MH, Denenberg JO, Langer RD, Kaplan RM, Fronek A. Epidemiology of chronic peripheral venous disease. In: Bergan JJ, editor. The vein book. Burlington: Elsevier Academic Press; 2007. p. 27–37.
30. O'Donnell TF. Lessons from the past guide the future: is history truly circular? J Vasc Surg. 1999; 30(5):775–86.
31. Merchant RF, Pichot O. Long-term outcomes of endovenous radiofrequency obliteration of saphenous reflux as a treatment for superficial venous insufficiency. J Vasc Surg. 2005;42:502–9.
32. Vasquez MA, Munschauer CE. Clinical and surrogate outcomes from the new radiofrequency catheter: an experience of 700 limbs. In: Greenhalgh R, editor. Vascular and endovascular challenges update. Bodmin: MPG Books Ltd; 2010. p. 425–33.
33. Mayo Clinic. Varicose veins. 2011. http://www.mayoclinic.com/health/varicose-veins/DS00256. Accessed 28 Oct 2011.
34. Mayo Clinic. Peripheral artery disease (PAD). 2010. http://www.mayoclinic.com/health/peripheral-arterial-disease/DS00537. Accessed 28 Oct 2011. Mayo Foundation for Medical Education and Research.
35. Carr SC. Current management of varicose veins. Clin Obstet Gynecol. 2006;49(2):414–26.
36. Neglén P, Thrasher TL, Raju S. Venous outflow obstruction: an underestimated contributor to chronic venous disease. J Vasc Surg. 2003;38:879–85.
37. Meissner MH, Eklöf B, Smith PC, Dalsing MC, DePalma RG, Gloviczki P, Moneta G, Neglén P, O'Donnell T,

Partsch H, Raju S. Secondary chronic venous disorders. J Vasc Surg. 2007;46(suppl S):68S–83.
38. Raju S, Neglén P. High prevalence of nonthrombotic iliac vein lesions in chronic venous disease: a permissive role in pathogenicity. J Vasc Surg. 2006;44:136–44.
39. Porter JM, Rutherford RB, Clagett GP, Cranley JJ, O'Donnell TF, Raju S, Zierler RE, Browse N, Nicolaides A. Reporting standards in venous disease. J Vasc Surg. 1988;8:172–81.
40. Paraskevas P. Femoral vein duplication: incidence and potential significance. Phlebology. 2011;26:52–5.
41. Neglén P, Hollis KC, Raju S. Combined saphenous ablation and iliac stent placement for complex severe chronic venous disease. J Vasc Surg. 2006;44:828–33.
42. Neglén P, Hollis KC, Olivier J, Raju S. Stenting of the venous outflow in chronic venous disease: long-term stent-related outcome, clinical, and hemodynamic result. J Vasc Surg. 2007;46:979–90.
43. Neglén P, Raju S. Intravascular ultrasound scan evaluation of the obstructed vein. J Vasc Surg. 2002;35:694–700.
44. Lurie F, Creton D, Eklöf B, Kabnick LS, Kistner RL, Pichot O, Schuller-Petrovic S, Sessa C. Prospective randomized study of endovenous radiofrequency obliteration (closure procedure) versus ligation and stripping in a selected patient population (EVOLVeS Study). J Vasc Surg. 2003;38(2):207–14.
45. Caradice D, Mekako AI, Hatfield J, Chetter IC. Randomized clinical trial of concomitant or sequential phlebectomy after endovenous laser therapy for varicose veins. Br J Surg. 2009;96:369–75.
46. Min RJ, Khilnani N, Zimmet SE. Endovenous laser treatment of saphenous vein reflux: long-term results. J Vasc Interv Radiol. 2003;14(8):991–6.
47. Monahan DL. Can phlebectomy be deferred in the treatment of varicose veins? J Vasc Surg. 2005;42:1145–9.
48. Theivacumar NS, Dellagrammaticas D, Mavor AI, Gough MJ. Endovenous laser ablation: does standard above-knee great saphenous vein ablation provide optimum results in patients with both above- and below-knee reflux? A randomized controlled trial. J Vasc Surg. 2008;48:173–8.

Reflux Management

4

Daniel F. Geersen and Eric Mowatt-Larssen

Contents

Abstract

The most common cause of chronic venous disease (CVD) is reflux. Reflux is abnormal blood flow direction resulting from venous valve dysfunction. In the lower extremity thigh and calf, abnormal flow is from proximal to distal in deep or superficial veins, or deep to superficial in perforator veins. Reflux is most often primary (unknown etiology and not present at birth), is less often secondary (known cause like thrombosis or trauma), and is rarely congenital. This chapter will discuss how to manage symptomatic venous reflux disease.

4.1 Introduction

The most common cause of chronic venous disease (CVD) is reflux. Reflux is abnormal blood flow direction resulting from venous valve dysfunction. In the lower extremity thigh and calf, abnormal flow is from proximal to distal in deep or superficial veins, or deep to superficial in perforator veins. To account for a normal valve closure time, reflux is defined by consensus opinion to be 0.5 s for veins generally, with the exception of the femoropopliteal deep system, where the value is 1.0 s [1]. Reflux is most often primary (unknown etiology and not present at birth), is less often secondary (known cause like thrombosis or trauma), and is rarely congenital.

Obstruction, typically from thrombosis, is also an important cause of CVD. Anatomic

D.F. Geersen, MPAP, PA-C
Division of Vascular Surgery, Duke University Medical Center, Durham, NC, USA
e-mail: daniel.geersen@duke.edu

E. Mowatt-Larssen, MD, FACPh, RPhS (✉)
Pacific Street 757, Suite C-2, Monterey, CA 93940, USA
e-mail: eric.mowatt.larssen@gmail.com, veinspecs@gmail.com

E. Mowatt-Larssen et al. (eds.), *Phlebology, Vein Surgery and Ultrasonography*,
DOI 10.1007/978-3-319-01812-6_4, © Springer International Publishing Switzerland 2014

Table 4.1 Common venous discomfort symptoms

Tingling
Aching
Burning
Muscle cramps
Swelling
Throbbing
Heaviness
Itching
Restless legs
Tiredness
Fatigue

obstructions, such as vein compression from an artery, as in May-Thurner syndrome, or even a tumor, can also cause CVD. Some unfortunate patients may have combined reflux and obstruction, which produces worse symptoms than either condition alone. Both reflux and obstruction in the infrainguinal lower extremity are accurately diagnosed by duplex ultrasound, and this test is essential to management of potential CVD patients.

This chapter will discuss how to manage symptomatic venous reflux disease. Not all reflux causes symptoms, and not all reflux should be treated. The differential diagnosis of potential venous symptoms will be discussed. Then the principles of conservative and procedural management will be outlined.

4.2 Differential Diagnosis

CVD can manifest itself in a variety of ways. The hallmark symptoms of CVD are pain, discomfort, spider veins, reticular veins, varicose veins, swelling, skin changes, and leg ulcers. Table 4.1 outlines common venous discomfort complaints. Pain, discomfort, and swelling symptoms typically worsen with extremity dependence (i.e., standing) as the day progresses, since reflux is activated by gravity. The symptoms are also worse when the weather is warm, as a result of venous dilatation. Symptoms usually improve with extremity elevation or compression. Swelling, skin changes, and ulcers typically start at the ankle area, where ambulatory venous pressure is highest, but may progress proximally up the calf and thigh.

Table 4.2 outlines differential diagnostic considerations for lower extremity pain and discomfort. Tables 4.3 and 4.4 outline the differential diagnoses of unilateral and bilateral leg swelling, respectively. Table 4.5 outlines the differential diagnosis of leg ulcers. Skin changes in the ankle area are often due to chronic venous insufficiency, but each skin sign has a differential diagnosis of its own, and dermatology consultation should be considered if chronic venous insufficiency cannot be ruled in. Leg ulcers can also be caused by skin cancer, or venous ulcers can become malignant [2]. It is not clear from the literature when to biopsy, but skin biopsy should be considered for leg ulcers which do not heal despite appropriate management and

Table 4.2 Differential diagnosis of lower extremity pain and discomfort

Deep or superficial venous thrombosis
Peripheral arterial disease
Iliocaval obstruction
Pelvic congestion syndrome
Proximal venous reflux (i.e., branches of the internal iliac vein)
Vascular malformation
Nutcracker syndrome
Chronic compartment syndrome
Neuralgia (i.e., sciatica)
Complex regional pain syndrome
Restless legs syndrome
Musculoskeletal (i.e., muscle/tendon/ligament sprain, muscle pain, osteoarthritis, rheumatoid arthritis)
Cellulitis

Table 4.3 Differential diagnosis of unilateral leg swelling

Chronic venous insufficiency
Deep venous thrombosis
Iliocaval obstruction
Lymphedema
Lipedema
Baker's cyst
Cellulitis
Orthopedic trauma

Table 4.4 Differential diagnosis of bilateral leg swelling

Bilateral chronic venous insufficiency
Congestive heart failure
Pulmonary hypertension
Protein-losing nephropathy
Liver cirrhosis
Obesity

Table 4.5 Differential diagnosis of leg ulcer

Venous ulcer
Peripheral arterial disease
Neuropathic ulcer
Pressure ulcer
Skin cancer

patient compliance and for nonhealing leg ulcers in unusual locations.

More advanced CVD, measured as increased CEAP class, is associated with more areas of reflux. Saphenous reflux is common in all CEAP classes. The prevalence of perforator and deep venous reflux increases with increasing CEAP class [3]. The most common pattern of saphenous reflux involves the great saphenous vein (GSV) (Fig. 4.1). Reflux in the small saphenous vein (Fig. 4.2) or anterior accessory GSV (Fig. 4.3) is also common. However, crossover involvement occurs, and each patient with suspected CVD merits a duplex ultrasound to determine if they meet the typical pattern [4]. Non-saphenous reflux (Fig. 4.4) occurs in around 10 % of patients [5].

Venous symptoms can also be caused by venous sources other than lower extremity reflux or obstruction. Iliocaval obstruction should be considered in patients with venous symptoms with minimal or no reflux on infrainguinal ultrasound. Pelvic congestion syndrome can present with pelvic pain or varicosities or lower extremity varicosities which can be followed with ultrasound above the inguinal ligament. A vascular malformation usually presents at birth or puberty (due to hormonal changes) and can also be suggested by unusual anatomy seen on ultrasound. Reflux of tributaries of the internal iliac vein can cause varicosities on the buttocks or pelvic areas.

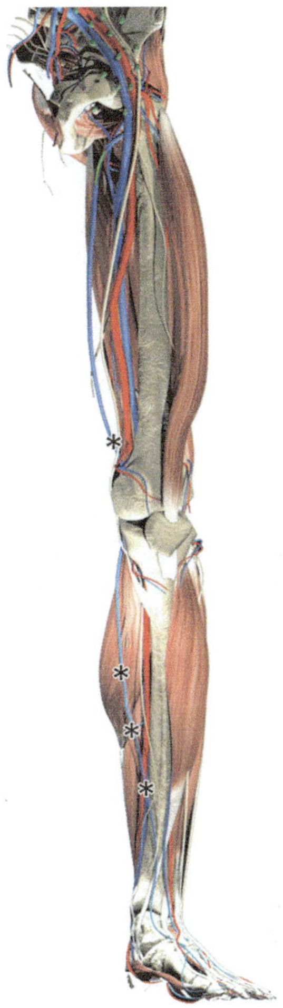

Fig. 4.1 The classic great saphenous vein (*asterisk*) pattern

4.3 Medical Management

Multiple conservative measures have been recommended for patients with CVD, including compression, leg elevation, exercise, diet and weight loss, and analgesics. Compression options include elastic compression stockings, inelastic bandaging, and pneumatic compression. Prescription strength compression stockings start at 20–30 mmHg (Class 1) and are followed by 30–40 mmHg (Class 2), 40–50 mmHg (Class 3), and 50+ mmHg (Class 4). In general, compression at 20–30 mmHg seems effective for symptomatic varicosities, while 30–40 mmHg is preferred if tolerated for those with venous ulcers

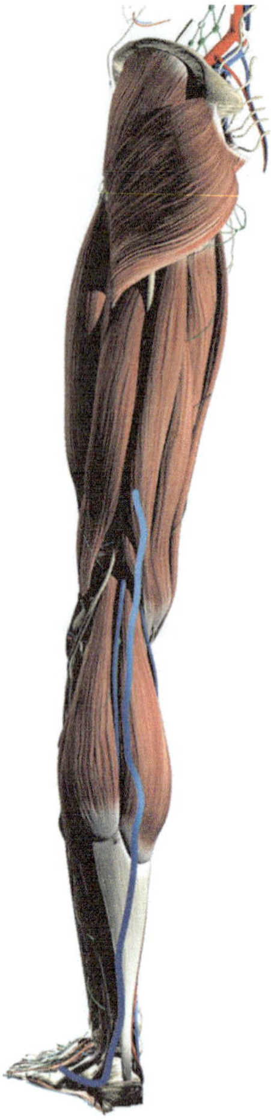

Fig. 4.2 Classic small saphenous vein reflux pattern

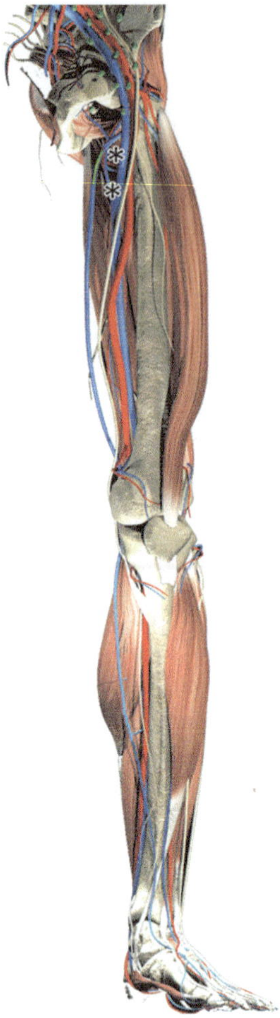

Fig. 4.3 The anterior accessory great saphenous vein (*asterisk*), when present, runs superficial to the femoral vessels

or leg swelling [1]. Knee-high length is often used due to greater ease in getting the stocking on, but thigh and pantyhose styles are also available. Compression therapy improves symptoms and quality of life in patients with simple symptomatic varicosities, but it does not reverse disease [6]. In patients with venous ulcers, compression accelerates healing and reduces ulcer recurrence risk [7]. Compression has not been shown to reduce varicosity recurrence rates or slow disease progression [6].

Compression therapy is contraindicated in patients with significant peripheral arterial disease, congestive heart failure, or active infection at the site. Patient compliance and difficulty getting the stocking on can be a major problem, so providers should carefully explain the benefits to patients. Interventional ablation of symptomatic reflux is more effective in improving quality of life than compression and lifestyle modification [8]. Despite the data, third-party payers often require a "trial" of conservative measures, such as compression, before ablation can be performed.

Exercise has been advocated under the hypothesis that making the calf muscle stronger, even in the presence of malfunctioning venous valves from reflux, may improve overall calf muscle pump function. In patients with venous ulcers, improving ankle range of motion and muscle strength improves venous hemodynamic parameters but has not yet been clearly shown to affect clinical outcomes [9].

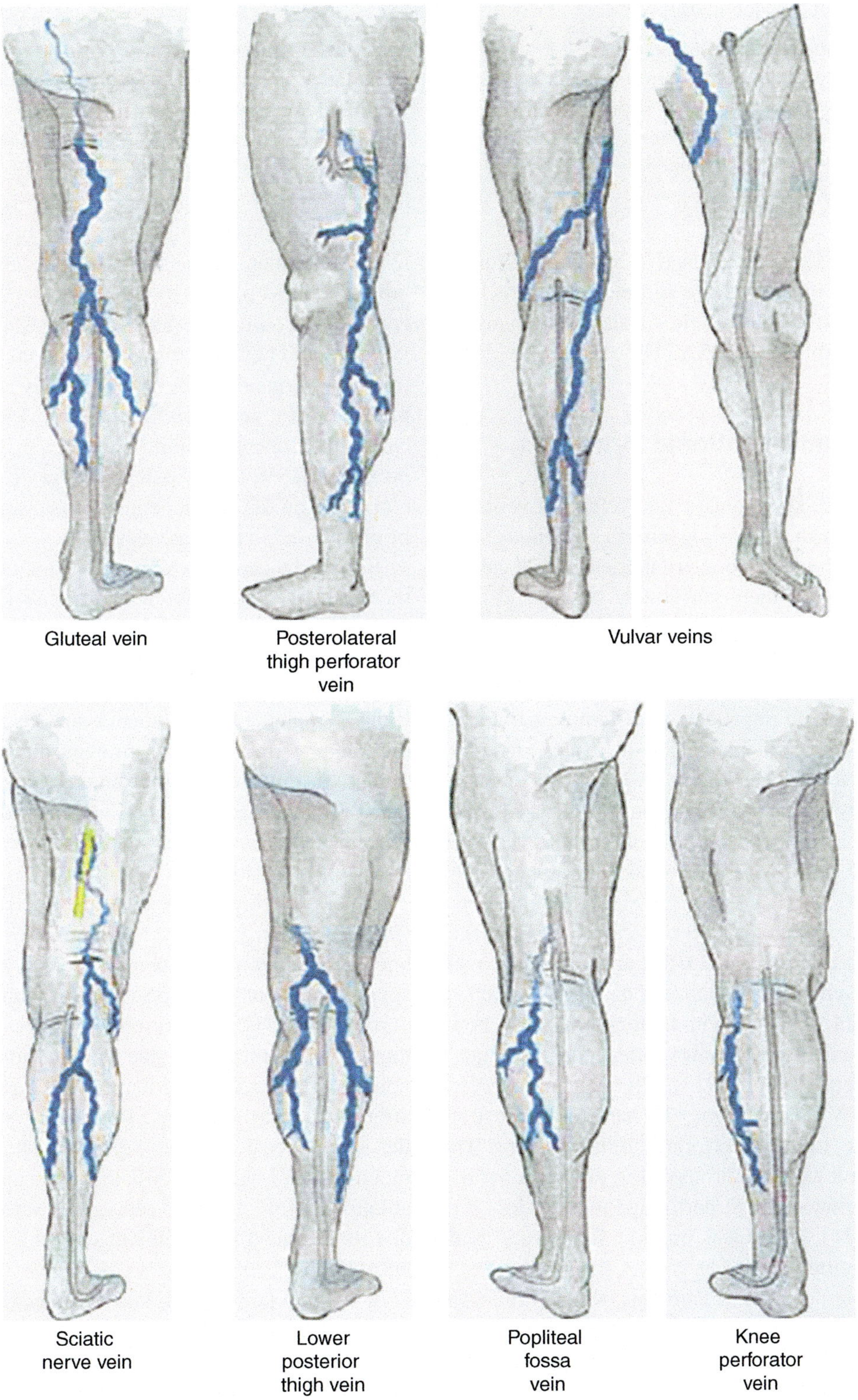

Fig. 4.4 Non-saphenous vein reflux patterns (Used with permission) [5]

Table 4.6 Venoactive medicines

Horse chestnut seed extract (aescin)
Flavonoids – rutosides, diosmin, hesperidin
Micronized purified flavonoid fraction (MPFF)
French maritime pine bark extract
Calcium dobesilate, naftazone
Benzarone

Table 4.6 lists venoactive medicines. Studies on these medicines are limited, none are FDA approved for venous reflux disease, and many are not available in the USA [1].

4.4 Interventional Strategies

In general, symptomatic and refluxing veins are treated in the following order: saphenous, then epifascial (saphenous tributaries and localized varicosities), then perforator veins, and then deep veins. This order is based upon assessment of benefits and risks. Ablation of symptomatic saphenous reflux has been shown to improve quality of life in patients with symptomatic varicosities [10]. In patients with healed or active ulcers, it has been shown to reduce ulcer recurrence by 25 % at 4 years, from 50 to 25 % [11]. It is not clear if saphenous ablation improves ulcer healing rates, with positive and negative results reported [11, 12].

Incompetent perforator vein (IPV) management is controversial. IPVs are associated with worse venous disease, based on CEAP score [3]. The clinical benefit with treatment of IPVs, however, has not been shown independent of saphenous vein treatment [13]. Clinical improvement after IPV treatment may be hard to demonstrate because isolated perforator reflux is rare. The ankle blowout syndrome of a leg ulcer with a nearby incompetent perforator was described in 1953 [14]. Consensus opinion still favors treatment in this setting [1].

Some deep vein treatments, such as iliocaval stenting for obstruction or gonadal vein ablation for pelvic congestion syndrome, carry a high benefit at low risk. Other deep vein disease treatments, such as those for mixed obstruction and reflux, carry significant morbidity and require specialized skills, allowing performance only at specialized centers.

Relative contraindications to superficial vein treatment include severe medical comorbidities which limit patient quality of life benefits from treatment. Inability to walk reasonably (i.e., at least 5 min/h) may increase clot risk with treatment. Although the opinion has been challenged, treatment of the superficial system in the presence of deep venous obstruction is generally considered contraindicated, since the superficial system could be functioning as collateral circulation [15]. Acute thrombosis is generally a contraindication to superficial treatment, except in cases like saphenofemoral junction ligation of proximal GSV thrombosis in order to reduce embolization risk. Anticoagulation, however, can be considered in this case as well.

Some advocate concomitant instead of staged therapies of saphenous and epifascial systems. The main benefit of the concomitant strategy is that the patient can be treated in one session, resulting in a faster improvement in quality of life, although the improvement is not sustained in the longer term [16]. This strategy may be particularly useful for patients who travel a long distance for their appointments, who lack the time for repeated visits, or who are undergoing ambulatory phlebectomies.

Others advocate staged treatments. After GSV ablation, attached varicosities often become smaller, and some disappear [17]. Even small saphenous vein (SSV) reflux sometimes corrects after GSV ablation [18]. Presumably these improvements are due to reduction of the volume of reflux moving distally into these veins after successful ablations. Remaining varicosities are then easier to treat [19]. Some have even recommended waiting 4 months after saphenous ablation before treating remaining varicosities due to less need for treatment with this waiting period [20].

It is important for patients to understand that any chronic venous disease management strategy does not cure vein disease, but can often make a big difference in clinical endpoints such as quality of life and ulcer recurrence. Still, varicosity or ulcer recurrence remains a risk. The patient who presents with recurrent chronic venous disease needs a reassessment, including duplex ultrasound, to determine the cause of recurrence before a successful treatment strategy can be implemented.

4.5 Alternative Strategies

Some advocate treatment of the superficial tributaries before the saphenous in many cases. The saphenous-first strategy was based on a pathophysiologic model that reflux begins at saphenous-deep junctions, such as the saphenofemoral junction, and then progresses distally gradually, usually over several years. More recent ultrasound studies challenge that belief [21]. Based on this new information, some advocate treating the refluxing tributaries and localized varicosities first, before the refluxing saphenous vein, in many cases. Retrospective data on this technique, termed ASVAL (ambulatory selective varices ablation under local anesthesia), is intriguing [22].

An additional challenge to the standard saphenous then tributaries model comes from some who advocate disconnecting points where reflux crosses from deep to saphenous (like the saphenofemoral junction) or from saphenous to *epifascial* (like the saphenous-tributary junction) but to otherwise preserve these refluxing veins in order to preserve venous drainage and thus prevent disease recurrence [23]. CHIVA (for the French, "cure conservatrice et hemodynamique de l'insuffisance veineuse en ambulatoire" and in English, "conservative hemodynamic treatment for chronic venous insufficiency") utilizes surgical ligations for disconnection [24]. CHIVA has been shown in two randomized, controlled trials to reduce recurrence in comparison to surgical high ligation and stripping [25, 26].

4.6 Ablation Techniques

Thermal (endovenous laser or radiofrequency), surgical (high ligation with or without stripping), and chemical (ultrasound-guided foam sclerotherapy) are all safe and effective techniques to ablate a symptomatic saphenous vein. There are few studies comparing clinical endpoints between these options. The American Venous Forum and Society for Vascular Surgery recommend thermal ablation as first choice in a consensus opinion because it is minimally invasive and has similar or better early-term results, and equivalent midterm results, as surgery [1]. Techniques for ultrasound-guided foam sclerotherapy are rapidly improving, but results are not yet as good as those seen with thermal ablation and surgery [1].

Ablation techniques for epifascial veins include chemical (sclerotherapy with or without ultrasound guidance) and surgical (microphlebectomy or powered phlebectomy) [19]. Chemical ablation is fully reviewed in Chap. 11 and surgical techniques in Chap. 12. Thermal ablation (laser or radiofrequency), reviewed in Chap. 10, can also be used in some cases if the vein is straight and long enough for technical success, but this technique is less commonly used for these veins [19].

Surgical endoscopic perforator surgery (SEPS), thermal ablation, and ultrasound-guided foam sclerotherapy are all technically successful therapies for incompetent perforating veins [1]. Some deep vein problems, such as iliocaval obstruction and pelvic congestion syndrome, are now also amenable to endovascular treatments. Other deep vein diseases require sophisticated techniques like valvuloplasty or even venous bypass, which are performed only at specialized centers.

Conclusions

Venous disease occupies a wide spectrum of severity and possible treatments. The keys to success remain the same: identify the source of the symptoms; treat in order to achieve a durable improvement in quality of life for patients; and minimize venous disease recurrence. The history of phlebology is far from written. New technologies, instrumentation, and knowledge of the subject continue to alter our understanding of the disease.

References

1. Gloviczki P, Comerota A, Dalsing M, Eklof B, Gillespie D, Gloviczki M, Lohr J, McLafferty R, Meissner M, Murad M, Padberg F, Pappas P, Passman M, Raffetto J, Vasquez M, Wakefield T. The care of patients with varicose veins and associated chronic venous diseases: clinical practice guidelines of the Society for Vascular Surgery and the American Venous Forum. J Vasc Surg. 2011;53:2S–48.
2. Miller DR, Enoch S, Williams DT, Price PE, Harding KG. Value of wound biopsy in chronic venous ulceration. Phlebology. 2004;19:65–8.
3. Labropoulos N. Clinical correlation to various patterns of reflux. Vasc Endovascular Surg. 1997;31:242–8.
4. Obermayer A, Garzon K. Identifying the source of superficial reflux in venous leg ulcers using duplex ultrasound. J Vasc Surg. 2010;52:1255–61.
5. Labropoulos N, Tiongson J, Pryor L, Tassiopoulo AK, Kang SS, Mansour MA, Baker WH. Nonsaphenous superficial vein reflux. J Vasc Surg. 2001;34:872–7.
6. Palfreyman SJ, Michaels JA. A systematic review of compression hosiery for uncomplicated varicose veins. Phlebology. 2009;24 Suppl 1:13–33.
7. Motykie GD, Caprini JA, Arcelus JI, Reyna JJ, Overom E, Mokhtee D, et al. Evaluation of therapeutic compression stockings in the treatment of chronic venous insufficiency. Dermatol Surg. 1999;25:116–20.
8. Michaels JA, Campbell WB, Brazier JE, Macintyre JB, Palfreyman SJ, Ratcliffe J, et al. Randomized clinical trial, observational study and assessment of cost effectiveness of the treatment of varicose veins (REACTIV trial). Health Technol Assess. 2006;10:1–196.
9. Padberg FT, Johnston MV, Sisto SA. Structured exercise improves calf muscle pump function in chronic venous insufficiency: a randomized trial. J Vasc Surg. 2004;39:79–87.
10. Mowatt-Larssen E, Shortell C. Truncal vein ablation for laser: radial firing at high wavelength is the key? J Vasc Endovasc Surg. 2010;17:217–23.
11. Barwell JR, Davies CE, Deacon J, Harvey K, Minor J, Sassano A, et al. Comparison of surgery and compression with compression alone in chronic venous ulceration (ESCHAR study): randomized controlled trial. Lancet. 2004;363:1854–9.
12. Zamboni P, Cisno C, Marchetti F, Mazza P, Fogato L, Carandina S, De Palma M, Liboni A. Minimally invasive surgical management of primary venous ulcers vs compression treatment: a randomized clinical trial. Eur J Vasc Endovasc Surg. 2003;25:313–8.
13. O'Donnell TF. The present status of surgery of the superficial venous system in the management of venous ulcer and the evidence for the role of perforator interruption. J Vasc Surg. 2008;48:1044–52.
14. Cockett FB, Jones DE. The ankle blow-out syndrome: a new approach to the varicose ulcer problem. Lancet. 1953;1:17–23.
15. Labropoulos N, Volteas N, Leon M, Sowade O, Rulo A, Giannoukas AD, Nicolaides AN. The role of venous outflow obstruction in patients with chronic venous dysfunction. Arch Surg. 1997;132:46–51.
16. Carradice D, Mekako AI, Hatfield J, Chetter IC. Randomized clinical trial of concomitant or sequential phlebectomy after endovenous laser therapy for varicose veins. Br J Surg. 2009;96:369–75.
17. Monahan D. Can phlebectomy be deferred in the treatment of varicose veins? J Vasc Surg. 2005;42:1145–9.
18. Markovic J, Shortell C. Endovenous laser ablation: strategies for treating multilevel disease. Perspect Vasc Surg Endovasc Ther. 2009;21:73–81.
19. Mowatt-Larssen E. Management of secondary varicosities. Semin Vasc Surg. 2010;23:107–12.
20. Vasquez MA, Wang J, Mahathanaruk M, Buczkowski G, Sprehe E, Dosluoglu HH. The utility of the Venous Clinical Severity Score in 682 limbs treated by radiofrequency saphenous vein ablation. J Vasc Surg. 2007;45:1008–15.
21. Bernardini EB, De Rango P, Piccioli R, et al. Development of primary superficial venous insufficiency: the ascending theory. Observational and hemodynamic data from a 9-year experience. Ann Vasc Surg. 2010;24:709–20.
22. Pittaluga P, Chastanet S, Rea B, Barbe R. Midterm results of the surgical treatment of varices by phlebectomy with conservation of a refluxing saphenous vein. J Vasc Surg. 2009;50:107–18.
23. Mowatt-Larssen E, Shortell C. CHIVA. Semin Vasc Surg. 2010;23:118–22.
24. Franceschi C, Zamboni P. Principles of venous hemodynamics. New York: Nova Biomedical Books; 2009.
25. Carandina S, Mari C, De Palma M, Marcellino MG, Cisno C, Legnaro A, Liboni A, Zamboni P. Varicose vein stripping vs haemodynamic correction (CHIVA): a long term randomised trial. Eur J Vasc Endovasc Surg. 2008;35:230–7.
26. Pares JO, Juan J, Tellez R, et al. Stripping versus the CHIVA method: a randomized, controlled trial. Ann Surg. 2010;251:624–31.

Part II

Vein Testing

Ultrasound Physics

5

Frank R. Miele

Contents

F.R. Miele, MSEE
Pegasus Lectures, Inc., Forney, TX, USA
e-mail: fmiele@pegasuslectures.com

Abstract

Success in phlebology is predicated on the quality and accuracy of the ultrasound imaging and Doppler data pre-intervention, during intervention, and post-intervention. In order to avoid errors, image quality must be optimized, Doppler must be performed and interpreted correctly, and artifacts must be recognized and minimized. These requirements are met often through manipulation of scanning technique as well as changing instrument control settings. Taken together, these requirements designate that both foundational physics and ultrasound instrumentation must be well understood to ensure high-quality patient care. As such, the starting point for phlebology is a treatment in ultrasound physics and instrumentation.

5.1 Introduction

Success in phlebology is predicated on the quality and accuracy of the ultrasound imaging and Doppler data pre-intervention, during intervention, and post-intervention. In order to avoid errors, image quality must be optimized, Doppler must be performed and interpreted correctly, and artifacts must be recognized and minimized. These requirements are met often through manipulation of scanning technique as well as changing instrument control settings. Taken together, these requirements designate that both foundational physics and ultrasound instrumentation must be well understood to ensure high-quality

E. Mowatt-Larssen et al. (eds.), *Phlebology, Vein Surgery and Ultrasonography*,
DOI 10.1007/978-3-319-01812-6_5, © Springer International Publishing Switzerland 2014

patient care. As such, the starting point for phlebology is a treatment in ultrasound physics and instrumentation.

5.2 Ultrasound Physics and Ultrasound Basics

5.2.1 Sound Wave Parameters

Understanding ultrasound physics and instrumentation requires a brief review of sound and wave parameters. Sound is a mechanical wave, implying a physical interaction between the ultrasound (the wave) and tissue (the medium). It is precisely the mechanical interaction which allows for ultrasound image generation. As the sound waves propagate through the body, the physical interactions result in changes to the wave characteristics which are then processed to produce an image. Since varying the initial signal characteristics affects the characteristics of the returning signal, we start by discussing the basic wave parameters. By alternately compressing and rarefying the particles of the medium, sound waves propagate through the medium. The number of compression rarefaction pairs per second is referred to as the frequency (Fig. 5.1). Thus, a 5 MHz wave compresses and rarefies the molecules of a medium five million times per second. The distance between the compressions is referred to as the wavelength.

With respect to ultrasound, the wavelength is an extremely important parameter as the wavelength affects both the type of reflection that occurs as well as the axial resolution of the image. As depicted in Fig. 5.2a, b, within the same medium, higher frequencies result in shorter wavelengths while lower frequencies result in longer wavelengths.

Acoustic Power and Intensity

The power of the wave relates to the pressure developed within the tissue. In order to produce the sound waves, a piezoelectric transducer is excited by an electrical signal, referred to as the transmit voltage. Higher transmit voltages produce higher acoustic pressure fields, increasing the strength of the reflected signal as well as increasing the maximum depth of penetration. Of course, because of the physical interaction with the medium, a higher acoustic pressure potentially increases the risk of causing tissue damage (referred to as a bioeffect). The parameter that is measured to assess both the ability to improve signal strength and the risk of inducing a bioeffect is the intensity. The intensity is a measure of the distribution of the power per unit area, as

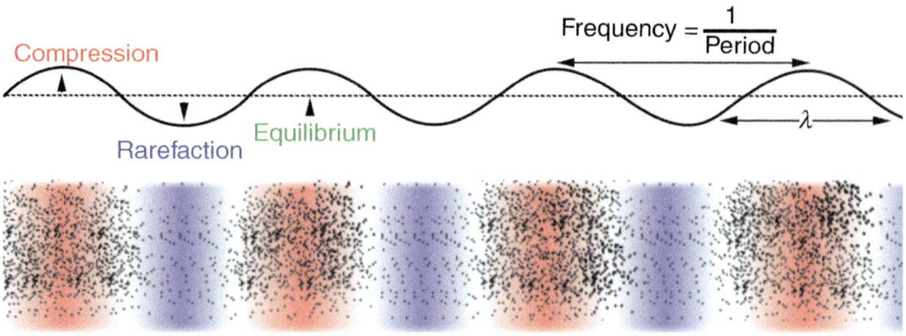

Fig. 5.1 Sound waves (longitudinal wave) propagate through compression and rarefactions of the medium

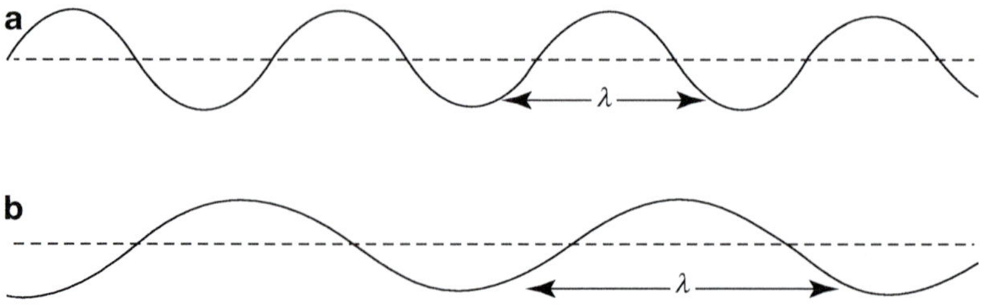

Fig. 5.2 (**a**) Higher frequency and shorter wavelength. (**b**) Lower frequency and longer wavelength

indicated by Eq. 5.1. Higher intensities increase sensitivity and penetration but also increase the risk of causing thermal bioeffect (an increase in temperature that can cause protein denaturing leading to cell death) and mechanical bioeffects referred to as cavitation (a rapid phase transition which creates cavities that can implode within the tissue).

$$\text{Intensity} = \text{Power}/\text{Area} \tag{5.1}$$

Propagation Velocity and Roundtrip Time

Another important wave parameter is the propagation velocity. The propagation velocity is the speed at which a wave travels through a medium and is determined by the properties of the medium. In essence, more dense tissues tend to be stiffer (higher bulk modulus) which results in higher propagation velocities. Ultrasound machines start with a simplified assumption that sound travels at 1,540 m/s (1.54 mm/μs). Based on this assumption and simple application of the distance equation, the time for sound to travel 1 cm in the body is calculated to be approximately 6.5 μs. Since ultrasound imaging is based on signal reflection, the roundtrip effect must be taken into account, which implies that 13 μs are required for each 1 cm of imaging depth (2 cm roundtrip travel) (Fig. 5.3). Of course, when the actual speed of sound varies significantly enough from the assumed 1,540 m/s, error exists with the displayed image (portraying structures too shallow when higher than the assumed speed and too deep when slower than the presumed speed).

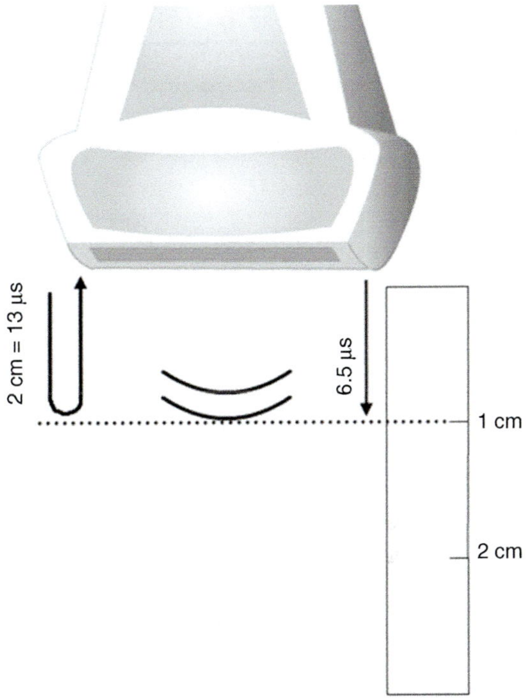

Fig. 5.3 Roundtrip effect and imaging travel time per centimeter (Reprinted from "Essentials of Ultrasound Physics: the Board Review Book," by F. R. Miele, p. 327. Copyright 2008 by Miele Enterprises, LLC. Reprinted with permission)

Reflection

Reflection from tissues is dependent on geometric and acoustic properties. Geometrically, when the reflecting surface is large and smooth with respect to the wavelength, a very angle-dependent type of reflection, specular reflection, occurs. When the surface is rough relative to the wavelength, the much less angle-sensitive (back) scattering occurs. Finally, when the reflecting structures are small relative to the wavelength (as occurs with red blood cells), Rayleigh scattering occurs. Note that reflection from a needle is highly specular and hence highly angle dependent. For specular reflection, the ideal angle is an incident angle of 0° (which implies that the beam direction is perpendicular to the reflecting structure) (Fig. 5.4).

As the angle increases (the beam direction relative to the reflective surface becomes more acute), an increasing percentage of the reflected energy is lost, decreasing the ability to visualize the reflecting structure. Eventually, at large enough incident angles, the reflecting structure will not be at all visualized. This change in visualization as a result of angle-dependent reflection is referred to as anisotropy. Practically speaking, this fact has ramifications when dealing with ultrasound-guided needle procedures. The ideal incident angle of 0° is generally not possible. By using a shallower entrance approach, the incident angle remains smaller and the needle is generally better visualized. The incident angle can be somewhat manipulated by rocking the transducer

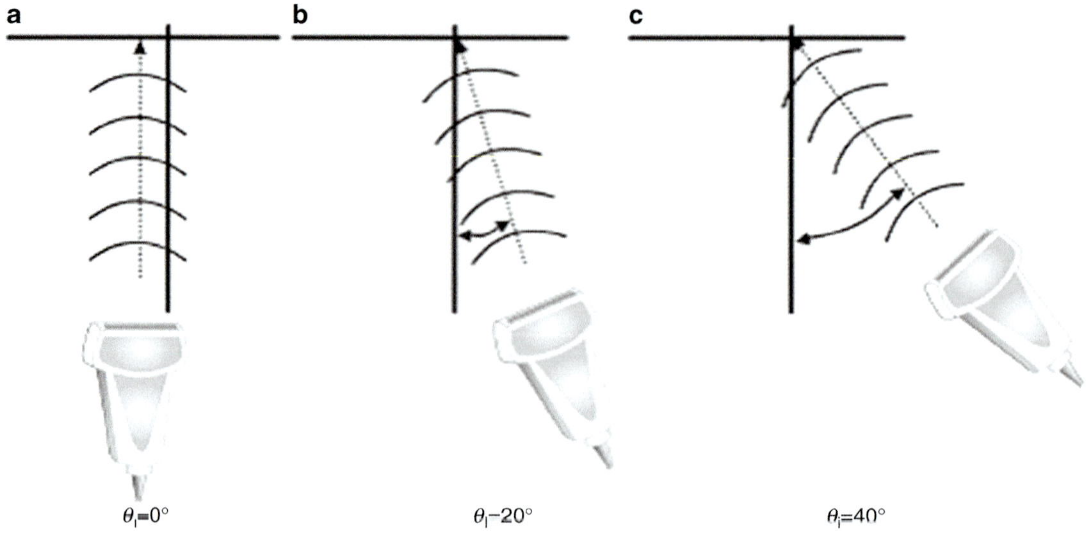

Fig. 5.4 Incident angle (Reprinted from "Ultrasound Physics & Instrumentation," by F.R. Miele, p. 147. Copyright 2006 by Miele Enterprises, LLC. Reprinted with permission)

(what is sometimes referred to as heel-to-toe rocking) and/or by changing the electronic B-mode steering (for those systems that offer this capability). Note that the ability to adequately visualize tendons and nerves is also very angle dependent.

Percentage Reflection and Acoustic Properties

The percentage of the sound wave energy that reflects at a boundary between two media is determined by the disparity between the acoustic properties of the adjoining tissues (Eq. 5.2). This property is referred to as the acoustic impedance. The acoustic impedance of a medium is directly proportional to the density and the propagation velocity of the medium. At a boundary between two mediums, when a large mismatch (difference) in acoustic impedances exists, the percentage of the sound energy reflected is high. Of course, as more energy reflects from a particular point, there is less energy to insonify the inferior tissues (lower transmission). When the impedance mismatch is smaller, less reflection (and hence more transmission) occurs. It is important to note that higher impedance mediums do not imply high reflection percentages. As specified in the equation, the amount of reflection is related to the difference in impedances such that transitioning from a high to a low impedance, or from a low to a high impedance, results in large reflections. When the sound wave transitions from a high impedance medium to another high impedance medium, very little reflection occurs. Similarly, when the sound wave propagates from a medium with a low acoustic impedance to another medium with a low impedance, very little reflection occurs. This fact explains why fresh thrombus comprised primarily of red blood cells of the same acoustic properties may not be visualized whereas older clot, especially when calcified, generally presents with a very echogenic appearance.

$$\%\text{Reflection} = \left((Z_2 - Z_1) / (Z_2 + Z_1) \right)^2 \qquad (5.2)$$

Application of the reflection equation is useful in predicting and understanding the acoustic appearance of various tissue structures. Relative to the acoustic impedance of muscle, the acoustic impedance of tendon and bone is quite high, resulting in very strong reflection (hyperechoic images). In comparison, fat has a lower acoustic impedance than muscle and therefore tends to produce lower acoustic echoes. Acoustically, blood appears relatively "homogenous" such that the blood pool itself typically produces very little reflection (hypoechoic). Note that when fluid-filled cystic structure is insonified, the boundary of the fluid represents a very large acoustic impedance mismatch and hence produces a strong echo; however, when the fluid itself is homogenous, no reflection occurs, and hence, no internal echoes are visualized (anechoic). At the other extreme from fluids, metallic structures such as needles and surgical clips represent very high impedances. Relative to the lower impedance of the surrounding tissue, the high impedance of these metallic objects results in very large reflection percentages and, hence, very strong bright echoes.

For ultrasound-guided needle procedures, visualization of nerves is obviously very important. Sonographically, nerves commonly have a honeycomb appearance in cross section, which translates to a striated appearance longitudinally. The explanation for this appearance, of course, is explained by the reflection equation (Eq. 5.2) in conjunction with the properties of nerves. A nerve consists of a bundle of fascicles. The bundle is encased with the epineurium, and each fascicle is encased by perineural connective tissue. The nerve fascicles generally appear hypoechoic surrounded by more hyperechoic perineural connective tissue. The epineurium is also echogenic.

5.2.2 Transducers, Absorption, and Resolution

Ultrasound transducers are created from piezoelectric materials. Piezoelectric materials convert mechanical stress (such as occurs with mechanical vibration from sound waves) into electrical energy (voltage). These materials also exhibit "reciprocity" which means that the same crystal can convert electrical energy into mechanical energy. Transducers operate over a range of frequencies, referred to as the transducer bandwidth as depicted in Fig. 5.5. This bandwidth allows for imaging at different frequencies without swapping transducers as well as allowing for different operating frequencies for different ultrasound modalities (i.e., imaging at

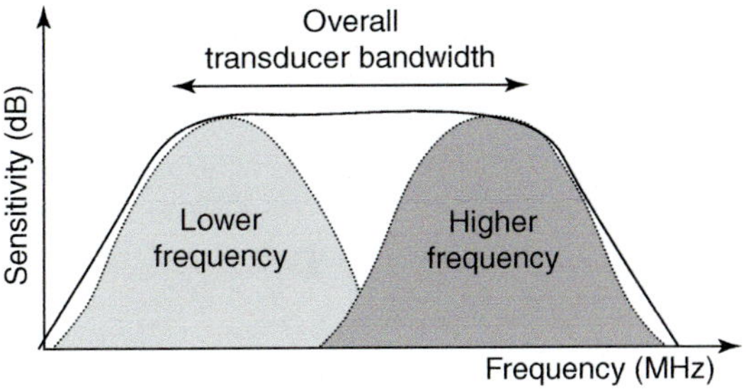

Fig. 5.5 Bandwidth (Reprinted from "Essentials of Ultrasound Physics: the Board Review Book," by F.R. Miele, p. 327. Copyright 2008 by Miele Enterprises, LLC. Reprinted with permission)

5 MHz while performing Doppler at 3.0 MHz). High-frequency ultrasound generally has the advantage of superior axial (depth), lateral (side by side), and elevation (slice thickness) resolution. The disadvantage of high-frequency imaging is significantly less penetration as a result of increased absorption (the conversion of sound energy into heat within the tissue). Absorption rates increase exponentially with increasing transmit frequency and increasing depth, implying that using even slightly higher frequencies can significantly decrease penetration and signal strength at deeper imaging depths. Broadband transducers offer the flexibility without having to change out transducers of transmitting with lower frequency for improved sensitivity and penetration at greater depths as well as transmitting at higher frequencies for improved resolution for shallower imaging.

Transducers can be constructed from single crystals (referred to as pencil probes, pedofs, or Doppler only) or multiple elements to form phased arrays. Phased array transducers consist of different form factors including:

Sectors, which bring the image to a point designed for rib access and used generally in cardiac imaging although also used for transcranial and, sometimes, abdominal imaging

Curved linears, which produce broad near field by a curved surface, generally used on the abdomen and for invasive transducers such as transrectal and transvaginal

Linears, which have a large flat surface ideal for contact with relatively flat surfaces such as the

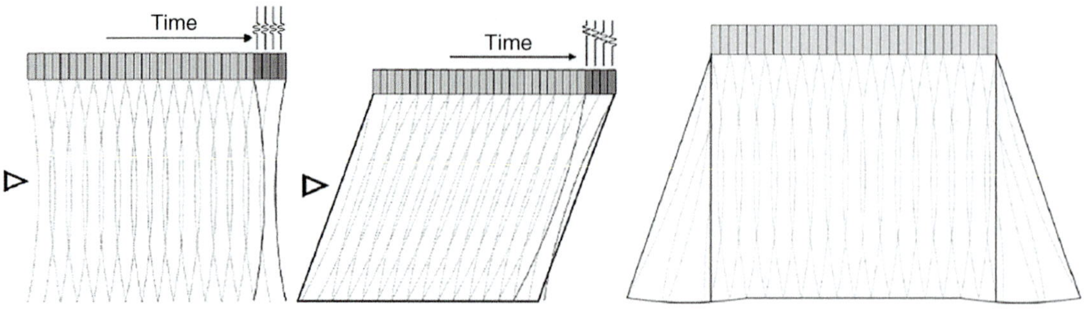

Fig. 5.6 Linear transducer imaging formats (Reprinted from "Ultrasound Physics & Instrumentation," by F.R. Miele, pp. 277–279. Copyright 2006 by Miele Enterprises, LLC. Reprinted with permission)

neck, arms, and legs. Linear transducers have three different imaging formats including unsteered, steered, and trapezoidal (Fig. 5.6)

5.2.3 Linear Phased Arrays

Since venous imaging is performed primarily with linear phased arrays, we will emphasize the functionality of linear arrays. Linear images are produced by activating a group of elements, referred to as the aperture, to produce a single beam. Generally the same aperture is then used to receive over time the returning echoes. Based on the depth setting, the system determines the required receive time, referred to as the pulse repetition period (PRP) before transmitting the next line. Recall that 13 μs is required for each cm of imaging depth such that the PRP is simply the imaging depth multiplied by 13 μs/cm. Once the required "listen" time has transpired, the system activates another group of elements to produce the next acoustic beam and the process is repeated until the user-specified region of the patient is scanned. The frequency at which the lines can be transmitted, the pulse repetition frequency (PRF) is equal to the reciprocal of the pulse repetition period (PRP). Once the entire region is scanned, the system goes back to the beginning and repeats the process, creating the next frame of data. The time required to acoustically produce a frame is simply calculated as the time required to produce a line (the PRP) multiplied by the number of lines that constitute the frame. The reciprocal of the frame time is the frame frequency, commonly referred to as the frame rate. The frame rate is one of the predominant determinants of the ability to resolve changes in time, or the temporal resolution. Higher frame rates imply better temporal resolution. Higher frame rates can be achieved by minimizing the time required to produce the frame. Clearly narrowing the image and decreasing the depth setting decrease the frame time and improve temporal resolution.

5.3 Ultrasound Imaging

5.3.1 Operating Frequency

Changing the transmitted wave parameters can have significant impact on the image quality and clinical value of the data acquired. As already mentioned, most modern systems offer broad bandwidth transducers that allow the user to select the operating frequency. Typically, the frequency range for linear transducers is between about 2.5 MHz and about 15 MHz. This range is too broad for any one transducer and is generally covered by either two or three different transducers (i.e., a specific vendor may offer broadband linear transducers with frequency ranges of 2.5–7, 5–12, and 8–15 MHz). For imaging, the general rule for operating frequency selection is to choose the highest frequency that still results in adequate penetration. Following this rule ensures that resolution is optimized while still presenting adequate signal above noise thresholds. Practically speaking, there can only be general and not specific rules about appropriate frequency selection for conventional imaging, since attenuation with depth varies from patient to patient.

5.3.2 Transmit Power

For deeper imaging, as occurs with deeper vessels on large patients, the transmit power should be increased. For the superficial venous system, the transmit power can generally be reduced from the maximum without compromise of image quality.

5.3.3 Transmit Focus

A third important system setting which affects sensitivity is the transmit focus or foci. When imaging superficially with only one focus, the focus should be set at the depth of vein or artery being assessed. For deep veins when inadequate sensitivity is a potential issue, the focus should be set just slightly deeper than the vein of interest since, for deeper imaging depths, the highest beam intensity is generally shallower than the focal depth. Using multiple foci improves the lateral resolution and sensitivity over the focal range and in general is very useful for venous imaging. The downside of using multiple foci is that image acquisition slows, decreasing the frame rate, hence, degrading temporal resolution.

5.3.4 Signal and Gain

The visualization of grayscale signals on the screen is the result of a complex interaction between multiple systems and environmental settings including the receiver gain, time gain compensation (TGC), compression settings, monitor contrast and brightness, and the ambient lighting of the room. Before discussing the approach to setting the system controls, it is imperative to first discuss the ultrasound signal relative to the light perception of the human eye. First, there is a need for signal amplification since even the highest amplitude signals reflecting from the body are too small to be adequately visualized. The system control, known as "receiver gain," is basically a multiplier that increases the amplitude of all received signals. TGC is also receiver gain but differs in how the gain is applied. Unlike the receiver gain that multiplies all signals, TGC is depth dependent. Signals that are received from deeper depths arrive later in time and generally require more amplification than signals from shallower depths. TGC allows for the image to be subdivided into zones based on depth, and then different amplification applied to each of these zones to compensate for the varying attenuation.

5.3.5 Signal and Compression

Reflected ultrasound signals span a very large range of intensities (referred to as the "signal dynamic range"). Reflections from mediums such as nerves, tendons, bones, and calcifications tend to be of very high amplitude as a result of the large acoustic impedance mismatches relative to the surrounding tissues. Conversely, reflections from within blood, fluids, and fresh thrombus tend to be of low amplitude as a result of the relative acoustic impedance homogeneity. The dynamic range of these reflected signals often spans 80 or even 100 dB (a factor in amplitude of 10,000:1 and 100,000:1). The human eye for a given ambient light is capable of detecting less than 36 dB (fewer than 64 shades of gray). The result is that the dynamic range of reflected signals from diagnostic ultrasound far exceeds the dynamic range of the human eye. This fact illustrates why compression must be employed in displaying ultrasound images. As the name suggests, compression reduces the dynamic range by mathematically remapping the wider range of signal amplitudes to a smaller range of signal amplitudes. The problem is, that by compressing the dynamic range of reflected signals, it is more than conceivable that some information may be lost and an important differentiation between tissue types may be missed (i.e., an

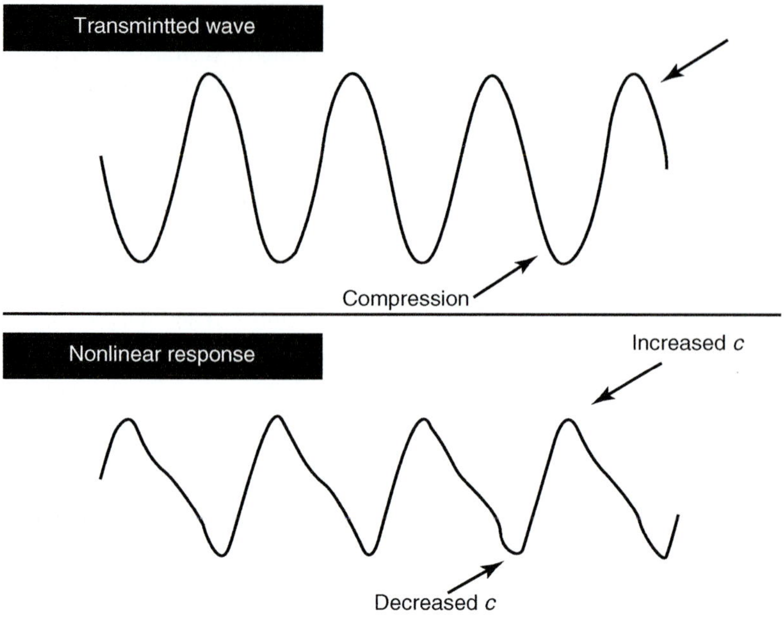

Fig. 5.7 Distortion of wave producing harmonic energy (Reprinted from "Ultrasound Physics & Instrumentation," by F. R. Miele, p. 664. Copyright 2006 by Miele Enterprises, LLC. Reprinted with permission)

inability to differentiate a mass from surrounding normal tissue or an inability to visualize a thrombus from the surrounding blood pool).

In light of the potential to not visualize important signals, ultrasound systems are designed with multiple compression maps. The names of the compression function vary relative to system manufacturers, but this function is generally called compression, grayscale, dynamic range, or post-processing. Regardless of the function name, the various compression settings map the signal strengths to differing brightness levels. Since the maps compress the signals nonlinearly, each setting changes the appearance of the image grayscale, potentially masking or unmasking a thrombus or mass visualized or not visualized at a different setting.

5.3.6 Signal and Ambient Light

Ultimately, the image is presented on a display monitor. The monitor should be calibrated relative to the ambient light. In brighter ambient light, the monitor brightness must be increased so that low-level signals are displayed with an appropriate brightness so as to be presented above the visual threshold.

5.3.7 Harmonic Imaging

The imaging technique discussed up to this point has assumed conventional, fundamental imaging. With fundamental imaging, the transmit frequency band and the receive frequency band are the same. Since the latter part of the 1990s, second harmonic imaging has revolutionized ultrasound. For harmonic imaging, the system transmits at a lower frequency band, referred to as the fundamental, and then receives and processes signals at twice the fundamental signal frequency, referred to as the second harmonic. In order to operate over such a wide frequency range, the transducers used for harmonic imaging require very broad bandwidth. When processing the returning echoes, the system applies a filter to "look at" just the second harmonic bandwidth, explicitly attempting to eliminate signal with frequencies in the transmit bandwidth.

Harmonic signals are generated in tissue because of a nonlinear response of the tissue to the compression and rarefaction induced by the sound waves. During compression, the density of the tissue molecules increases, resulting in a slight increase in propagation speed. During rarefaction, the density decreases such that there is a slight decrease in the propagation velocity. In essence, the sound wave is distorted as it propagates through the tissue (Fig. 5.7) as some fundamental energy is converted into harmonic energy within the sound wave. Although the generated harmonics are not limited to second harmonics, as of now, ultrasound systems are not making use of progressively weaker higher order harmonics. The generation of harmonic energy is very nonlinear with the beam intensity (related to the parameter called the mechanical index [MI]). Slightly decreasing the beam intensity (a lower MI) results in significantly less harmonic signal generation. As a result, harmonic imaging is very sensitive to where the beam focus is placed in the image as well as to the overall transmit power used when imaging. The best harmonic imaging occurs with higher transmit power and near within the focal region (the area about the depth of the focus).

The primary benefit of harmonic imaging is a reduction of clutter artifacts. Since harmonic beams are inherently narrower than beams generated using fundamental imaging, lateral resolution is improved. Additionally, because the beam intensity is generally low in the near field before the beam has converged to the focus, harmonic generation is generally low in the near field. Since most imaging artifacts result from strong reflectors in the near field (referred to as clutter signals), lower-level harmonic signals in the near field result in fewer imaging artifacts, improving image quality. For deep imaging in which attenuation dominates, harmonic imaging is not recommended as harmonic generation drops precipitously with lower beam intensities.

5.3.8 Compound Imaging

Compound imaging (also known as Sono CT or Crossbeam Technology) generally results in improved image quality. There are two primary components to compound imaging: frame averaging and varying steering angles between averaged frames. By averaging frames, the signal-to-noise ratio is improved as long as any changes in the region of interest occur slowly relative to the frame acquisition rate. In cases where the signal is changing slowly, the signal in each of the "*n*" frames are in phase such that adding together the frames results in the signal amplitude increasing by a factor "*n*." For example, adding nine signals, each with an amplitude of 0.1 V, would result in a combined signal with an amplitude of 0.9 V. In contrast, the noise (which exists in every image) is random from frame to frame. When the noise from each of the nine frames is averaged, the noise amplitude also grows, but at a slower rate. In fact, the noise generally grows at the rate of the square root of the number of frames used in the average ($\sqrt{n}$). Using the same example, imagine that the noise level is 1 nanovolt (nV); averaging nine frames together would result in the noise becoming bigger by the square root of nine, or 3×1 nV = 3 nV. Therefore, the signal grew nine times larger whereas the noise grew only three times as large, implying that the signal-to-noise ratio increased by a factor of 9, 3, or 3 times. In other words, averaging improves the signal-to-noise ratio by the square root of the number of samples in the average.

As already mentioned, in addition to averaging, compound image varies the image steering from frame to frame. Recall that specular reflection is very angle dependent. Combining this fact with the fact that most imaging artifacts are caused by specular reflection, it should be clear that compound imaging results in artifacts tend to "average out." The net result is that compound imaging generally results in images with better signal-to-noise (improved sensitivity) and fewer artifacts.

5.3.9 Artifacts

Ultrasound imaging is based on a series of assumptions. Whenever one or more of these assumptions are violated, artifacts exist. Some of the many assumptions made by ultrasound include:

- The speed of sound is 1,540 m/s (equivalent to 13 μs for sound to travel 2 cm, or image 1 cm).
- Sound travels only down to a structure and back and does not reverberate between structures.
- Sound travels in a straight line such that the beam path is "straight."
- Attenuation is never so significant so that deeper structures are still adequately insonified.

- Attenuation is relatively uniform so that no regions are insonified with higher intensities than other regions (at the same depth).
- The image plane is infinitesimally thin so that structures in front or behind the imaging plane are not presented in the image.

Speed error occurs when the true speed of sound propagation through a tissue is higher or lower than the assumed 1,540 m/s. When sound travels through a region faster than 1,540 m/s, the region appears to be "thinner" than reality and inferior structures are drawn too superficially. Likewise, when the speed of sound is slower than 1,540 m/s, the region appears "thicker" than reality and inferior structures appear too deep in the image. This error can sometimes make a needle appear to bend within am image, referred to as the "bayonet sign."

Reverberation occurs when sound does not take the simple path of traveling down to, and back from, a specular reflecting structure, but instead takes multiple trips between two specular structures. In the simple cases, reverberation artifacts show the reverberating structures multiple times with uniform spacing within the image. In more complex cases, as occurs when there are more than two specular reflectors, the spacing between the artifactual structures within the image will not be uniform, indicative of the more complex reverberating paths. The most complex situations exist when reverberation occurs by structures superior to a hypoechogenic region. As the sound is reverberating between the specular reflectors, multiple reflections are created by the intervening tissue. However, because of the increased path length increasing the attenuation, the signal generated from the tissue is relatively low level. This low-level reverberation signal now combines with the hypoechogenic signal from the actual depth, creating a faint gray signal in a region that should appear black. This is often why vessels appear to have thrombus when, in reality, the vessel is completely free of material. Reverberation can also be a useful artifact when dealing with ultrasound-guided needle procedures. The specular nature of the needle often leads to reverberation, making identification of the needle within the image easier.

The artifact of refraction occurs when the sound beam is bent away from straight. Refraction (as specified by Snell's Law) occurs when a sound beam encounters a specular interface between two mediums of differing propagation speeds at an incident angle other than zero degrees. The result of refraction is that structures are laterally translated in the image. This artifact sometimes gives the appearance of structures side by side where only one structure actually exists.

Shadowing and enhancement artifacts are both attenuation related. Shadowing occurs when there is excessive attenuation (either through increased absorption, reflection, or refraction) such that structures below are not adequately insonified. The result is a region of dropout aptly named an "acoustic shadow." Conversely, enhancement occurs inferior to a region in which less attenuation occurs relative to surrounding tissues. Both of these artifacts are useful in helping distinguish characteristics of the superior tissue. Calcifications and fibrous tissues are generally accompanied by acoustic shadowing whereas blood and cystic structures are often accompanied by enhancement.

Limits to lateral resolution can be problematic when performing ultrasound-guided needle procedures. For two-dimensional (2D) images, the elevation plane represents the image "slice thickness." In a 2D image display, there is no dimension dedicated to depicting the elevation plane. Hence, any reflecting structure(s) in front of or behind the desired image plane will be presented as if in plane (Fig. 5.8). The following figure illustrates how limited elevation resolution can make it appear as if a needle has been successfully inserted into a vessel. From an imaging standpoint, needle location within the vessel can be ascertained by slowly rotating the transducer from a longitudinal to a transverse view of the vessel. If the needle is within the vessel, the needle will be visualized within the image of the vessel throughout rotation. If the needle is in front of or behind the vessel, the needle will be visualized crossing out of the vessel wall.

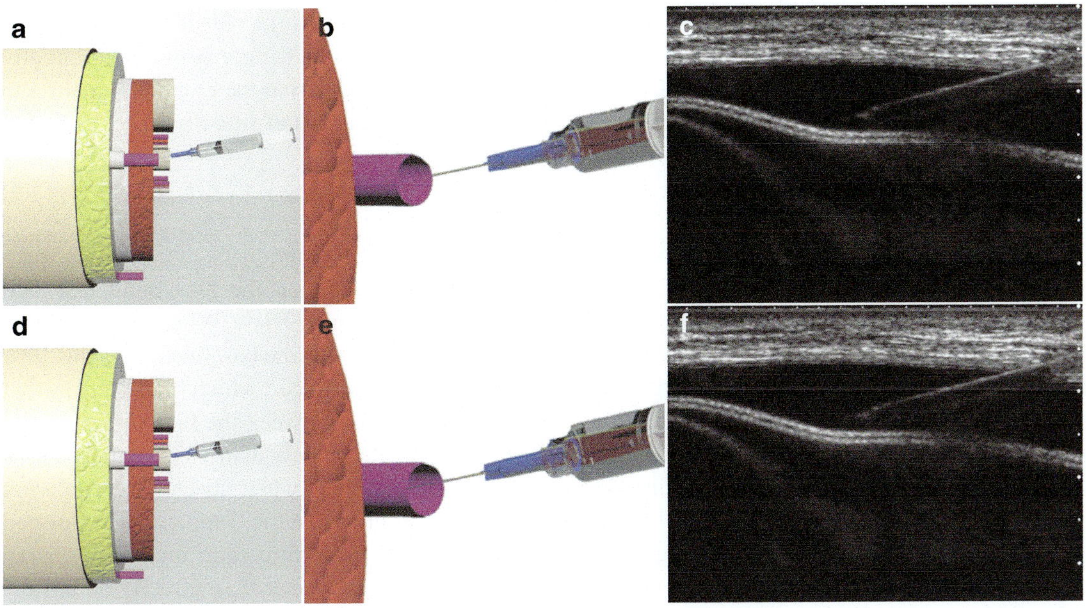

Fig. 5.8 Elevation artifact. (**a**) Vessel in longitudinal view. (**b**) Vantage point with image rotated. (**c**) Ultrasound with needle that appears to be in vessel. In parts a–c, the needle misses the vessel entirely. (**d**) The same image with the needle appearing to be in the vessel. (**e**) Vantage point with image rotated showing the needle actually within the vessel. (**f**) Ultrasound showing needle that appears to be in vessel. Parts d–f demonstrate a needle that is actually within the vessel, but the ultrasounds (shown in **c** and **f**) appear identical. Rotating the image slightly is important to confirm needle placement

5.4 Spectral Doppler

5.4.1 Doppler Theory and Basics

As discussed, B-mode imaging presents data based on the amplitude of the reflected echoes. The amplitude is representative of the varying acoustic properties within the tissues scanned. Unlike B-mode imaging, spectral Doppler is a non-scanned modality implying that the data is acquired by transmitting repeatedly in the same location. As a non-scanned modality, spatial information is sacrificed to generate velocity information. Therefore, the spectral Doppler signal strength is still represented by grayscale (like B-mode), but the horizontal axis of the display now represents elapsed time and the vertical axis represents velocity toward and away from the steered beam (line) from the transducer.

The velocity information is obtained by application of the Doppler Effect. The Doppler Effect is essentially a perceived change in frequency as the result of a compression or decompression of the wavelength of a wave which results from relative motion between the wave source and an observer. When the relative motion between source and observer decreases the separation distance, the wavelength decreases, giving the perception of a higher frequency. When the relative motion results in an increase in separation between source and observer, the wavelength increases, giving the perception of a lower frequency. The Doppler Effect is familiar to most people as the varying pitch that occurs in proximity to a fast-moving sound source such as a high-speed train or motorcycle. The detected shift in frequencies, referred to as the Doppler shift, is a function of the parameters which affect the relative motion (both velocity and angle) and the parameters that determine the wavelength (operating frequency and propagation velocity) as given in the Doppler equation (Eq. 5.3):

$$f_{\text{Doppler}} = (2f_o * v * \cos(0)) / c \quad (5.3)$$

f_o = operating (transmit) frequency
v = velocity of blood
0 = Doppler angle
c = speed of sound

5.4.2 Doppler Shift Detection

In order to determine velocities within the body, the ultrasound system transmits a signal at a known radio frequency range (typically from 1.6 MHz to as high as 10 or 12 MHz depending on the system and transducer). The ultrasound system then subtracts the transmit frequency from the frequency of the returning echoes, essentially "leaving" the Doppler frequency shift. Notice, however, that the Doppler equation indicates that the detected Doppler shift is dependent on the cosine of the Doppler angle (the angle formed between the steered Doppler beam and the flow direction) with maximal Doppler shifts detected at 0 and 180°. When the Doppler angle is less than 90°, the returning frequency is higher than the transmitted frequency and a positive Doppler shift is detected. Conversely, if the Doppler angle is greater than 90°, the returning frequency is lower than the transmitted frequency and a negative Doppler shift is detected. The important realization is that unless the Doppler angle is 0° or 180°, the system does not detect the full Doppler shift. As the Doppler angle approaches 90°, the Doppler shift converges to 0.

5.4.3 Angle Correction, Velocity, Direction, and Acceleration

As with most vascular applications, when the full Doppler shift is not detected, angle correction is generally employed. The user applies angle correction by aligning the flow indicator through the PW sample volume (gate) shown on the screen with the perceived flow direction. Through application of basic geometry, the system determines the Doppler angle, calculates the cosine of the Doppler angle, and corrects the partially detected Doppler frequency shifts. Since Doppler yields velocity information, the correction is essentially applied by manipulating the Doppler equation to be expressed in terms of velocity as

$$v = (c * f_{\text{Doppler}}) / (2f_o * \cos(0)) \quad (5.4)$$

As previously mentioned, the Doppler spectrum displays time on the horizontal axis and velocity on the vertical axis. When spectral invert is not on, flow above the baseline represents flow "toward" the transducer, which really means that the angle formed between the flow direction and the steered beam is less than 90°. Similarly, flow below the baseline (when spectral invert is not activated) implies that the Doppler angle (formed between the flow direction and the steered Doppler beam is greater than 90°. By definition, acceleration (Eq. 5.5) is change in velocity per time. Therefore, in addition to velocity measurements, acceleration and deceleration can also be assessed from a Doppler spectrum:

$$\text{Acceleration} = \text{Change in velocity} / \text{Change in time} \quad (5.5)$$

5.4.4 Optimal Operating Frequency

Unlike the reflection from tissues, reflection from blood is based on the very weak reflective mechanism of Rayleigh scattering. The result is that Doppler techniques (both spectral and color Doppler) are susceptible to errors because of inadequate sensitivity. The amount of back scattering increases with increasing frequency. This increase in reflectivity is the result of the "size increase" of the red blood cells relative to the decreasing wavelength. This fact intimates that better Doppler would be achieved by using a higher operating frequency. Paradoxically, with the exception of superficial Doppler imaging, the exact opposite is true. For most Doppler imaging, stronger Doppler signals are achieved by using a lower, not a higher, operating frequency. This paradox is explained by the realization that not only does scattering increase with a higher frequency, but that attenuation through absorption also increases with increasing frequency. In fact, since the absorption rate increases exponentially with increasing frequency, the increased attenuation using higher transmit frequencies well exceeds the increase in reflectivity, thereby resulting in weaker Doppler signals. Therefore (unless performing superficial Doppler) Doppler should be performed at the lowest frequency possible. Practically speaking, superficial imaging implies a depth of approximately 1–2 cm or shallower. Figure 5.9 indicates the ideal operating frequency based on Doppler depth. Notice that deeper than 3 cm, the Doppler frequency should be below 3 MHz.

When an inappropriately high Doppler frequency is used, the Doppler signal intensity decreases, potentially leading to underestimation of the true peak velocity and, in extreme cases, no detection of flow. When the transmit power is set to maximum (100 %) and the Doppler receive gain has to be increased so as to visualize the spectrum amidst strong speckle noise, the sensitivity limit is being reached, and the operating frequency should be lowered if possible.

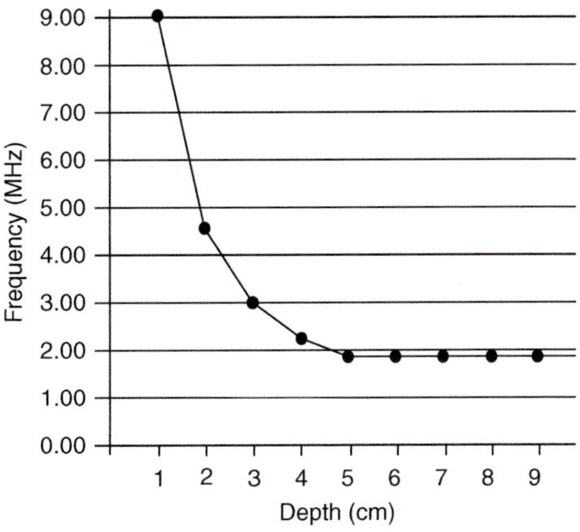

Fig. 5.9 Ideal Doppler operating frequency based on depth (Reprinted from "Ultrasound Physics & Instrumentation," by F.R. Miele, p. 534. Copyright 2006 by Miele Enterprises, LLC. Reprinted with permission)

5.4.5 Wall Filters

With both spectral and color Doppler, wall filters are necessary to reduce the very high amplitude clutter signals resulting from slowly moving structures such as vessel walls, movement related to patient respiration, and transducer motion. Relative to the amplitude of the blood signals, these clutter signals are enormous such that without wall filtering, these clutter signals would saturate the electronics and dwarf the desired blood signals. The baseline of the spectral display corresponds to no Doppler shift detected. No detected Doppler shift can be the result of no flow, poor angle to flow, poor sensitivity, or artifacts which obscure the Doppler signal, such as shadowing from excessive attenuation. Notice that there is a "black band" about the baseline in which no signal is presented. The width of the black band represents the velocity range over which the spectral Doppler wall filters are eliminating Doppler signals. For venous imaging, the spectral wall filters are generally set very low (typically 50 Hz or lower). If the wall filters are set too high, low-velocity flow may not be displayed, giving a false impression of no flow in a patent vessel.

5.5 Color Doppler

5.5.1 Color Doppler Basics

Color Doppler has similarities with B-mode imaging and with spectral Doppler. Like B-mode imaging, spatial dimensions are portrayed. Like spectral Doppler, velocity information is displayed. However, color Doppler is different from both spectral Doppler and B-mode imaging since amplitude information (signal strength) is not directly displayed.

Color Doppler generates a mean velocity estimate at each point within the color box scan region. Since a mean estimate requires taking an average of multiple samples, a color display line cannot be generated from a single acoustic line (a single transmit pulse). Unlike the simplest case of B-mode imaging in which a single transmit (acoustic line) is required to produce a single display line, for color, an entire packet of acoustic lines must be transmitted in the same direction, in order to generate a single color display line. As a result of the increased number of transmitted lines, the time required to create a color frame increases significantly, generally resulting in degraded temporal resolution. Since the temporal resolution with color Doppler is typically poor, scanning techniques such as narrowing the color box width, cropping the color box depth, and potentially decreasing color packet size or decreasing the color line density become important to optimize frame rate.

5.5.2 Optimizing Operating Frequency

As discussed at length in the spectral Doppler section, the appropriate frequency for color Doppler operation is highly depth dependent. Shallower than 1–2 cm, higher frequencies result in stronger color Doppler signals. Deeper than 3 cm, especially when sensitivity is an issue, the lowest possible operating frequency should be used to ensure adequate sensitivity. Using too high an operating frequency at deeper depths can result in loss of color filling and, in the worse cases, an inability to detect the presence of flow.

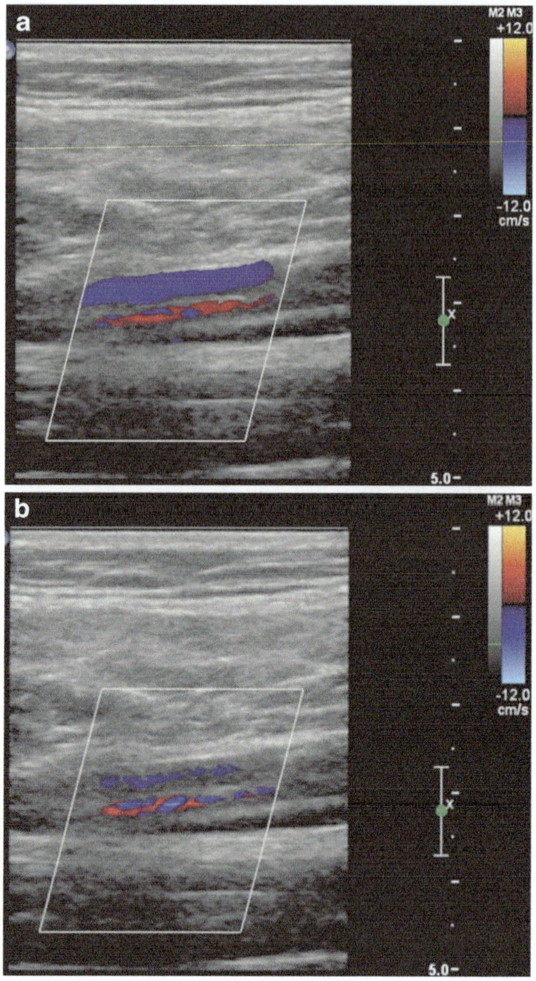

Fig. 5.10 (**a**) High color priority image. (**b**) Low color priority image

5.5.3 Color Priority and Color Gain

As already mentioned, color Doppler does not directly display signal amplitude. There are however indirect methods of determining whether or not the color receiver gain is adequately set. To understand these methods, it is important to realize that color Doppler displays color signals based on color signal thresholds. At each specific location within the color image, if the color signal amplitude exceeds a specific threshold, color is displayed. If instead the signal is weaker than the specific amplitude threshold, no color is displayed so that grayscale values are presented. Since an individual pixel cannot represent both tissue and flow, if both flow and grayscale values simultaneously exist, the threshold determines when color is displayed versus when the grayscale value is presented. Most systems provide a user control to specify the color priority which determines at what level the tissue signal must be below to allow color to be displayed. A high color priority implies that color is generally given priority unless the grayscale amplitude is very high (Fig. 5.10a). A low color priority implies that color is given a lower priority so that even moderate-level grayscale values will potentially take priority over displaying color (Fig. 5.10b).

When the receiver gain is set too low, the amplitude of the color signal for many pixels within the flow region will be below the color threshold, resulting in color dropout. Since the

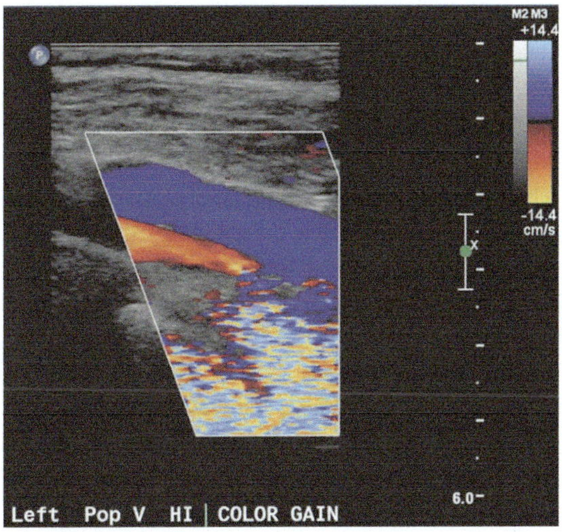

Fig. 5.11 Color speckle from excessive color gain

lack of flow is generally recognized by sonographers, the problem is detected and the color gain is increased. Determining when overgaining exists is more complicated. In the near field, overgaining generally presents differently than overgaining in the far field in which sensitivity becomes an issue. When imaging superficially, color overgaining results in color bleed over regions of tissue at the flow boundaries. Imaging a vessel, the color bleed occurs more commonly and more excessively at the posterior wall. This phenomenon is the result of limited axial resolution sometimes referred to as the "color tail."

For deeper color imaging, especially when close to penetration limits, setting the correct color gain is slightly more complex. Since optimal sensitivity is required for deeper imaging, setting the gain too low can result in inadequate color filling, as the lower-level echoes can drop below the amplitude threshold required to display color. The technique for setting the color gain is to increase the color gain until color speckle (noise) appears within the color box in regions where flow does not exist (Fig. 5.11). Then the color gain should be decreased until the color speckle just disappears from the non-flow regions. At this setting, the color gain is set for optimal sensitivity. When color speckle is apparent within the image (in regions where flow does not exist), the color gain is set incorrectly too high.

5.5.4 Color Scales and the PRF

The color scales are an alternative name for the pulse repetition frequency (PRF). The PRF specifies the maximum mean velocity that can be displayed before aliasing occurs. The PRF is simply the reciprocal of the time between transmit pulses, or the pulse repetition period (PRP). As discussed in the imaging section, the speed of sound is assumed to be 1,540 m/s equivalent to 13 μs of travel time for each centimeter of imaging depth (6.5 μs for each centimeter of tissue through which the sound must travel). For a specific depth, the minimum PRP is calculated by multiplying the imaging depth in cm by the assumed 13 microseconds per cm travel time. For example, with an imaging depth of 4 cm, the PRP and the PRF are calculated as follows:

This calculation illustrates that for an imaging depth of 4 cm, the ultrasound system can transmit and receive approximately 20,000 beams (lines) per second or 20,000 samples per second. Recalling the Nyquist criterion, the maximum detectable frequency is half of the sample rate. Therefore at a depth of 4 cm, the highest detectable mean Doppler shift is 10 kHz. If the mean frequency shift exceeds half of the PRF, color aliasing occurs. By employing the Doppler equation, the mean frequency shifts can be presented as mean velocities. Using the color bar of Fig. 5.12 as a reference, notice that the color scales (PRF) are set to ±65 cm/s. For Doppler angles less than 90°, flow with mean velocities below 0 cm/s will be presented as hues of blue through green. If the mean velocity exceeds 0 cm/s, aliasing occurs which implies that the color will wrap first to hues of red followed by shades of orange.

5.5.5 Decreasing the Color Scales

Consider an imaging situation in which the maximum detectable mean velocity is 50 cm/s, and the mean flow velocity is only 5 cm/s. Clearly, in order to better appreciate flow velocity gradients about this low mean, you would need to lower the color scales. How does the system "lower" the color scales? From the above calculation, it is

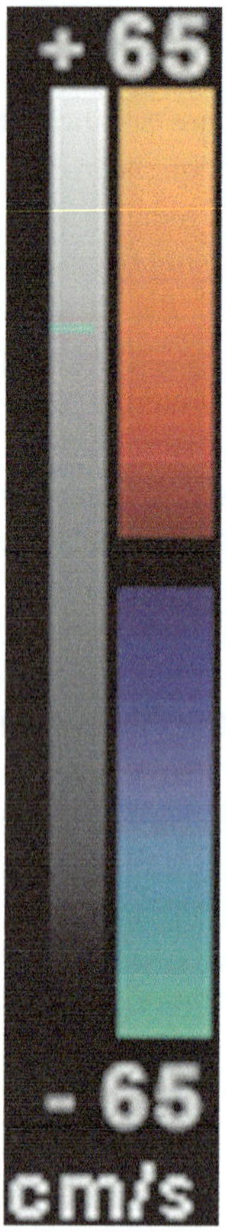

Fig. 5.12 Color bar

evident that increasing the PRP decreases the PRF. One method of increasing the PRP is to simply increase the color box depth. However, this approach makes very little sense, as the color box would now be displaying color in regions deeper than the region of interest. Instead, when the scales are decreased from the maximum possible, the system simply increases the PRP by adding in "dead time" between transmit events. In essence, the system transmits the pulse, waits the required time for the pulse to reach and to return from the maximum imaging depth, and then simply does nothing for a period of time, the dead time, before repeating the process. Since the dead time increases the PRP, the PRF is decreased.

5.5.6 Color Wall Filters

Referring to Fig. 5.12, notice that the center of the color bar has a "black band." The center of this black band represents the color baseline. The span of the black band above and below the center represents the color wall filters. Both spectral and color Doppler require wall filters to reduce the very large clutter signals from slowly moving structures such as vessel walls and transducer movement so that the lower amplitude signals from the blood are not obscured. The baseline represents no Doppler shift detected. No detected shift can be the result of no flow, poor angle to flow, poor sensitivity, or artifacts which obscure the color signal such as shadowing. The width of the black band represents the range of mean velocities eliminated by the wall filters.

With all ultrasound systems, changing the color PRF (scales) also changes the wall filters. In essence, the color wall filters are a percentage of the PRF. When the color scales are decreased, the color wall filters also decrease. Similarly, when the color scales are increased, the color wall filters also increase. The implication is that when trying to detect very low velocity flow, the color scales must be lowered so as to lower the color wall filters. If the color scales are set too high, the corresponding high wall filters may eliminate the signals from the low velocity flows, resulting in no low velocity flow presented in the image. It is valuable to stress that changing the color scales automatically changes the color wall filters on all ultrasound systems.

In addition to the corresponding change of wall filters with change in color scales, some systems allow the user to adjust how aggressively the wall filters attenuate the lower mean velocity flow signals. When the wall filters are set to "high," the system increases the percentage of the color scales to which the wall filters attenuate. With wall filters set less aggressively, the percentage to which the wall filters attenuate decreases. The systems that have this additional control generally display an indication on the

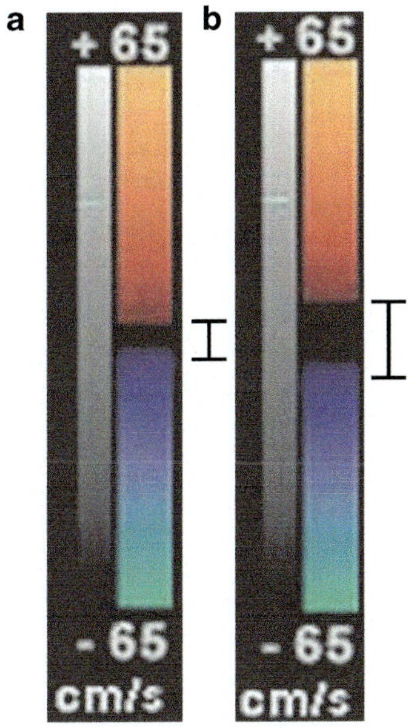

Fig. 5.13 (**a**) Low wall filters. (**b**) High wall filters

screen indicating the wall filter setting (i.e., "WF: High"). For some ultrasound systems, the filter behavior can be easily identified by assessing the width of the black band of the color bar. As displayed in Fig. 5.13a, notice that the band is narrower since the wall filter was set to "low," whereas in Fig. 5.13b, notice that the black band is wider since the wall filter was set to "high."

5.5.7 Color Power Doppler

Power Doppler, also referred to as energy Doppler, color angio, or color power angio, is another flow detection technique. Although power Doppler presentations often look "similar" to conventional color Doppler imaging, there are some significant differences. First, power Doppler encodes the presence of flow based on signal amplitude, not based on the detected frequency shift. This fact implies that there is no velocity information given, either in terms of speed of the flow or direction of the flow. The different color hues presented on the color bar for power Doppler therefore correlate to signal strength. Stronger signals are encoded with colors higher up the color bar, and lower intensity signals are encoded as colors closer to the bottom of the color bar. Since velocity information is not detected or presented, color Doppler is not concerned with the optimizing for frame rate or aliasing. As such, power Doppler is usually used in conjunction with averaging which allows for greater sensitivity to low flow states. Power Doppler also has the advantage of being less angle sensitive than color Doppler imaging. In essence, power Doppler is a very useful tool for detecting flow in low flow states, especially when the Doppler angle would be poor for conventional color Doppler imaging. Also, although standard power Doppler does not present flow velocity information, some ultrasound systems offer a hybrid technique which combines power Doppler with color Doppler to yield directional power Doppler.

Conclusion

The application of ultrasound, the instrumentation, and the techniques used to optimize imaging are all based on physics. Physics explains the steps required for optimization, the methodology for recognizing and interpreting artifacts, and the approach required to be certain that the appropriate clinical conclusion is reached. Whereas this book deals primarily with the clinical and physiologic aspects of phlebology, it is sincerely hoped that this brief physics overview serves as a starting point for developing a greater understanding in the best practices, methodologies, and procedures performed.

Ultrasound for Reflux 6

Joseph A. Zygmunt Jr.

Contents

Abstract

The use of ultrasound in diagnosing deep vein thrombosis remains important today with venous thromboembolism being the leading cause of preventable in-hospital death. The use of ultrasound for diagnosing DVT has come to overshadow its use for treating superficial venous disease. Duplex ultrasound is one of the most highly operator-dependent imaging modalities, the accuracy of which completely depends on the person performing the scan. Since this modality is so operator dependent, there is a need for additional information, especially for understanding of the key underlying concepts of chronic venous disease, presentation, and the factors inherent to its pathology. Additionally it is extremely important to understand proper technique for performing the exam as well as common errors and artifacts. Continued use of standardized terminology and techniques will help to reduce confusion and give better clarity to the information gathered with duplex ultrasonography before, during, or after treatment of chronic venous insufficiency.

6.1 Introduction

Vascular diagnosis took an important step forward in the 1980s with the use of Doppler and ultrasound. Advancing our knowledge of deep venous system anatomy and pathology were important early contributors, Cranley,

J.A. Zygmunt Jr., RVT, RPhS
Covidien Vascular Therapies,
Global Clinical Education, San Jose, CA, USA
e-mail: veinz@aol.com

E. Mowatt-Larssen et al. (eds.), *Phlebology, Vein Surgery and Ultrasonography*,
DOI 10.1007/978-3-319-01812-6_6, © Springer International Publishing Switzerland 2014

Strandness, and others. Steve Talbot, notably, began using duplex ultrasound in the diagnosis of deep vein thrombosis (DVT), its first use in venous disease [1–3]. Prominent in the advancement of our understanding of venous Doppler signals and flow characteristics were, among others, van Bemmelen and Strandness [4]. At the time, venous thrombosis and its complications, most notably pulmonary embolism, were the primary indications for the use of ultrasound. The emphasis was placed on the use of ultrasound as the standard diagnostic tool for deep vein thrombosis, to replace venography which is more invasive. Interestingly, during this time, "venous Doppler" was a commonplace term. For many years ultrasound was used as a rule-out DVT study, as superficial venous testing was all but nonexistent in mainstream medicine. The use of ultrasound in diagnosing deep vein thrombosis remains important today, as was highlighted recently when the Surgeon General stated that the incidence of deep vein thrombosis is a "national crisis," with greater than 600,000 Americans diagnosed annually, and further, with venous thromboembolism being the leading cause of preventable in-hospital death [5, 6]. The use of ultrasound for diagnosing DVT has come to overshadow its use for treating superficial venous disease.

The early adopters of phlebology, with a focus on chronic venous disease (CVD), or in more advanced stages, chronic venous insufficiency (CVI), spurred an intensified interest in the superficial venous system [7]. Expanding the practice of phlebology, Michael Schadeck performed the first ultrasound-guided sclerotherapy injection in 1984, which he later published in 1986 [8]. He was followed shortly thereafter by others [9, 10]. In the decade that followed, repeatable duplex ultrasound studies led to the enrichment of knowledge and understanding of the saphenous networks [11]. Descriptions of the saphenous vein, its compartment, and other works created a groundswell of interest in phlebology, eventually leading to the advancement of treatment techniques, including the development of thermal ablation of the saphenous vein [12–14].

6.2 Diagnostic Ultrasound Protocols

As noted above, DVT and knowledge of DVT ultrasound techniques are widely understood both in the USA and abroad. Those credentialed in vascular ultrasound (i.e., Registered Vascular Technologists [RVT] and Registered Vascular Specialists [RVS]) are certified to perform deep venous duplex examinations [15, 16]. Although the skill set of using ultrasound to gather images and flow information transfers nicely to insufficiency testing, the knowledge base is not as widespread, and, consequently, many RVTs and RVSs have done little, if any venous insufficiency testing. In April of 2010, Cardiovascular Credentialing International released a new ultrasound credential, the Registered Phlebology Sonographer (RPhS), to designate proficiency with venous reflux testing and its application to phlebologic sciences. Although the technique is reproducible and noninvasive, as with any ultrasound modality, it is extremely operator dependent. Therefore, the quality and quantity of information gathered during an insufficiency examination can vary widely and be influenced by the training and experience of the sonographer [17]. The vascular division of the Intersocietal Accreditation Commission (ICAVL), among other national organizations, has established guidelines for diagnostic testing, including separate protocols for DVT and venous insufficiency [18]. The major differences between DVT and venous insufficiency (or insufficiency) protocols are described below.

6.2.1 DVT (and Deep System) Documentation Protocol

For DVT, the primary goal is to determine the presence or absence of intraluminal thrombus, as demonstrated by compressibility of the vein walls. This

Table 6.1 Vascular testing protocol: DVT

Transverse gray scale	Spectral wave forms
CFV, SFJ (prox GSV)	Right and left CFV
Prox, mid, and distal FV	
Pop V	Pop V
Post tib V	
Peroneal V	
Additional images as needed	
Additional as per protocol	Additional as per protocol

Table 6.2 Vascular testing protocol: reflux (insufficiency)

Transverse gray scale	Spectral wave forms
CFV	CFV
SFJ	SFJ
Mid FV	FV
GSV	GSV
Pop V	Pop V
SSV	SSV
Additional images as needed	Suspected areas of reflux
Additional as per protocol	Additional as per protocol

is accomplished with application of external probe pressure on the vein to compress it and have wall-to-wall approximation. This is best done with a transverse B-Mode (or gray scale) approach. Documentation can be accomplished with split screen or with side-by-side still digital images or cine loop clips of the coaptations. The entire length of the target vein needs to be imaged, typically at 3 cm intervals. However, representative documentation is captured at specific sites to include: common femoral vein, saphenofemoral junction (SFJ), proximal mid- and distal femoral vein, popliteal vein, posterior tibial veins, and peroneal veins. Spectral waveforms of flow—phasicity and augmentation—are required at the right AND left common femoral veins and popliteal vein. Other images are required in the following circumstances: in the presence of disease, or as per written protocol, which typically calls for additional images to fully document the presence of disease; to understand the location and length of thrombus if found; and in the interrogation of the anterior tibialis, iliacs, profunda femoris, great saphenous vein (GSV), small saphenous vein (SSV), gastrocnemius, and soleal veins as necessary. Listed in Table 6.1 are the basic DVT requirements. Additional aspects could include an evaluation using color and power Doppler flow imaging, which will vary according to individual lab protocols.

6.2.2 Reflux (or Insufficiency) Documentation Protocol

For an insufficiency protocol, the goal is to determine the presence and pattern of venous reflux. Although DVT testing is not the primary goal, evaluating the deep system for thrombosis is still a critical aspect. This is an abbreviated exam compared to a full DVT protocol, but the insufficiency protocol includes some DVT-type determinations. Evaluation for DVTs is performed at the following locations: common femoral, SFJ, proximal great saphenous, mid-femoral, popliteal, and SSV. If a DVT is found, the typical protocol calls for a conversion to a standard DVT protocol in order to more fully document the DVT.

After this abbreviated DVT protocol, the reflux study continues to include spectral wave forms (typically using release of distal augmentation in the standing position, cuff inflators) of the following deep and superficial vessels: common femoral (right AND left), SFJ, femoral vein, great saphenous vein in multiple locations (from three to five sites), popliteal vein, and SSV (at least two sites). Other images are required in the following circumstances: the presence of disease or as per written protocol which typically calls for additional images to fully document the presence of disease; to understand the location and length and pattern of reflux if found; and in the interrogation of the varicose veins, perforators, and other veins suspected of reflux (according to written protocol). Listed in Table 6.2 are the basic insufficiency requirements. Additional aspects could include an evaluation using color and power Doppler flow imaging, which will vary according to individual lab protocols. Most significantly and covered in another section of this chapter is the creation of a venous reflux map, which is becoming the standard procedure in most dedicated vein treatment centers.

6.3 Deep System Considerations

Although CVD is related to saphenous insufficiency and varicose veins, deep system analysis cannot be overlooked due to the significance of hemodynamics and overload. A recent consensus document from the International Union of Phlebology (UIP) suggests the underappreciated nature of deep system disease, including some interesting new trends and findings:

Partial correction of venous defects may have enormous influence on the clinical state.

Axial reflux is poorly tolerated by the skin and subcutaneous tissues of the lower extremity and deserves surgical correction. Axial deep vein reflux need not be corrected as the initial step when deep and superficial refluxes coexist.

Correction of post-thrombotic reflux can be achieved by direct repair when the proximal valve has not been destroyed.

Early restoration of iliac vein patency at the time of acute iliofemoral thrombophlebitis has shown improved long-term results and is becoming the norm.

It is now recognized that iliac vein obstruction is ubiquitous and is often present in silent form in the general population. In symptomatic (CEAP clinical 3–6) primary and post-thrombotic CVI patients, such lesions are present in >90 % when examined with intravascular ultrasound (IVUS) [19].

Further, when performing reflux testing on the deep system, particular attention needs to be paid to the deep system valves in the infra- and supra-saphenic positions in relation to a saphenous junction (i.e., SFJ or saphenopopliteal junction [SPJ] [Fig. 6.1]). Kostas et al. define reflux in the deep system as the "presence of reflux in any deep venous segment distal to the level of the common femoral vein and at least 1 cm away from the saphenofemoral or saphenopopliteal junctions where there was coexistent reflux at these sites" [20]. Others have described the segmental deep system reflux at the SFJ or SPJ as being actually a "siphon effect," due to the suction created by the incompetent saphenous and varicose reservoir [21, 22]. This suggests that with the removal of the refluxing segment's reservoir, the segmental deep insufficiency will correct, which has been seen in this author's personal experience. Further, in the recent UIP consensus document on Duplex Reporting after Varicose Vein Treatment, there are clear recommendations that the deep system "should be examined in both the lying and standing position to check for residual obstruction and reflux, respectively" [23].

With these concepts in mind, one can appreciate the importance of the DVT exam, and further, how the insufficiency evaluation of the deep venous system is equally important. In this regard, augmentation techniques are important and will be covered more fully later, but van Bemmelen clearly describes that "diastolic function of valves is clinically more important," and goes on to state, "Valves refluxing while the patient is in the erect position may seem competent when the patient is in the supine position" and "Manual compression of the supine limb proximal to the transducer site did not result in closure of the valve but rather *in reflux during the entire compression…*" [4]. Those ideas can be distilled into the following practical information by this author: compression distal to the valve being tested is preferred; proximal compression should be avoided, with the exception of Valsalva for evaluation of the common femoral vein and SFJ; and a cuff device is more standardized and reproducible when compared to a hand augmentation.

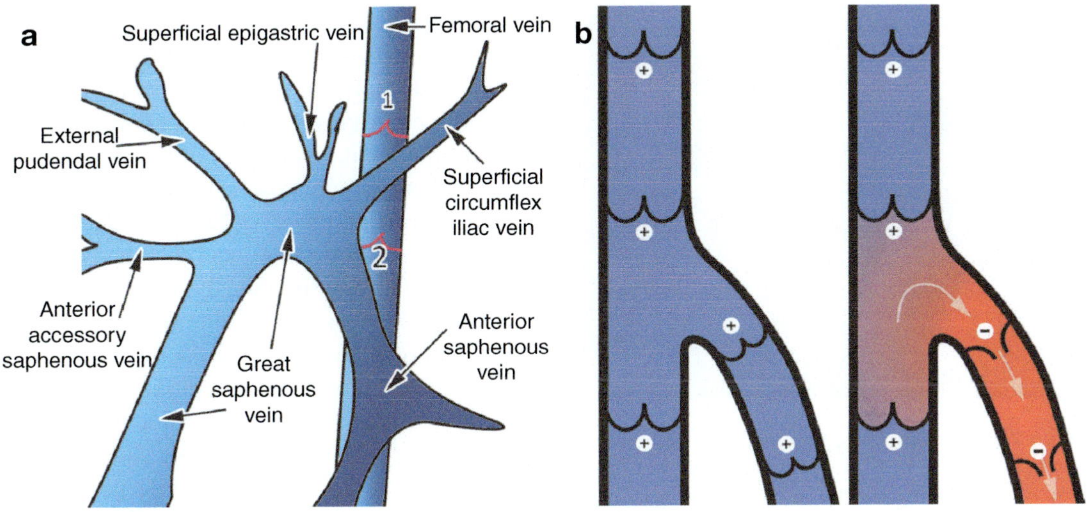

Fig. 6.1 (**a**) Illustration of the branches of the saphenous vein. The saphenous vein arch contains the space between the preterminal valve and the terminal valve. (**b**) The varicose reservoir below an incompetent segment reflux near a junction can create false deep vein reflux

6.4 Saphenous and Superficial Venous System General Considerations

The amount of information currently available on superficial venous anatomy and testing techniques has been vastly expanded over the past two decades. The following section will cover such aspects as terminology, overview of key anatomy, reflux, and factors that affect reflux reproducibility including augmentation techniques.

6.4.1 General Anatomy Basics

Although anatomy was covered more fully in an earlier chapter, understanding of some key anatomic facts assists the sonographer not only in gathering information during a diagnostic reflux exam but also in understanding and interpreting the results, so that clinical correlation and appropriate next steps can be considered.

Superficial veins are divided into saphenous and epifascial veins. Saphenous veins run in an "Egyptian eye" visible on transverse ultrasound (Fig. 6.2). As opposed to arteries, which bifurcate, veins are generally described from a normal flow direction, and therefore distal veins form a confluence (or union) with other veins, becoming larger as we move proximal or towards the heart. Regarding terminology, the generally accepted terms of great saphenous vein (GSV), and small saphenous vein (SSV), though ubiquitous in the phlebology community, are not yet well adopted in general medicine or by newcomers entering the field who still might inappropriately refer to the "L" lesser saphenous vein, or "superficial" femoral vein. The concept of a junctional "area," sometimes referred to as the "saphenous arch" for the saphenofemoral junction (SFJ), includes a length of the saphenous vein that includes the preterminal valve.

Some general terms in the current language making their way into our diagnostic reports

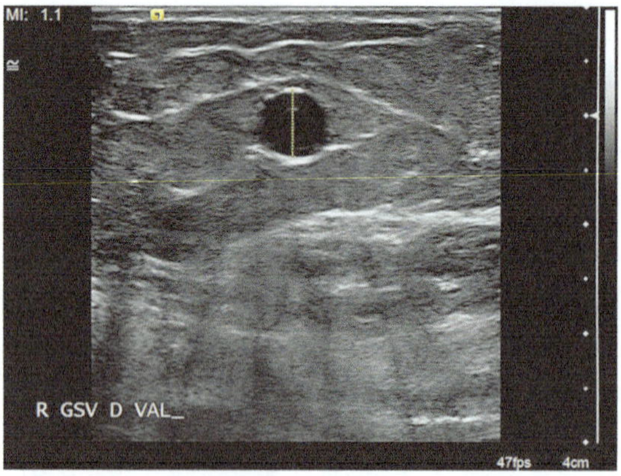

Fig. 6.2 Saphenous veins, by consensus definition [37], run in saphenous "eyes." In this image, the black "pupil" (saphenous vein) is enclosed in the hyperechoic "globe" (fasciae) above and below the vein

are: *agenesis* for either non-development of a vein or for varying degrees of incomplete development of a vein, *aplasia* being more severe than *hypoplasia*, and *atrophy* for a wasting away of a normal vein. Also, key points are that a *venous aneurysm* is a local dilation of a vein >50 % than the normal adjacent vein [24]. A true "duplication" of the great saphenous vein is one that occurs in the saphenous canal at an incidence of approximately 2 % and is much lower than previously reported [25]. As described in the UIP posttreatment document, venous measurements should be "performed in the transverse veins and the outer diameter should be measured (including the vein wall)…. the saphenous trunk should be measured at a site where there is no focal (or aneurysmal) dilation of the trunk….for the GSV trunk, measurements…should be made 3 cm below the saphenofemoral junction (SFJ)" [23].

We also now appreciate the presence of the three compartments of the leg (N1 deep, N2 saphenous, and N3 epifascial), as well as the saphenous ligament, which is not present in conjunction with the epifascial tributaries. Additionally, though chronic venous disease is predominantly related to saphenous reflux, the diagnostic investigator will need to appreciate that approximately 9 % of CVD patients will have non-saphenous reflux patterns [26]. Unfortunately, pelvic symptoms related to CVD are often missed. Awareness of this category of non-saphenous reflux patterns can serve to refocus the clinician on pelvic issues. Finally with regard to anatomy, a reminder that the posterior tibial perforators (previously Cockett's) connect the posterior tibial veins to the posterior accessory saphenous vein of the leg (previously posterior arch vein) and *not to the distal great saphenous vein itself*. Though not fully inclusive, these key points on anatomy and terminology should be kept in mind while performing diagnostic ultrasound for reflux; they will be invaluable for recognition and reporting.

6.4.2 Considerations on Reflux

The definition of reflux was made by Labropoulos et al., stating that abnormal retrograde flow and valve closure times for the superficial venous system in excess of 0.5 s defines pathologic reflux [7, 27]. For the femoropopliteal segment, 1.0 s is the cutoff. Further, reflux is related to fluid hemodynamics and typically involves a change in compartment (i.e., deep system [N1] leaking out into the superficial compartment [N2] or into the epifascial compartment [N3]). Even after several decades of reflux testing, there is no standardization in method or technique, but there are some relative consistencies. Some consider the "absolute quantitative" determination of reflux as a fool's errand because there are so many factors that affect the amount, rate, and volume of reflux at any given time. Repeatability and reproducibility are compelling discussion points in reflux testing and have recently been investigated. Repeatability is the variability of the measurements obtained by one person while measuring the same item repeatedly, versus reproducibility, which is the variability in measurement caused by differences in operator behavior (i.e., between different sonographers). As presented recently at the American Venous Forum meeting, several key conclusions were drawn: "Repeatability of duplex ultrasound in detection of venous reflux is high; reproducibility of this test is sufficient and can be improved by educational intervention; testing patients at different times of day, in different positions, and using different reflux-provoking maneuvers significantly decreases reliability" [28]. In order to achieve the most accurate, reliable, and reproducible diagnostic testing results, the sonographic investigator needs to be aware of these factors and their impact, especially the reasons for false negatives. Some of these key factors will be explored further in this chapter. To emphasize the point, although these variables have influence, most clinicians with a phlebologic interest follow a set of "standardized" techniques that maximize accuracy and minimize variability. It should be noted that there is high confidence in these methods. Further, it is suggested that anyone performing reflux testing should adopt these techniques and clearly describe methods used in reporting, or any variations that occur on an individual case-by-case basis.

6.4.3 Time of Day

Although intuitively we understand that standing is a better position to test reflux than supine, does the time of day a reflux study is performed really have an impact? The Investigating Venous disease Evaluation and Standardization of Testing (INVEST) study suggests that including the time of day that testing was performed should be part of the reporting process, and this author agrees. If we think about the effects of gravity on reflux, it makes sense that the longer a patient is standing, the greater the impact of reflux. Also, it makes sense that while sleeping in bed, equilibration and normalization occurs. These considerations align with the general pattern of symptoms being worse with prolonged standing and relieved with rest and elevation. In one study, patients who work third shift (overnight) were considered outliers and eliminated from statistical analysis in its published data [29]. Further, this study reveals specifics of increased swelling, increased reflux in general, and especially reflux in perforators, as noted in afternoon examinations when compared to morning examinations. The changes in perforator reflux from abnormal to normal were stumbled upon during morning reexaminations to verify reflux prior to perforator interventions scheduled first thing in the morning. Varying results were noted when compared to the study performed the preceding afternoon. Others have described this variability [11, 30]. Ironically, no consensus on time of day for performing scans has been agreed upon. It is impractical to perform all studies in either the morning or afternoon. As stated above, the best line of thought is to realize this variability exists, especially when results do not match symptoms or clinical findings (false negatives), and to include time of day in the dictated report as suggested in the INVEST study.

6.4.4 Patient Position

As previously mentioned, reflux requires a pressure gradient, and this is not only typically related to compartment, but is also gravity dependent. Therefore, position of the patient is a key variable in the reflux determination process. Purists in the phlebology community adamantly defend the concept of standing evaluation for venous reflux [31–33]. The recent UIP document on posttreatment evaluation echoes this sentiment, "When assessing superficial veins, patients should be examined in the standing position where possible." The INVEST study, though carried out using both standing and non-standing positions, indicates the "position of the patient" should be a part of the report. Typically, reflux evaluation in the standing position is performed on the non-weight-bearing leg to avoid effects of muscular systole on venous flow.

6.4.5 Augmentation Techniques

Venous flow in the lower extremity is a slow flow state and normally an orchestrated combination of the foot, calf, and thigh muscle pumps working with respiratory changes, intra-abdominal pressures, and valves to produce a ratchet-like movement of blood from the distal limb to the heart in the standing patient. When it comes to diagnostic testing, the examiner needs to augment flow for evaluation of patency and, especially, reflux. The systolic portion of the augmentation mimics muscular contraction normally pushing blood central, while the diastolic phase is when we seek to measure reflux (retrograde flow), for a period of ascribed time, 0.5 s in the superficial system. There are several methods that can be used for systolic augmentation, depending on which diastolic observation of reflux will be described. It should be noted that a systolic reflux is a significant finding, suggesting a proximal deep obstruction (i.e., a systolic reflux of the SPJ can be seen with a femoral vein obstruction).

Valsalva Maneuver

As recently reported, a "standardized Valsalva maneuver….consists of forced exhalation into a special tube system that measures expiratory pressure" at set parameters [23]. This technique and its parameters, while cumbersome, are highly reproducible. However, because a reflux wave cannot proceed downward through a healthy valve, they "cannot be used to assess reflux in veins distal to competent valves." This key point needs to be emphasized; Valsalva is only accurate to the level of the first competent valve. Because this is not clearly understood, the author suggests only using Valsalva at the common femoral vein or SFJ. Additionally, when using Valsalva without the standardization techniques outlined in the UIP documents, patient instruction and performance variability are the most likely variables to be non-reproducible.

Active Dorsiflexion, Plantar Flexion, and Parana Maneuvers

These methods to augment flow involve slight movement of the patient to elicit calf systole in a more physiologic similar manner. In each of these techniques, the challenge is with patient movement while holding the probe stationary on the vein being examined. These techniques are very helpful when extrinsic pressure from edema may alter venous capacitance and flow.

Manual Distal Compression

Although this is the most commonly used method, distal compression is best when applied over the capacitor (varicose bed) that is connected to the vein being tested. Due to the inherent differences in hand size, strength, force delivered, etc., there are increased differences in reproducibility for quantitative reflux determinations. To determine if reflux is simply present or absent, this method is effective. As noted earlier, proximal compression should be avoided as a method of augmentation.

Standardized Cuff Inflation-Deflation Method

Although some consider it cumbersome, this method is the most reproducible and repeatable augmentation method for duration of reflux and should be preferred over manual or proximal compression [34]. Typically, this technique involves placement of a cuff on the calf that can be rapidly inflated and, after a short pause, rapidly deflated, mimicking a highly repeatable distal hand squeeze. Many units have variable pressure settings that are most often set in the 80–120 mmHg range.

To summarize "augmentation," for reproducible and repeatable findings, a standardized Valsalva maneuver (for proximal sites only) and standardized cuff inflation-deflation methods are preferred, though in most settings these standardized methods are not commonly used. Additionally, understanding the limitations or concerns of other techniques is advised, as well as avoidance of proximal compression.

6.5 Capacitance of the Venous Segment

When considering the positive or negative determination of reflux, 0.5 s is a relatively straightforward concept. It is essential to understand the capacitance of the distal venous segment, and

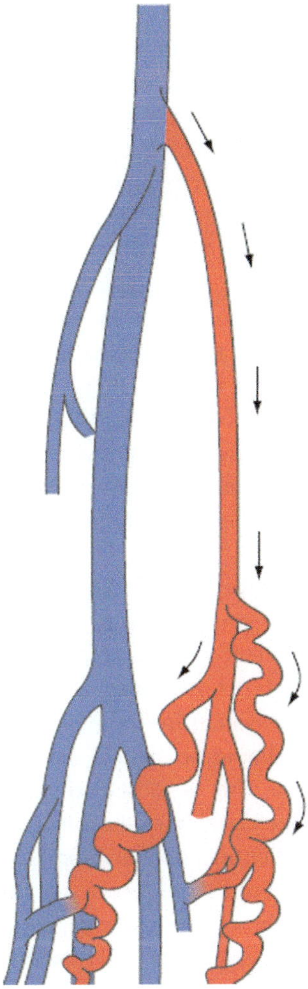

Fig. 6.3 In the "varicose bed" (distal network of varices), the size and extent of this "capacitor" greatly influences the reflux curve

especially the variability of the varicose bed. The distal bed, or capacitor, has a major impact on the determination of the refluxing volume, peak reflux velocity, the flow duration, or other quantitative factors (Fig. 6.3), where the varicose bed (capacitor) is noted in red. Labropoulos best describes this conundrum, writing that "when a large incompetent vein empties into a small capacitor, peak vein velocity is high, but duration is short. When the refluxing vein is small and the capacitor is large, velocity is low and retrograde flow (RF) duration is long….and no definite conclusions can be made" [27]. Therefore, the shape of a reflux curve is nondiscriminatory with regard to the severity, extent of disease, or correlation with the CEAP classifications. Repeated compression or augmentation in quick succession will empty the "distal capacitance" resulting in less flux (forward flow) and reduced reflux. Allowing time for venous refilling following a distal compression is required for a more accurate assessment. A few other factors that can influence reflux include venous tone, venous distensibility or vessel compliance, temperature, hydration, and length of time standing.

In general, in order to maximize accuracy of the interpretation of results and correlation to clinical presentation, the preceding concepts need to be understood by the investigative sonographer.

6.6 The Superficial Reflux Examination

In the most practical of approaches, a vein map to describe the path of reflux can be the most valuable tool in understanding a patient's pathology and assist in formulation of a treatment plan. This concept has become well accepted [35, 36]. Further, in addition to a dictated report, a visual map is becoming a common practice. Vein mapping involves the knowledge of several ultrasound anatomic markers and other tips known to the experienced phlebology sonographer:

"h" vein: One of the most common patterns involves the "h" vein presentation in which a large epifascial branch is noted coming off the saphenous trunk [37]. The specific location of the branch may be higher or lower along the course of the GSV, and anterior or posterior, but this appears to be the most common presentation.

Alignment sign: The GSV is located more posterior on the medial aspect of the thigh than most novices assume. In a fair number of cases, this leads to misidentification of the anterior accessory saphenous vein (AAGSV) as the great saphenous. The alignment sign denotes the presence of the deep vessels of the thigh under the proximal section of the AAGSV (Fig. 6.4) [37]. If scanning the true

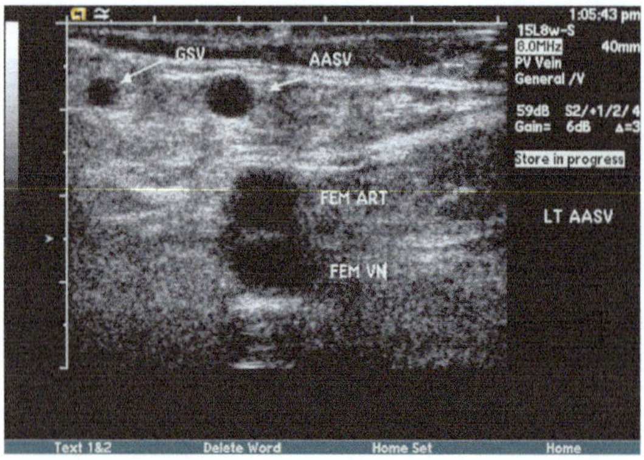

Fig. 6.4 Alignment sign. The anterior accessory great saphenous vein (*AASV*) runs anterior (above in this image) the femoral vein and artery in transverse ultrasound view. By consensus definition [37], the alignment sign differentiates the AASV from the great saphenous vein (*GSV*), which runs medial to the AASV

GSV as one moves distally from the junction to the knee, the deep veins should move lateral from the field of view on the sonographic image.

Color flow is not a crutch: Although color flow is helpful for identification of reflux, understanding how color is produced is critical to understanding severity of reflux. Since reflux of less than 0.5 s is considered normal, almost every vein can have a snapshot in time (i.e., frozen digital image) when "red" for reflux is present. The question is more related to how long that red lasts. Therefore, reflux determinations (and documentation) should be performed using spectral analysis, in the long axis with optimal angle (45–60 °) (Fig. 6.5).

Vein size and reflux: When tracing reflux, changes in size of the saphenous vein is a key finding. It is typical for a saphenous vein to change size where pressure (and reflux) enters or leaves the saphenous canal. Special attention should be paid to areas where the saphenous trunk undergoes a change in size, especially at the level of a large tributary or a perforating vein.

Perforators are either exit or reentry points for reflux: Perforators allow for the transmission of high pressure from N1 to the lower pressure N2 or N3 compartments. One must appreciate that once reflux occurs and the blood falls, it needs to re-enter the deep (N1) compartment, and that many distal perforators are actually reentry perforators. Reentry perforating veins may disappear or diminish in size with the removal of an incompetent saphenous system, as the hydrostatic overload is removed [30]. Recent updates include a definition of a pathologic perforator, which, in addition to outward flow, needs to be adjacent to an active or healed ulcer [7].

Serial assessment of the GSV is recommended: If reflux is found at one level of the saphenous (GSV or SSV) and not another, investigation between these two points is required in order to understand the pathology involved in the change noted between the two locations [11]. Without the use of serial investigation, a complete understanding of reflux along the course of the entire saphenous vein (great or small) is not possible.

Vein diagram for GSV in thigh: Since a vast majority of vein therapy is currently directed at incompetence of the great saphenous vein in the thigh, *at minimum*, a vein map of the saphenous system from the inguinal crease to the knee should be created during diagnostic evaluation. This is most easily facilitated by use of a technical worksheet (Fig. 6.6).

Saphenous identification and pre-scan: Due to some difficulties in proper identification of either of the saphenous veins, a "midsection" approach is suggested. By placing the transducer at either mid-thigh or mid-calf along the path of the corresponding saphenous vein, the saphenous compartment is most easily identifiable within the canal. Through a quick prescan of the proximal and distal segments of the compartment by transverse approach, a preliminary understanding of the anatomy can be appreciated and more fully investigated as the diagnostic scan progresses.

Heel on ground: Preferred patient position is standing, with the leg being examined externally rotated with the patient's weight on the contralateral leg. Care should be taken that the heel is on the ground, especially on the leg being tested, so that calf contraction (muscular systole) is avoided as is seen when the heel is lifted.

Sourcing reflux and crossover patterns: Recently described, a "sourcing" technique can be employed to detect the superficial reflux routes with ulceration [38]. This approach

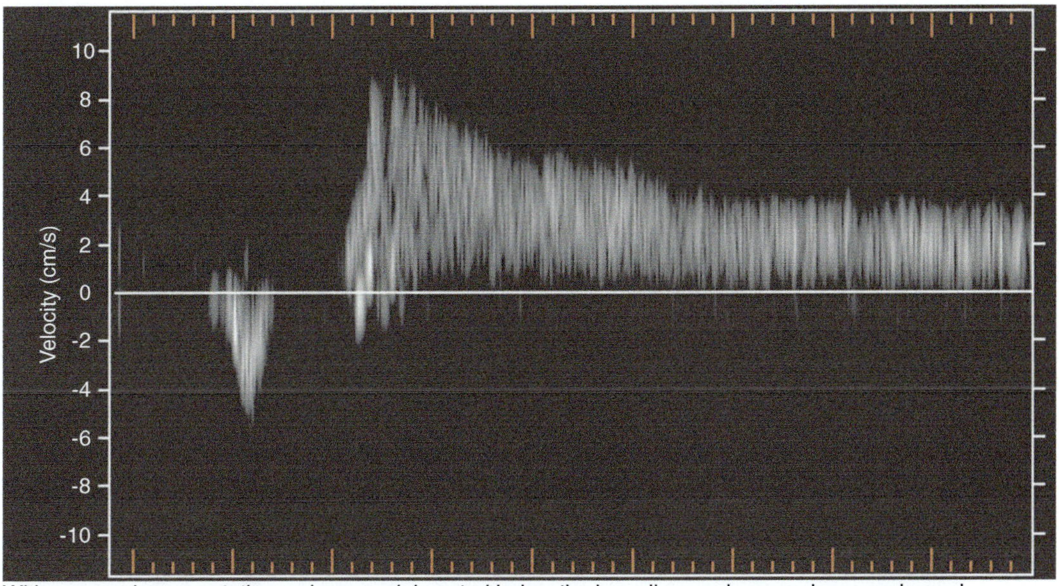

With a normal augmentation a sharp peak is noted below the base line, and upon release prolonged reverse flow is noted above the line on the spectral traching

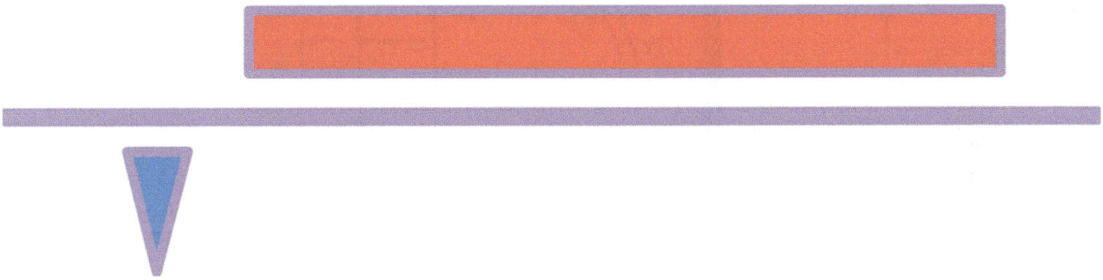

If the spectral curve was "displayed" with color, the normal augmentation is blue, and short in duration, while reflux is red and prolonged

Fig. 6.5 Color flow as related to spectral curve

needs to also be employed for varicose ulcers, and especially for non-saphenous varices. Additionally, the understanding of axial and crossover patterns has been clarified. Crossover reflux was noted in 46 %, of lateral ulcers while it was only seen in 11 % of medial ulcers. Furthermore, 20 % of patients with venous ulcers have no visible varicose veins.

Non-junctional GSV reflux: Reflux can develop proximally, distally, or along the course of the GSV [39]. "Refluxes are often found below competent terminal valves, especially in youngsters, and in up to 67 % of patients, saphenous reflux exists without SFJ (26–67 %) or saphenopopliteal junction incompetence (42 %)" [40]. Therefore, although junctional investigation is important, the concept of serial investigation along the course of the saphenous vein cannot be overlooked, as distal reflux is often present below a normal junction.

6.7 Segmentation of the Saphenous Mapping: Technique Suggestions

The basics of performing a duplex examination have been previously described [11, 31]. The supine position can produce both false-positive

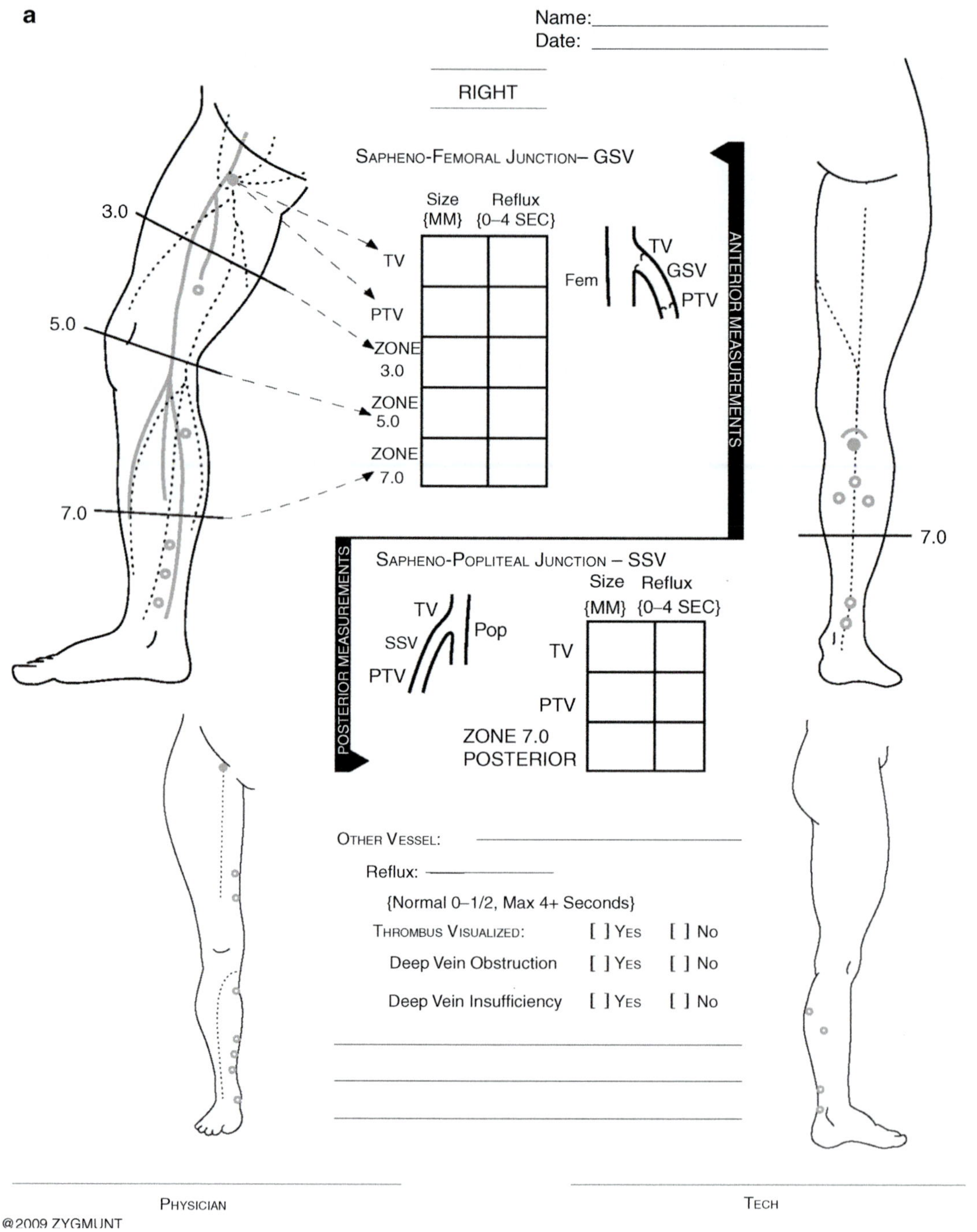

Fig. 6.6 Duplex worksheet for CVI examination [11]

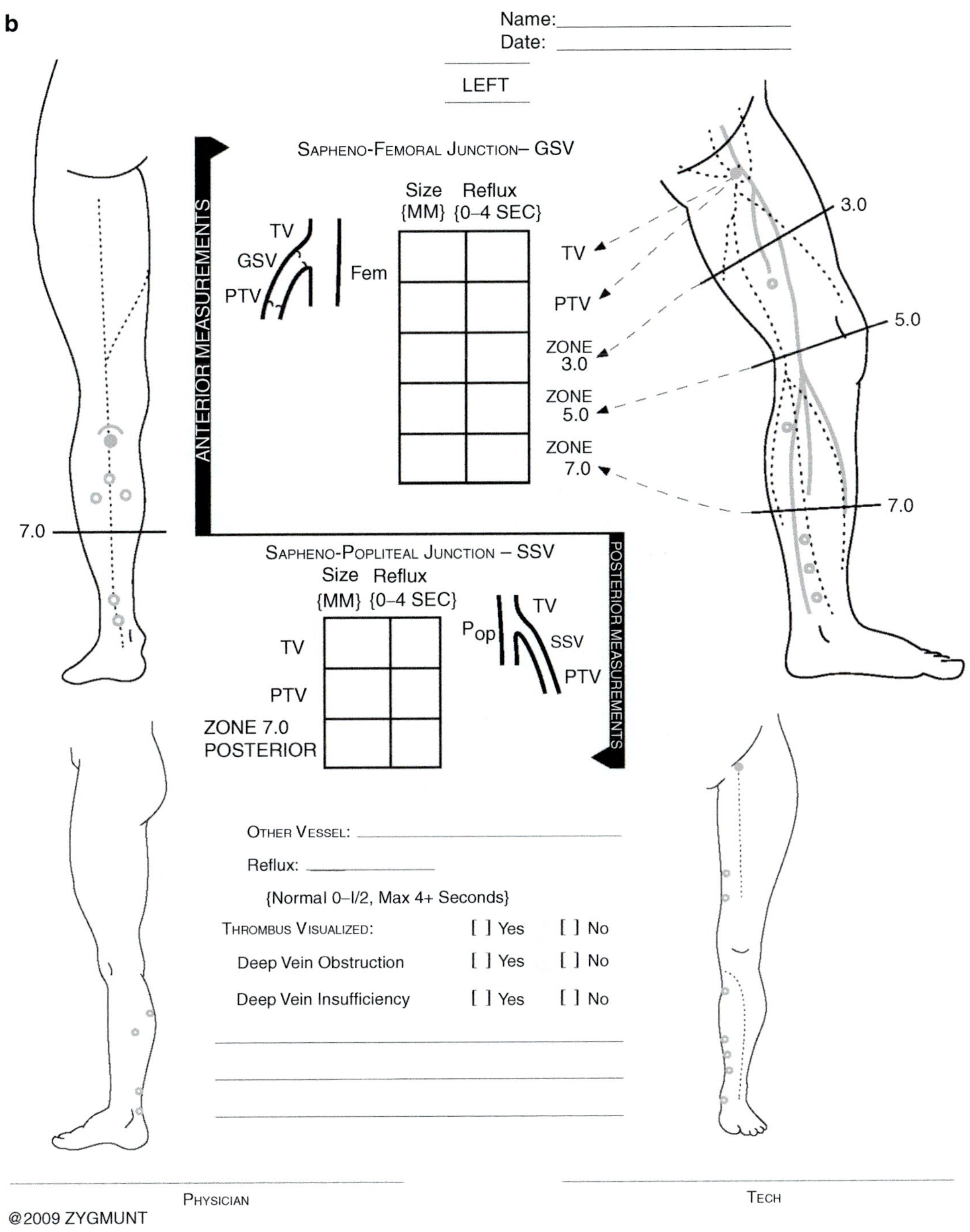

Fig. 6.6 (continued)

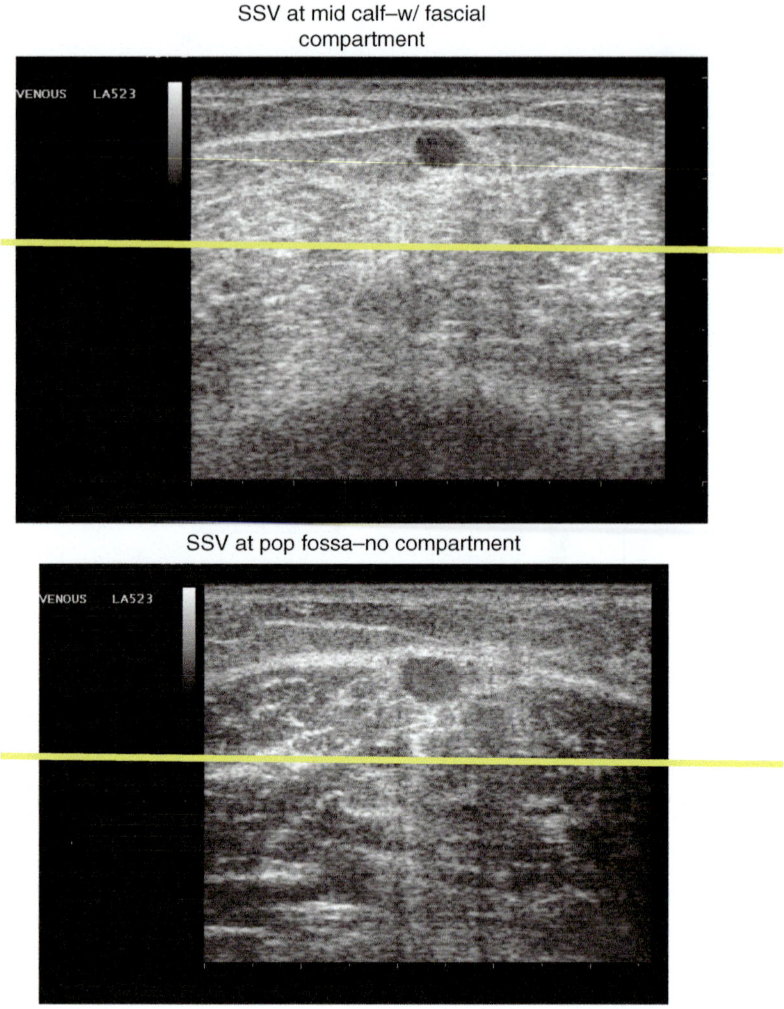

Fig. 6.7 SSV and fascia. The image above is from the mid-calf and defines the wide fascia space in which the SSV resides. The image below is from the popliteal crease which shows the thinning of the fascial compartment at that level

and false-negative results [7]. Also, the advantages of distal augmentation were previously discussed; however, the key to performance for a newbie (and others) is focusing on steps or protocol that can sometimes be lost in the excitement of tracing large varices or other interesting anatomic findings. For this reason, a "segmentation" approach is often employed.

The initial step is a physical inspection of the legs for visible signs of the patient's condition. This examination should be performed with the patient standing in order to fully appreciate the magnitude of any bulging vessels.

The (SSV) and posterior calf are easily accessed. Scanning should proceed on the non-weight-bearing leg with the patient standing. Investigation and identification of the SSV is best achieved at mid-calf (Fig. 6.7). In the mid-calf area, the saphenous compartment is thicker and easily seen. This compartment thins significantly as one approaches the popliteal fossa, making its identification more difficult and misidentification of the SSV more likely. Following the investigation of the SSV, paying particular attention to crossover routes and incompetence of the SPJ, a quick scan of the lateral calf is done to check the lateral accessory SSV. Next, scanning should move up to the posterior thigh for interrogation of the cranial extension and its variants, including the Giacomini vein.

Figure 6.7 SSV at mid-calf is easily identified in the compartment due to the size of the compartment, SSV in proximal calf is harder to identify as the saphenous compartment is thinner and harder to identify, thus making correct identification of the SSV more difficult.

In the next segment, the patient is repositioned to stand facing the investigator with the leg externally rotated and investigation of the non-weight-bearing leg is carried out. The great saphenous vein investigation can be segmented into the thigh and the leg, while notes on a technical worksheet could be made separately to reinforce the segmentation concept. In the thigh, as in the calf, identification of the GSV at mid-thigh, where the compartment is easily appreciated, is a good starting point. A pre-scan, up and down the thigh, as described recently, is recommended. Focusing first on the saphenous canal, evaluation of the GSV is completed. A 50 % rule is suggested for evaluation of tributaries and branches (i.e., if the branch or tributary is not at least 50 % the size of the saphenous vein at that point, it may be less important to trace out and indicate on the worksheet). Evaluation of the (AAGSV) and posterior accessory saphenous (PAGSV) are completed next, with the goal of understanding perforators, and anatomic patterns and vessels in the epifascial space (above the canal).

The GSV in the leg is the next focus of the segmented approach. At this time, the continuity of the GSV from ankle to thigh, especially in the area at or just below the knee, is important to evaluate. In many cases the GSV demonstrates aplasia or hypoplasia frequently in the proximal calf just below the knee. It is very important to note if the distal GSV does not connect to the posterior tibial perforators, as these perforators drain the PAGSV of the leg (previously the posterior arch vein). Perforators are an area of particular interest in the advanced venous patient (C4–6).

The final segmental step would be evaluation for non-saphenous reflux sources. The typical mindset for this segment is to question whether the information gathered up to this point fully correlates with the clinical signs and symptoms, and whether additional pathology (reflux) has yet to be identified.

Especially for someone new to reflux diagnostics, this segmentation approach allows for compartmentalization of the testing protocol for speed, efficiency, and accuracy.

Conclusion

Duplex ultrasound is one of the most highly operator-dependent imaging modalities [41]. The accuracy of duplex ultrasound is based on the experience and technical skill of the person performing the scan as well as the patient's cooperation. Since the modality is highly operator dependent, this reinforces the necessity of understanding the key underlying concepts of chronic venous disease: its pathology, presentation, and the factors inherent in its pathology as well as an increased awareness of testing techniques that can introduce error in measurement and diagnosis. The improvements since the mid-1980s, with the introduction of ultrasound to vascular diagnosis, have been significant. Continued use of standardized terminology and techniques help to reduce inter-user variability and give better clarity to the information gathered with duplex imaging before, during, or after treatment of chronic venous insufficiency.

References

1. Talbot SR. Use of real-time imaging in identifying deep venous obstruction: a preliminary report. Bruit. 1982;6:41–2.
2. Sullivan ED, Peter DJ, Cranley JJ. Real-time B-mode venous ultrasound. J Vasc Surg. 1984;1:465–71.
3. Talbot S, Oliver M. Techniques of venous imaging. 2nd ed. Pasedena: Davies; 1992.
4. Van Bemmelen P, Bedford G, Beach K, Strandness DE. Quantitative segmental evaluation of venous valvular reflux with duplex ultrasound scanning. J Vasc Surg. 1989;10:425–31.
5. Arko FR, et al. Aggressive percutaneous mechanical thrombectomy of deep venous thrombosis – early clinical results. Arch Surg. 2007;142:513–9.
6. National Quality Forum. http://www.qualityforum.org/Publications/2006/12/National_Voluntary_Consensus_Standards_for_Prevention_and_Care_of_Venous_Thromboembolism__Policy,_Preferred_Practices,_and_Initial_Performance_Measures.aspx. Accessed Oct 2011.
7. Gloviczki P, et al. The care of patients with varicose veins and associated chronic venous diseases: clinical practice guidelines of the Society for Vascular Surgery

and the American Venous Forum. J Vasc Surg. 2011; 53:2S–48.
8. Schadeck M. Doppler et Echotomographies dans las sclerose des veines saphenes. Phlebologie. 1986;39: 697–716.
9. Knight R, Vin F, Zygmunt J. 10th Congress of the International Union de Phlebologie: ultrasound guidance of injections into the superficial venous system, Strasbourg, 1989. p. 334–41.
10. Parsi K. Catheter-directed sclerotherapy. Phlebology. 2009;24:98–107.
11. Zygmunt J. What is new in duplex scanning of the venous system. Perspect Vasc Surg Endovasc Ther. 2009;21(2):94–104.
12. Caggiatti A, Bergan JJ. The saphenous vein, derivation of its name and relevant anatomy. J Vasc Surg. 2002;35:172–5.
13. Caggiatti A, Ricci S. The long saphenous vein compartment. Phlebology. 1997;12:107–11.
14. Weiss RA. Endovenous techniques for elimination of saphenous reflux: a valuable treatment modality. Dermatol Surg. 2001;27:902–5.
15. RVT is the Registered Vascular Technologist credential of ARDMS. www.ardms.org. Accessed Oct 2011.
16. RVS is the Registered Vascular Sonographer credential of CCI. www.cci-online. Accessed Oct 2011.
17. Baker S, Willey B, Mitchell C. The attempt to standardize technical and analytic competence in sonography education. J Diagn Med Sonography. 2011; 27(5):203–11.
18. Revision to Venous Standards. http://intersocietal.org/vascular/main/vascular_standards.htm. Accessed Oct 2012.
19. Lurie F, et al. Invasive treatment of deep venous disease. A UIP consensus. Int Angiol. 2010;29:199–204.
20. Kostas T, Ioannou C, Touloupakis E, et al. Recurrent varicose veins after surgery: a new appraisal of a common and complex problem in vascular surgery. Eur J Vasc Endovasc Surg. 2004;27:275–82.
21. Creton D, Pare EC. Diameter reduction of the proximal long saphenous vein after ablation of a distal incompetent tributary. Dermatol Surg. 1999;25:394–8.
22. Somjec GM, Royle JP, Fell G. Venous reflux patterns in the popliteal fossa. J Cardiovasc Surg. 1992;33:85–91.
23. De Maeseneer M, et al. Duplex ultrasound investigation of the veins of the lower limbs after treatment for varicose veins – UIP consensus document. Eur J Vasc Endovasc Surg. 2011. doi:10.1016/j.ejvs.2011.03.013.
24. Caggiatti A, et al. Nomenclature of the veins of the lower limb; extensions, refinements and clinical application. J Vasc Surg. 2005;41:719–24.
25. Labropoulos N, et al. The distribution and significance of varicosities in the saphenous trunks. J Vasc Surg. 2010;51:96–103.
26. Labropoulos N, et al. Nonsaphenous superficial vein reflux. J Vasc Surg. 2001;34:872–7.
27. Labropoulos N, et al. Definition of venous reflux in lower extremity veins. J Vasc Surg. 2003;38:793–8.
28. Lurie F. Investigating venous disease evaluation and standardization of testing. In: Proceedings of the American Venous Forum, San Diego, 2011.
29. Tarrant G, Clarke J. Differences in venous function of the lower limb by time of day: a comparison of chronic venous insufficiency between an afternoon and a morning appointment by duplex ultrasound. J Vasc Ultrasound. 2008;32:187–92.
30. Meissner MH, et al. The hemodynamics and diagnosis of venous disease. J Vasc Surg. 2007;46(suppl):4S–24.
31. Coleridge_smith P, et al. Duplex ultrasound investigation of the veins in chronic venous disease of the lower limbs, UIP consensus document. Part I: basic principles. Eur J Vasc Endovasc Surg. 2006;31:83–92.
32. Neuhardt D, et al. Differences in saphenous vein reflux detection according to patient positioning. Proceedings of the Union de Phlebologie conference. Monaco, 2009, abstract #0079.
33. Foldes M, et al. Standing versus supine positioning in venous reflux evaluation. J Vasc Tech. 1991;15(6): 321–4.
34. Yamaki T, et al. Comparison of manual compression release with distal pneumatic cuff maneuver in ultrasonic evaluation of superficial venous insufficiency. Eur J Vasc Endovasc Surg. 2006;32:462–7.
35. Blomgren L, et al. Changes in superficial and perforating vein reflux after varicose vein surgery. J Vasc Surg. 2005;42:315–20.
36. Labropoulos N, Leon N, Kwon S. Study of venous reflux progression. J Vasc Surg. 2005;41:291–5.
37. Cavezzi A, et al. Duplex ultrasound investigation of the vein in chronic venous disease of the lower limbs: UIP consensus document. Part II: anatomy. Eur J Vasc Endovasc Surg. 2006;31:288–99.
38. Obermeyer A, Garson K. Identifying the source of superficial reflux in venous leg ulcers using duplex ultrasound. J Vasc Surg. 2010;52:1255–61.
39. Pittaluga P, et al. Classification of saphenous refluxes: implications for treatment. Phlebology. 2008;23:2–9.
40. Bernardini E, et al. Development of primary superficial venous insufficiency: the ascending theory. Observational and hemodynamic data from a 9 year experience. Ann Vasc Surg. 2010;24:709–20.
41. Medicare information. http://www.cms.hhs.gov/medicare. Accessed Oct 2011.

Ultrasound for Phlebology Procedures

7

Diana L. Neuhardt

Contents

D.L. Neuhardt, RVT, RPhS
CompuDiagnostics, Inc., Phoenix, AZ, USA
e-mail: dneuhardt@compudiagnostics.com

Abstract

The goal of this chapter is to provide a basic explanation for using an ultrasound imaging device in its dual role for therapeutic imaging. Direct visualization with ultrasound gave way to the development of minimally invasive venous therapies. Endovenous thermal ablation and chemical ablation are becoming the preferred treatments for superficial venous valvular reflux disease. Compelling successful outcomes, early recovery, and low complication rates have ignited interest in using less invasive methods in lieu of the traditional open surgical methods. The text is targeted for phlebology treatments, though many of the fundamentals can be applied to other modalities of intervention requiring ultrasonic guidance. These skills are unique compared to those used for diagnostic ultrasound visualization, that is, ultrasound used as a tool to aid in treatment of chronic venous insufficiency.

7.1 Introduction

There is no disputing the vital role ultrasound technology has served for the growth of phlebology. Within the diagnostic arena, duplex ultrasound has become the gold standard for the evaluation of chronic venous insufficiency of the lower extremities. Once a mainstay, venography has largely been replaced. Historically, venous duplex studies of the lower extremities were aimed at the diagnosis of deep vein thrombosis.

E. Mowatt-Larssen et al. (eds.), *Phlebology, Vein Surgery and Ultrasonography*,
DOI 10.1007/978-3-319-01812-6_7,

The genesis of venous "mapping" fully expanded the potential of diagnostic ultrasound to examine both the deep and superficial venous systems, particularly in the study of venous valvular hemodynamics and reflux detection.

Direct visualization with ultrasound gave way to the development of minimally invasive venous therapies. Endovenous thermal ablation and chemical ablation are becoming the preferred treatments for superficial venous valvular reflux disease. Compelling successful outcomes, early recovery, and low complication rates have ignited interest in using less invasive methods in lieu of the traditional open surgical methods.

We recognize our expanded knowledge of venous disease by virtue of the advancement and refinement of duplex ultrasound instrumentation. As the equipment expanded into digital sophistication, the technical knowledge and experience must be applied proportionally to maximize our diagnostic results and therapeutic outcomes. Specifically, the diagnostic nuances, clinical background, and therapeutic applications that involve phlebology are specialty focused. Ultrasound sonography visualization during therapeutic interventions has unfolded numerous options for minimally invasive treatments. Accordingly, ultrasound training expertise must be expanded to be inclusive of the applied skills for pre-, peri-, and post-phlebologic treatments.

The goal of this chapter is to provide a basic explanation for using an ultrasound imaging device in its dual role for therapeutic imaging. The text is targeted for phlebology treatments, though many of the fundamentals can be applied to other modalities of intervention requiring ultrasonic guidance. These skills are unique compared to those used for diagnostic ultrasound visualization, that is, ultrasound used as a tool to aid in treatment of chronic venous insufficiency.

7.2 Ultrasound Instrumentation

Ultrasound manufacturers have been downplaying the complexity of the ultrasound device through packaging design. Many non-trained users buy into promotions touting ease of use, affordability, and portability. Nowhere to be found in the description is one important detail, namely, that ultrasound technology is both operator based and operator dependent and is completely reliant on the individual's experience and skill to use the device. Without such knowledge the ultrasound device is without value. Additionally, the overall engineering design characteristics of the equipment will affect the variability one has during therapeutic interventions. Duplex ultrasound systems, regardless of size or specific use, require a thorough understanding of Doppler physics and the scientific principles applied to ultrasound within the human body. These topics are covered in Chap. 5. Ultrasound quality can be obtained only by users who have applied diligent study and practice. In addition, the ultrasound image one can attain is equally dependent on the caliber of the instrument being used.

Much of the focus of this chapter will pertain to the use of ultrasound as a tool specific to therapeutic interventions. The greater understanding one has either as an ultrasound user or observer, the easier the therapeutic intervention will be. Additionally, a comprehensive knowledge of the lower extremity venous system and its relation to anatomy (structure) and physiology (flow) will impact outcomes. Other structures will be visualized from the skin line, and these include subcutaneous fat, arteries, muscles, tendons, and nerves. Ultrasound users must be familiar with normal and abnormal ultrasound findings within the region of interest.

Within a relatively short time span, phlebology ultrasound technology progressed from static images to what is referred to today as "real-time" imaging. Crude handheld Doppler listening devices have also evolved. Radical breakthroughs occurred for all specialties in ultrasound when engineers discovered how to integrate the two technologies of Doppler and imaging into one device; hence the term *duplex* was coined. Doppler physics combined with imaging created simultaneous real-time information for the user, and this is particularly useful in application to blood vessels. Further technology expanded with the introduction of color Doppler. A basic understanding of the scientific theories applied to an ultrasound scanner will provide a basis for obtaining best ease of use.

With the application of an acoustic medium (gel) and a transducer to touch the skin, sound waves are transmitted from the ultrasound scanner. Brightness of the returning echo forms the basis for B-mode, gray scale imaging. Such images (pixels) displayed are subject to manipulation of the sound waves through soft tissue. This basic concept is important as sound waves are reflected and displayed uniquely and are influenced by whatever lies between the skin and the targeted image.

The ultrasound imaging transducer, or probe, one selects will determine the depth range that can be examined. Higher-frequency transducers (i.e., ranging 10.0–17 MHz) are designed to look in the near field (close to the skin) to identify structures such as the superficial venous anatomy and/or facilitate needle access or guidance. Lower-frequency transducers (i.e., ranging 4.5–7.5 MHz) permit visualization at lower depths and are selected when evaluating the deeper structures and may be necessary in larger or obese patients. For most phlebology interventions, a high-frequency linear transducer is necessary. A multi-frequency transducer would be a versatile option, a statement addressed in further text. Additionally, the ultrasound images are visibly displayed on a screen/monitor. When selecting equipment, the monitor should be ample in size for good visualization and have swivel features as well. This obviates the need to move the equipment during the procedure, as the monitor can be adjusted to greatest visible acuity.

7.3 Ultrasound Training

The use of ultrasound for phlebology techniques requires technical skill. The training and expertise necessary for individuals who utilize ultrasound will vary relative to application of use. One resource to acquire such skill can be found through the American College of Phlebology (http://www.phlebology.org/) which offers ultrasound fellowship training opportunities specific to venous diagnostic and therapeutic applications. Other training opportunities may include regional ultrasound courses or rotational fellowships. Targeted study and practice are necessary to obtain experience and confidence in one's ability. Though the intent may be to examine venous structures, these are not the only anatomical features identified on routine examination or visualization. Imaging from the skin line will identify subcutaneous fat, muscle, tendons, arteries, nerves, joint spaces, periarticular bursae, and bone.

Professional medical societies, such as the American College of Radiology (ACR), recommend that "physicians responsible for diagnostic ultrasound examinations should be able to demonstrate familiarity with the anatomy, physiology, and pathophysiology of those organs or anatomic areas that are being examined" [1]. Statements from The American College of Surgeons (ACS) are that "physicians performing ultrasound examinations and ultrasound-guided procedures must be familiar with the principles of ultrasound physics and the indications, advantages, limitations, performance, and interpretation of the ultrasound examinations" [2]. Further criteria of "personnel performing ultrasound (under the supervision of the surgeon) require they must be appropriately trained and certified and their performance regularly evaluated within the framework of the quality improvement process" [2].

Credentialing for ultrasound users can be obtained through independent bodies such as Cardiovascular Credentialing International (http://www.cci-online.org/) or the American Registry of Diagnostic Medical Sonographers (http://www.ardms.org/). The examination of Registered Phlebology Sonographer (RPhS) is directly linked to individuals performing phlebology diagnostic and therapeutic ultrasound and would be a worthwhile achievement. Local state and government regulations exist regarding not only the individuals performing diagnostic ultrasound but also the accreditation of the ultrasound facility. Many private insurers also restrict reimbursement for ultrasound usage based on a variety of factors. Overall these variable policies may directly impact those using ultrasound within a medical facility.

7.4 Instrumentation Settings

In many instances, phlebology treatments are performed within an ambulatory location. Most phlebology procedures utilize visualization with ultrasound which may include a means to obtain needle guidance for sclerotherapy, percutaneous access, regional anesthesia placement (tumescent), or device placement. To facilitate optimal visualization, the ultrasound equipment settings should be enhanced for the specific application of use. In contrast to diagnostic applications which require high dynamic ranges (decibel [dB]) to differentiate tissue characteristics, settings for highly reflective objects (needles, man-made objects) which have increased specular reflection are best identified with low dynamic ranges. Adjusting the depth specific to the shallow field of view will inherently enlarge the target. In addition, movement of the focal zone settings (when applicable) to a height in line with the target level will enhance visualization as well. Once settings have been established, a preset application can be configured and stored for the specific task of therapeutic guidance.

Successful ultrasound-guided needle placement relies on a combination of ultrasound principles, many centered on the design of a linear high-frequency transducer. To visualize objects, the transducer interface must have good contact with the skin with generous gel placement. Once a target is obtained, the transducer must be steadied and remain fixed in an absolute parallel position along the skin line, with care to avoid applying pressure onto the skin which may inadvertently compress the vein. Views in the long or short axis of the transducer can be selected though, and depending on the technical task, a specific view may have greater advantages. In addition, there are situations unique to each patient, including vein depth and vein wall characteristics, to which the specific technical applications will be modified based on skill and experience. These details will be discussed in further text.

7.5 Pre-procedural Mapping/Assessment

A pre-procedural therapeutic "mapping" in this chapter applies to a patient who has had a recent detailed duplex diagnostic examination, which excluded acute deep vein thrombosis. The prior mapping also determined the presence of superficial venous reflux or a grossly incompetent perforating vein. When performing a sonographic examination for pre-endovenous therapy planning, the individual gathering information must recognize what types of veins are amenable and/or ideal for correction/treatment of saphenous reflux. Of importance are the reflux point and variations of the saphenous vein within the saphenous sheath. Reflux is detected more frequently in the great saphenous vein (GSV) when compared to the small saphenous vein (SSV), though the prevalence of SSV reflux may be underestimated due to investigative technique [3, 4].

The variability of venous anatomy compounds the importance of an experienced sonographer, as there are other saphenous veins which may be selected for ablation as well if abnormalities were detected. In particular, when mapping the GSV, there are common patterns to anticipate. The GSV commonly will pierce (exit) the saphenous fascia into the superficial fascia in the mid-thigh, above the knee, or below the knee. It has been described within the International Union of Phlebology (UIP) Consensus Document on Anatomy as one of three anatomical patterns, and these include Type "I" pertaining to a GSV trunk with normal diameter throughout the length of the saphenous compartment without large parallel tributaries, Type "H" wherein the GSV trunk is present throughout the saphenous compartment with a parallel tributary that is greater in diameter than the GSV, or Type "S" in which the GSV leaves the saphenous fascia and (exits) pierces the superficial fascia and continues as the primary flow channel of the GSV (now in the superficial fascia), though a very small vein may be in the saphenous fascia (hypoplastic) or no vein will remain in the saphenous fascia (aplastic) [5].

In contrast to the GSV anatomy, the small saphenous vein (SSV) remains in its fascia boundary for its entire length from the lateral margin in the foot to the termination proximal. The complex anatomical variability of the termination of the SSV may create some technical challenges in mapping the SSV. According to the UIP Consensus Document on Anatomy, the SSV may terminate at the popliteal, the gastrocnemius, the distal femoral vein, or may have no termination. With no termination, the SSV will continue proximally as either a thigh extension or as the Giacomini vein [5]. Venous duplex hemodynamic detail will be useful information, particularly whether the Giacomini vein or thigh extension will be targeted for treatment. Often these vessels may transfer reflux from more proximal incompetent veins, such as the GSV, thigh perforators, or pelvic draining veins to the SSV. Sparing distal saphenous veins may be indicated, based on hemodynamic assessment. The SSV may also have duplications of various lengths within the compartment. In particular, the preoperative mapping of the SSV may include an evaluation to determine which comprehensive treatment strategy will be necessary to correct reflux patterns.

7.6 Thermal Ablation

Thermal ablation of the saphenous vein involves placing a device (catheter or fiber) within the lumen at the point of access and passing the device tip to a proximal location specific to treatment. With this in mind, the sonographer must take note of any vein segments which are tortuous or which may have valve sinus segments that may prevent or hinder passage of guide-wires or endovenous thermal devices. Skin burns during thermal ablation have been reported, and recommended vein distance from skin is at least 1.0 cm. A vein distance less than 1.0 cm should be noted so adequate anesthesia can be strategically applied within the tissue to create greater vein depth [6]. The access site selection will be influenced by the anatomic location of the saphenous trunk as the vein distance from the skin is an important constraint. Though access below the knee may be more desirable, if the GSV exits the saphenous fascia in the mid-thigh, the site selection is more or less predetermined by the patient's individual anatomy. In addition, when arterial structures are in anatomic close proximity to the selected vein segment, there may potentially be a complication risk for formation of arteriovenous fistula [7]. Thus, it would be prudent to avoid planning treatment to veins that are within these specific areas. A venous "pre-procedural mapping" should be completed with details such as the relative diameter measurements, the course of the saphenous vein segment to be treated, and other relevant details including vein depth and the precise intended proximal tip placement. Suffice it to say, this thorough survey is undertaken to streamline the procedure and anticipate details that may require innovative skills or techniques during the procedure.

The pre-procedural sonographic mapping will expose other particulars about the saphenous vein and may include aspects of the wall thickness. When patients have had previous thrombosis or sclerotherapy, the vein wall may appear thickened, which may hamper needle access. With these details, a micro-insertion needle will be beneficial to penetrate the aberrant vein wall. Pre-procedural mapping may also discern evidence for a large perforating vein forming a direct link from the saphenous vein to the deep venous system. This detail is critical as passage of a thermal device from the saphenous vein may inadvertently route into the deep system via the perforating vein. Curtailing this mishap can be aided by the pre-procedural mapping to avoid the perforator as the device nears this dangerous detour. Some facilities will utilize a protocol for skin markings with indelible ink drawn along the course of the vein as the predetermined "mapping" of the vein to be treated. The skin markings/mapping may be helpful to expedite vein location during the interventional process.

When a mapping is performed to plan treatment of an incompetent perforating vein, a diagnostic assessment of the perforating vein may be required to assure the precise treatment location has been selected. Perforating veins are typically measured by their distance from the patient's heel.

7.7 Chemical Ablation

Chemical ablation procedures are often referred to as ultrasound-guided injection sclerotherapy. This method was first published in 1989 but gained greater acceptance in 1995 when first presented by Juan Cabrera, MD [8]. The use of foam sclerotherapy, which is injections into abnormal veins under ultrasound guidance, has gradually gained acceptance by many phlebologists [9]. The foam is created by "Tessari's" method, mixing one part sclerosant liquid and four parts gas, which produces a stable foam consistency.

The use of ultrasound-guided sclerotherapy (UGS) has many practical considerations. The application of ultrasound visualization during UGS (chemical ablation) ensures accurate guidance and placement of the catheter or direct needle punctures into the vein, absolute avoidance of catastrophic intra-arterial injections, and control of the foam distribution within the vein to modify or adapt the volume being injected. With skill and expertise, foam sclerotherapy can successfully ablate saphenous truncal and non-truncal reflux. The primary use for ultrasound-guided injection is the precise placement of sclerosant into the abnormal vein and observation of the high contrast foamed sclerosant. Veins that are resistant to treatment, or previously injected, can be re-treated with foam sclerotherapy injections.

Foamed sclerosant can easily be visualized as hyperechoic bubbles present in the target vein (Fig. 7.1). Successful foam placement is typically followed by venous spasm. Foam injection is therefore typically halted well before the deep system (i.e., some use 5 cm distal in the case of the saphenofemoral junction), since the foam can progress proximally during venous spasm. Calf muscle contractions to dilute any significant amount of foam seen in the deep venous system can be effected to minimize deep vein adverse events. Any extravasation outside the vein can also be seen and the injection halted. Chapter 11 details further particulars of sclerotherapy.

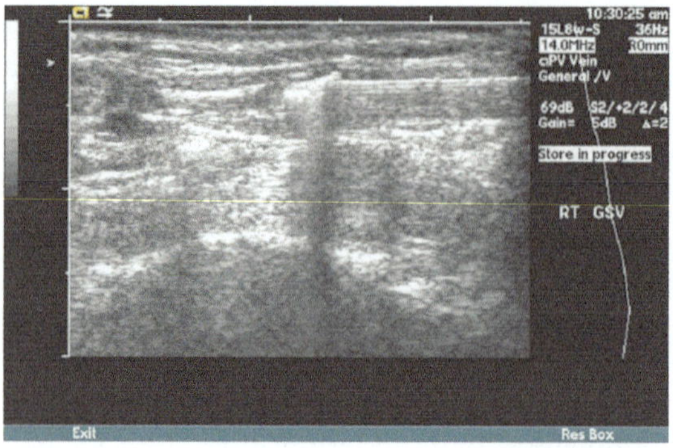

Fig. 7.1 Foamed sclerosant can be seen as hyperechoic bubbles present in the target vein

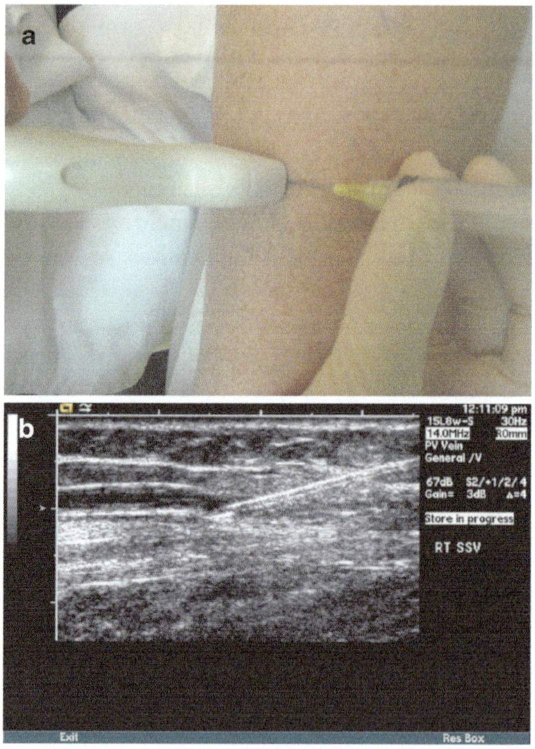

Fig. 7.2 A long-axis ultrasound view allows needle visualization where the needle goes through the skin (**a**, *above*) to the target vein (**b**, *below*)

There are advantages to using a transverse target position for needle access along the long axis of the transducer. The long axis provides for needle identification from the onset of needle introduction into the skin with guidance directly to the target (Fig. 7.2a, b). Manipulation of the image target close to the transducer edge is

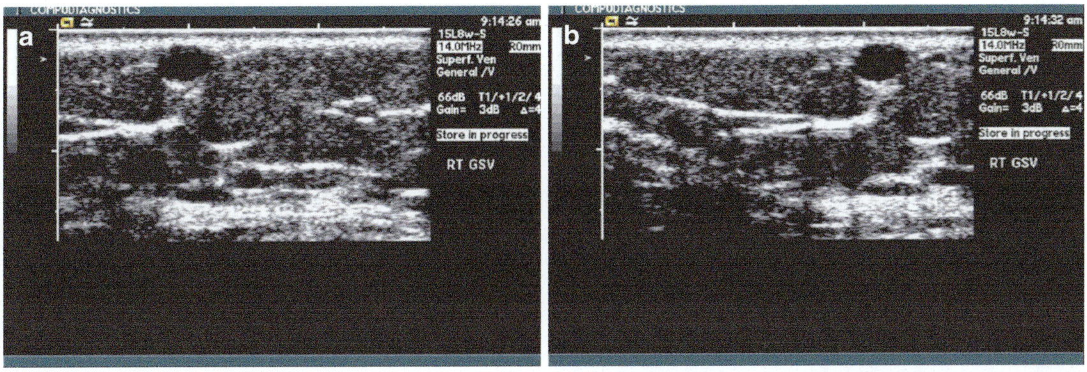

Fig. 7.3 (**a**) Transverse grey-scale image of target vein 2 cm from the needle. (**b**) Manipulating the transducer medial will reduce the target distance to 1 cm

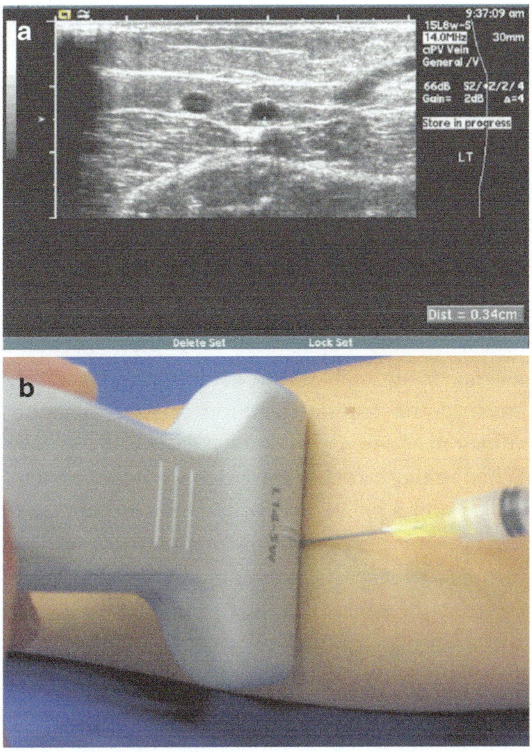

Fig. 7.4 The transverse image of the target vein is placed at the center of the ultrasound screen (**a**, *above*) and the needle is introduced in direct line with the target (**b**, *below*)

helpful, as the distance for the needle to travel through tissue is minimized (Fig. 7.3). For optimal visualization, the needle must be kept in the absolute center of the ultrasound transducer beam. The short axis is preferred by some sonologists based on previous training and experience. A transverse target is selected and is positioned into the center of the screen's image (Fig. 7.4a). Needle access along the center of the transducer is obtained in direct line with the target below (Fig. 7.4b). The disadvantage to this method is non-visualization of the needle tip until it reaches the target.

7.8 Venous Access Principles

The critical role of ultrasound for a preoperative mapping of the saphenous vein to be ablated includes the determination of an access site. The access site selection is not random, but rather it is based on knowledge of multiple extenuating factors. Consideration for the site insertion should favor proper ergonomics, as the technique for access may be a time commitment. It will be helpful to know exactly how the patient will be positioned and plan accordingly with aids available to overcome details such as body habitus or back comfort issues that may arise. The selection process favors a vein at an area closer to the skin, as the technical aspect of venipuncture is less challenging in the near field when compared to a steep angle (Fig. 7.5a, b). Vein diameter must be suitable for successful vein cannulation, as smaller caliber veins (<2 mm) pose the need for greater technical skill. Successful vein access can also be hampered by vasospasm related to a patient's cool body temperature. A warming blanket and a heating pad are useful aids to encourage vasodilatation. Imposed gravity and tourniquets are useful strategies to increase vein diameter.

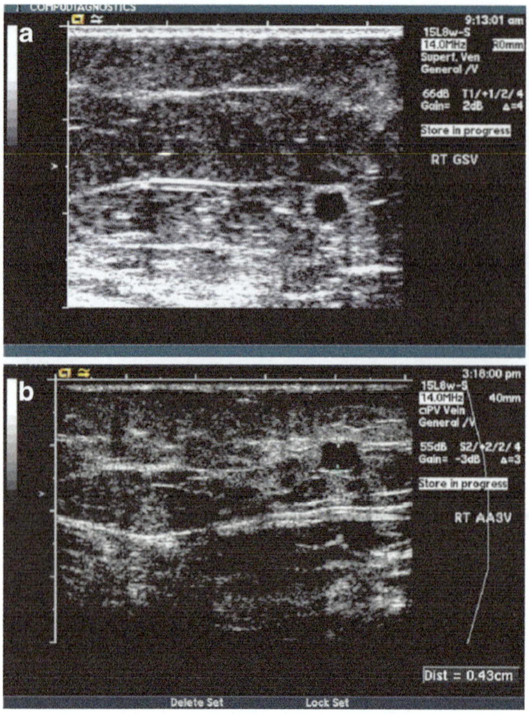

Fig. 7.5 More superficial veins (**b**, *below*) are easier to access than deeper veins (**a**, *above*)

When feasible, keeping the patient sitting upright may also maximize vein caliber, encouraging dilatation. Local application of 2 % nitroglycerin ointment on the intended access skin site (refer to package guidelines insert for use and/or contraindications of product) has been reported to increase vein diameter and reduce vasospasm. Application has been reported to increase vein diameter as much as 69 % [10].

The access site presumes the vein proximally is fully patent and free from vein kinking or obstructions to permit the passage of a thermal device. Hematoma and excessive bleeding may be minimized by avoiding vein access in regions drained by large perforating veins. Large diameter veins, particularly in the upper thigh, are influenced greatly by the patient's leg position. Repositioning the patient's leg may decrease any vein kinking or stretching that may thwart device passage.

The access site designated is also affected by other considerations in the case of thermal ablation. Endovenous catheters and fibers vary in length, thus care must be taken during planning

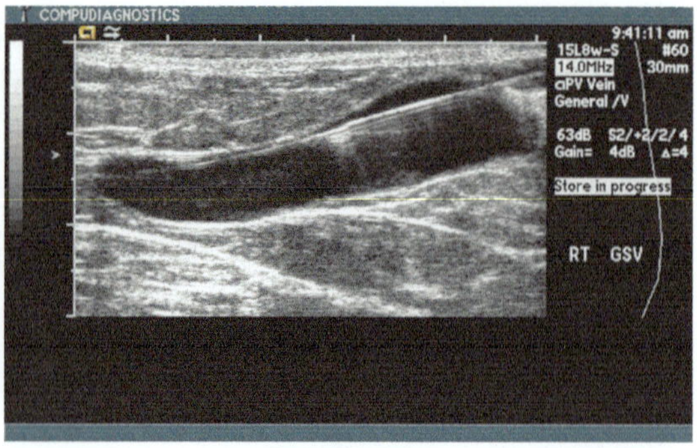

Fig. 7.6 Access to the saphenous vein can be routed

so the type of thermal device used will be generous enough to adequately cover the span of the mapped vein distance. The manufacturers of thermal devices have guidelines for the upper and lower limits of vein diameters as well, thus the ultrasound technologist must be cognizant of these specific recommendations during the mapping for treatment.

Every patient will be unique as to the treatment vein length and access site chosen. However, since the thermal device is controlled by the user, access to the saphenous vein can, in some instances, alternatively be routed via a large tributary in the parallel position to the saphenous vein or in a region not conducive to heat (Fig. 7.6). When in these zones, the thermal device can simply be non-activated to avoid untoward effects to the skin or nerves. Ultrasound is an excellent resource to visualize structures other than veins. Based on its anatomical proximity, the saphenous nerve for the below-knee GSV and the sural nerve (SN) for the SSV are at greatest risk for injury during intervention in the distal calf. Sural and saphenous nerve injury may be reduced by ultrasound visualization to avoid this proximity during intervention (see further text under post-procedural complications).

7.9 Venous Access with Seldinger Technique

Once a suitable vein access site is chosen, the patient's lower extremity undergoes a sterile prep and drape according to the physician's routine. After an application of adequate gel is placed

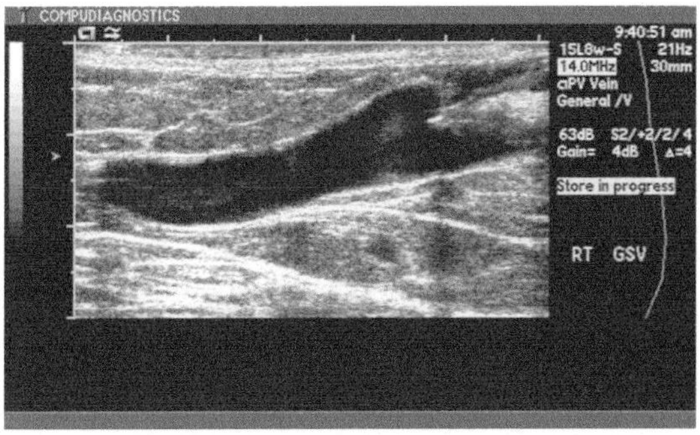

Fig. 7.7 Vein "tenting," with a needle pushing the superior vein inferiorly, is visible at the right side of the image

onto the ultrasound transducer interface, a sterile sleeve is positioned over the surface so the transducer can be used freely during the procedure. Care is taken to reduce air trappings within the sleeve, which can introduce ultrasound artifact and hamper visualization.

Percutaneous vein access is achieved with sonographic guidance. The technique for access can be with the ultrasound transducer positioned in a longitudinal or a transverse view, and skill for either method for access improves with repetition. It is imperative the transducer be maintained in an absolute parallel position on the skin. Manipulation of a needle in three dimensions is often easier to facilitate with a longitudinal view, particularly for the access, wire, and sheath placement. Visualization of the needle tip is imperative to insure a precise puncture into the vein. Soft tissue motion is not a reliable method and, simply stated, is a blind technique. Instead, rely on the real-time ultrasound visualization to successfully guide the needle to the target. Fix attention to identification of the tip of the needle and less emphasis on the length of the needle. Needle enhancement is optimized with high contrast ultrasound settings (i.e., decreased dynamic range [dB]). When the needle is placed along the long axis of the transducer (longitudinal view), needle identification is achieved from the onset of needle introduction into the skin. As the needle tip is advanced through the soft tissue toward the anterior wall of the target vein, "tent" the wall to ensure the needle and ultrasound image are within the same plane (Fig. 7.7). Successful vein penetration is achieved with slight pressure of the needle. For optimal visualization, the needle must be kept in the absolute center of the ultrasound transducer beam.

The short axis approach is preferred by some sonologists based on previous training and experience. A transverse (short axis) target is selected and is positioned into the center of the screen's image. Needle access along the center of the transducer is obtained in direct line with the target below. The disadvantage to this method is non-visualization of the needle tip until it reaches the target. Once the tip is visualized, "tent" the anterior wall for vein puncture and proceed through the vein walls. With either method of access into the vein, brisk back bleeding may not be readily observed because of low pressure. Once vein entry (access) is obtained under ultrasound guidance, a guide-wire is placed. A tapered vessel combination introducer/dilator is threaded over the guide-wire.

7.9.1 Thermal Tip Placement

The thermal device is threaded through the sheath and is positioned in the saphenous vein. The use of real-time ultrasound imaging aids in accurate placement of the thermal tip. Artifacts, such as trapped air bubbles, can often hinder optimal visualization of the thermal tip. Manipulation with forward and backward movement of thermal tip may help to validate accurate position with certainty. Views in multiple ultrasound planes are encouraged. Passage of the thermal device can be hampered by tortuous venous pathways, venous valve leaflets, and webbing. Repositioning the patient's lower extremity or manipulation of the device with skin pressure are both effective, in most instances, to permit passage proximally. Verify with ultrasound in transverse views to confirm the device is within the vein's lumen. Painful passage of the device through the vein may indicate the device has penetrated the wall and is extravascular or has detoured via a perforating vein.

Placement of the thermal tip may be somewhat subjective and is influenced according to which saphenous vein is being treated and at the juncture of the reflux point. The type of thermal device being utilized may also influence the

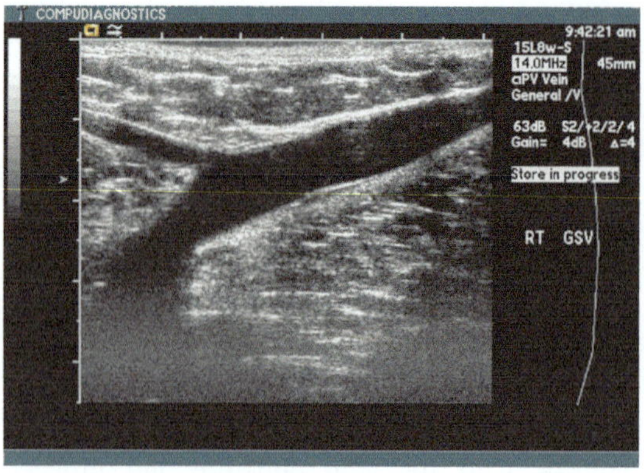

Fig. 7.8 The superior epigastric vein in this image is the smaller diameter vein moving diagonally to the left and up from the larger great saphenous vein

placement distance used, as there are relative heat transfer differences between optically generated laser energy and radiofrequency energy. Both thermal devices share the same goal of treatment: to deliver sufficient thermal energy to the vein wall to produce permanent occlusion, fibrosis, and eventual sonographic disappearance of the vein.

An important thermal positioning landmark for the GSV is the superficial epigastric vein (SEV) (Fig. 7.8). Placement of the thermal tip *inferior* to the SEV and approximately 2 cm from the common femoral vein (CFV) is recommended by many device manufacturers. Preserving flow from the SEV allows for pelvic drainage and may discourage coagulation propagation from the GSV into the CFV. Strategies for thermal tip placement of other saphenous veins in the thigh, such as the anterior accessory great saphenous vein, will vary depending on the patient's anatomy and the reflux point. Vein caliber, skin distance, and reflux lengths will warrant individualized treatment strategies.

As previously discussed, the complex variations of the termination of the SSV may create some technical challenges in thermal tip placement. The variants in termination may present some ambiguity in relation to the precise ultrasound-directed thermal tip strategy. Ultimately, the curvature of the termination entry and reflux point will serve as the ultrasound landmark for tip placement. In all cases, the thermal tip must be clearly visible and free of deep venous contact.

7.9.2 Tumescent Anesthesia

Once the thermal tip is placed and the landmark for accurate recognition is established, the application of anesthetic fluid is accomplished with ultrasound guidance. The technique relies on fluid hydrodissection and separation of the perivenous plane, which enables anesthesia tissue infiltration in a targeted manner. Once the anesthesia is sufficiently placed, the fluid also facilitates extrinsic compression (exsanguination) of the vein wall to reduce the size of the vessel. The fluid also creates a heat sink to absorb the temperature increase created by the thermal device.

The chief benefit of ultrasound real-time visualization is the directed needle placement for precise regional anesthesia application. However, there are several technical challenges when using ultrasound during this step of the procedure, including the inherent nature of fluid movement and application. This dynamic process introduces ultrasound imaging artifacts which may hinder optimal visualization of the needle and the thermal device. Air bubbles mixed within the anesthetic fluid, though benign in the soft tissue, wreak havoc on ultrasound beams. Take care to minimize any air bubbles in the application of the anesthesia which may have mixed with the fluid during anesthesia within the IV tubing. Because of ultrasound artifact considerations, one can understand why the thermal tip is positioned prior to administering the tumescent anesthesia. Use of a lower-frequency transducer or increased power settings may help to overcome artifact obstacles.

Transverse or longitudinal ultrasound views may be used to place tumescent anesthesia depending on provider preference. Using both views (i.e., longitudinal moving up the extremity, and transverse back down to double-check the extremity) will be of double benefit. Circumferential placement of the tumescent fluid is best confirmed in transverse orientation (Fig. 7.9).

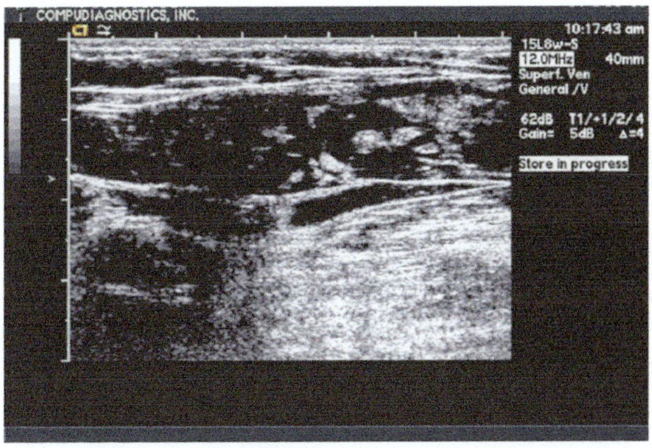

Fig. 7.9 Tumescent fluid (hypoechoic), seen here in transverse view, is circumferential around the bright (hyperechoic) thermal ablation device

The thermal ablation is completed once the device has been successfully pulled back at the appropriate speed and removed from inside the vein. The benefit of skilled direct visualization during treatment to reduce risks and complications cannot be overstated.

7.9.3 Post-procedural Follow-up

Completion of ultrasonography documents patency of the deep venous system and efficacy of superficial venous ablation. While it is completely gratifying to obtain treatment success, some patients do encounter treatment failure. Additionally, there are reported complications following venous procedures, including deep vein thrombosis and superficial thrombophlebitis [11]. Early intervention is critical and begins with identification, which may require new or additional therapy. Interval follow-up will reassure the patient and monitor timely progress. The frequency of vein recurrence is due to several factors of the disease, thus ultrasound surveillance after treatment is warranted and suggested. The ultrasound examiner should possess a comprehensive knowledge of potential complications and expected outcomes. Gradual shrinkage of the treated veins over a course of 6–9 months will result in their eventual disappearance from ultrasonic detection.

Duplications of the deep venous system are common, including the femoral vein of the thigh, popliteal, and calf veins. The significance of these duplications includes possible missed deep vein thrombosis (DVT) on examination, especially post-sclerotherapy follow-up. Unique flow patterns may potentiate thrombus in one or more of duplicated vessels.

7.9.4 PASTE (Post Ablation Superficial Thrombus Extension)

Though care is given to thermal tip placement, thrombus extension/propagation can be a complication of treatment (Fig. 7.10a, b) [12]. The extent of the thrombus into the deep venous system is monitored by careful follow-up with ultrasound. The timing of ultrasound follow-up in the posttreatment period is controversial, but this author recommends 3–7 days. Ultrasound following treatment may reveal the presence of hyperechogenicity resembling organizing thrombus. The thrombus extends beyond the border of treatment from the saphenous vein. Patients presenting with these findings are typically asymptomatic (see Chap. 18 for further discussion).

7.9.5 Nerve Injury

Reported adverse events following thermal ablation of the SSV suggest a higher rate of nerve injuries, although arguably there is less data regarding SSV treatment compared to the GSV. Based on its anatomical proximity to the SSV, the SN is at greatest risk for injury during intervention in the distal calf [12]. Paresthesia and dysesthesia, though usually transient, are the manifestations of damage to the SN. The SN is a sensory nerve and supplies the skin of the posterolateral aspect of the distal calf, lateral malleolus, lateral foot, and toe. Motor fibers and unmyelinated autonomic fibers have been discovered within the SN up to 4.5 % [13]. Based on this evidence, care must be taken to avoid SN complications.

Ultrasound is an excellent resource to visualize structures other than veins. Ultrasound images are not selective. In other words, imaging from

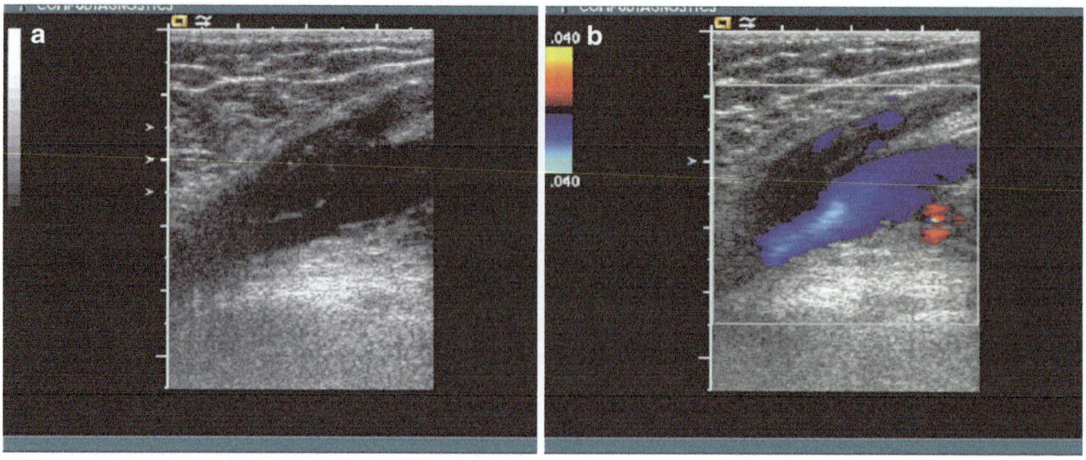

Fig. 7.10 Thrombus extension after vein ablation is seen in *gray scale* (**a**) and Doppler (**b**) is the area without *blue flow*

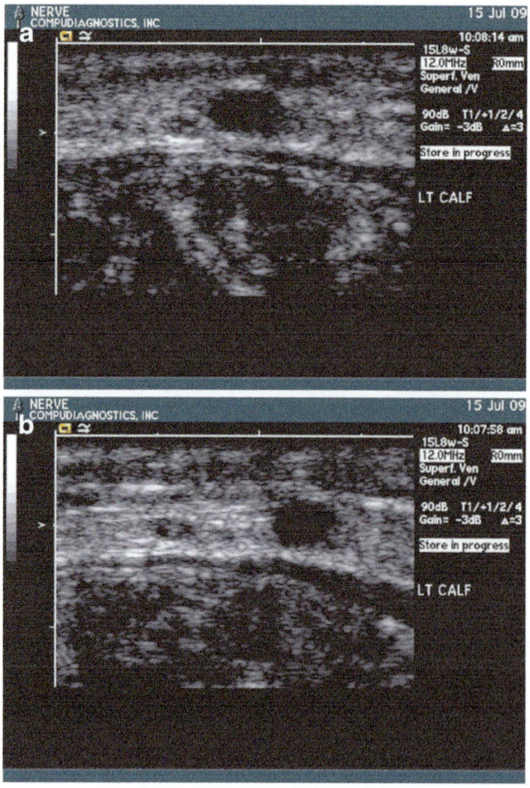

Fig. 7.11 The small saphenous vein (hypoechoic) is visible at the proximal calf (**a**, *above*), and the sural nerve is visible close to the left of small saphenous vein at the distal calf (**b**, *below*)

the skin line demonstrates subcutaneous fat, muscle, tendons, arteries, veins, nerves, joint space, periarticular bursae, and bone. Identification of the SN by ultrasound may allow one to safely gain vein access for phlebology treatments.

Though variation exists, the SN is best visualized in the distal calf/ankle region. A high-frequency linear transducer is used to identify the SSV in transverse orientation. Immediately adjacent to the SSV is the SN, a round structure with mixed internal hypoechogenic characteristics. Movement of the transducer along the skin line will demonstrate the variable proximity of the SN to the SSV (Fig. 7.11a, b). Identification of the SN in the mid- to lower calf may assist in determining the most advantageous point for percutaneous venous access. With ultrasound detection, the area in which the SN is closest to the SSV should be avoided.

Dr. Stefano Ricci of Rome, Italy, was among the first to describe the ultrasound anatomic features of the nerve structures in the popliteal fossa, including the sciatic, peroneal, and tibial nerves [13, 14]. Dr. Ricci's profound description of the sciatic nerve is "always visible, never seen" and serves as a reminder to phlebologists to expand their use of ultrasound to include the identification of nerves. Awareness of the visualization techniques to identify nerves, their location, and proximity to the vein to be treated may reduce the risk of nerve injury [14]. This information may be considered in planning treatment for patients who undergo venous procedures, including endovenous thermal ablation and ultrasound-guided sclerotherapy.

7.10 Summary

Ultrasound-directed minimally invasive procedures have become the cornerstone for the venous practitioners. A successful approach to treating patients with venous disease includes the use of duplex ultrasound and careful evaluation pre-, peri-, and post-treatment. Critically important factors in venous assessment are the quality of the ultrasound imaging prior to device utilized and the qualifications of the sonographic examiner. In the future, it is likely that the new generations of venous surgeons/phlebologists/sonographers will need to be proficient at numerous venous treatments as well as clinical sonography. Clinical sonography will be tailored to the individual patient and vital to the treatment process. Accordingly, ultrasound training expertise must be expanded to include the applied skills for pre-, peri-, and post-phlebologic treatments.

References

1. ACR–SPR–SRU Practice Guideline for Performing and Interpreting Diagnostic Ultrasound Examinations, Resolution 7, Revised 2011. http://www.acr.org/Quality-Safety/Standards-Guidelines/Practice-Guidelines-by-Modality/Ultrasound. Last accessed 28 Nov 2013.
2. Surgical Technology – 31, Ultrasound Examinations by Surgeons. Bulletin of the American College of Surgeons, vol.83, no. 06, 1998.
3. Engelhorn CA, Engelhorn AL, Cassou MF, Salles-Cunha SX. Patterns of saphenous reflux in women with primary varicose veins. J Vasc Surg. 2005; 41:645–51.
4. Neuhardt DL, Salles-Cunha SX, Morrison N. Prevalence and patterns of small saphenous vein reflux. J Vasc Ultrasound. 2009;33:19–22.
5. Cavezzi A, Labropoulos N, Partsch H, Caggiati A, Myers K, Nicolaides A, Smith PC. Duplex ultrasound investigation of the veins in chronic venous disease of the lower limbs – UIP consensus document part II. Anatomy. Eur J Vasc Endovasc Surg. 2006; 31:288–99.
6. Kundu S, Luri F, Millward S, Padberg F, Vedantham S, Elias S, Khilnani N, Marston W, Cardella J, Meissner M, Dalsing M, Clark T, Min Robert J. Recommended reporting standards for endovenous ablation for the treatment of venous insufficiency: joint statement of the American Venous Forum and the Society of Interventional Radiology. J Vasc Surg. 2007;46:582–9.
7. Vaz C, Matos A, Oliveira J, Nogueira C, Almeida R, Mendonca M. Iatrogenic arteriovenous fistula following endovenous laser therapy of the short saphenous vein. Ann Vasc Surg. 2009;23(3):412.
8. Knight RM, Vin F, Zygmunt JA. Ultrasonic guidance of injections into the superficial venous System. In: Davy A, Stemmer R, editors. Phlebolgie 89. Paris: John Libby Eurotext; 1989. p. 339–41.
9. Cavezzi A, Tessari L. Foam sclerotherapy techniques: different gases and methods of preparation, catheter versus direct injection. Phlebology. 2009;24:247–51.
10. Hogue RS, Schul MW, Dando CF, Erdman BE. The effect of nitroglycerin ointment on great saphenous vein targeted venous access site diameter with endovenous laser treatment. Phlebology. 2008;23:222–6.
11. Merchant RF, Pichot O, Closure Study Group. Long-term outcomes of endovenous radiofrequency obliteration of saphenous reflux as a treatment of superficial venous insufficiency. J Vasc Surg. 2005;42:402–509.
12. Wright D, Morrison N, Recek C, Passariello F. Post Ablation Superficial Thrombus Extension (PASTE) into the common femoral vein as a consequence of endovenous ablation of the great saphenous vein. Acta Phlebol. 2010;11:59–64.
13. Sankar D, Bhanu P, et al. Variant formation of sural nerve and its distribution at the dorsum of the foot. Int J Anat Var. 2009;1:33–4.
14. Ricci S. Ultrasound observation of the sciatic nerve and its branches at the popliteal fossa: always visible, never seen. Eur J Vasc Endovasc Surg. 2005; 30:659–63.

Physiologic Testing

8

Julianne Stoughton

Contents

J. Stoughton, MD, FACS
Department of Vascular Surgery,
Massachusetts General Hospital, Boston, MA, USA
e-mail: jstoughton@partners.org

Abstract

Noninvasive physiologic testing is often underutilized and should be recognized as being complementary to duplex scanning in a variety of clinical scenarios. The duplex scan can give important anatomic information, but the measurement of the severity of hemodynamic reflux or obstruction cannot be quantified. Plethysmography allows for an objective analysis of treatment outcome, objective assessment of individual's progress over time, prediction of successful outcomes, evaluation of the role of collaterals before treatments, functional evaluation of calf muscle pump, measurement of effectiveness of compression therapy, and better noninvasive assessment of proximal obstruction. This chapter discusses several physiologic tests for venous disease.

8.1 Introduction

Physiologic testing has been available for many years, yet its clinical application has been underutilized. Venous duplex evaluation has become the standard of care to evaluate the venous anatomy for conditions such as deep venous thrombosis, yet there are still many situations where additional information is helpful in the management of patients with venous disease. Plethysmography measures the volume changes of the leg while in various positions and while performing certain maneuvers. The testing reveals information

E. Mowatt-Larssen et al. (eds.), *Phlebology, Vein Surgery and Ultrasonography*,
DOI 10.1007/978-3-319-01812-6_8, © Springer International Publishing Switzerland 2014

about the patient's physiologic condition. When combined with ultrasound evaluation, this can be an important clinical tool, especially in those cases of advanced disease or complicated clinical situations. In addition to allowing a quantitative assessment of reflux (in the deep and superficial system), this technology is superior to duplex testing in evaluating for proximal obstruction, evaluating calf muscle pump function, and assessing the importance of venous collaterals prior to superficial ablative treatments. Plethysmography can also predict the long-term prognosis, and the patient's clinical status can be accurately and objectively followed over time. The data from venous duplex and plethysmography is complementary, and this combination is a more complete evaluation as our understanding of venous disease continues to progress [1–5].

8.2 Anatomy

Plethysmography (or measurement of volume change) is considered to be an accurate assessment of total venous volume in the limb, as the volume of the arterial inflow is generally considered to be nearly constant. The lower extremity venous system consists of the deep veins draining the muscle compartments, the superficial veins draining the skin and subcutaneous tissue outside the muscular fascia, and the perforator veins which connect the two systems.

In the upright position, as the venous blood returns to the heart against gravity, the muscle pump is essential to propel the blood upward toward the heart. The one-way valves within the deep, superficial, and perforator veins keep flow in an inward and cephalad direction. Above the inguinal ligament there are pelvic veins which drain the abdominal and pelvic organs which continue to drain toward the inferior vena cava and finally drain into the right atrium of the heart.

8.3 Types of Plethysmography

Historically, several different instruments were developed to indirectly measure the changes in the venous volume of the limb.

Impedance plethysmography (IPG) measures skin impedance, which indirectly correlates to measurement of volume. This technology is not often used due to the fact that measurement of impedance in the skin is affected by other factors such as electrolyte concentration and hematocrit. Photoelectric plethysmography (PPG) has been used somewhat in clinical practice; however, this test provides only a qualitative assessment of blood volume. This PPG technology utilizes photo-sensors and an infrared light-emitting diode applied to the skin. Blood volume in the leg can be related to the intensity of the reflected light in the underlying tissue, but this technology is limited to assessment of the cutaneous layer, which can be inaccurate. This technology can be used to measure the arterial or venous changes in the limb and is still commonly used for measurements of arterial toe pressures (see later ABI discussion). A more direct measure of venous volume consists of a strain-gauge plethysmography (SGP) which consists of a band wrapped around the limb. The amount of stretch in the circumferential band can be converted by calibration into volume measurements. This technology is limited by measurement errors due to variable positioning of the device on the limb and from changes in temperature [1–3].

The most widely used form of plethysmography in clinical practice is air plethysmography (APG) which utilizes a large inflated cuff around the entire lower leg and directly measures changes in volume. This measures a larger area and can be directly calibrated to assess the blood volume over the entire length of the calf.

8.4 Physiologic Principles

The function of the venous system is to store and transport blood (mostly against gravity) toward the heart. As the collapsible veins are filled, they are very distensible. The pressure in nearly empty veins is quite low, but as the veins become more distended, the pressure becomes greater per unit of volume. Venous flow depends upon an adequate muscular contracture and a series of competent valves, as well as a small pressure gradient to help overcome gravity. Respiratory variations influence the venous flow while supine, but these changes are not significant while in the upright position. The competent valves prevent retrograde flow by dividing the hydrostatic column of blood into compartments. The most accurate measure of venous insufficiency is an assessment of ambulatory venous pressure (AVP), which is an invasive measure of pressure taken in a dorsal foot vein. Because venous pressure correlates fairly well with volume changes, the less invasive measure of volume change with plethysmography has been used to help quantify the degree of venous insufficiency.

Although duplex scanning can assess the anatomic locations of refluxing segments, it is impossible to quantify the global amount of reflux in a limb. Plethysmography measures the rate of venous refilling when the patient stands up. Total venous volume (VV) is assessed after a plateau is reached, and the time to reach 90 % of total volume is assessed. These measures meet at a point where the veins have filled to 90 % providing a venous filling index (VFI) measured in mL/s. Normal limbs with competent valves have very slow venous refilling and thus a lower venous filling index (usually <2 mL/s). By contrast, if there is a significant amount of reflux in the limb, the VFI is higher (i.e., 20 mL/s) [2].

Muscular contraction is essential for propelling the blood upward, and this ejection fraction (EF) can be quantified as the amount of blood removed with a single muscle pump (ejection volume [EV]) divided by the total VV). After multiple muscular contractions are done in rapid succession, the venous system is considered as empty as possible. The volume remaining in the leg is called the residual volume (RV). The residual volume fraction (RVF) is the RV divided by the VV, and this correlates well with measurements of ambulatory venous pressure (AVP) [1].

In addition, venous outflow from the leg can be quantified using plethysmography by inflating a tourniquet proximally. The VV builds as the arterial inflow continues to enter the leg until the venous pressure equals that of the tourniquet. Once this pressure is reached, the tourniquet can be released and the VV in the calf should rapidly diminish due to the pressure gradient. If there is proximal obstruction, the outflow fraction (OF) of the leg is reduced. OF is calculated by assessing the volume of blood ejected from the leg in the first second after the tourniquet is removed (V1), divided by the total venous capacity (VC) of the leg. Maneuvers can also be performed by compressing the proximal great saphenous vein (GSV) prior to removal of the tourniquet. This maneuver eliminates the GSV from the available outflow veins: thus, one can calculate the amount of outflow that goes through the deep system separately. The superficial system should carry no more than 10 % of the venous outflow from the leg. If the superficial veins contribute more than 10 % to the outflow of the leg, they should not be ablated in the patient with deep venous obstruction as they are most likely important sources of venous collaterals.

Proximal venous obstruction can be *quantitatively* evaluated using this form of physiologic testing. Each patient should be evaluated bilaterally for venous outflow obstruction prior to reflux testing in order to prevent changes due to reactive hyperemia. In centers where venous duplex evaluation is unavailable, the 1 s venous outflow measure may be a reasonable screening alternative for symptomatic patients.

8.5 Techniques of Outflow Testing

VO is evaluated with the patient in the supine position with the knee slightly flexed and leg elevated. The APG cuff is applied to the calf, inflated to a baseline of 6 mmHg, and calibrated. A thigh tourniquet/cuff is applied above this, yet not inflated. Baseline evaluation is performed prior to inflation of the thigh tourniquet, and then the thigh cuff is inflated to 70 mmHg and maintained as the venous pressure in the calf rises. Once the calf vein pressure reaches the 70 mmHg pressure in the tourniquet, the curve reaches a plateau which is designated as the venous capacitance (VC). The proximal GSV can be compressed manually by applying pressure at the saphenofemoral junction prior to deflation of the thigh cuff. Following rapid deflation of the thigh cuff, the venous emptying begins which is measured by the APG cuff on the calf. Rapid emptying implies an open proximal venous system, whereas a slower outflow curve implies proximal obstruction. After 1 s of venous emptying, the change in venous volume (V1) is calculated. VO fraction is calculated by dividing the V1 by the VC. The test is usually repeated with and without GSV compression in order to assess the outflow contributions of the superficial and deep system. Normal outflow fraction at 1 s should be over 35 % with the superficial vein compressed and over 40 % in normal legs without superficial vein compression. In patients with deep venous obstruction, this can be a critical objective method to evaluate the importance of superficial venous collaterals to the outflow of the leg prior to making any decisions on venous ablation therapy [3–5].

8.6 Assessing Proximal Conditions Indirectly by Doppler

Normally, there is a combination of pulsatile and respirophasic flow patterns noted within the proximal veins of the lower extremity. Some pathologic conditions such as pulmonary hypertension, right heart failure, and tricuspid or pulmonary valve dysfunction can alter the pulsatility of the vein. Proximal venous obstruction can lead to a decrease in respirophasicity as noted by duplex. Flow pattern evaluation by Doppler must be evaluated and compared bilaterally in order to pick up subtle changes. Asymmetric flow patterns at the common femoral vein level should be investigated further, yet the absence of change does not entirely rule out obstruction. Combining data from duplex findings and bilateral plethysmographic assessment of VO can help detect clinically significant proximal venous obstruction.

8.7 Techniques of Reflux Testing

The principles of reflux testing can be applied to all types of plethysmography, yet this discussion will concentrate on the APG. The exam begins with the patient in the supine position with the leg elevated in order to obtain a baseline volume without any venous filling. A calibration is performed once prior to the exam by injecting a known quantity of air into the bladder/cuff in order to make direct measurements of volume changes during the exam. Once the baseline (empty) volume is assessed with the leg elevated, the patient is asked to stand up without putting any weight on the leg being tested. This maneuver allows the veins to fill by gravity without any muscular contraction. The curve will show a rise in volume in the calf which can demonstrate the degree of thigh-to-calf reflux in the leg. If a tourniquet is applied above the knee, the test will demonstrate the amount of reflux within the deep system only. Without a tourniquet, this will show the combination of deep and superficial vein reflux within the leg. The slope of the venous filling curve demonstrates the degree of reflux, and parameters, such as the VFI, are measured as the average filling rate at a point where 90 % of the filling has been achieved. The VV is the total volume achieved after complete filling in the standing position. Normal veins should fill more slowly (<2 mL/s), whereas legs with incompetent veins will fill more rapidly due the reflux in the deep and/or superficial systems.

With the venous volume maximally full in the dependent position with the muscles relaxed, the patient is asked to stand on the leg and perform a single "toe-up" maneuver in order to empty the calf veins. The EV is the amount of volume ejected from the calf during the single calf pump. As discussed previously, the amount of EV divided by the total VV in the leg is the EF.

Normal individuals are able to eject at least 60 % or greater with a calf muscle pump contraction, whereas patients with poor calf emptying are found to empty less than 40 %. Patients with orthopedic issues including arthritis, neurologic deficits, or other nonvascular problems which limit muscular contracture show poor EF. If the patient has large calf varicosities which are not emptied with muscular contracture, or large incompetent perforator veins, they may also exhibit poor emptying with calf contracture. Finally, if there is severe proximal venous obstruction, there may be slower venous emptying, therefore making the EF lower than expected.

The next step in reflux examinations includes repetitive calf pump contractions, having the patient perform 10 successive toe-up maneuvers. This will show slightly more emptying than the single EV, and the volume at the end of the last muscular contraction is termed the residual volume (RV). This volume is compared with the total VV and expressed as the residual volume fraction (RVF). The leg is kept in the dependent position, non-weight bearing, until it has refilled to the original VV. Finally, the patient is placed back into the supine position to empty the veins back to the original baseline.

8.8 Indications/Roles for APG

When performing superficial venous surgery, the reduction in ambulatory venous hypertension can be significant. The postoperative effect can be symptomatic relief and ulcer healing. Plethysmography has been used prior to and after superficial venous interventions to demonstrate physiologic success [1]. Although most achieved improvement in physiologic measures, some did not become normalized even after intervention. Patients with residual deep venous reflux, deep venous obstruction, or persistent incompetent perforators are less likely to show complete correction in venous function following superficial surgery. When a patient's postoperative venous function has not fully normalized, additional procedures might be recommended. Failure to normalize VFI has been found to result in more rapid recurrence. Plethysmographic assessment might help to improve outcomes and help to guide a more aggressive approach in patients who have a higher risk of recurrent disease.

Following correction of reflux, the APG testing usually shows improvement in all measures except for the calf muscle pump, which is unchanged. APG testing can also assess the effect of compression therapy and help guide management to improve outcomes.

It is hard to predict outcomes for patients with advanced venous disease who have duplex findings of partial deep venous obstruction and superficial venous reflux. These patients should undergo physiologic testing prior to making decisions about prognosis of surgical intervention.

8.9 Summary of Venous Physiologic Testing

Noninvasive physiologic testing is often underutilized and should be recognized as being complementary to duplex scanning in a variety of clinical scenarios. The duplex scan can give important anatomic information, but the measurement of the severity of hemodynamic reflux or obstruction cannot be quantified. Plethysmography allows for an objective analysis of treatment outcome, objective assessment of individual's progress over time, prediction of successful outcomes, evaluation of the role of collaterals before treatments, functional evaluation of calf muscle pump, measurement of effectiveness of compression therapy, and better noninvasive assessment of proximal obstruction.

8.10 Ankle-Brachial Arterial Pressure Testing

Although not a detailed segmental evaluation of the lower extremity arterial inflow, the Ankle-Brachial Index (ABI) can be used as a normalized, reproducible assessment of the patient's blood pressure in the lower extremity as compared to the systemic blood pressure. Both the dorsalis pedis (DP) and posterior tibial (PT) vessels should be measured in each leg, and both arm brachial pressures are obtained. The highest pressure in each ankle is divided by the highest of the arm brachial pressures to give an index. The ABI can be used to correlate with the degree of peripheral arterial disease, and in general, the values of the ABI can be used to predict likelihood of healing and severity of symptoms (Table 8.1).

One limitation to the measurement of lower extremity ABI is the presence of calcified, non-compressible vessels. Patients with diabetes mellitus often have non-compressible vessels; therefore, they can have falsely elevated pressures. The size of the cuff used to obtain the pressure measurement should also be appropriate

Table 8.1 Relationship of ABI to degree of PAD and symptomatology

ABI	Degree of PAD	Symptoms
0.97–1.25	None	None
0.75–0.96	Mild	Minimal claudication
0.50–0.74	Moderate	Claudication
<0.50	Severe	Severe claudication
<0.30	Critical	Rest pain, poor healing, ischemic ulcers/ tissue loss

for the size of the limb. In an oversized limb, a smaller cuff will yield falsely elevated measurements of the pressure. The width of the pressure cuff used on any limb should be 20 % wider than the diameter of the limb for the most accurate measurements. In diabetic patients, the use of a toe-brachial index (TBI) is considered to be more accurate assessment of the arterial pressure. The toe pressures are obtained using a PPG on the distal toe with a small toe cuff applied proximally to measure the pressure. TBI is usually >0.8 in the normal individuals, 0.2–0.5 in patients with claudication, and <0.2 in patients with critical or severe PAD (rest pain, likely poor healing, or tissue loss).

References

1. Meissner MH, Moneta G, Bernand K, Gloviczki P, Lohr J, Lurie F, Mattos M, McLafferty R, Mozes G, Rutherford R, Padberg F, Sumner D. The hemodynamics and diagnosis of venous disease. J Vasc Surg. 2007;46:4S–24.
2. Park UJ, Yun WS, Lee KB, Rho YN, Kim YW, Joh JH, Kim DI. Analysis of the postoperative hemodynamic changes in varicose vein surgery using air plethysmography. J Vasc Surg. 2010;51:634–8.
3. Van Rij A, Jianq P, Solomon C, Christie R, Hill G. Recurrence after varicose vein surgery: a prospective long-term clinical study with duplex ultrasound scanning and air plethysmography. J Vasc Surg. 2003;38(5):935–43.
4. Christopoulos D, Nicolaides AN, Szendro G. Venous reflux. Br J Surg. 1988;75:352–6.
5. Lurie F, Rooke T. Evaluation of venous function by indirect non-invasive testing (plethysmography). In: Gloviczki P, editor. Handbook of venous disorders. 3rd ed. London: Hodder Arnold; 2009.

Conventional and Cross-Sectional Venography

9

Charles Y. Kim and Carlos J. Guevara

Contents

C.Y. Kim, MD (✉)
Division of Vascular and Interventional Radiology,
Duke University Medical Center,
Durham, NC, USA
e-mail: charles.kim@duke.edu

C.J. Guevara, MD
Division of Vascular and Interventional Radiology,
Department of Radiology,
Duke University Medical Center,
Durham, NC, USA
e-mail: carlos.guevara@duke.edu

Abstract

Conventional venography has long been considered the gold standard for evaluation of the venous system. This exam is performed in an angiography suite using real-time X-ray imaging (fluoroscopy) to visualize intravenously injected iodinated contrast media. Digital subtraction angiography (DSA) is a technique that allows depiction of only the venous structures of interest by "subtracting" out the nonvascular structures, such as bone. This greatly improves visualization of intravascular contrast material. Cross-sectional venography, comprised of CT venography and MR venography, has the unique advantage of allowing visualization of any obstructing masses or other extrinsic structures that impact the venous system. The entire central venous system can be evaluated by injection through a central venous catheter or a single peripheral IV at any site using indirect imaging. MRV is the preferred method for evaluation of the central veins because the excellent signal intensity generated by gadolinium agents allows excellent visualization with indirect injection. With time-resolved MRA, the contrast bolus can be visualized passing through the vasculature in real-time manner, which allows excellent evaluation of collateral veins and routes of preferential blood flow. High-spatial resolution imaging can also be performed, allowing accurate characterization of lesions. This chapter discusses

E. Mowatt-Larssen et al. (eds.), *Phlebology, Vein Surgery and Ultrasonography*,
DOI 10.1007/978-3-319-01812-6_9, © Springer International Publishing Switzerland 2014

conventional and cross-sectional venography with a focus on particular disease processes.

9.1 Introduction

Ultrasound, conventional venography, computed tomographic venography (CTV), and magnetic resonance venography (MRV) are the primary imaging modalities used to assess venous anatomy, functionality, and pathology. Common indications for venous imaging include concerns for deep venous thrombosis (DVT), venous reflux disease, pelvic congestion syndrome, venous malformations, and steno-occlusive disease. The underlying etiology of the venous abnormality may also be determined, such as congenital variant anatomy, tumor-related mass effect or invasion, and venous compressions syndromes (May-Thurner syndrome, Paget-Schroetter syndrome, nutcracker syndrome, etc.). Each modality offers different advantages and disadvantages and should be chosen based on the indication for imaging and individual patient considerations. Determination of the optimal imaging modality requires an understanding of the strengths and weaknesses of each modality, prioritization of the pathologic findings needed to make or exclude a specific diagnosis, and identification of pertinent factors, such as renal function, which may impact the choice of imaging. Not infrequently, more than one imaging modality may be required to obtain full physiologic and physical information necessary for diagnosis and treatment planning. In this chapter, we will review conventional venography, CTV, and MRV. Venous ultrasound will be covered in a separate chapter.

9.2 Conventional Venography

Conventional venography has long been considered the gold standard for evaluation of the venous system. This exam is performed in an angiography suite using real-time X-ray imaging (fluoroscopy) to visualize intravenously injected iodinated contrast media. Digital subtraction angiography (DSA) is a technique that allows depiction of only the venous structures of interest by "subtracting" out the nonvascular structures, such as bone. This greatly improves visualization of intravascular contrast material (Fig. 9.1).

Conventional venography requires an IV or catheter to be inserted into the venous system of interest. The access site must be distal to the vein(s) of concern; for example, to image the entire venous system of the leg, the IV must be inserted into a foot vein. Iodinated contrast, which is much denser than blood, is injected into the IV or catheter. During the injection, the operator utilizes fluoroscopy to visualize and record the flow of contrast through the veins. During the study, the operator can focus on areas of interest, using various techniques to alter flow dynamics, such as the use of tourniquets, varied arm or leg positioning, and additional venipuncture sites. Furthermore, if deemed necessary, the venous access site can be used to perform endovascular interventions if deemed appropriate at that time. Since iodinated contrast can worsen renal function in patients with renal impairment, the renal function should be documented prior to performing this procedure [1]. At our institution, a serum creatinine level above 2.0 mg/dL would be a relative contraindication for conventional venography. Furthermore, there is a significant incidence of allergic reactions to contrast agents, and therefore a careful history should be performed. In cases of minor allergic reaction, such as hives, a corticosteroid premedication regimen is often used.

Conventional venography is considered to be the gold standard for venous imaging, particularly for the diagnosis of DVT and venous stenosis [2, 3]. Validation of all other imaging modalities has historically been based upon comparison to conventional venography. For imaging small veins and branches, the superior spatial resolution of conventional venography renders it superior to all other modalities [4]. Conventional venography can readily diagnose venous thrombosis and venous disease throughout the body. Because conventional venography allows visualization of the flow dynamics of the contrast bolus, collateral venous flow in the setting of venous obstruction is very well

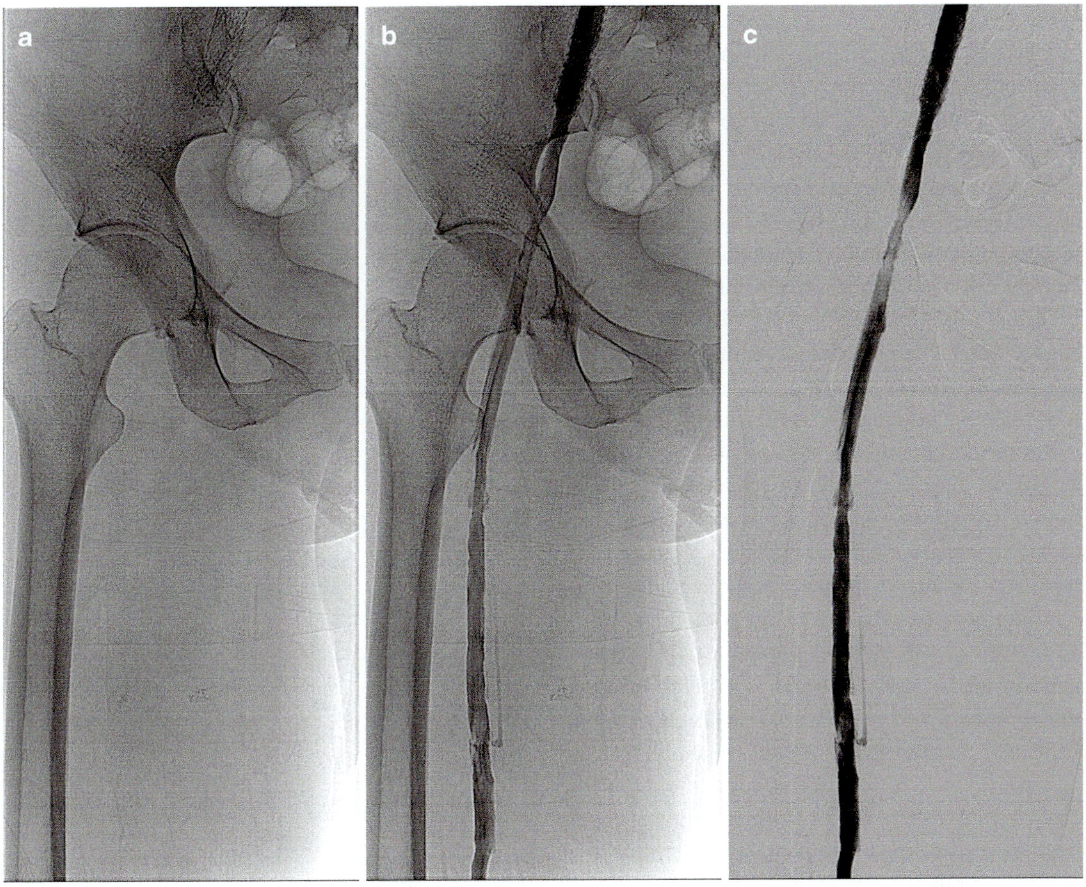

Fig. 9.1 DSA images of the femoral vein. (**a**) Immediately before contrast injection, an X-ray "mask" image is obtained. (**b**) Imaging is performed during injection of contrast into a vessel. (**c**) A subtraction image is created by "subtracting" the mask image from the injection image, which greatly improves visualization of the contrast-filled blood vessel

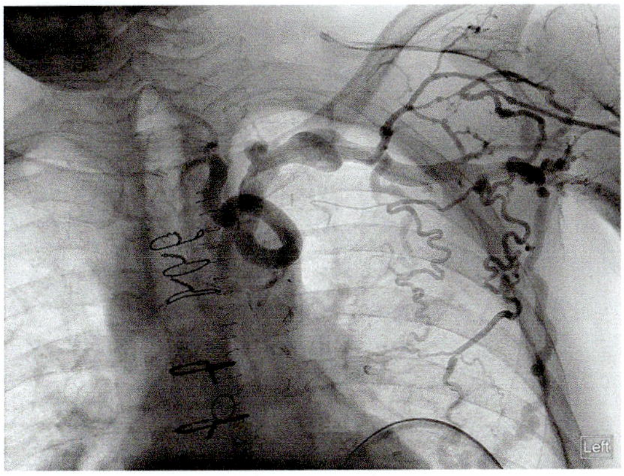

Fig. 9.2 Collateral veins are well demonstrated with conventional venography of this patient with a left brachiocephalic vein occlusion

demonstrated (Fig. 9.2). This is particularly helpful for determining the hemodynamic significance of a venous stenosis and chronicity of any obstructive pathology. Furthermore, repeat imaging with altered extremity positioning (i.e., provocative maneuvers) can be utilized to recreate symptoms, such as thoracic outlet syndrome. Stenosis, reflux, incompetent valves, and reversal of flow are also well evaluated with conventional venography. Venous mapping for hemodialysis access planning is commonly performed with conventional venography, given the ability to rapidly and easily visualize the configuration of the upper extremity venous system. Another advantage of conventional venography is the ability to perform endovascular therapies at the time of diagnosis. Conventional venography can be tailored specifically for each patient with excellent flexibility for problem solving.

The primary disadvantage of conventional venography is its invasive nature. Because injection of contrast into a vein results in opacification of the associated draining veins in their physiologic direction of flow (typically towards the heart), a vein in the affected extremity must be accessed as distally as possible. In patients with suspected DVT or stenosis, arm or leg swelling is the typical presenting symptom, and thus accessing veins in edematous hands and feet can be extremely challenging. Furthermore, pedal vein access in diabetic patients poses a significant infection risk. In general, there is a 2 % chance of IV or catheter-induced DVT with venipuncture [3]. Iodinated contrast is, by far, the most commonly used contrast agent for conventional venography, although, in rare circumstances, gadolinium or carbon dioxide can be used as the contrast agent. Another disadvantage of conventional venography is that visualization of an opacified vein is highly dependent upon the concentration of contrast. When imaging veins near the IV insertion site, a high concentration of contrast can be easily achieved. However, as the contrast bolus travels centrally into larger veins, progressive contrast dilution occurs, which can limit visualization of the more centrally located vein(s). This problem is markedly worsened in the setting of stenotic or occluded veins, where visualization of the vein(s) central to the lesions can be difficult to impossible when distant from the IV. Furthermore, only the veins in the direct line of flow from the IV access site to the right atrium will be opacified with contrast. This requires multiple access sites if multiple venous distributions are in need of imaging. For example, evaluation of the bilateral pelvic veins requires bilateral lower extremity IVs. A technical disadvantage of conventional venography is inflow artifact, which is the disturbance of the contrast column by non-opacified blood flowing into the opacified vein from a branch vein (Fig. 9.3). This can cause the appearance of a filling defect or stenosis. Careful inspection of a questionable filling defect on sequential frames should demonstrate some degree of subtle fluctuation of the margins of this abnormality in the setting of such inflow artifact. In patients with a mild allergy to iodinated contrast, a corticosteroid premedication regimen should be administered. A history of anaphylactic reaction to iodinated contrast is often considered an absolute contraindication. Adequate renal function is necessary, unless the patient has end-stage renal disease [1]. Conventional venography uses ionizing radiation to generate the images, and the dose can vary widely based on the indication.

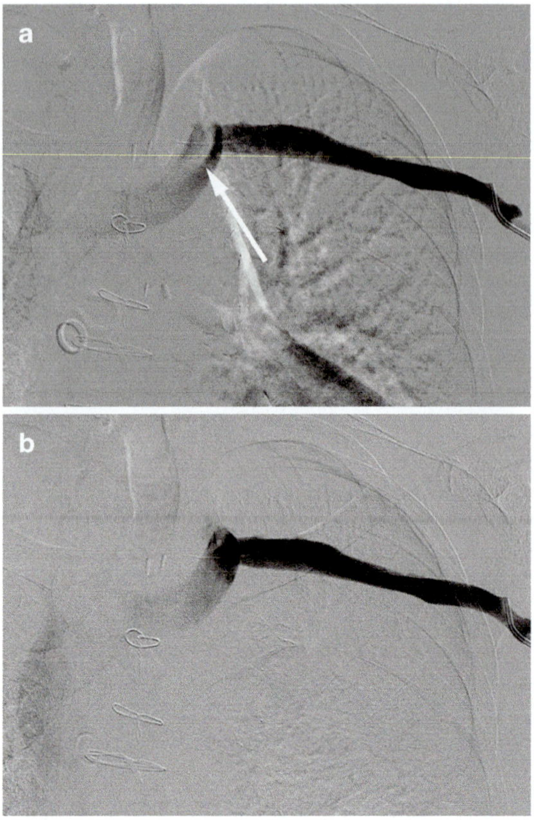

Fig. 9.3 Inflow artifact on a left upper extremity conventional venogram. (**a**) In this subtraction image, there appears to be a filling defect (*arrow*) in the left brachiocephalic vein. (**b**) However, a subsequent frame from this set of images reveals absence of a filling defect, which was caused by inflow of non-opacified blood via the left internal jugular vein

In summary, while conventional venography is considered the gold standard imaging modality for venous imaging, it is not typically utilized as first-line imaging for evaluating venous pathology.

Conventional venography is often used in cases where endovascular therapy is anticipated, such as acute venous thrombosis (for thrombolysis) or venous stenosis requiring angioplasty or stenting. If other modalities have failed to diagnose an underlying venous process with certainty, then conventional venography can be used to obtain a definitive diagnosis. Some centers still utilize conventional venography as first-line imaging for upper extremity venous mapping for surgical hemodialysis access planning. If the patient has tenuous renal function or anaphylaxis to iodinated contrast, then special measures or alternative imaging modalities should be considered.

9.3 Computed Tomographic Venography

Computed tomography (CT) is well established as a method for three-dimensional imaging of the human body. CT images are generated based on the varying densities of different tissues. CT angiography (CTA), although well established as an excellent modality for imaging the arterial system, can also be used specifically for imaging the venous system (CT venography [CTV]). Both direct imaging and indirect imaging techniques can be used. Direct imaging entails injecting iodinated contrast in the venous distribution of interest and acquiring images as the contrast flows from the IV to the right atrium (Fig. 9.4). Indirect imaging entails injection of contrast into any vein (or central venous catheter), waiting several minutes to allow the contrast to reach the heart, recirculate through the arterial system, and back into the venous system [5]. Image acquisition is then performed as the contrast has opacified the venous system in its second pass (Fig. 9.5). By doing so, all veins in the body may potentially be imaged with a single injection, but at the expense of marked dilution of the injected contrast, which may limit or prohibit visualization of the vein(s) of interest. CTV image acquisition is the fastest of any modality, but it is performed with a set protocol with little flexibility.

Currently, multidetector CT scanners are typically used, which allows rapid scanning of areas of interest with minimal motion artifact due to breathing, etc. Although an 18–20 gage IV is ideal for automated power injection of contrast, a smaller IV with hand injection may be adequate for many cases. For imaging of the thoracic central veins, the patient needs to be able to hold their breath for a short period of time. As with conventional venography, appropriate renal function is required and a history of potential allergy should be elicited. A large body habitus can limit imaging quality due to attenuation of the radiation beam. Metallic implants such as prosthetic joints cause substantial "streak artifact" which

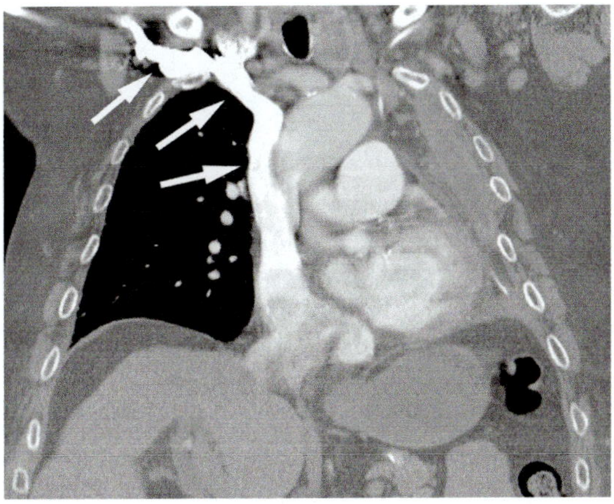

Fig. 9.4 Direct CTV image from a right arm venous injection. Note the extremely dense contrast in the right-sided central veins (*arrows*), but without significant opacification of any other veins

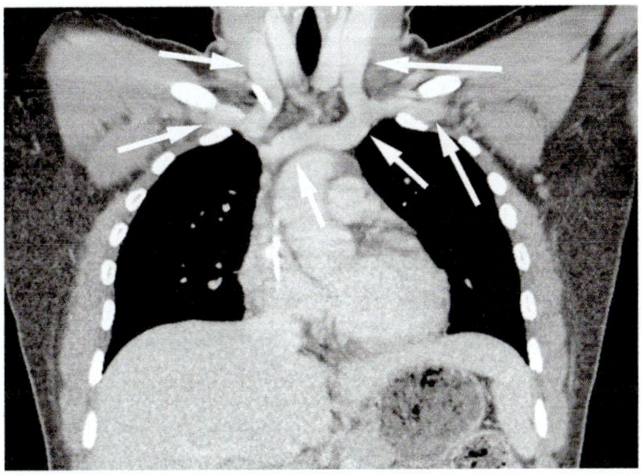

Fig. 9.5 Indirect CTV image from a right arm venous injection. The opacification of the right-sided central veins is much less dense, but all veins in this image are opacified (*arrows*)

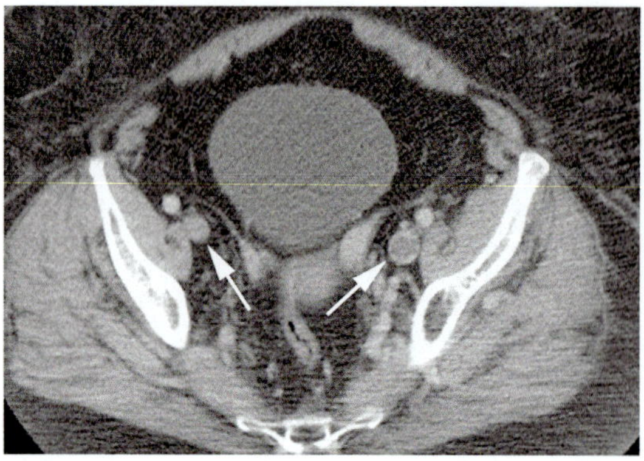

Fig. 9.6 CTV image showing an acute DVT in the left external iliac vein. This manifests as a filling defect (less density than expected due to the absence of intravenous contrast). Additionally, the clot is expansile, resulting in a larger diameter compared to the contralateral external iliac vein. *Arrows* denote the bilateral external iliac veins

can obscure visualization of the nearby venous structures. Appropriate protocols should be developed to obtain the greatest contrast opacification of the desired venous system.

The largest body of literature supporting CTV is for the detection of lower extremity DVT, often performed concurrently with pulmonary arterial imaging [6]. With this form of imaging, intravenous contrast is injected into an upper extremity IV, and pulmonary arterial imaging is first obtained to detect the presence of pulmonary emboli. A few minutes after contrast injection, the abdomen, pelvis, and lower extremities are then scanned for the presence of DVT (indirect imaging) [6, 7]. With this technique, CTV of the lower extremities has been shown to have a very high sensitivity and specificity for detection of DVT. However, due to the radiation dose and questionable incremental yield when the CTA reveals pulmonary embolism, this dual CTA/CTV protocol is no longer commonly used. The classic imaging finding for DVT is an occlusive filling defect which causes expansion of the vein (Fig. 9.6). In areas where a significant amount of fat surrounds the vein, acute DVT often causes increased density of the fat, termed "fat stranding." Peripheral to the DVT, lower extremity edema is often present, as manifested by diffuse fat stranding, skin thickening, and thickening of subcutaneous septa. However, lower extremity

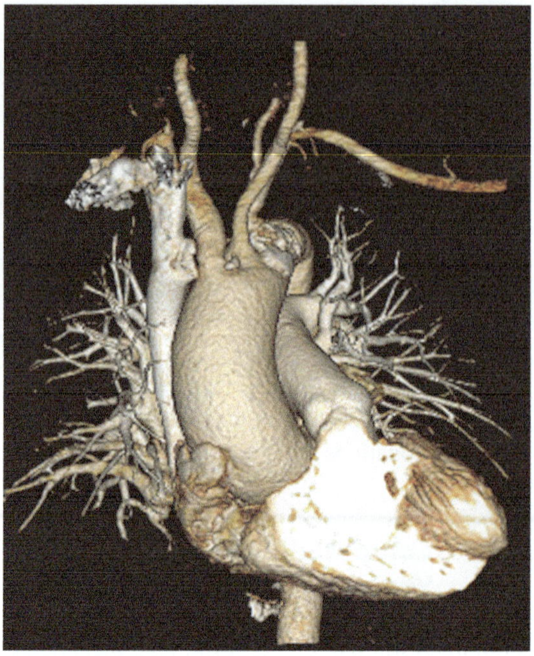

Fig. 9.7 Three-dimensional processed CTA image

edema is a nonspecific finding which can be caused by numerous other causes, such as volume overload, hypoalbuminemia, and others. Varicose veins can also be fairly well visualized, and thus, CTV has been reported to have significant utility for preoperative planning [8, 9]. CTV can also be helpful for evaluating central venous pathology. Occlusions and stenosis of the central veins can be well-depicted, as are any associated obstructive masses.

Advantages of CTV include three-dimensional reconstruction and multiprojectional reconstruction which allow excellent evaluation of venous pathology and the presence of collateral veins [9]. Using specialized software, structures not of interest (bones and organs) can be removed from the image (Fig. 9.7). Any structural abnormalities impacting the venous system are well evaluated with CT, allowing diagnosis of masses and normal variant anomalies. Additionally, nonvascular pathology may be revealed, providing an alternate or additional diagnosis. Using indirect imaging, the entire bilateral venous system can be evaluated with a single contrast bolus under ideal conditions.

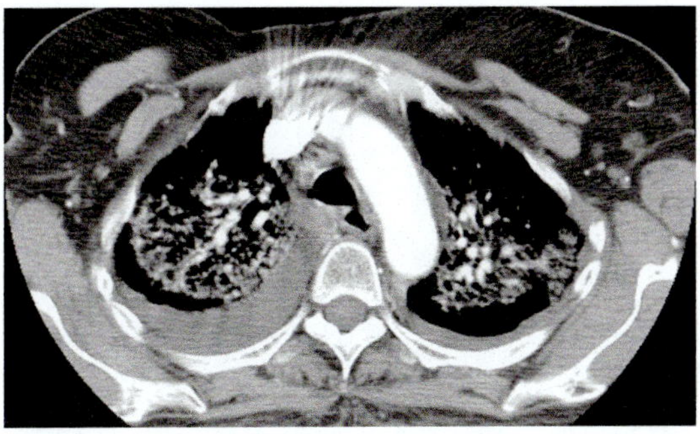

Fig. 9.8 Streak artifact caused by a high concentration of contrast in the superior vena cava. This star-like artifact obscures visualization of the adjacent structures

The primary disadvantage of indirect CTV is the low level of venous opacification, which may not be adequate for diagnosing certain types of venous pathology, particularly intraluminal pathology. To the contrary, while direct CTV provides excellent venous opacification in the injected venous pathway, inflow artifact predisposes this method to false-positive studies. Additionally, with direct CTV of an upper extremity, the contralateral upper extremity veins and lower extremity veins will not be visualized. While utilization of both direct and indirect CTV in the same study will help alleviate these disadvantages, a double dose of radiation is required. Although the ionizing radiation dose to the lower extremities is generally of little concern in terms of carcinogenesis, the organs in the thorax and abdomen are more radiation sensitive, and thus radiation dose becomes of more significant concern for imaging these areas. And finally, the concentration of contrast in the vein may be excessive to the point that streak artifact occurs with associated image degradation (Fig. 9.8).

CTV can, in experienced centers, provide valuable diagnostic information of the venous system for a variety of indications. Because of the limitations as discussed above, CTV is not typically a first-line imaging modality. However, in cases where surrounding structures are important to the diagnosis, and when high spatial resolution is crucial, CTV can provide excellent diagnostic information without need for other adjunct studies.

9.4 Magnetic Resonance Venography

Magnetic resonance imaging (MRI) combines an extremely strong magnet to align the polar molecules in the body with repetitive radiofrequency pulses to alter the alignment. The resulting differences in electromagnetic signal are then processed into an image. Numerous technical parameters can be adjusted to optimize visualization of any type of tissue in the body. For visualization of blood, both contrast-enhanced techniques as well as non-contrast techniques can allow excellent visualization of vessels (Fig. 9.9). When contrast is used, gadolinium-based agents are by far most common.

The physics involved in MRI are complex and multiple textbooks have been dedicated to explain

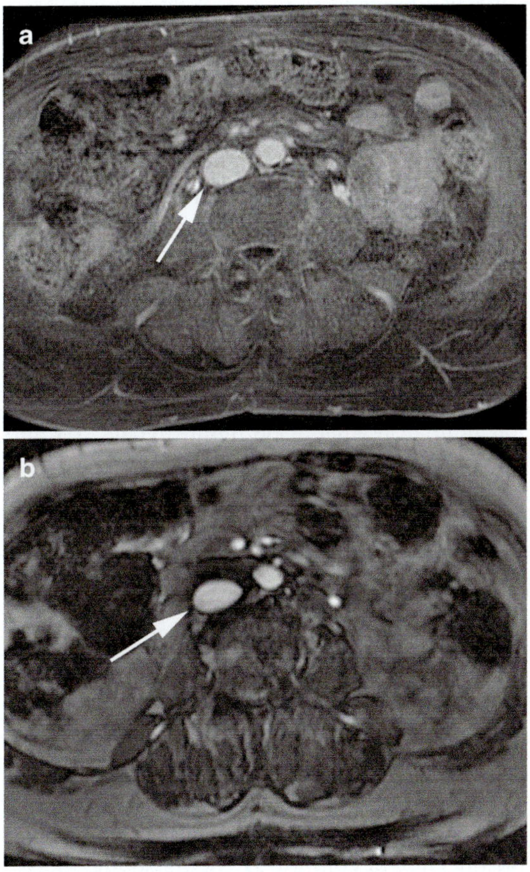

Fig. 9.9 MRV through the inferior vena cava (*arrow*). (**a**) Contrast enhanced. (**b**) Non-contrast

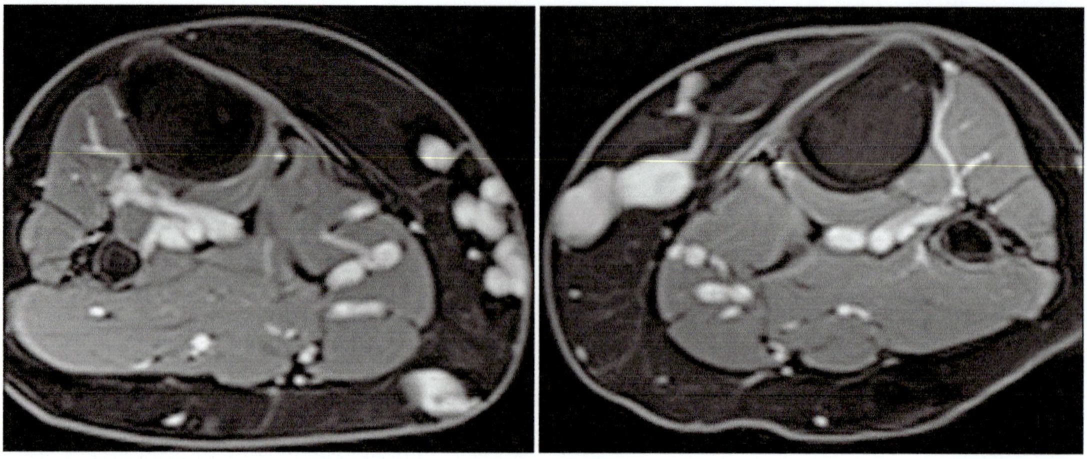

Fig. 9.10 Contrast-enhanced MRV of the thighs with a blood-pool agent allows excellent venous visualization with high detail

the technology behind it. An extremely strong magnet is the basis of this imaging modality, typically in the range of 1.5–3 Tesla (T) strengths. Dedicated coils, specialized apparatus placed upon the body, are used to maximize signal detection for the various body parts. During imaging, patients need to lie motionless in the supine position within the magnet, or else the image quality will be significantly degraded. For imaging of the chest and abdomen, intermittent breath-holding is necessary. Although numerous gadolinium-based agents can be used for MRV, the use of a blood-pool agent may be best suited for venous imaging (Fig. 9.10). This agent, by virtue of albumin binding, is retained in the intravascular space markedly longer than regular gadolinium agents. By this principle, the contrast is more highly concentrated in veins, which allows superior venous imaging quality. Furthermore, due to its long intravascular retention time, timing of image acquisition in relation to the time of contrast injection is no longer a difficult task, and prolonged imaging can be performed which can markedly improve spatial resolution. Another helpful technique for venous imaging is time-resolved MRA, which is characterized by the rapid acquisition of three-dimensional image datasets at three- to five-second time intervals over the course of several minutes after the injection of contrast. By doing so, the images can be viewed in a real-time manner, which allows visualization of the flow dynamics, similar to conventional venography (Fig. 9.11). This can provide valuable physiologic information of the venous system. Numerous non-contrast MRA techniques are available, which work via varying mechanisms, and thus have varying advantages and disadvantages. Currently, the most popular non-contrast techniques include "time-of-flight" and "steady-state free precession" pulse sequences, which result in high signal in the blood vessels. Due to the risk of nephrogenic systemic fibrosis, discussed in further detail later in the chapter, an appropriate glomerular filtration rate is needed if gadolinium-based contrast is going to be used. According to the Federal Drug Administration guidelines, an estimated glomerular filtration rate of less than 30 mL/min/1.73 m^3 is a contraindication to administration of gadolinium contrast.

MRV has been shown to be highly sensitive and specific for imaging the veins, using both contrast-enhanced and non-contrast techniques. While contrast-enhanced MRV is considered the gold standard for imaging arteries and veins, non-contrast MRV can provide excellent imaging of medium to large vessels. The vast majority of venous distributions implicated in venous pathology have been studied with MRV, with excellent results. The detection of DVT using either non-contrast or contrast-enhanced techniques in the lower extremities and pelvis has been reported to be highly sensitive and specific

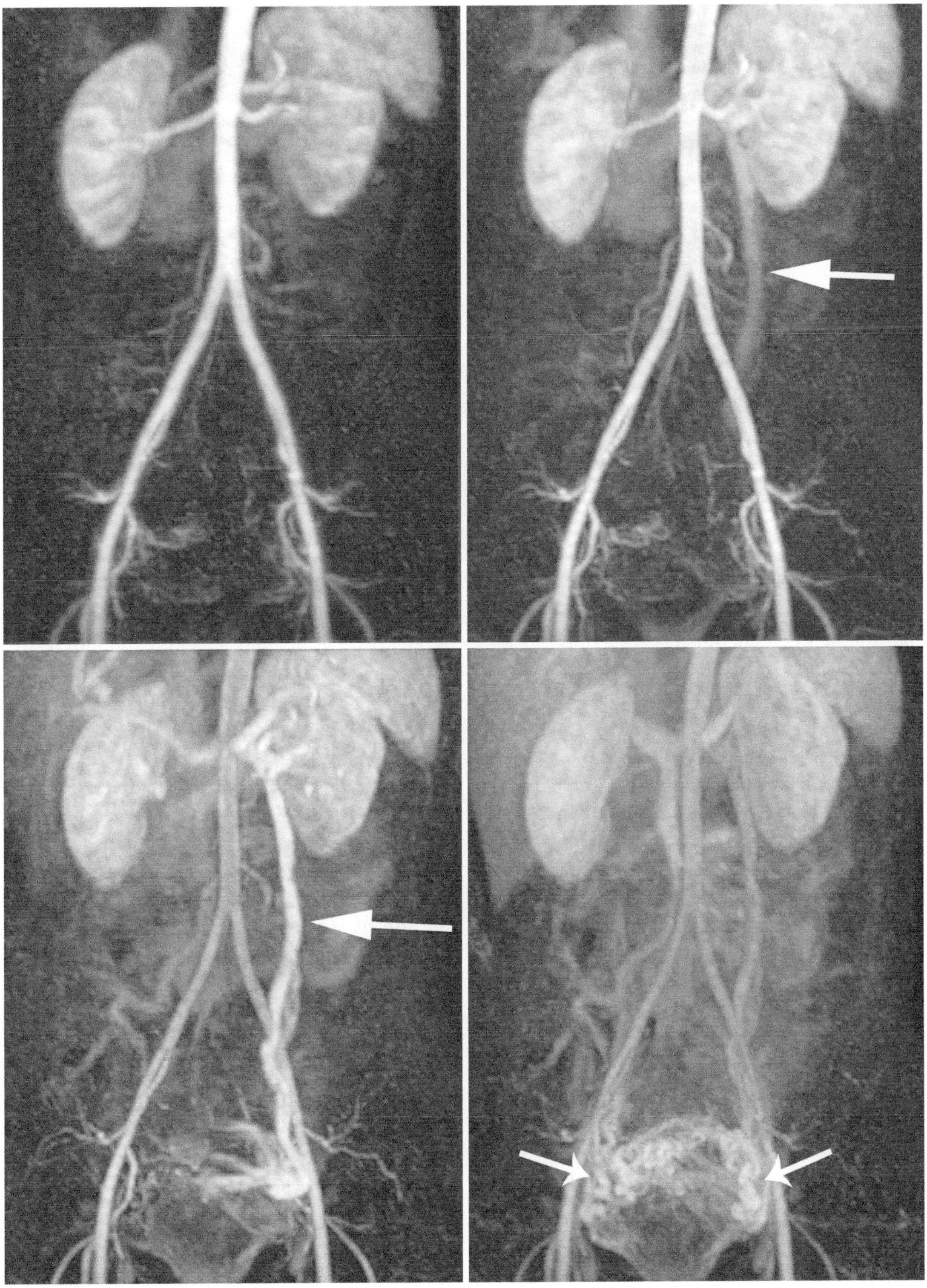

Fig. 9.11 Time-resolved MRV of the abdomen and pelvis allows visualization of the blood flow dynamics. (**a**) Arterial phase image. (**b**, **c**) Venous phase images demonstrate progressive opacification of the left ovarian vein (*arrow*) towards the ovaries, which is in the wrong direction. (**d**) Late venous phase images demonstrate opacification of periuterine venous varices (*arrows*). This constellation of findings is compatible with pelvic congestion syndrome

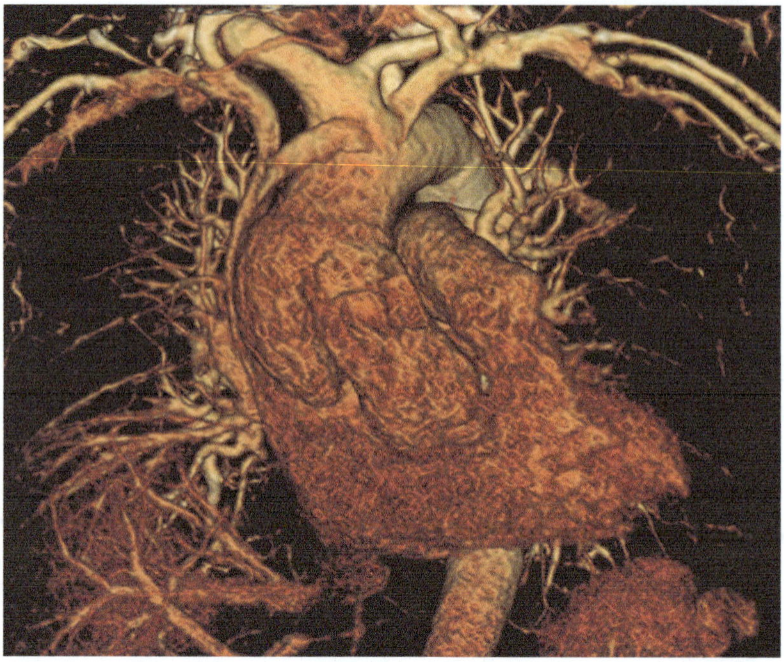

Fig. 9.12 Three-dimensional processed MRA image

compared to conventional venography and ultrasound. Detection of stenoses and occlusions of the upper extremity and central venous system are all well evaluated with contrast-enhanced MRV, with accuracy rivaling conventional venography [10]. Time-resolved MRV is a particularly helpful technique, allowing for detection of indirect signs of pathology that can confirm ambiguous diagnoses, such as the presence of retrograde flow in a vein or well-developed venous collateral veins [11, 12]. Contrast-enhanced MRV has also proven to be nearly equally as helpful as conventional venography in the evaluation of varicosity development, post-thrombotic changes, and evaluation of saphenous veins for bypass procedures [13].

MRV conveys numerous advantages. Similar to CTV, MRV allows for three-dimensional imaging throughout the body (Fig. 9.12) [14]. Certain MRV sequences allow evaluation of anatomy as well as physiology. Therefore, pathology causing mass effect on the venous system can be well evaluated. If the patient's renal function is inadequate for gadolinium administration, non-contrast techniques can be used to evaluate flow, although some of these techniques are prone to certain artifacts. Contrast-enhanced MRV eliminates many of the artifacts encountered in non-contrast MRV sequences and, for this reason, is preferred over non-contrast techniques. Numerous different pulse sequences and protocols can be customized to provide highly specific information, including physiologic information, if the differential diagnosis is well tailored. For example, the direction of flow as well as velocity of flow can be ascertained. These MR pulse sequences are the subject of intense research investigation, with a constant outpouring of techniques. For venous imaging, the use of targeted molecular agents is becoming a frequent topic of research, for example, to directly image various components of thrombus. And finally, the electromagnetic radiation used with MR is considered to be harmless, unlike the ionizing radiation used with conventional and CTV.

While MRV can provide an abundance of information, a number of disadvantages intrinsic to MRI must be kept in mind. The extreme strength of the magnetic fields makes it dangerous to image patients with pacemakers and certain cerebral vascular clips. Not only can the magnet cause movement and dislodgement of certain magnetic implants, it can also cause generation of an electric circuit within certain

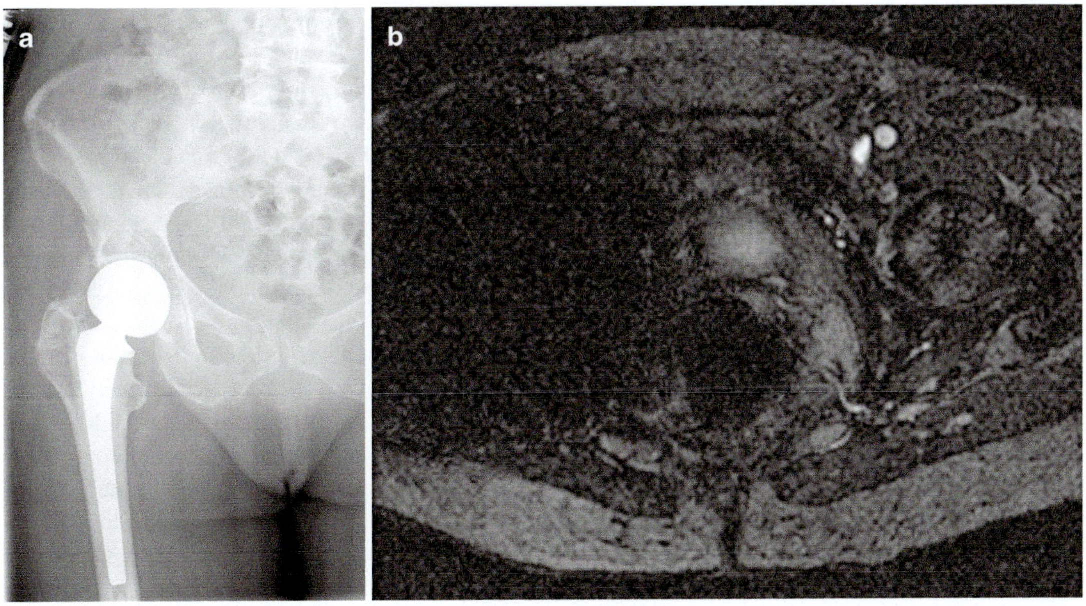

Fig. 9.13 Metallic susceptibility artifact due to a hip prosthesis. (**a**) Frontal radiograph of the pelvis shows a right-sided metallic hip prosthesis. (**b**) On the right side of the pelvis, there is a loss of MR signal in a large region surrounding the hip, due to the presence of the metallic prosthesis. This prevents visualization of the right common femoral artery and vein, while the left common femoral artery and vein are easily visible

metallic objects which can cause electric dysfunction and generation of high temperatures which can cause thermal injury. In most metallic implants, the circuit generated in the metallic implant is harmless, but causes disruption of signal of surrounding tissues, preventing visualization of surrounding structures, termed "metallic susceptibility artifact" (Fig. 9.13). For this reason, vessels containing vascular stents often are poorly evaluated due to this metallic susceptibility artifact. Currently, metallic clips, stents, and other implants have been made to be MR compatible, given the growing popularity of this technology, which render the implant safe and with lesser degrees of susceptibility artifact. The hollow tube within which patients must lay is more long and narrow than with CT, and thus claustrophobia is a much more significant concern. Many patients that suffer from claustrophobia are unable to lie still for the duration of the exam and therefore the exam may need to be terminated prematurely. Furthermore, the imaging time can be lengthy. Typical duration of imaging is from 20 to 45 min, but can be significantly longer. Non-contrast sequences are relied upon when patients cannot receive gadolinium contrast, but are prone to artifacts that can simulate thrombi or occlusion. As with administration of iodinated contrast agents for CT and conventional venography, adequate renal function is also required for administration of gadolinium-based contrast agents. However, the risk is completely different. Renally impaired patients who receive gadolinium are at risk for development of nephrogenic systemic fibrosis (NSF), which is an untreatable systemic disorder of the skin and connective tissues. Therefore, patients with a low glomerular filtration rate (GFR) of less than 30 mL/min/1.73 m^3 should not receive gadolinium [15]. MRV is quite expensive and not readily available in all locations.

MRV, as a three-dimensional imaging technique, is often favored over CTV due to its lack of ionizing radiation and the ability to achieve superior venous conspicuity than CTV [6]. Numerous studies have demonstrated that MR techniques are as good as ultrasound and conventional venography in various venous distributions [16]. Anatomic and physiologic data are well evaluated with this modality. In patients with renal impairment who cannot receive iodinated or gadolinium-based contrast, several non-contrast techniques can be used.

9.5 Considerations in Renally Impaired Patients

Patients with renal insufficiency or renal failure can pose a unique challenge when venous imaging is required. The potential risks of various contrast agents in renally impaired patients must be weighed against the benefits gained from its administration. Therefore, one must be aware of the alternative imaging options along with their strengths and weaknesses. It should go without saying that ultrasound is the ideal modality for patients with renal dysfunction because administration of contrast media is not necessary. However, when conventional or cross-sectional venography is needed, several principles should be taken into consideration.

Conventional venography and CTV require the intravenous injection of iodinated contrast. Iodinated contrast has been associated with the development of contrast-induced nephrotoxicity in a dose-dependent relationship. This nephrotoxicity typically entails a transient elevation of serum creatinine levels, occurring within several days of contrast administration, and resolving within a few weeks. When high doses of contrast are used in patients with severe renal insufficiency, progression to end-stage renal disease may potentially occur. Although contrast-induced nephropathy can rarely develop in patients with normal renal function, this phenomenon is of significant concern for patients with renal insufficiency. At many centers, a creatinine of less than 1.6–2.0 mg/dL is considered within acceptable limits for iodinated contrast administration. However, when the creatinine level is above this threshold, consideration should be given to minimizing contrast and use of alternative imaging modalities. CTV typically utilizes an injection of approximately 120–150 mL of iodinated contrast. The amount of contrast utilized for conventional venography depends on the anatomic part of the body studied as well as the indication. For a directed examination of a single venous distribution, a study can be performed with as little as 10–20 mL of contrast [4]. However, for a comprehensive examination with intervention, up to 200 or even 300 mL of contrast may be needed. It should be noted that in dialysis-dependent patients with end-stage renal disease, iodinated contrast can be administered without concern because renal function has already been lost. However, the risk of volume overload is still present as with any fluid administration in renal failure patients.

MRV can be performed with gadolinium-based contrast agents, which pose a completely different concern in patients with renal impairment. Herein, the concern is for development of nephrogenic systemic fibrosis (NSF), which is a rare systemic disorder characterized by progressive and irreversible fibrosis of skin and connective tissues [15]. Currently, no treatments have been shown to be effective, and this disorder can lead to significant disability related to loss of mobility across joints. NSF also occurs in a dose-dependent manner, but has been documented to occur only in patients with a glomerular filtration rate less than 30 mL/min/1.73 m^3 [15]. Because the link between NSF and gadolinium was only recently discovered in 2006, the actual pathophysiology is not well understood. The American College of Radiology has issued the guideline that renal function be evaluated prior to receiving gadolinium-based contrast, and patients with a GFR less than 30 should not be administered gadolinium-based contrast.

9.6 Imaging for Specific Venous Indications

9.6.1 Deep Venous Thrombosis

Deep venous thrombosis (DVT) is one of the most common reasons for imaging of the venous system. Typically, one or more of a number of predisposing factors are present, such as prolonged immobility, hypercoagulability, and/or recent surgery. DVT can cause significant lower extremity swelling, which can be painful and limit mobility. Even worse, DVT can result in substantial long-term morbidity if post-thrombotic syndrome results. However, the most feared sequela of DVT is pulmonary embolism, which can be fatal.

Currently, duplex ultrasound of the lower extremities is the first-line imaging modality for suspected DVT, demonstrating an excellent sensitivity and specificity for detection of DVT. However, ultrasound typically cannot provide reliable imaging of the inferior vena cava (IVC) and pelvic veins. Furthermore, patients with casts or large postoperative lower extremity incisions may not be able to be imaged at all with ultrasound: the latter, because compression maneuvers are required for the accurate detection of DVT, and pain or wound contamination may not allow performance of such compression with the ultrasound probe. For this reason, alternative imaging modalities may be required.

Although conventional venography was historically the gold standard for detection of lower extremity DVT, it is now rarely performed. As mentioned previously, IV insertion into edematous feet may be difficult or impossible in this patient population who often present with significant lower extremity edema. MRV and CTV both provide excellent alternative imaging modalities, with high sensitivity and specificity for detection of DVT [4, 10]. For patients with renal insufficiency, non-contrast MRV is an excellent technique, with nearly equivalent accuracy as contrast-enhanced MRV. Patients with contraindications for MR can undergo contrast-enhanced CTV if their renal function is adequate. In all modalities, the presence of an intraluminal filling defect is characteristic of DVT (Fig. 9.14). Expansion of the vein is present in acute DVT, due to clot expansion. Associated subcutaneous and perivascular edema is also typically present. With MRI, T2 pulse sequences are extremely sensitive to the presence of edema, which assists in determining the chronicity of DVT. Chronic DVT tends to present as intraluminal webs, nonocclusive wall-adherent filling defects, wall thickening, diffuse venous narrowing, or venous occlusion.

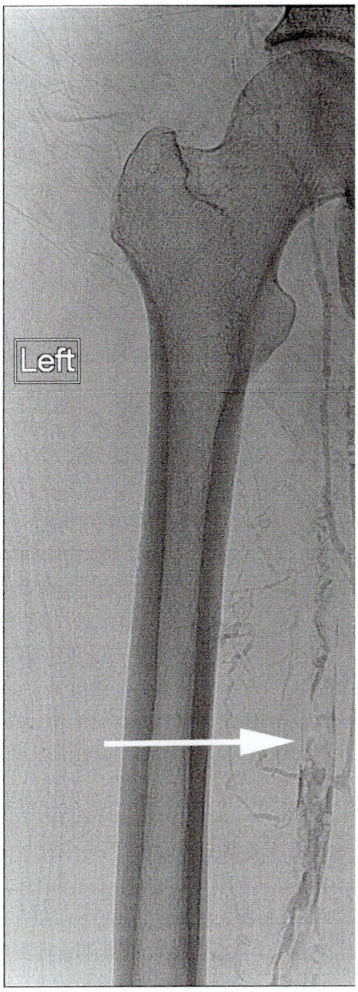

Fig. 9.14 Conventional venogram of the leg demonstrating an occlusive filling defect (*arrow*) in the left femoral vein consistent with acute DVT

9.6.2 May-Thurner Syndrome

May-Thurner syndrome is characterized by compression of the left common iliac vein by the overlying right common iliac artery causing outflow obstruction with resulting left lower extremity DVT. The compression is thought to be present at a young age; over time, the chronic vibratory pulsation incites an intimal hyperplasia response in the compressed segment of vein, with resulting progressive stenosis. Because of the slow and chronic nature of this process, as the stenosis becomes hemodynamically significant, collateral veins to the contralateral iliac veins and

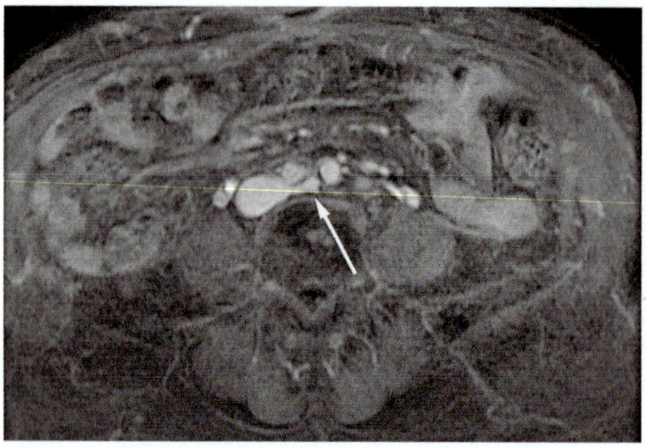

Fig. 9.15 MRV showing compression of the left common iliac vein (*arrow*) by the right common iliac artery, as can be seen with May-Thurner syndrome

to the IVC enlarge over time. These collateral veins are an important imaging finding. When the flow is slow enough, spontaneous thrombosis can occur, particularly when the patient is subject to other risk factors for DVT, such as a hypercoagulable state. May-Thurner syndrome is more common in females and tends to present in the third to fifth decades of life. In addition to DVT, May-Thurner syndrome has also been associated with left-sided venous reflux disease which is often refractory to various treatments.

Imaging for May-Thurner syndrome can be performed with ultrasound, MRV, CTV, and conventional venography. Frequently, ultrasound is the initial imaging modality. In the setting of acute presentation, unilateral left lower extremity DVT is typically encountered with thrombus throughout the entire sonographically evaluable venous system (usually popliteal vein, femoral vein, and common femoral vein). This finding, along with the appropriate clinical history, should prompt further imaging with CT or MR to determine the extent of thrombosis. Both CT and MR can accurately depict the extent of thrombosis. MRV is often preferred because this study can be performed with or without intravenous contrast, while CT requires the use of intravenous contrast as well as ionizing radiation [17]. Both modalities can provide adequate spatial resolution to visualize a stenosis of the left common iliac vein and mass effect of the overlying right common iliac artery (Fig. 9.15). In the setting of acute DVT, the left lower extremity veins are typically thrombosed to the origin of the left common iliac vein. While CT often allows superior spatial resolution, the contrast density is typically quite poor. In the non-acute setting, sequelae of chronic or prior DVT are typically present in the left lower extremity venous system.

Conventional venography is not typically performed purely for diagnostic purposes, but is more commonly performed for therapy when a high index of suspicion exists based on clinical history, ultrasound, and cross-sectional imaging. It can also be used together with intravascular ultrasound. Endovascular therapy begins with thrombolysis, typically via popliteal vein access site, using mechanical and or pharmacologic means. After mechanical or catheter-directed thrombolysis is performed, venography should demonstrate a focal stenosis at the origin of the left common iliac vein as it courses between the right common iliac artery anteriorly and the lumbar vertebral body posteriorly. Venous collateralization is often also typically seen because the chronic compression of the left common iliac vein allows ample time for formation of alternative pathways for venous drainage. The first-line management in the majority of cases is endovascular therapy, typically involving thrombolysis followed by angioplasty and stenting of the left common iliac vein stenosis, with subsequent anticoagulation.

9.6.3 Superficial Lower Extremity Reflux Disease

Diagnosis and preoperative imaging work-up of superficial venous reflux disease is typically performed with duplex ultrasound, which provides excellent structural and physiologic information. However, obstructive central pathology and occult perforating veins may predispose patients to a higher risk of recurrent disease. For these reasons, alternative imaging modalities may be sought for imaging the lower extremities in the setting of superficial venous reflux disease.

Obstructive pathology related to superficial reflux disease is most commonly present in the abdomen or pelvis. Etiologies include

May-Thurner syndrome, IVC or iliac vein DVT, intrinsic venous stenosis/occlusion, lymphadenopathy, or other abdominopelvic masses compressing the veins. For all of these pathologies, MR and CT venography are both the optimal modalities for evaluating these associated structures. Retrograde ovarian vein flow has also been associated with recalcitrant superficial reflux disease in women and, as described above, is best evaluated with time-resolved MRV. And finally, congenital anomalies can be evaluated with both CT and MR venography. Conventional venography can identify the presence of obstructive pathology, but often cannot provide additional information as to the nature of the obstruction, which can have an impact on the treatment choice.

Complex venous anatomy and occult perforating veins have been considered best evaluated with conventional venography. However, this modality requires insertion of at least one distal lower extremity IV. Direct CT and MR venography via a pedal vein can provide excellent diagnostic information, but again, suffers from the drawbacks of a distal lower extremity IV. CT and MR venography via conventional indirect techniques is generally inadequate in terms of level of venous opacification and spatial resolution to visualize fine perforating veins. However, MRV with use of a blood-pool gadolinium contrast agent to visualize such small caliber veins has proven to be highly promising (Fig. 9.10).

9.6.4 Venous Thoracic Outlet Syndrome

Thoracic outlet syndrome describes symptomatic compression of the subclavian artery, vein, or brachial plexus by bony and soft tissue structures as they exit the thoracic outlet. Most commonly, the involved compressive structures involve the clavicle, first rib, a cervical rib, and/or scalene muscles. Thoracic outlet syndrome causes neurogenic symptoms by compressing the brachial plexus-related nerves in 90–95 % of cases. The subclavian vein is compressed sufficiently to cause symptoms in 5–10 % of cases. Compression of the subclavian artery is the rarest, accounting for approximately 1 % of cases. The term "Paget-Schroetter syndrome" is used when acute thrombosis of the subclavian vein occurs in the setting of venous thoracic outlet syndrome.

Physical exam findings of arm swelling, upper chest varices, and a sensation of arm heaviness, exacerbated with arm abduction (provocative maneuvers), typically raise the suspicion of venous thoracic outlet syndrome. The imaging work-up of venous thoracic outlet syndrome has three primary components: (1) identification of venous thrombosis, which would require thrombolysis prior to any other treatment, (2) imaging findings to make the diagnosis of venous thoracic outlet syndrome, and (3) determination of the offending structures causing the venous compression for preoperative planning.

Duplex ultrasound is excellent for the detection of upper arm and axillary vein DVT; however, detection of subclavian vein DVT can be difficult, based on its location relative to the overlying clavicle which can prevent its visualization. Contrast-enhanced CT and MR venography are also very good for detection of subclavian vein thrombosis; injection of contrast via the ipsilateral arm is preferred because direct and indirect imaging can be performed. Conventional venography is the gold standard for demonstration of DVT. Furthermore, when DVT is present, catheter-direct thrombolysis is considered the appropriate first-line therapy prior to operative intervention.

The actual diagnosis of thoracic outlet syndrome requires the demonstration of luminal stenosis or occlusion of the subclavian vein at the thoracic outlet. Frequently, the site of stenosis is at the junction of the clavicle and first rib. Due to the chronic nature of this disease, collateral veins must be demonstrated, which helps to differentiate from spontaneous subclavian vein thrombosis from a different cause. Dynamic provocative maneuvers should be used to recreate the positioning that induces maximal symptoms in the patient. Typically, this involves imaging in the neutral arm position, followed by imaging with the arm in abduction. This is easily performed with conventional venography. The classic finding is

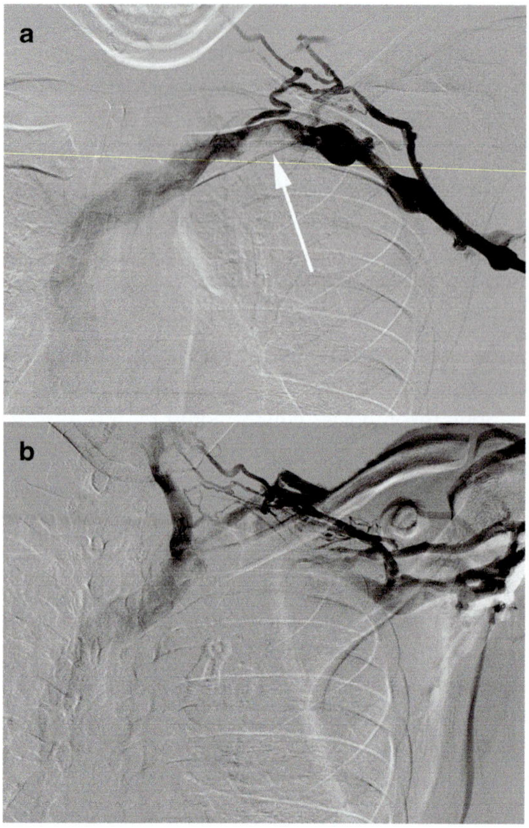

Fig. 9.16 Conventional venogram of the left arm demonstrating venous thoracic outlet syndrome. (**a**) In neutral position, a significant stenosis is present at the junction of the clavicle and first rib with well-developed collaterals (*arrow*). (**b**) With left arm abduction, there is complete occlusion of the left subclavian vein with markedly increased filling of collateral veins and the left internal jugular vein

the development or exacerbation of the stenosis with abduction along with more pronounced filling of developed collateral veins [18] (Fig. 9.16). However, it must be kept in mind that up to 40 % of normal patients can have some degree of subclavian vein compression with abduction: in these normal patients, however, collateral veins are typically not present. MRV is also well suited for provocative maneuvers with repeat imaging. Using time-resolved MRV, the collateral veins are well evaluated. A fraction of the usual dose can also be utilized, which allows repeat imaging with the same total dose. Imaging with a blood-pool gadolinium agent with a long retention time is also well suited to such repeat-imaging studies because the contrast stays intravascular for an extended period of time. CT venography is suboptimal for repeated imaging due to the doubling of radiation dose and washout of contrast which may require a double dose.

Identification of the offending structural etiology is best achieved with MR or CT venography due to their excellent ability to demonstrate nonvascular structures [18]. CT is arguably the best imaging modality for depiction of bony structures, with moderately good depiction of muscles and ligaments. MRI is, without a doubt, superior for demonstration of muscles, nerves, and ligaments, with bony structures being moderately well demonstrated. Because any bony involvement tends to be simple to detect, with soft tissue structure involvement being more challenging, MRI is preferred as the modality for detection of compressive structures.

Because MR is able to answer all three crucial components to thoracic outlet syndrome imaging, MR is, overall, the preferred modality for imaging work-up of thoracic outlet syndrome. Conventional venography is often used for confirmation and thrombolysis when indicated.

9.6.5 Pelvic Congestion Syndrome

Pelvic congestion syndrome (PCS) is chronic pelvic pain caused by incompetent ovarian veins, with associated venous reflux. Typically, only the left ovarian vein is involved. This is thought to be due to the fact that the left ovarian vein originates from the left renal vein, which is a very high-flow vein. On the other hand, the right ovarian vein originates from the IVC, which has a significantly lower flow rate.

Several noninvasive modalities are used to detect PCS, including ultrasound, CT, and MRI. Ultrasound is optimally performed using a combination of transabdominal and transvaginal approaches. With transvaginal views, periuterine varices and dilated arcuate veins are often seen with PCS. With transabdominal views, reversed flow in the left ovarian vein is sought. However, the transabdominal approach can be markedly limited or impossible due to obesity and bowel gas.

Conventional angiography is currently considered the gold standard for the detection of PCS [19]. Contrast is injected through a catheter selectively positioned in the left ovarian vein. Dilation of the left ovarian vein with retrograde flow and periuterine varices is consistent with pelvic congestion syndrome. However, this procedure is time consuming, invasive, and necessitates the use of ionizing radiation. Furthermore, the injection of contrast into the origin of the ovarian veins alters the normal physiologic hemodynamics within the veins, potentially making conventional angiography less specific. Conventional venography is typically utilized only when the diagnosis of pelvic congestion syndrome is highly suspected based on the clinical exam and/or other imaging modalities because endovascular occlusion of the pathologic ovarian vein is highly successful in alleviating symptoms.

CT or MRI performed at one phase of contrast (static imaging) is sometimes used for the detection of PCS. This technique relies on the detection of ovarian vein dilation and early filling of the ovarian veins, although neither can accurately determine whether flow is anterograde or retrograde. Furthermore, pelvic veins tend to dilate under certain situations, such as prolonged standing or coitus. Therefore, while lying prone for CT or MRI, abnormal ovarian veins with incompetent valves may be non-dilated and therefore may not be detected on static CT or MRI. Time-resolved MRA has been shown to be extremely helpful by virtue of being allowing visualization of flow direction in the left ovarian vein [18] (Fig. 9.11). This technique is theoretically more sensitive than CT or static MR due to the ability to visualize actual reflux in non-dilated veins, and more specific, because the direction of flow can be easily determined regardless of ovarian vein dilation. Furthermore, nutcracker syndrome (left renal vein entrapment syndrome), caused by compression of the left renal vein by the superior mesenteric artery, can cause PCS by obstructing the left renal vein outflow. This can be detected with CT and MRI and can alter the treatment. And finally, since pelvic pain is the primary symptom of patients with pelvic congestion syndrome, the ability to evaluate other causes of pelvic pain would be ideal; MRI happens to be an outstanding imaging modality for diagnosis of pelvic pain in women, such as leiomyomas, endometriosis, and adenomyosis. For these reasons above, MRA with a time-resolved sequence is the preferred method for imaging in PCS.

9.6.6 Superior Vena Cava Syndrome

Stenosis and occlusion of the superior vena cava (SVC) is most commonly intrinsic, caused by central venous catheters, thrombus, and arteriovenous hemodialysis access fistulas, but can also be caused by extrinsic compression or invasion by malignancies such as lymphoma and metastatic lung cancer. SVC compromise impairs drainage of the head and arms, resulting in swelling in these areas. When severe and acute, laryngeal edema with airway compromise can occur, which is an acute emergency. Obstruction of other central veins of the chest (brachiocephalic vein, internal jugular vein, and subclavian veins) will also cause swelling of the associated distributions. Collateral veins will eventually develop, and symptoms will decrease over time (Fig. 9.3).

Initially, ultrasound can be obtained to evaluate the upper extremity and internal jugular veins; however, the SVC, brachiocephalic veins, and subclavian veins are unreliably imaged. Conventional venography has been considered the gold standard, but requires puncture of a peripheral arm or neck vein. Often, due to swelling, this requires puncture of a deep vein in the upper arm using sonographic guidance: either the basilic, brachial, or cephalic vein. Venography performed from the arm does not typically allow visualization of the internal jugular veins or the contralateral subclavian or brachiocephalic veins. Thus, multiple access sites may be required. In the setting of a stenosis, occlusion, or thrombus, endovascular therapies may be immediately employed at the time of diagnosis.

Cross-sectional venography has the unique advantage of allowing visualization of any obstructing masses or other extrinsic structures. Furthermore, the entire central venous system can be evaluated by injection through a central venous catheter or a single peripheral IV at any site using indirect imaging. MRV is the preferred method for evaluation of the central veins because the excellent signal intensity generated by gadolinium agents allows excellent visualization with indirect injection [12]. With time-resolved MRA, the contrast bolus can be visualized passing through the vasculature in real-time manner, which allows excellent evaluation of collateral veins and routes of preferential blood flow. High-spatial resolution imaging can also be performed, allowing accurate characterization of lesions. Due to the image acquisition time, breath-holding is required for high-spatial resolution images. In severely compromised patients, this can be difficult to impossible. CTV of the central veins has also been shown to be useful. The spatial resolution is superior to MRA, and soft tissue characterization is superior, which can be useful for diagnosing any compressing masses or associated lung tumors. Furthermore, the extremely rapid acquisition time requires only a brief breath-hold. However, the contrast opacification during indirect imaging is not nearly as robust as with MR, and direct imaging can result in substantial mixing artifacts with non-opacified blood. Furthermore, a significant ionizing radiation dose to the thorax is required.

References

1. Ellis JH, Cohan RH. Reducing the risk of contrast-induced nephropathy: a perspective on the controversies. AJR Am J Roentgenol. 2009;192(6):1544–9.
2. Sidhu PS, Alikhan R, Ammar T, Quinlan DJ. Lower limb contrast venography: a modified technique for use in thromboprophylaxis clinical trials for the accurate evaluation of deep vein thrombosis. Br J Radiol. 2007;80(959):859–65.
3. Katz DS, Hon M. Current DVT imaging. Tech Vasc Interv Radiol. 2004;7(2):55–62.
4. Won YD, Lee JY, Shin YS, Kim YS, Yoon SA, Kim YS, Hahn ST, Park SC, Kim YO. Small dose contrast venography as venous mapping in predialysis patients. J Vasc Access. 2010;11(2):122–7.
5. Krishan S, Panditaratne N, Verma R, Robertson R. Incremental value of CT venography combined with pulmonary CT angiography for the detection of thromboembolic disease: systematic review and meta-analysis. AJR Am J Roentgenol. 2011;196(5):1065–72.
6. Ciccotosto C, Goodman LR, Washington L, Quiroz FA. Indirect CT venography following CT pulmonary angiography: spectrum of CT findings. J Thorac Imaging. 2002;17(1):18–27.
7. Lin YT, Tsai IC, Tsai WL, Chen MC, Lin PC, Chan SW, Chen CC. Comprehensive evaluation of patients suspected with deep vein thrombosis using indirect CT venography with multi-detector row technology: from protocol to interpretation. Int J Cardiovasc Imaging. 2010;26 Suppl 2:311–22.
8. Jung SC, Lee W, Chung JW, Jae HJ, Park EA, Jin KN, Shin CI, Park JH. Unusual causes of varicose veins in the lower extremities: CT venographic and Doppler US findings. Radiographics. 2009;29(2):525–36.
9. Min SK, Kim SY, Park YJ, Lee W, Jung IM, Lee T, Ha J, Kim SJ. Role of three-dimensional computed tomography venography as a powerful navigator for varicose vein surgery. J Vasc Surg. 2010;51(4):893–9.
10. Ruehm SG, Zimny K, Debatin JF. Direct contrast-enhanced 3D MR venography. Eur Radiol. 2001; 11(1):102–12.
11. Kim CY, Miller Jr MJ, Merkle EM. Time-resolved MR angiography as a useful sequence for assessment of ovarian vein reflux. AJR Am J Roentgenol. 2009;193(5):W458–63.
12. Kim CY, Merkle EM. Time-resolved MR angiography of the central veins of the chest. AJR Am J Roentgenol. 2008;191(5):1581–8.
13. Müller MA, Mayer D, Seifert B, Marincek B, Willmann JK. Recurrent lower-limb varicose veins: effect of direct contrast-enhanced three-dimensional MR venographic findings on diagnostic thinking and therapeutic decisions. Radiology. 2008;247(3):887–95.
14. Butty S, Hagspiel KD, Leung DA, Angle JF, Spinosa DJ, Matsumoto AH. Body MR venography. Radiol Clin North Am. 2002;40(4):899–919.
15. Prince MR, Zhang HL, Prowda JC, Grossman ME, Silvers DN. Nephrogenic systemic fibrosis and its impact on abdominal imaging. Radiographics. 2009; 29(6):1565–74.
16. Vogt FM, Herborn CU, Goyen M. MR venography. Magn Reson Imaging Clin N Am. 2005;13(1): 113–29, vi.
17. Wolpert LM, Rahmani O, Stein B, Gallagher JJ, Drezner AD. Magnetic resonance venography in the diagnosis and management of May-Thurner syndrome. Vasc Endovascular Surg. 2002;36(1):51–7.
18. Demondion X, Herbinet P, Van Sint Jan S, Boutry N, Chantelot C, Cotten A. Imaging assessment of thoracic outlet syndrome. Radiographics. 2006; 26(6):1735–50.
19. Ganeshan A, Upponi S, Hon LQ, Uthappa MC, Warakaulle DR, Uberoi R. Chronic pelvic pain due to pelvic congestion syndrome: the role of diagnostic and interventional radiology. Cardiovasc Intervent Radiol. 2007;30(6):1105–11.

Part III

Superficial Vein Therapy

Endovenous Thermal Ablation

10

Mark N. Isaacs

Contents

Abstract

Prior to the introduction of endovenous ablation, surgery was considered the only effective treatment option for venous insufficiency caused by saphenous venous reflux. Lack of patient acceptance and discouragingly high rates of varicose vein recurrence have led to efforts to find less traumatic, more cost-effective, and more successful methods of treatment. Two such methods include endovenous chemical and endovenous thermal ablation. Endovenous thermal ablation will be discussed in this chapter. When compared to traditional surgery, these treatment methods are associated with a faster patient recovery and may prevent recurrent varicose veins due to neovascularization. The use of perivenous tumescent anesthesia has largely eliminated the adverse effects that were associated with earlier generations of equipment and protocols.

10.1 Introduction

Reflux from the deep system into the great and small saphenous veins is recognized as the major cause of varicose veins in the saphenous tributaries. Prior to the introduction of endovenous ablation, surgery was considered the only effective treatment option for venous insufficiency caused by this type of venous reflux. Lofgren and colleagues felt that surgery could be effective if every abnormal junction between the deep system

M.N. Isaacs, MD, FACPh, FAAFP, RPhS
Vein Specialists of Northern California,
Walnut Creek, CA, USA
e-mail: misaacs@veinspec.com

E. Mowatt-Larssen et al. (eds.), *Phlebology, Vein Surgery and Ultrasonography*,
DOI 10.1007/978-3-319-01812-6_10, © Springer International Publishing Switzerland 2014

and the refluxing vein along with all refluxing tributaries could be meticulously exposed and eliminated [1, 2]. Other studies, however, have shown a high rate of recurrent reflux, generally thought by contemporary reviewers to be due to neovascularization [3–6].

Lack of patient acceptance and discouragingly high rates of varicose vein recurrence have led to efforts to find less traumatic, more cost-effective, and more successful methods of treatment. Two such methods include endovenous chemical and endovenous thermal ablation. Endovenous thermal ablation will be discussed in this chapter while endovenous chemical ablation will be covered in Chap. 11. While cryotherapy technically could be considered thermal ablation (and there are studies in the literature addressing this method of treatment), this form of therapy is not commonly accepted in the medical community and will not be described in this chapter.

In endovenous thermal ablation, a catheter threaded into the refluxing vein generates an extreme temperature resulting in damage to the inner aspect of the vein wall and obliteration of the vein lumen. Attempts to utilize endovenous thermal energy to ablate the abnormal great saphenous vein date back to at least the 1950s when a "monoactive" electrode was introduced in Eastern Europe and later modified to a "biactive" electrode a decade later [7]. These early catheters were usually passed from the surgically ligated saphenofemoral junction distally to the ankle. Electrically generated heat was monitored by the surgeon's hand on the skin surface. Though short-term results in eliminating reflux were encouraging, there was a high rate of complications due to thermal damage to adjacent tissues.

10.2 Endovenous Radio-Frequency Ablation

In the late 1990s and early 2000s, two methods of heat catheter treatment emerged: endovenous radiofrequency ablation (ERA) and endovenous laser ablation (ELA). ERA, the first method to gain Food and Drug Administration (FDA) approval in the USA, was introduced by the VNUS Medical Technologies Company of Sunnyvale, California (later acquired by Covidien). The Closure Plus™ and Restore™ catheters had sheathed fans of electrodes at their tips utilizing a computer-controlled bipolar generator. Unlike earlier electrode-type catheters, these catheters allowed for instantaneous monitoring of impedance and vein wall temperature. Feedback loop circuitry maintained thermal energy in the vein wall within specified parameters during continuous pullback, providing controlled heating adequate to denature collagen in the vein wall.

Early published results of treatment trials revealed problems with thermal injury to skin and adjacent nerves causing necrosis and paresthesias, clinical thrombophlebitis, and propagation of thrombus into the femoral vein [8]. The treatment protocol was modified to begin treatment 2 cm from the actual saphenofemoral junction and to include subcutaneous fluid injection. The later introduction of perivenous tumescent anesthesia largely eliminated heat-related complications and the need for general anesthesia (see Sect. 10.7).

Problems with char developing on the electrodes, slow pullback speed, and the need for a cumbersome compression wrap during treatment led to the VNUS Company to develop a new generation of radio-frequency catheters (ClosureFast™) that utilize segmental ablation. The elimination of fragile electrodes and the need for elastic compression have made the ClosureFast™ the leading radio-frequency catheter in the USA (Figs. 10.1 and 10.2).

The Olympus Celon RFITT™ from Olympus Medical Systems of Hamburg, Germany, is an alternative system that has yet to be FDA approved for use in the USA.

10.3 Endovenous Laser Ablation

The first report of the use of laser for ELA was in 1999 from Dr. Boné in Spain [9]. This was followed by two reports in the American literature describing treatment of the great saphenous vein

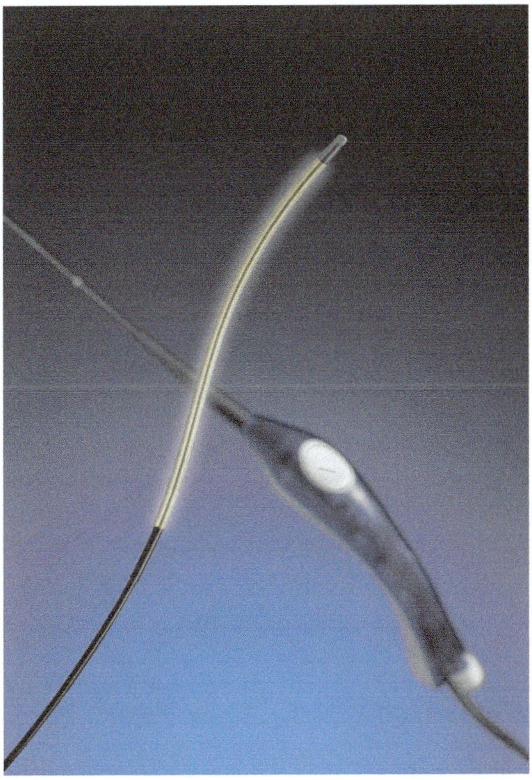

Fig. 10.1 The ClosureFast™ radio-frequency catheter (Copyright ® Covidien. Used with permission)

utilizing an 810 nm diode laser from Diomed and a 600 μm laser fiber (Fig. 10.3) [10, 11]. Since then, a number of lasers with different wavelengths have been introduced for endovenous laser treatment of both the great and small saphenous veins, often with accompanying reports purporting to show a therapeutic advantage of the newly introduced wavelength [12–15]. The suggestion is that higher wavelengths target water over hemoglobin, leading to fewer side effects (see discussion under Sects. 10.8 and 10.9) [16, 17].

The technique initially used during the FDA trials for ELA involved pulses of laser energy at specified intervals during pullback. With time, the technique was modified to employ continuous pullback with energy calculated as joules per linear centimeter. Unlike the ERA catheter, laser fibers have no feedback loop control, and the energy delivered to the vein wall is a function of both the power setting used and the pullback speed.

10.4 Patient Selection

Patient selection and preoperative evaluation are the same for both methods of endovenous thermal ablation. Both rely heavily on an accurate ultrasound evaluation of the superficial venous system, making the role of the ultrasonographer crucial. The recommended protocol for diagnosing and mapping reflux in the superficial system is different from the traditional protocol for evaluation of the deep veins [18]. For this reason, it is highly desirable for the treating physician to become appropriately credentialed in doing this examination or to work with a technician with demonstrated experience and skill.

The vast majority of patients with venous insufficiency have reflux in the great saphenous and/or the small saphenous vein. The extent of reflux in these veins must be meticulously mapped prior to treatment along with refluxing tributary veins and perforators. Indeed, it might be theorized that the disappointing rates of success reported with surgery in past decades had as much to do with the unavailability of adequate ultrasound mapping as with the treatment method itself. While an alternative strategy has adherents (mostly in Europe) [19, 20], the majority of phlebologists in the USA believe that the most effective treatment for long-term elimination of superficial venous insufficiency is to ablate all incompetent junctions with the deep system along with all major pathways of reflux [3, 8].

The ideal candidate for endovenous thermal ablation is the patient with a single, principle route of reflux that is relatively straight and easily accessible directly or via a tributary by percutaneous puncture or by limited surgical exposure. The patient with an enlarged, refluxing great or small saphenous vein is ideal. Patients with isolated abnormal tributary veins, often the anterior or posterior circumflex vein, are also candidates if the proximal portion of the vein is straight enough for the catheter to pass easily. Reflux from incompetent perforators can also be treated, though this technique requires experience and skill in order to precisely maneuver the catheter/fiber tip to the perforator junction. Patients with multiple routes of reflux also can be treated,

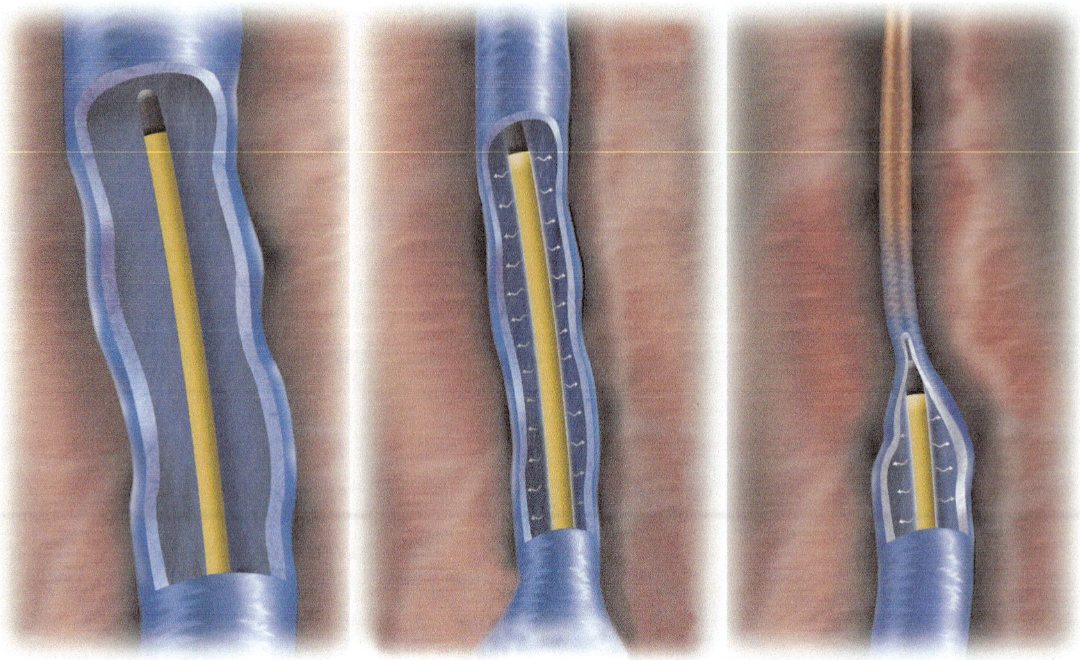

Fig. 10.2 Radio-frequency endovenous thermal ablation with the ClosureFast™ catheter (Copyright ® Covidien. Used with permission)

though more than one treatment session might be required, both for logistical reasons and because superficial veins tend to spasm once one vein has been traumatized.

While the use of the original Closure Plus™ catheter was limited to veins with a diameter of 2–12 mm, no such size limitation exists for either the ClosureFast™ or laser fibers. While a vein may look extremely large when the patient is upright, the combination of supine position and tumescent anesthesia empties the vein enough to dramatically reduce the vein diameter.

10.5 Contraindications

Contraindications include allergy to local anesthetic used in tumescent solution, an implanted device that could be affected by radio frequency, complete anatomic or thrombotic obstruction in the vein to be treated, and recent or active thromboembolic disease. Deep vein occlusion in which the superficial veins form a collateral route of circulation is a major contraindication if the vein to be treated is a major pathway for venous return.

Relative contraindications include morbid obesity, pregnancy, nursing, significant hypercoagulopathy, nonambulatory status, peripheral arterial disease, lymphedema, and disease states that could inhibit adequate healing such as uncontrolled diabetes mellitus.

10.6 Mechanisms of Action

The original VNUS Closure Plus™ catheter directly heated tissue surrounding the active electrode to a temperature of 85 °C utilizing resistance to RF current. At this temperature, collagen denaturation and contraction cause vein shrinkage. Ideally, subsequent endothelial damage causes a fibrotic reaction, eventually occluding the vein lumen. The introduction of subfascial tumescent anesthesia virtually eliminated early problems with heat-related damage to adjacent tissues [22]. Available since 2006, the VNUS ClosureFast™ segmental ablation catheter utilizes an increased target temperature of 120 °C.

There is some controversy regarding the mechanism of heat generation by laser fibers. Theoretically, lower wavelength lasers (810, 940, 980 nm) target hemoglobin, while higher wavelength lasers target water. It has been suggested from in vitro studies that hemoglobin-targeting lasers are more likely to generate diffuse, high temperatures and steam bubbles that affect a larger surface area of vein wall compared to water-targeting lasers [23]. Conversely, it has been proposed that it is precisely this lack of hemoglobin targeting in a 1,320 nm laser that results in less postoperative pain and ecchymosis [24]. Whatever the mechanism, both types of laser will damage the endothelial lining of the vein, thereby initiating a process of fibrosis that eventually occludes the vein lumen.

10.7 Procedure

ERA and ELA are both endovenous thermal ablation methods, and they have many procedural steps in common. Once comprehensive ultrasound mapping of the sources and routes of reflux is accomplished, patient consent is obtained as it would be with any medical procedure. Though the risks of endovenous ablation are far lower than equivalent surgery, the procedure is not without significant potential morbidity, and a thorough informed consent process is essential [12–16].

While some phlebologists with surgical training choose the operating room as the setting for the procedure, endovenous ablation can be accomplished safely and expeditiously in the outpatient setting. A table that allows adjustments in height and body angle is desirable. The room should be large enough to allow the presence of the ultrasound machine, the ERA or ELA equipment, at least one assistant, and a large table upon which a sterile field can be established. The presence of a sonographer to facilitate direct visualization of the target veins is highly desirable, though some advanced practitioners choose to hold the ultrasound probe with one hand while manipulating the catheter with the other. Preoperative marking on the skin of the vein to be treated along with any deep vein junctions may be helpful. A low dose of a short-acting oral sedative medication such as alprazolam 0.5–1.0 mg may help the patient relax and thereby help prevent vein spasm.

Patient positioning depends on the vein to be treated. For the great saphenous vein and/or its major tributaries, the patient is usually positioned supine with the leg externally rotated. Some operators elevate the leg in order to ensure that blood is emptied from the vein lumen as much as possible, but there is no evidence that this position yields better results or reduces complications. For the small saphenous vein, the patient is positioned prone with a pillow under the feet for comfort. The skin is scrubbed with antiseptic solution and a sterile field is established in the usual fashion. Care must be taken to make sure the ultrasound probe is covered with a sterile condom and that sterile ultrasound gel is used. Since veins may move relative to the skin surface during patient positioning on the table, a brief ultrasound exam to reidentify the target vein is advisable.

Ideally, the catheter should be inserted at the most distal site at which reflux is documented in order to achieve optimum results from the initial treatment [11]. In reality this may be difficult due to the tortuous anatomy of distal segments or inadvisable due to the close proximity of the saphenous nerve to the great saphenous vein below the knee and the sural nerve to the small saphenous vein in the lower third of the calf. While some practitioners feel that adequate tumescent anesthesia protects against damage to an adjacent nerve [14, 17–23], many practitioners choose to insert the catheter at or just below the knee in the case of the great saphenous and at or above the mid-calf in the case of the small saphenous. The actual technique of insertion depends on the kit being used, the recommendations of the equipment manufacturer, and the experience of the operator. Most kits include a J-wire that is inserted through a needle followed by an introducer threaded over the J-wire.

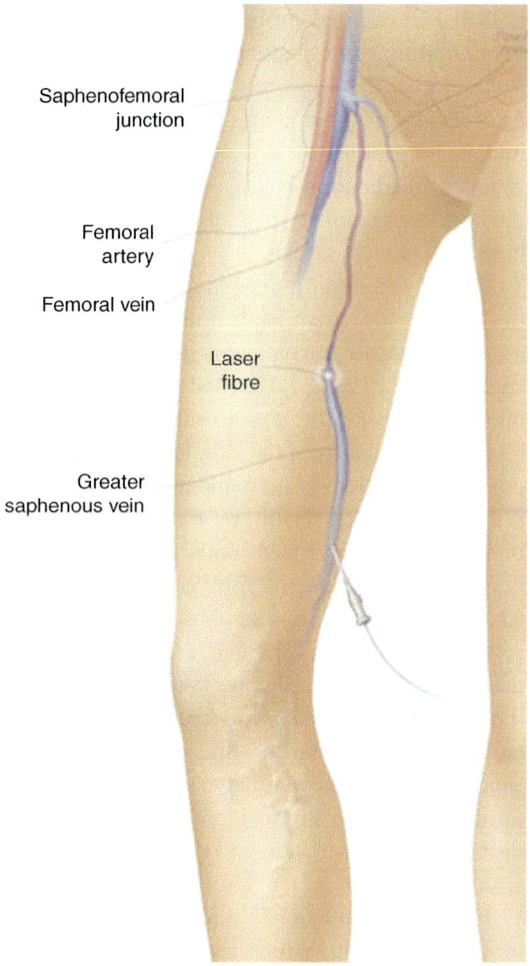

Fig. 10.3 Endovenous laser fiber ablating the great saphenous vein (Photo courtesy of AngioDynamics, Inc.)

The catheter or fiber is then threaded through the introducer.

With experience, percutaneous puncture of the vein under direct ultrasound visualization is almost always possible, though occasionally a small cutdown might be necessary. Superficial infiltration of the skin with local anesthetic is the only anesthesia required. Whether the ultrasound image is transverse or longitudinal during the puncture is a matter of preference, but once the radio-frequency catheter or laser fiber is introduced into the lumen of the vein, the probe should be held longitudinally to follow the course of the catheter as it is advanced toward the deep vein junction.

While early protocols called for the catheter or fiber tip to be positioned close to the deep vein junction, two factors have altered the thinking about positioning. An early study of ERA showed a disturbingly high incidence of thrombus extending from the area of treatment through the junction into the deep vein lumen, in one case causing a true deep vein thrombosis with resulting pulmonary emboli [8]. Also, it became clear with experience, as well as from surgical literature on varicose vein recurrence [5, 25], that preserving normal routes of drainage of high tributaries from the groin and abdomen into the proximal saphenous trunk (in the case of the great saphenous) helps prevent recanalization and neovascularization. While this concept is hard for some surgeons to accept given the traditional emphasis on ligation flush to the deep vein, positioning the catheter 1–2 cm from the deep vein junction or below the junction of the superficial epigastric vein is now the accepted norm in most centers (Fig. 10.4) [11].

Once the catheter is correctly positioned (Fig. 10.5), the next step is the intrafascial infiltration of tumescent anesthetic. As has been previously stated, general anesthesia for endovenous ablation is neither necessary nor recommended due to the increased risk of heat-related damage to adjacent tissue structures and the risk of DVT due to lack of early ambulation. Properly administered tumescent solution not only provides adequate anesthetic effect for patient comfort but also acts as a heat sink to prevent transmission of thermal energy beyond the immediate zone of the vein wall. An additional benefit of perivenous anesthetic fluid is the resulting compression of the treated vein, allowing better contact between the endovenous catheter tip and the vein wall. Even very large diameter veins can be adequately compressed using this technique. The most commonly used solutions are 0.1 and 0.2 % lidocaine with sodium bicarbonate added as a buffer. The addition of epinephrine prolongs the anesthetic effect by reducing absorption. The recommended maximum dose of lidocaine with epinephrine is 7 mg/kg, but higher doses are reported to be safe. A solution of 0.1 % lidocaine can be made by diluting 100 cc of 1 % lidocaine with 900 cc of

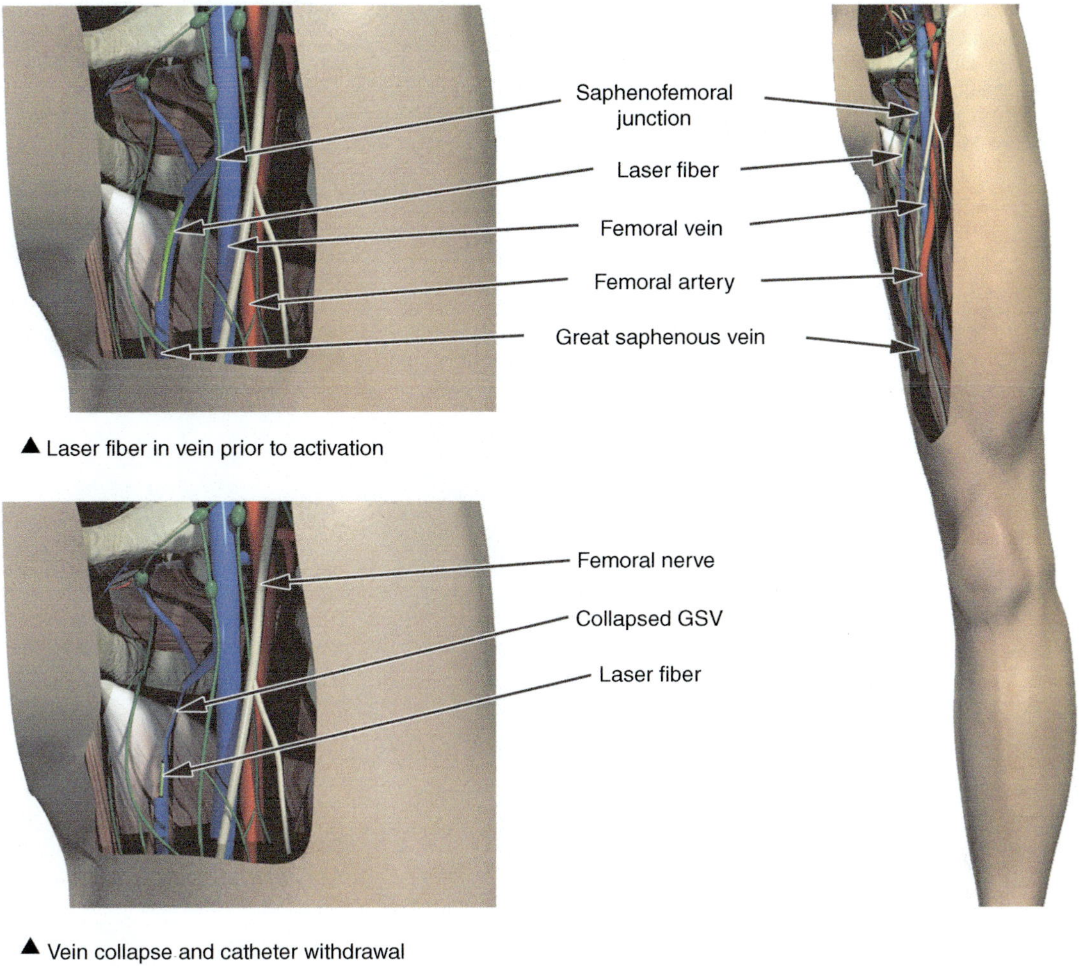

Fig. 10.4 Endovenous catheter tip shown advanced to just distal to the superficial epigastric vein, approximately 2 cm from the deep vein junction

normal saline, then adding 10 cc of 8.4 % sodium bicarbonate.

Of all the skills necessary to perform endovenous thermal ablation, infiltration of tumescent anesthesia is probably the hardest for the beginner to learn. Briefly, the injecting needle is advanced under ultrasound guidance until the tip looks like it is just contacting the vein wall closest to the skin surface. When fluid is then injected, it will be seen to be contained within a distinct compartment superficial to the vein but deep to the subcutaneous layer. Whether a pump is used or the injection is done manually, the needle is advanced within the fluid pocket along the length of the vein until the entire vein segment, including the area of the deep vein junction, is infiltrated. Should it be necessary to advance the needle deep into the catheter or fiber, care must be exercised to avoid causing damage by direct contact between the sharp needle tip and the catheter or laser fiber.

Figure shows the great saphenous vein in longitudinal view with the injecting needle within the plane of the saphenous fascia as fluid is being injected. The second image is a transverse view of the same vein several minutes after injection. As is illustrated, though the anesthetic fluid is initially injected superficial to the vein wall but deep to the fascia, it soon spreads circumferentially to completely surround the vein within the fascial

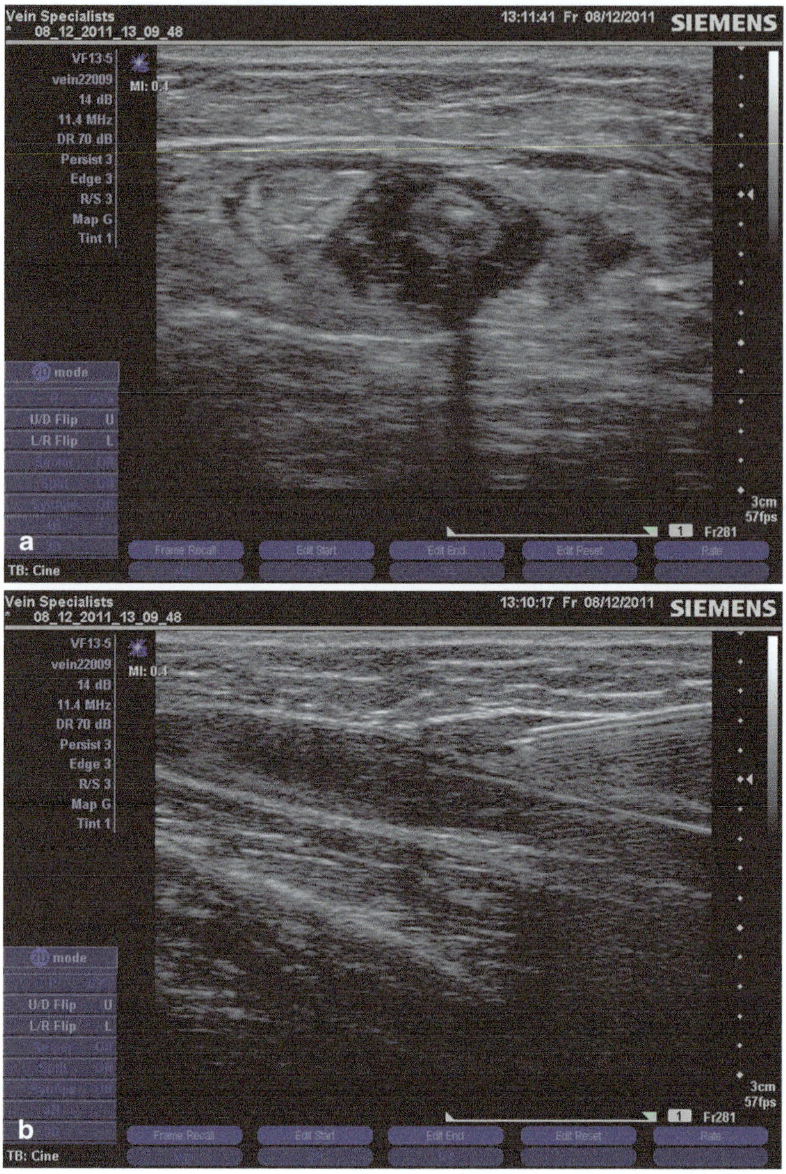

Fig. 10.5 Diagnostic ultrasound images showing catheter placement during endothermal venous abiation. (**a**) Transverse view. (**b**) Longitudinal view (Courtesy: Mark N. Isaacs)

compartment. This method of tumescent anesthetic injection is more effective in providing complete anesthesia for the patient, as well as in absorbing heat, than non-intrafascial subcutaneous infiltration of larger volumes of fluid.

After the administration of the tumescent anesthetic, but before ablation is begun, there is the opportunity to use ultrasound-guided sclerotherapy to treat refluxing distal segments and tributaries. Either foam or liquid sclerosant can be used for this purpose, though foam is considered to be more effective. Foam does carry some risk, however, of drifting into the catheterized portion of the vein and obscuring the ultrasound view of the catheter, and at this time, foam is considered an "off-label" use of FDA-approved sclerosant. It is also perfectly reasonable to treat these additional veins at a later date by either sclerotherapy or phlebectomy.

Anesthetic is usually injected at the deep vein junction last, yet this is the area that will be ablated first. Because anesthetic can take several minutes to be fully effective, it is wise to delay briefly before starting the endovenous ablation procedure. It is also advisable to use either digital pressure or pressure from the ultrasound probe over the vein to be ablated at the site of the catheter tip in order to compress the vein around the catheter and to prevent flow of hot blood products proximally into the deep vein or into unanesthetized tributaries.

The actual ablation procedure varies depending on the equipment being used. If the ERA ClosureFast™ catheter is being used, the manufacturer recommends that the proximal portion of the vein be treated using double heat applications. Some operators also use this technique in any segment where the vein is unusually dilated and at junctions with incompetent perforator veins. Given that the RF generator automatically regulates the catheter tip temperature and times each segmental ablation, the pullback rate does not otherwise vary.

The rate of ELA pullback, on the other hand, varies depending on the power output of the laser, the type of fiber, and the philosophy of the person doing the procedure. There is general agreement in the literature, however, that a certain threshold energy must be delivered in order to adequately ablate the inner vein wall. The range of this threshold is thought to be approximately 60–70 Joules (J) per linear centimeter for the commonly used 810 nm wavelength. Fluence (J/cm^2) has been proposed as a more accurate indicator of energy delivery, but variable vein diameter and the effect of tumescent anesthetic on vein size make fluence impractical as a guideline outside of the research setting. Calculating J/linear cm is simple given that 1 J equals 1 W-s. If the laser being used generates 14 W and the total time spent ablating a 20 cm segment of vein after doing a continuous pullback is 100 s, then:

$$\mathrm{J/cm} = (14\ \mathrm{W} \times 100\ \mathrm{s}) / 20\ \mathrm{cm} = 70$$

Put another way, to calculate the appropriate pullback rate to achieve 70 J/cm energy delivery for a 14 W laser:

$$(14\,\mathrm{W} \times 10\,\mathrm{mm/cm}) / (70\,\mathrm{W}\ \ \mathrm{s/cm}) = 2\,\mathrm{mm/s}$$

Both ERA and ELA have been used successfully to close incompetent perforators. While some reports advocate threading the catheter or fiber into the superficial portion of the perforator itself, the simpler method is to thoroughly ablate the segment of vein into which the incompetent perforator is refluxing. Limited "spot welding" of this type can be very successful in treating incompetent perforator veins and should be considered even in the absence of truncal vein reflux from the saphenofemoral or saphenopopliteal junction.

Once ablation is completed, compression is applied with a graduated compression stocking and/or a compression wrap. In theory, compression promotes deep vein circulation, limits "trapped" blood in the healing vein that might later have to be removed, and decreases inflammation, pigmentation, and pain. Surprisingly, however, little evidence exists in the medical literature to prove that compression is helpful or even necessary. Despite this, the use of compression following ablation is common in the medical community based on a consensus of opinion. Non-stretch wraps and graduated compression hose in the 20–30 and 30–40 mmHg classes have been used. The length of time that compression is used is controversial and a matter of individual opinion. The interval described in studies varies from 3 days to 6 weeks.

As with the issue of compression, the recommended interval before follow-up ultrasound is done varies. Some people do a follow-up within days to make sure there is no thrombus extending into the deep vein system, but this complication is rare when proper ablation procedure is followed. Furthermore, there is considerable disagreement as to whether the most common form of deep vein thrombus, a "hanging chad" thrombus (thrombus barely extending into the deep vein lumen), really requires treatment with anticoagulants at all. Anticoagulation therapy is far from risk-free, and it is yet to be determined in which situations the risk of complications from thrombus in the deep vein following ablation outweighs the risk of anticoagulant treatment. Should a thrombus be noted that is not free floating and is barely within the deep vein lumen, one acceptable approach is to follow the patient with frequent serial ultrasound examinations and to withhold treatment unless the thrombus is seen to be extending. For the experienced operator, following a patient with a routine post-procedure course, it is reasonable to wait 4–8 weeks before assessing the results with ultrasound.

The traditional advice for bed rest and leg elevation that used to be routine after vein surgery has no place in post-endovenous ablation care. Early post-procedure ambulation and daily leg exercise are felt to decrease the risk of deep vein thrombosis, speed healing, and decrease pain. Indeed, inability to ambulate is considered a relative contraindication to doing the procedure at all.

Whether ERA or ELA is used to accomplish endovenous ablation, successful completion of the procedure is, for most patients, only the first step in the process of eliminating troublesome vein dysfunction. Remaining large tributaries, superficial dilated reticular veins, and telangiectasia may cause continued symptoms along with cosmetic deformity unless treated. Endovenous thermal ablation should be considered only one part of a comprehensive treatment plan that is likely to include other modalities such as ambulatory phlebectomy and sclerotherapy. "Success," as it is usually defined in studies as vein occlusion, may have little in common with the patient's notion of success.

10.8 Efficacy: ELA

Assessing the efficacy of ELA is complicated by the presence of multiple variables including wavelength, type of pullback (continuous vs. pulsed), energy delivered, use of compression, use of tumescent anesthetic, and the type of fiber. Since the initial studies published in 1999 and 2009 [10] using an 810 nm diode laser, additional studies have appeared in the medical literature using a bewildering variety of wavelengths including 808, 940, 980, 1,320, 1,470, and 1,500 nm. Purported advantages of various wavelengths have been proposed based on the theoretical target chromophore (hemoglobin vs. water), and spirited debate has existed regarding the need or lack of need for contact between the laser fiber tip and the vein wall. Some critical skepticism regarding these various claims might be warranted given underlying legal patent issues and the fact that many of these studies were funded by laser companies with a vested interest in the outcome. In general, it can be stated that there is no definitive evidence from prospective, blinded, multicenter trials that any one wavelength has a better long-term outcome than any other. When adequate energy is delivered, long-term occlusion rates are in the range of 97–99 % no matter what wavelength is used. Likewise, there is no clear evidence that long-term results vary with the type of fiber used. There is some indication from the literature and from anecdotal evidence, however, that higher wavelengths may result in lower rates of immediate post-procedure pain and ecchymosis [12, 23].

When compared to equivalent surgery, ELA has been shown to be equally effective at eliminating saphenous reflux at 1 year, but ELA was associated with a faster return to work and normal activity [26]. Patient satisfaction, cosmesis, and vein symptom scores were not significantly different between the groups at 1 year in this study.

10.9 Efficacy: ERA

A review of ERA results by Gohel and Davies includes a table of success rates defined as lack of recanalization of treated vein segments. Meta-analysis of the original VNUS Closure™ procedure using the earlier generation of ERA catheter showed an early success rate of 89 % dropping to 80 % at 5 years. A large prospective 4-year follow-up study showed similar results, but interestingly, the reported improvement in pain, fatigue, and edema exceeded the rate of success as defined by sonographic findings.

A study of ERA done with the contemporary VNUS ClosureFast™ segmental catheter showed lack of reflux in the treated vein in 99.7 % at 3 months and 95.7 % at 36 months. An additional 3.1 % were reported to show blood flow without reflux at 36 months. Relative to the earlier catheter, the ClosureFast™ also shows efficacy in veins with a diameter larger than the previously recommended limit of 12 mm.

The results of a multicenter trial sponsored by VNUS® demonstrated reduced pain, tenderness, and ecchymosis compared to 980 nm endovenous bare tip laser in the 30 days following endovenous ablation, though long-term success as measured by a venous clinical severity score and quality of life score was not significantly different.

10.10 Complications and Adverse Events

The obvious concern in using endovenous thermal ablation is that heat generated in an effort to ablate the abnormal vein may also damage adjacent structures such as nerves or skin. Indeed, even when a feedback loop was employed in the original VNUS Closure catheter to keep heat within specified parameters, early studies showed a significant incidence of paresthesia when either the saphenous or sural nerve was close to the treated vein wall [8]. The anatomic relationship between the saphenous nerve and the great saphenous vein is highly varied, and unless tumescent anesthesia is used, damage to the saphenous nerve with either method of endovenous thermal ablation is likely in at least a small percentage of cases. When tumescent anesthesia is used, the incidence of true nerve injury is well below 1 %, though temporary dysesthesia is more common.

Bruising is common following ablation and may be due to either trauma from the tumescent anesthesia needle or from vein perforation during ablation. Such bruising may appear dramatic to the patient but will resolve without any specific intervention. Likewise, soreness and mild swelling in the area of the vein ablation is not unusual after the anesthetic wears off, but extreme pain or edema warrants investigation to rule out deep vein thrombosis. High rates of "phlebitis" appear in some studies, but given that the procedure is, by its nature, a cause of inflammation within the vein, it is difficult to assess how phlebitis is differentiated from anticipated soreness.

The reported incidence of DVT varies from 0 % to more than 7 %. While no study looks specifically at risk factors for DVT, careful reading of the methodology in various studies indicates that possible variables include how DVT is defined, the level of scrutiny with ultrasound, the use of tumescent anesthesia vs. general anesthesia, encouragement of early ambulation, catheter tip placement, the technique of ablation used, and the experience of the operator. In studies in which the catheter/fiber tip is kept at least 1 cm from the deep vein junction and tumescent rather than general anesthesia is used allowing early ambulation, the DVT rate after treatment of the great saphenous vein is almost always 0 % for both ERA and ELA. A study of ELA in the treatment of the small saphenous vein, however, showed a 5.7 % rate of DVT on early duplex follow-up despite the use of adequate perivenous tumescent anesthesia and careful positioning of the fiber tip. None of these patients had any adverse effect from these conservatively defined DVTs.

Patients should be warned to expect discoloration in skin overlying extremely superficial, dilated varicose veins. Such discoloration may be due to reactive hyperpigmentation in patients with certain skin types but is more often due to hemosiderin from red blood cells trapped in the fibrosing vein. Areas of "trapped" blood may be drained in weeks following the procedure using local anesthetic and a large gauge needle in order to relieve discomfort, limit skin staining, and speed healing.

ELA carries an additional risk to the staff that should be mentioned. Inadvertent firing of the laser while outside the patient's body can cause damage to unprotected eyes either directly or indirectly from reflections. Class 4 laser hazard precautions are mandatory, including the use of appropriate eyewear.

10.11 Summary

Demand from the public for minimally invasive treatment for varicose veins has increased dramatically as awareness of this option has increased. While endovenous thermal ablation was viewed initially with skepticism, there is now a wealth of evidence demonstrating the safety and effectiveness of both ERA and ELA. Further, when compared to traditional surgery, these treatment methods are associated with a faster patient recovery and may prevent recurrent varicose veins due to neovascularization. The use of perivenous tumescent anesthesia has largely eliminated the adverse effects that were associated with earlier generations of equipment and protocols. As impressive as these treatment methods are, however, they should be viewed as only one step in a comprehensive treatment plan based on the patient's goals and a thorough pretreatment evaluation that includes ultrasound mapping of all sources of reflux and abnormal venous flow. No one treatment method is ideal for all patients in all situations, and more often than not a combination of treatment methods is necessary to achieve the desired results.

References

1. Lofgren E, Lofgren K. Recurrence of varicose veins after the stripping operation. Arch Surg. 1971; 102:111–4.
2. Larson R, Lofgren E, Myers T, Lofgren K. Long-term results after vein surgery. Mayo Clin Proc. 1974; 49:114–7.
3. Bergan J, editor. The vein book. Amsterdam/Boston: Elsevier/Academic Press; 2007. p. 239–46.
4. Jones L, Braithwaite B, Selwyn D, Cooke S, Earnshaw J. Neovascularisation is the principal cause of varicose vein recurrence: results of a randomised trial of stripping the long saphenous vein. Eur J Vasc Endovasc Surg. 1996;12:442–5.
5. Fischer R, Linde N, Duff C, Jeanneret C, Chandler J, Seeber P. Late recurrent saphenofemoral junction reflux after ligation and stripping of the greater saphenous vein. J Vasc Surg. 2001;34(2):236–40.
6. Fischer R, et al. The unresolved problem of recurrent saphenofemoral reflux. J Am Coll Surg. 2002; 195(1):80–92.
7. Frantsev V, Ershov V, VestnNovoselets S. New electrodes for electrosurgical treatment of subcutaneous varicose veins. Khir Im I IGrek. 1973;110(5):115–7.
8. Chandler J, et al. Treatment of primary venous insufficiency by endovenous saphenous vein obliteration. Vasc Surg. 2000;34(3):201–14.
9. Boné C. Tratamiento endoluminal de las varices con laser de Diodo: Estudio preliminary. Rev Patol Vasc. 1999;5:35–46.
10. Navarro L, Min R, Boné C. Endovenous laser: a new minimally invasive method of treatment for varicose vein – preliminary observations using an 810 nm diode laser. Dermatol Surg. 2001;27:117–22.
11. Min R, Zimmet S, Isaacs M, Forrestal M. Endovenous laser treatment of the incompetent greater saphenous vein. J Vasc Interv Radiol. 2001;12(10):1167–71.
12. Proebstle T, Gul D, Kargl A, Knop J. Endovenous laser treatment of the lesser saphenous vein with a 940-nm diode laser: early results. Dermatol Surg. 2003;29(4):357–61.
13. Oh C, Jung D, Jang H, Kwon K. Endovenous laser surgery of the incompetent greater saphenous vein with a 980-nm diode laser. Dermatol Surg. 2003; 29(11):1135–40.
14. Goldman M, Mauricio M, Rao J. Intravascular 1320-nm laser closure of the great saphenous vein: a 6- to 12-month follow-up study. Dermatol Surg. 2004; 30(11):1380–5.
15. Pannier F, Rabe E, Rits J, Kadiss A, Maurins U. Endovenous laser ablation of great saphenous veins using a 1470 nm diode laser and the radial fiber – follow-up after six months. Phlebology. 2011;26:35–9.
16. Proebstle T, Moehler T, Gul D, Herdemann S. Endovenous treatment of the great saphenous vein using a 1320 nm Nd:YAG laser causes fewer side effects than using a 940 nm diode laser. Dermatol Surg. 2005;31(12):1678–84.
17. Kabnick L. Outcome of different endovenous laser wavelengths for great saphenous vein ablation. J Vasc Surg. 2006;43:88–93.
18. Coleridge-Smith P, Labropoulos N, Partsch H, Myers K, Nicolaides A, Cavezzi A. Duplex ultrasound investigation of the veins in chronic venous disease of the lower limbs – UIP consensus document. Parts 1 and 2. Phlebology. 2006;21(4):158–79.
19. Carandina S, et al. Varicose vein stripping vs haemodynamic correction (CHIVA): a long randomized trial. Eur J Vasc Endovasc Surg. 2008;35(2):230–7.
20. Franceschi C, Zamboni P, editors. Principles of venous hemodynamics. Hauppauge: Nova Biomedical Books; 2009.
21. Alam M, Nguyen T, editors. Treatment of leg veins. Philadelphia: Elsevier/Saunders; 2006. p. 59.
22. Weiss R, Weiss M. Controlled radiofrequency endovenous occlusion using a unique radiofrequency catheter under duplex guidance to eliminate saphenous varicose vein reflux: a 2-year follow-up. Dermatol Surg. 2002;28(1):38–42.
23. Proebstle T, Sandhofer M, Kargl A, Gul D, Rother W, Knop J, Lehr H. Thermal damage of the inner vein wall during endovenous laser treatment: key role of energy absorption by intravascular blood. Dermatol Surg. 2002;28(7):596–600.
24. Theivacumar N, Dellagrammaticas D, Mavor A, Gough M. Endovenous laser ablation: does standard above-knee great saphenous vein ablation provide optimum results in patients with both above and below knee reflux? A randomized controlled trial. J Vasc Surg. 2008;48(1):173–8.
25. Blomgren L, Johansson G, Dahlberg-AKerman A, Noren A, Brundin C, Nordstrom E, Bergqvist D. Recurrent varicose veins: incidence, risk factors and groin anatomy. Eur J Vasc Endovasc Surg. 2004; 27:269–74.
26. Darwood R, Gough M. Endovenous laser treatment for uncomplicated varicose veins. Phlebology. 2009; 24 Suppl 1:50–61.

Chemical Superficial Vein Ablation 11

Nick Morrison

Contents

N. Morrison, MD, FACPh, FACS, RPhS
Morrison Vein Institute, Scottsdale, AZ, USA
e-mail: nickmorrison2002@yahoo.com

Abstract

Sclerotherapy plays a fundamental role for nearly all patients in returning their legs to a healthier state: from the young female patient who comes to the practice with a few telangiectasias to the older patient with severe chronic venous insufficiency, leg ulcers, and resulting limited physical activities and whether using dilute liquid sclerotherapy for those tiny telangiectasias or ultrasound-guided foam sclerotherapy (UGFS) for the large incompetent truncal veins, tributaries, and perforators. Of the many patients presenting with telangiectasias to a phlebology practice and professing cosmetic concerns, only about 20 % will be found to have purely "cosmetic" vein problems once they are thoroughly screened and undergo duplex scanning. The others will have underlying venous incompetence contributing to the appearance of the telangiectasias, to a greater or lesser extent, and will require correction of the underlying venous disorder prior to sclerotherapy to treat the telangiectasias. This chapter discusses chemical ablation of superficial veins.

11.1 Introduction

Chemical ablation and sclerotherapy (liquid or foam) are interchangeable terms. Both will be used in this chapter. As the foundation of the phlebology practice, sclerotherapy will play a fundamental role for nearly all patients in

E. Mowatt-Larssen et al. (eds.), *Phlebology, Vein Surgery and Ultrasonography*,
DOI 10.1007/978-3-319-01812-6_11,

returning their legs to a healthier state: from the young female patient who comes to the practice with a few telangiectasias to the older patient with severe chronic venous insufficiency, leg ulcers, and resulting limited physical activities and whether using dilute liquid sclerotherapy for those tiny telangiectasias or ultrasound-guided foam sclerotherapy (UGFS) for the large incompetent truncal veins, tributaries, and perforators.

Of the many patients presenting with telangiectasias to a phlebology practice and professing cosmetic concerns, only about 20 % will be found to have purely "cosmetic" vein problems once they are thoroughly screened and undergo duplex scanning. The others will have underlying venous incompetence contributing to the appearance of the telangiectasias, to a greater or lesser extent, and will require correction of the underlying venous disorder prior to sclerotherapy to treat the telangiectasias.

11.2 Which Sclerosants to Use?

Currently the only sclerosing agents approved for use in the USA are hypertonic saline, sodium tetradecyl sulfate (STS), polidocanol, glycerin, and sodium morrhuate. It is important to bear in mind that the use of imported or compounded non-FDA-approved sclerosing agents may not only be illegal but also be against the policy of insurance carriers. The use of such agents may even constitute fraud if reimbursement is received on behalf of a patient from an insurance carrier, including Medicare. Additionally, the sclerosant concentrations and presence of impurities are at considerable variance when compared to manufactured products [1, 2]. Over and above the cost savings to be gained by using imported or compounded agents, the primary considerations should be patient safety first and medicolegal exposure for the practice.

Sclerotherapists should be thoroughly familiar with the appropriate concentrations and volumes of sclerosants and be prepared to handle any side effect or untoward sequelae. The incidence of postinjection adverse events, such as hyperpigmentation, telangiectatic matting, and ulceration, correlates directly with the strength of sclerosing agent, the pressure used to inject, and the volume used in each injection. The practitioner should have available a variety of sclerosing agents, the appropriate use of each being dictated by individual considerations, such as target vein size, how superficial the vein is, allergic history, skin type, and previous sensitivity.

11.3 Which Sclerosant for Which Veins?

11.3.1 Sclerotherapy: Indications and Contraindications

Visual sclerotherapy may be performed on most patients given their understanding of and commitment to a fully informed consent and, if indicated, a thorough duplex ultrasound scan to exclude underlying sources of venous incompetence. Indications may include veins from less than 1 mm to large varicosities, although the larger the diameter of the vein, the more appropriate other methods, such as microphlebectomy, may be. Even laser or light-based treatment advocates agree that sclerotherapy should generally be tried before proceeding to other noninvasive methods. Contraindications will include allergy to the sclerosant, arteriovenous fistula, previous nonallergic reaction to the sclerosant (e.g., cutaneous eruption or systemic reaction), pregnancy, infectious process in the target area, active venous thrombosis, and patient immobility.

Indications for UGFS have been reported to be the primary treatment of saphenous veins; extending the treatment of thermal ablation to segments of concern for nerve injury; treating saphenous and non-saphenous varicosities and recurrences after stripping or thermal ablation; ablation of perforating veins; and treatment of venous malformations [3], sciatic nerve varices [4], and perineal and pelvic veins [5]. Contraindications for UGFS are the same as for cutaneous sclerotherapy but may also include telangiectasias (increased risk of thrombosis, hyperpigmentation), known symptomatic right-to-left shunt, neurosensory adverse event following previous UGFS, history of migraine with aura (greater than 50 % of such patients have patent foramen ovale) [6], and confirmed or suspected thrombophilic condition (thrombosis prophylaxis may be indicated).

11.3.2 Sclerotherapy Technique

It is of primary importance to be thoroughly familiar with the theory of sclerotherapy, the risks, complications, and treatment of complications. Sclerotherapy is not difficult to learn, but some will learn more quickly than others. It is advisable to acquire the skills necessary for visual sclerotherapy before advancing to ultrasound-guided sclerotherapy. One should start by observing a skilled sclerotherapist, followed by practice on friends or volunteers and guided by a mentor. One can then graduate to "real" patients, at first doing sclerotherapy on larger veins alongside the mentor who, meanwhile, can be working on smaller veins, until the technique has been mastered. Limit these learning sessions to 30 min or so, as longer sessions will cause fatigue that will degrade performance. Clearly written protocols for sclerotherapy should be an integral part of every phlebology practice, so that every sclerotherapist delivers consistently safe and effective treatment.

As one gains sclerotherapy experience, personal preferences for syringes, needles, compression pads, etc. will become apparent. Some syringes have smoother pistons than others, and needle sharpness and durability will vary by manufacturer. A variety of needle sizes, from the larger caliber 22–27 gauge used during ultrasound-guided sclerotherapy to smaller caliber 30–33 gauge needles for telangiectasias, will be necessary to accommodate different size veins. Remember, a needle dulled by repeated use will be more painful for the patient and make it more difficult for the sclerotherapist to successfully inject a vein. Changing needles frequently will avoid such problems.

11.3.3 Visual Sclerotherapy

A standard patient examination room with good florescent or indirect sunlight is quite acceptable. Magnification with microsurgical loops, headgear, or simply "drugstore reading glasses" will aid in successful venous access. Both sclerotherapist and patient must each assume a comfortable position on a mechanically adjustable chair or table, respectively (Fig. 11.1). As the patient will likely be lying on a table for some time, comfort is very important. If the room temperature is

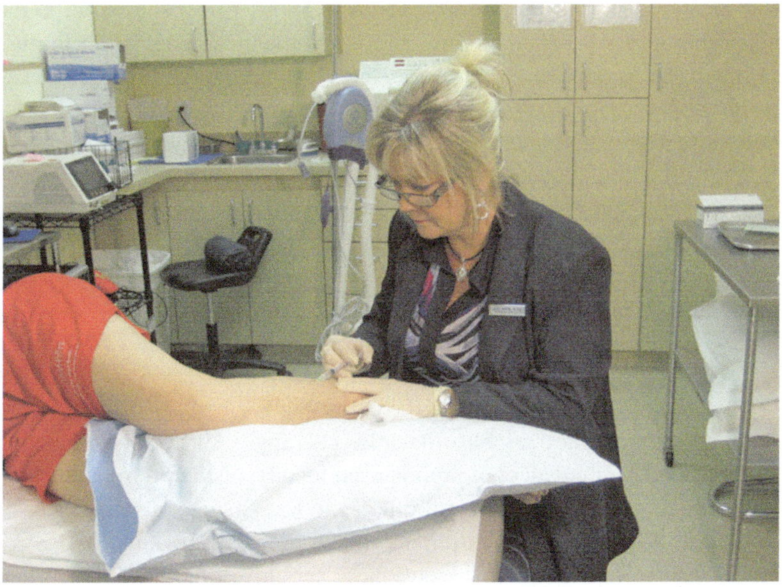

Fig. 11.1 Relative position of patient and sclerotherapist when done efficiently

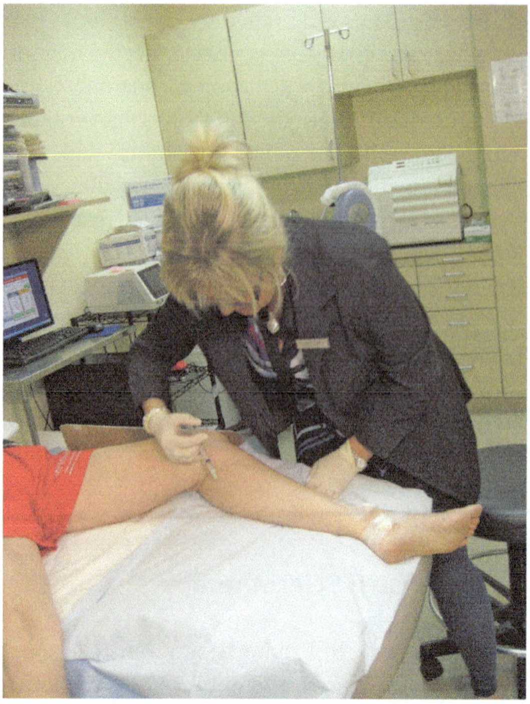

Fig. 11.2 Example of a poor ergonomic position

kept cool, a blanket over, or heating pad under, the patient will allow for patient comfort and improve vein visibility. For the sclerotherapist, adjustable chair height will help save muscle and joint strain during a long day of patient treatment. The sclerotherapist should attempt to achieve the most ergonomically optimal position (note sclerotherapist's position in Fig. 11.1) in order to maximize successful access to as many veins as possible. It is unlikely the sclerotherapist will "hit" every vein, no matter how skilled, but a sitting position that allows for relaxed large muscle groups will greatly enhance the function of fine muscle groups, which in turn will lead to more successfully injected veins. Starting with poor ergonomic positions (Fig. 11.2) will limit one's ability to inject veins successfully and lead to suboptimal results.

In some practices, the skin of the entire leg is prepped with alcohol prior to the sclerotherapy session; in others, an alcohol prep is used locally before each injection; and in still others, no prep is used at all. Infection is extremely uncommon following sclerotherapy, so practitioners should decide with which method they are most comfortable. According to infectious disease specialists, patients with foreign body implants, or those with underlying medical conditions that require antibiotic prophylaxis prior to invasive surgery or dental work, do not need such treatment prior to sclerotherapy.

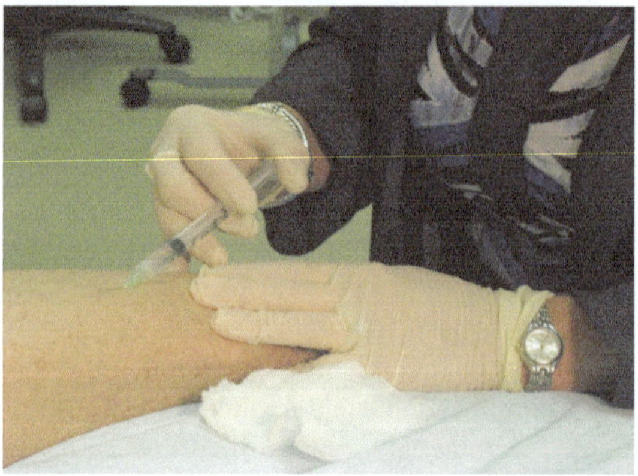

Fig. 11.3 To facilitate injections, along with stretching of the skin, a small gauge needle, such as 30–33 gauge, may be angled to augment access that is near parallel rather than perpendicular

To facilitate injections, along with stretching of the skin, a small gauge needle, such as 30–33 gauge, may be angled to augment access that is near parallel rather than perpendicular (Fig. 11.3). In order to limit side effects of telangiectatic matting and hyperpigmentation, it is generally considered better to make numerous injections using small volumes of sclerosant in larger syringes so the pressure generated is low (e.g., it is possible to generate much greater pressure with a TB syringe than a 3 or 5 mL syringe). Limiting each injection treatment area to 2–4 cm^2 may also reduce matting and hyperpigmentation.

11.4 From Liquid to Foam Sclerotherapy

Ultrasound-guided liquid sclerotherapy is considered by many to be ineffective in causing permanent vein sclerosis in large veins [7]. However, utilization of foam for large truncal veins has fundamentally changed conventional wisdom regarding successful chemical ablation of saphenous and large tributary veins. Good mid-term results have been reported following duplex-guided chemical ablation using foamed detergent sclerosants, compared to results from thermal and surgical ablation [8–10].

Foaming a detergent sclerosing agent changes the biological activity of the drug. While most would consider foaming a sclerosant to be an "off-label" use of an approved sclerosant, the drug in its foam form could be considered by regulatory agencies as unapproved. Of more practical importance is that a foamed sclerosant is much more potent than in liquid form, requiring less volume and concentration than in liquid form to successfully achieve vein sclerosis [11–13].

Side effects and complications of foam injection include sequestered coagulum, hyperpigmentation, telangiectatic matting, headache, visual disturbances, chest discomfort, and changes in neurologic or mental status [14].

11.4.1 Methods of Foam Production

Foam is produced by agitating a gas with a liquid detergent sclerosing agent, most commonly via a straight connector (Fig. 11.4) or three-way tap (Fig. 11.5), between two syringes containing the ratio of four parts gas to one part liquid, described by Tessari in 2000 [15]. Twenty to forty agitation cycles will produce durable microbubble foam.

Foam produced for injection should be durable enough to allow adequate time for injection of the microbubbles but should also break down

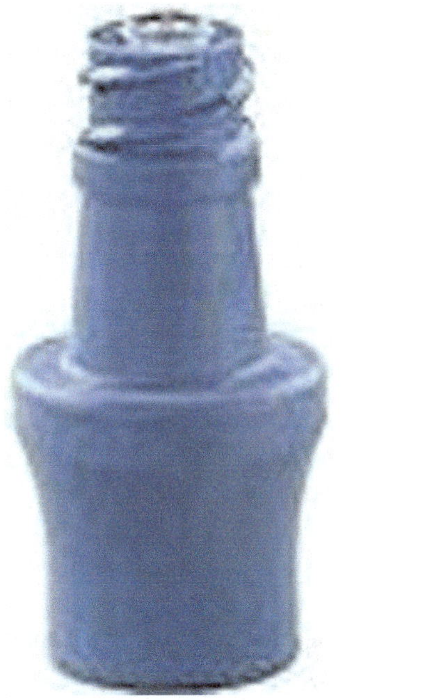

Fig. 11.4 Example of a straight connector

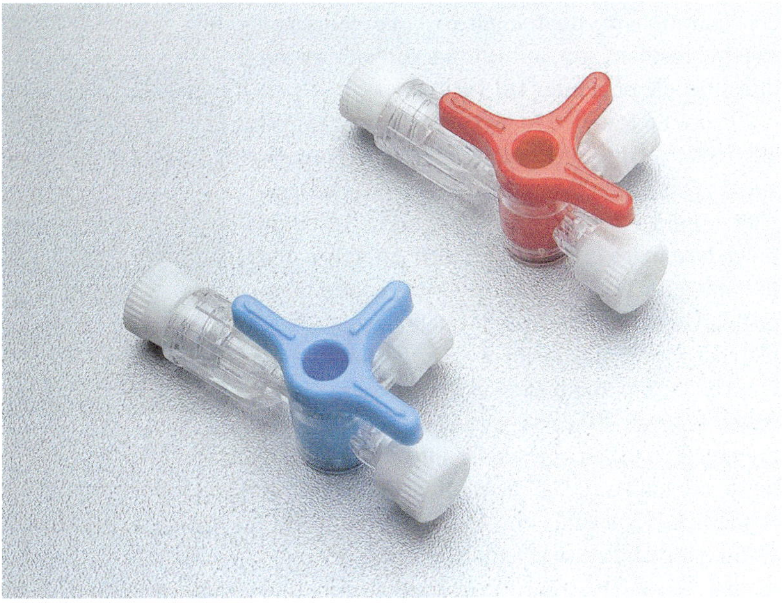

Fig. 11.5 Example of a three-way tap

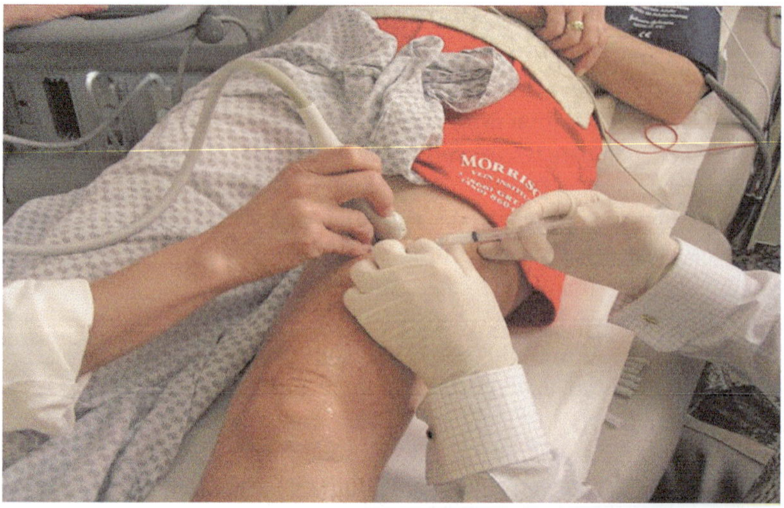

Fig. 11.6 For the direct needle injection method, however, enlisting the help of an assistant or sonographer is useful

quickly once injected to reduce the effects of gas embolization. Sterile or room air has been most commonly employed, but a more biocompatible gas such as carbon dioxide (CO_2) or a gas combining carbon dioxide and oxygen (O_2) may lead to fewer side effects due to greater solubility and less in vivo stability than air (limited gas embolization) [16–18].

The detergents used to create foam for sclerosis are sodium morrhuate, ethanolamine oleate, sodium tetradecyl sulfate (STS), and polidocanol, though most phlebologists utilize either polidocanol or STS. Foam can be prepared in various concentrations to treat small or large veins and can be instilled via indwelling catheter or by direct needle puncture [18, 19].

Ultrasound-guided foam sclerotherapy is usually performed by the practitioner alone, but the aid of an assistant to generate foam or a sonographer to image the target vein may make the entire procedure more efficient and time-effective. For the indwelling catheter method, the sclerotherapist can easily produce high-quality (small bubble size) foam and inject it into the target vein quickly before foam degradation occurs (large bubbles, lower efficacy, greater risk of adverse events). For the direct needle injection method, however, enlisting the help of an assistant or sonographer is useful (Fig. 11.6).

Imaging of the target vein may be in the longitudinal view (Fig. 11.7) or transverse view (Fig. 11.8). With the direct needle injection method, a transversely imaged target vein will make access easier. But for the catheter method, the longitudinal view may be more advantageous for cannulation. In Fig. 11.9 we see the technique

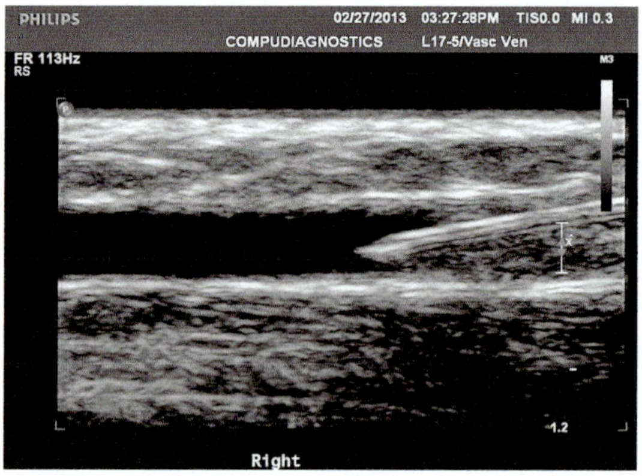

Fig. 11.7 Longitudinal view of target vein

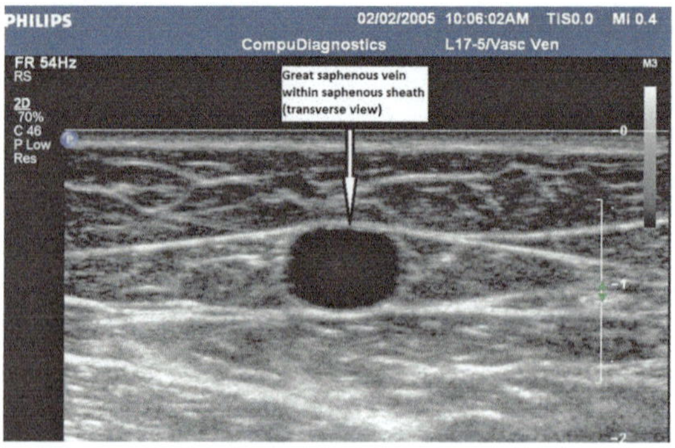

Fig. 11.8 Transverse view of target vein

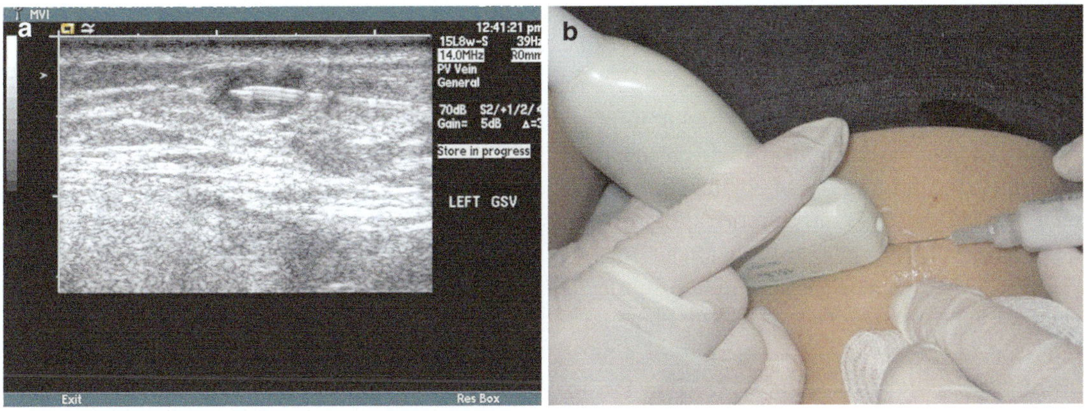

Fig. 11.9 Advancing the needle along the long axis of the ultrasound probe. (**a**) ultrasound image of needle course into target vein and (**b**) visual image of injection technique

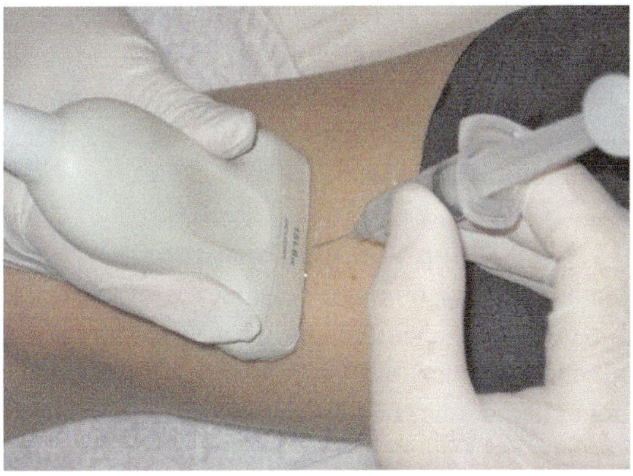

Fig. 11.10 Inserting the needle along the short axis of the ultrasound probe

of advancing the needle or catheter along the long axis of the ultrasound probe so that the needle is visualized all the way from the skin insertion site to the target vein. This is different than the "triangulation" technique typically favored by radiologists, wherein the needle is inserted along the short axis of the probe allowing visualization of the tip only when it arrives at the target vein (Fig. 11.10).

The volume of foam injected at each site is determined by the size of the treatment vein and the volume required to replace blood in the vein with foam but is usually limited to 0.5–3 mL. The total volume of foam used per treatment session is the subject of debate, as little data has been published regarding the volume of foam necessary to achieve successful vein sclerosis while limiting side effects. The upper limit of foam is generally considered to be 10 mL when utilizing air-based foam, while there is evidence that the use of biocompatible gas to produce foam allows for higher volumes to be injected safely [16, 20].

11.4.2 Efficacy of Foam Sclerotherapy

Efficacy trials have been conducted internationally [8, 21–26]. Successful ablation has been reported to range from 68 to 100 %, with follow-up from 1 month to 10 years, though interpretation of these results is difficult because of the differences in definitions of success, the use of surrogate markers (occlusion or narrowing of the treated vein, resolution of reflux), differing primary outcome markers (resolution of symptoms, improved quality of life scores, recurrent varices, ulcer healing), and the number of ultrasound-guided foam sclerotherapy sessions needed to achieve success, among others. Recently a consensus document has been published under the auspices of the Union Internationale de Phlebologie (UIP) in an attempt to standardize duplex reporting following treatment of lower extremity venous disorders [27].

It is also important to state that simply creating thrombosis of a target vein will likely not result in permanent occlusion of the vein. Damage to or destruction of the vein wall is necessary to ensure sclerosis [28]. It may be necessary to produce injury through the intimal layer into the media in order to achieve the desired destruction [29].

11.4.3 Methods to Improve Foam Sclerotherapy Efficacy

Various methods have been proposed to improve efficacy: agitation methods which enhance the durability and uniformity of foam [18, 30, 31], increased sclerosant concentration [22] or volume used [22, 32], indwelling catheter method [18, 33], foam production methods resulting in smallest bubble size possible [18], and leg elevation (for "empty vein") [34]. In spite of a number of well-conducted studies [22, 25, 35, 36] in a review of the published and unpublished data available in the world literature, Jia et al. [14] concluded that there exists insufficient data to determine the optimal volume of foam, optimal concentration, and optimal foam-producing method.

Recently, a method of catheter-directed foam sclerotherapy utilizing ultrasound-guided perivenous tumescent injection has gained interest for reported better efficacy [18, 33].

By increasing the direct contact of the sclerosing agent with the endothelium, foam production methods that create microbubbles of smaller size may add to the efficacy: first, by displacing blood as much as possible from the targeted vein and second, by greatly increasing the total surface area of the smaller bubbles to which the active sclerosant is attached, thereby increasing endothelial contact [23, 37, 38].

For similar reasons, leg elevation prior to the injection will also help clear blood from the vein, thus allowing greater sclerosant contact with the endothelium and less sclerosant mixing with and deactivation by blood.

11.4.4 Safety of Foam Sclerotherapy

Early reports regarding UGFS did not study safety aspects beyond local tissue reactions or venous thrombosis. Primarily because of concern about neurosensory adverse reactions following UGFS [39, 40], more recent reports have looked at such concerns more closely [16, 41–44]. Minor or major complications following foam sclerotherapy have almost uniformly been very limited in incidence and in duration [62]. The practitioner needs to be aware of these risks and their management in order to discuss risk-benefit decisions with patients regarding the use of UGFS.

Table 11.1 A list of side effects and adverse events reported to be associated with UGFS

Deep venous thrombosis (DVT)
Superficial thrombophlebitis (STP)
Localized perivenous tissue injury
Paradoxical embolism
Neurosensory effects
Respiratory effects

UGFS may have the potential for pulmonary, visual, and/or cerebral effects, particularly in a patient with a patent foramen ovale, or other right-to-left shunt, which may be more common in patients with varicose veins than in the general population [45] (Table 11.1).

11.4.4.1 Deep Venous Thrombosis

Data is lacking on the true incidence of DVT following liquid sclerotherapy. There appears to be a higher incidence of DVT following UGFS than is generally assumed following the use of liquid sclerosants, especially in foam sclerotherapy studies wherein patients are routinely examined for DVT by duplex scanning as opposed to duplex scanning only when warranted by symptoms [9, 22]

However, these thromboses most often involve calf veins that, if followed closely, are most often of limited clinical significance. Symptomatic or femoral-popliteal DVT remain rare, except in the smaller diameter duplicated femoral vein segment [46] or in Myers' study, veins larger than 5 mm in diameter [47]. There is conflicting in vitro evidence regarding sclerosant foam effect on coagulation [48, 49] and in vivo as well [50]. In the clinical setting, however, Hamel-Desnos has presented evidence that mirrors the author's experience: foam sclerotherapy can be successfully and safely performed on patients with documented thrombophilia with no increased risk of DVT, given prophylactic anticoagulation [51].

11.4.4.2 Superficial Thrombophlebitis

Superficial thrombophlebitis probably should be considered a direct consequence of treatment, unless thrombophlebitis extends beyond the region treated or if the inflammation is significantly worse than routinely observed. The incidence varies from less than 1–18 % in the literature probably because of individual interpretation of the clinical findings [52].

11.4.4.3 Perivenous Tissue Injury

Extravascular tissue injury with the use of UGFS has been reported to be less than 2 % likely because of the benign effects of foam extravasated in the perivenous tissue (significantly lower concentration). This is in contrast to the more damaging effects of some liquid sclerosants (typically three to four times the concentration of foam).

11.4.4.4 Paradoxical Embolism

A right-to-left shunt, present in 25–30 % of the general population, and perhaps even higher in patients with varicose veins [45], may allow emboli or degradation products released from damaged endothelium to pass to the arterial circulation and affect the microcirculation of any organ. Whether symptoms are related to particulate or bubble emboli or to endothelial destruction products (such as endothelin-1, a potent vasoconstrictor) is currently under investigation. What is known is that UGFS has the potential for nearly always rare and transient pulmonary, cardiac, visual, and/or cerebral effects, particularly in a patient with a patent foramen ovale or other right-to-left shunt.

A rare complication, thromboembolism has also been reported following UGFS when either a thrombus forms in and embolizes from a deep vein or a thrombus extension from a truncal or perforator vein embolizes. In the presence of a right-to-left shunt, the embolus can progress to the arterial circulation with variable sequelae depending on the location of the embolus.

11.4.4.5 Neurosensory Effects

Reports of significant adverse neurologic events are very few. Forlee et al. reported one case of stroke following varicose vein foam injection sclerotherapy [40]. The patient was subsequently found to have a very large patent foramen ovale. Also reporting neurologic events in patients, Ceulen et al. [39], Bush and colleagues [53], and Ma and Parsi [54] have also reported neurologic events in patients. Because of numerous anecdotal reports of similar events, the true incidence may not be as rare as is reported. The question could be whether all patients should be screened for right-to-left shunt prior to UGFS. The consensus opinion of international experts [55] is that these uncommon neurosensory effects do not justify such pre-sclerotherapy screening, since similar serious incidents have occurred following liquid sclerotherapy, thermal ablation, or surgical stripping [56–58].

It is imperative, however, that the practicing phlebologist has protocols to deal with such serious adverse events should one occur.

Transient visual disturbances, or scotomas, have been mentioned when evaluating adverse events following foam sclerotherapy. Frequencies of occurrence vary from 0 to 6 % following air-based foam injection, with most publications indicating a frequency around 1 % [14, 59]. Other events have been described in the literature. True migraine or ocular migraine is uncommon, but Gillet and colleagues found in a study of 20 patients with visual disturbances following UGFS that clinical features of migraine with aura were present in all patients, suggesting a strong association between visual disturbances following UGFS and migraine [60]. Since it has been established that twice as many patients (50 %) with a history of migraine with aura have right-to-left shunts as is seen in the normal population (25 %) [6, 61], it may be reasonable to expect that patients with a history of migraine with aura have an increased risk of suffering neurosensory events following UGFS.

11.4.4.6 Respiratory Effects

Acute respiratory difficulties are rarely reported in the literature but may be commonly seen in phlebologic practice. Chest tightness, transient shortness of breath, and dry cough have been described as uncommon or rare adverse events, but all appear self-limited [16].

11.4.4.7 Long-Term Effects: Pulmonary, CNS, Visual

Long-term adverse pulmonary effects such as pulmonary fibrosis are of theoretical concern but have not been identified. Such side effects have also been reported with liquid sclerosants. Pulmonary embolism is a concern, but its occurrence is rare and may relate more to other patient conditions than to the procedure itself [20, 63].

11.4.5 Foam Sclerotherapy: Methods to Improve Safety

Several methods have been proposed to improve the safety of foam sclerotherapy (Table 11.2).

The use of an indwelling catheter is thought to improve safety of UGFS by minimizing extravasation of foam (as seen with direct needle injection) and by allowing for immediate instillation of foam following production in order to deliver the highest quality of foam possible (no lag time between foam production and instillation as with direct needle injection) [64, 65].

Table 11.2 Proposed methods for improved safety

Indwelling catheter (balloon-tipped or open-ended)
Saphenofemoral junction occlusion
Limitations of volume
Low-silicone syringe
Non-air-based foam
Maneuvers to limit or prevent foam migration

When performing UGFS, a balloon-tipped catheter can be used to occlude the saphenofemoral or saphenopopliteal junction, theoretically preventing foam from entering the deep venous system. However, it has been shown [66–68] by ultrasound examination that foam is still seen in the deep system as having moved through myriad perforator veins. In fact, many phlebologists believe it is better to have foam gradually migrating into the deep venous system than to have a large bolus enter the central circulation when the occlusive balloon is deflated.

Limiting the volume of foamed sclerosant injected at any one time has been proposed as a method to minimize the risk of symptomatic bubble embolization [55, 69]. However, in studies of foam sclerotherapy with simultaneous monitoring using transthoracic echocardiography and transcranial Doppler, the author has shown that the use of even very small volumes of foam does not prevent foam migration to the central venous circulation or across a PFO (Fig. 11.11) [70].

It is presumed that the use of low-silicone syringes enhances foam stability, because silicone helps speed foam degradation. Thus, foam will remain of good quality longer with silicone-free or low-silicone syringes, allowing for more time to complete a successful injection [18, 30].

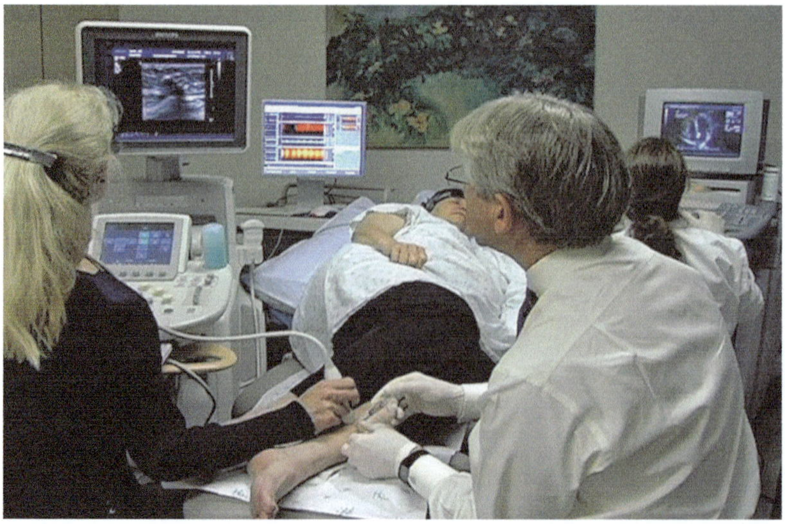

Fig. 11.11 In studies of foam sclerotherapy with simultaneous monitoring using transthoracic echocardiography and transcranial Doppler, the use of even very small volumes of foam does not prevent foam migration to the central venous circulation or across a PFO

The type of gas used to create the foam will also influence foam degradation. Tessari has shown that a gas combination of CO_2 and O_2 with 70 % CO_2 and 30 % O_2 to produce foam will result in more stable, longer-lasting foam than pure CO_2-based foam [71]. Because of its presumably more rapid dissolution, CO_2/O_2-based foam (70 % CO_2/30 % O_2 combination) has been shown by the author to be 7 and 40 times less likely, respectively, to produce side effects or complications compared to pure CO_2-based foam and air-based foam [44].

Maneuvers such as preinjection and/or postinjection leg elevation and limiting patient mobility for a few minutes immediately after injection were found to be ineffective in eliminating foam migration into the central circulation or, for that matter the arterial circulation in the presence of a right-to-left shunt [17].

However, in a study of a proprietary manufactured foam injected into patients with known right-to-left shunts, Regan et al. [42] noted no cardiac, neurologic, or visual field changes in patients undergoing foam sclerotherapy. It is uncertain whether to assume the findings of this study of a proprietary manufactured foam are similar for "home-made" foam used by most phlebologists. But the lack of evidence for serious long-term adverse events in spite of the huge worldwide experience with self-manufactured foam is reassuring [72].

11.5 Postoperative Care

Although Level 1 evidence for the use of postoperative compression is lacking, compression and early ambulation are regarded by many phlebologists as the cornerstones of successful postoperative management, no matter which modality of truncal vein ablation is chosen. Extrinsic compression using foam padding, short stretch and/or elastic bandages, compression hose, and early ambulation and return to normal activities all will likely help to minimize postoperative discomfort and avoid complications, such as deep venous thrombosis.

Conclusion

All published reports support UGFS as a reasonably safe method of superficial venous ablation. Efficacy, simplicity, economy, and serial applications have made UGFS an attractive and efficient treatment option. Side effects and complications of UGFS are nearly always transient and infrequent or rare. Evaluations of the use of foam sclerotherapy are ongoing and likely will result in more refined evidence-based guidelines that will address its indications and methods to enhance efficacy and ensure safety. Most investigators agree on the need for adequate training in this technique to reduce the risk of complications.

Acknowledgements The author gratefully acknowledges the contribution of Diana Neuhardt, RVT, of Compudiagnostics for her clinical assistance and provision of the excellent duplex images in this manuscript, as well as editing assistance provided by Adrienne Travis and Denise Bork.

References

1. Goldman MP. Sodium tetradecyl sulfate for sclerotherapy treatment of veins: is compounding pharmacy solution safe? Dermatol Surg. 2004;30:1–3.
2. Weiss R, et al. Absence of concentration congruity in six compounded polidocanol samples obtained for leg sclerotherapy. Dermatol Surg. 2011;37:812–5.
3. Yamaki T, Nozaki M, Sasaki K. Color duplex-guided sclerotherapy for the treatment of venous malformation. Dermatol Surg. 2000;26:323–8.
4. Ricci S, Georgiev M, Jawien A, Zamboni P. Sciatic nerve varices. Eur J Vasc Endovasc Surg. 2005; 29:83–7.
5. Tessari L. Foam Sclerotherapy Alcock Channel (P point) in pelvic varicose veins. In: 14th annual congress, Melbourne, Australia. Australasian College of Phlebology. 2011.
6. Carod-Artal FJ, et al. Prevalence of patent foramen ovale in migraine patients with and without aura compared with stroke patients. A transcranial Doppler study. Cephalalgia. 2006;26:934–9.
7. Ouvrey P, et al. Efficacy of polidocanol foam versus liquid in sclerotherapy of the great saphenous vein: a multicentre randomised controlled trial with a two-year follow up. Eur J Vasc Endovasc Surg. 2008;36(3):366–70.
8. Rabe E, Otto J, Schliephake D, Pannier F. Efficacy and safety of great saphenous vein sclerotherapy using standardised polidocanol foam (ESAF): a ran-

domised controlled multicentre clinical trial. Eur J Vasc Endovasc Surg. 2008;35:238–45.
9. Wright D, Gobin JP, Bradbury AW, et al. Varisolve® polidocanol microfoam compared with surgery or sclerotherapy in the management of varicose veins in the presence of trunk vein incompetence: European randomized controlled trial. Phlebology. 2006;21:180–90.
10. Rasmussen L, et al. Randomized clinical trial comparing endovenous laser ablation, radiofrequency ablation, foam sclerotherapy and surgical stripping for great saphenous varicose veins. Br J Surg. 2011;98: 1079–87.
11. Hamel-Desnos C, Desnos P, Wollmann JC, Ouvry P, Mako S, Allaert FA. Evaluation of the efficacy of polidocanol in the form of foam compared with liquid form in sclerotherapy of the greater saphenous vein: initial results. Dermatol Surg. 2003;19(12):1170–5.
12. Coleridge Smith P. Saphenous ablation: sclerosant or sclerofoam? Semin Vasc Surg. 2005;18(1):19–24.
13. Yamaki T, Nozaki M, Iwasaka S. Comparative study of duplex-guided foam sclerotherapy and duplex-guided liquid sclerotherapy for the treatment of superficial venous insufficiency. Dermatol Surg. 2004;30:718–22.
14. Jia X, Mowat G, Burr JM, Cassar K, Cook J, Fraser C. Systematic review of foam sclerotherapy for varicose veins. Br J Surg. 2007;94:925–36.
15. Tessari L. Nouvelle technique d'obtention de la sclero-mousse. Phlebologie. 2000;53:129.
16. Morrison N, Neuhardt DL, Rogers CR, McEown J, Morrison T, Johnson E, Salles-Cunha SX. Comparisons of side effects using air and carbon dioxide foam for endovenous chemical ablation. J Vasc Surg. 2008;47:830–6.
17. Morrison N. Foam sclerotherapy: how to improve results and reduced side effects. Phlebologie. 2008; 37:211–20.
18. Cavezzi A, Tessari L. Foam sclerotherapy techniques: different gases and methods of preparation, catheter versus direct injection. Phlebology. 2009;24:247–51.
19. Hamel-Desnos C, et al. Échosclerotherapie a la Mouse par Ponction-Injection Directe aL'Aiguille: Technique et Doses. J Mal Vasc. 2006;31(4):180–9.
20. Cabrera J, Cabrera Jr J, Garcia-Olmedo MA, Redondo P. Treatment of venous malformations with sclerosant in microfoam form. Arch Dermatol. 2003; 139:1409–16.
21. Cabrera J, Cabrera Jr J, Garcia-Olmedo MA. Treatment of varicose long saphenous veins with sclerosant in microfoam form: long term outcomes. Phlebology. 2000;15:19–23.
22. Myers KA, Jolley D, Clough A, Kirwan J. Outcome of ultrasound-guided sclerotherapy for varicose veins: medium-term results assessed by ultrasound surveillance. Eur J Vasc Endovasc Surg. 2007;33:116–21.
23. Frullini A, Cavezzi A. Sclerosing foam in the treatment of varicose veins and telangiectasias: history and analysis of safety and complications. Dermatol Surg. 2002;28:11–5.
24. Smith PC. Chronic venous disease treated by ultrasound guided foam sclerotherapy. Eur J Vasc Endovasc Surg. 2006;32:577–83.
25. Darvall K, et al. Duplex ultrasound outcomes following ultrasound-guided foam sclerotherapy of symptomatic primary great saphenous varicose veins. Eur J Vasc Endovasc Surg. 2010;40:534–9.
26. Stucker M, et al. Review of published information on foam sclerotherapy. Dermatol Surg. 2010;36:983–92.
27. De Maeseneer M, Pichot O, Cavezzi A, Earnshaw J, van Rij A, Lurie F, Coleridge Smith P. Duplex ultrasound investigation of the veins of the lower limbs after treatment for varicose veins – UIP consensus document. Eur J Vasc Endovasc Surg. 2011;42(1):89–102.
28. Fegan WG. Injection with compression as a treatment for varicose veins. Proc R Soc Med. 1965;58:874–6.
29. McAree B, et al. Comparative stability of sodium tetradecyl sulphate (STD) and polidocanol foam: impact on vein damage in an in-vitro model. Eur J Vasc Endovasc Surg 2012;43:721–725.
30. Wollman JC. Sclerosant foams: stabilities, physical properties and rheological behavior. Phlebologie. 2010;39:208–17.
31. Eckmann DM, Kobayashi S, Li M. Microvascular embolization following polidocanol microfoam sclerosant administration. Dermatol Surg. 2005;31: 636–64.
32. Bhogal RH, et al. Can foam sclerotherapy be used to safely treat bilateral varicose veins? Phlebology. 2012;27(1):19–24..
33. Parsi K. Catheter-directed sclerotherapy. Phlebology. 2009;24:98–107.
34. Bergan J, Pascarella L, Mekenas L. Venous disorders: treatment with sclerosant foam. J Cardiovasc Surg (Torino). 2006;47:9–18.
35. Hamel-Desnos C, Ouvry P, Benigni J-P, Boitelle G, Schadeck M, Desnos P, Allaert F-A. Comparison of 1 % and 3 % polidocanol foam in ultrasound guided sclerotherapy of the great saphenous vein: a randomised, double-blind trial with 2 year-follow-up. "The 3/1 study". Eur J Vasc Endovasc Surg. 2007; 20:1–7.
36. Ceulen RP, Bullens-Goessens YI, Pi-VAN de Venne SJ, Nelemans PJ, Veraart JC, Sommer A. Outcomes and side effects of duplex-guided sclerotherapy in the treatment of great saphenous veins with 1 % versus 3 % polidocanol foam: results of a randomized controlled trial with 1-year follow-up. Dermatol Surg. 2007;33:276–81.
37. Wollman JC. The history of sclerosing foams. Dermatol Surg. 2004;30:694–703.
38. Van Deurzen B, Ceulen R, et al. Polidocanol concentration and time affect the properties of foam used for sclerotherapy. Dermatol Surg. 2011;37:1448–55.
39. Ceulen R, et al. Microembolism during foam sclerotherapy of varicose veins. N Engl J Med. 2008; 35:8–14.
40. Forlee MV, Grouden M, Moore DJ, Shanik G. Stroke after varicose vein foam injection sclerotherapy. J Vasc Surg. 2006;43:162–4.

41. Guex JJ, et al. The French polidocanol study on long-term side effects: a survey covering 3,357 patient years. Dermatol Surg. 2010;36:993–1003.
42. Regan J, et al. Clinical significance of cerebrovascular gas emboli during polidocanol endovenous ultra-low nitrogen microfoam ablation and correlation with magnetic resonance imaging in patients with right-to-left shunts. J Vasc Surg. 2011;53:131–8.
43. Gillet J-L, et al. Side-effects and complications of foam sclerotherapy of the great and small saphenous veins: a controlled multicentre prospective study including 1025 patients. Phlebology. 2009;24:131–8.
44. Morrison N, et al. Incidence of side effects using carbon dioxide-oxygen foam for chemical ablation of superficial veins of the lower extremity. Eur J Vasc Endovasc Surg. 2010;40:407–13.
45. Wright DD. High prevalence of right-to-left shunt in patients with symptomatic great saphenous incompetence and varicose veins. J Vasc Surg. 2010;51:104–7.
46. Neuhardt D. Incidence of deep vein thrombosis in a duplicated femoral vein following Foam USG of the GSV. Abstract: first days of phlebology. Parma. 2006.
47. Myers K, Jolley D. Factors affecting the risk of deep venous occlusion after ultrasound-guided sclerotherapy for varicose veins. Eur J Vasc Endovasc Surg. 2008;20:1–4.
48. Parsi K, et al. In vitro effects of detergent sclerosants on coagulation, platelets and microparticles. Eur J Vasc Endovasc Surg. 2007;34:731–40.
49. Parsi K, et al. The lytic effects of detergent sclerosants on erythrocytes, platelets, endothelial cells and microparticles are attenuated by albumin and other plasma components in vitro. Eur J Vasc Endovasc Surg. 2008;36:216–23.
50. Hamel-Desnos C, Desnos P, et al. In vivo biological effects of foam sclerotherapy. Eur J Vasc Endovasc Surg. 2011;42(2):238–45.
51. Hamel-Desnos C, Gillet J-L, Desnos P, Allaert F. Sclerotherapy of varicose veins in patients with documented thrombophilia: a prospective controlled randomized study of 105 cases. Phlebology. 2009;24:176–82.
52. Thomasset SC, et al. Ultrasound guided foam sclerotherapy: factors associated with outcomes and complications. Eur J Vasc Endovasc Surg. 2010;40:389–92.
53. Bush RG, Derrick M, Manjoney D. Major neurological events following foam sclerotherapy. Phlebology. 2008;23:189–92.
54. Ma RWL, Parsi K, et al. Three cases of stroke following peripheral venous interventions. Phlebology 2011;26:280–4.
55. Breu FX, Guggenbichler S. 2nd European consensus meeting on foam sclerotherapy. Tegernsee, Germany. VASA. Eur J Vasc Med 2008;37:S37–71.
56. Hanisch F, Müller T, Krivokuca M, Winterholler W. Stroke following variceal sclerotherapy. Eur J Med Res. 2004;9:282–4.
57. Caggiati A, Franceschini M. Stroke following endovenous laser treatment of varicose veins. J Vasc Surg. 2010;51:218–20.
58. Harzheim M, Becher H, Klockgether T. Brain infarct from a paradoxical embolism following a varices operation. Dtsch Med Wochenschr. 2000;125:794–6.
59. Morrison N. Studies on safety of foam sclerotherapy. In: Bergan JJ, Chang V, editors. Foam sclerotherapy. London: Royal Society of Medicine Press Ltd; 2008.
60. Gillet JL, et al. Pathophysiology of visual disturbances occurring after foam sclerotherapy. Phlebology. 2010; 25:261–6.
61. McCandless RT, et al. Patent foramen ovale in children with migraine headaches. J Pediatr. 2011; 159(2):243–7.
62. Bradbury A, et al. Ultrasound-guided foam sclerotherapy is a safe and clinically effective treatment for superficial venous reflux. J Vasc Surg. 2010; 52(4):939–45.
63. Wright D, et al. Polidocanol microfoam does not cause remote sclerosis in the lung. Poster presentation: ACP 23rd annual congress. Palm Desert. Nov 2008.
64. Broderson JP, Geismar U. Catheter-assisted vein sclerotherapy: a new approach for sclerotherapy of the greater saphenous vein with a double-lumen balloon catheter. Dermatol Surg. 2007;33:469–75.
65. Kolbeln T, Hinchliffe R, Lindbladn B. Catheter-directed foam sclerotherapy of axial saphenous reflux: early results. Phlebology. 2007;22:219–22.
66. Parsi K. Venous gas embolism during foam sclerotherapy of saphenous veins despite recommended treatment modifications. Phlebology. 2011;26:140–7.
67. Hill D, et al. Assessment of techniques to reduce sclerosant foam migration during ultrasound-guided sclerotherapy of the great saphenous vein. J Vasc Surg. 2008;48:934–9.
68. Ceulen R, et al. Blocking the saphenofemoral junction during ultrasound-guided foam sclerotherapy: assessment of a presumed safety-measure procedure. Eur J Vasc Endovasc Surg. 2010;40:772–6.
69. Yamaki T, et al. Multiple small-dose injections can reduce the passage of sclerosant foam into deep veins during foam sclerotherapy for varicose veins. Eur J Vasc Endovasc Surg. 2009;37(3):343–8.
70. Morrison N, Neuhardt D. Foam sclerotherapy: cardiac and cerebral monitoring. Phlebology. 2009;00:1–8.
71. Tessari L, Cavezzi A, Rosso M, Cabrera Garrido A. Variables in foam sclerotherapy: literature and experimental data. Aust NZ J Phlebol. 2008;11(1):83–4.
72. Gillet J-L. Neurological complications of foam sclerotherapy: fears and reality. Phlebology. 2011; 26:277–9.

Surgical Techniques 12

Marc A. Passman

Contents

M.A. Passman, MD
Section of Vascular Surgery and Endovascular Therapy, University of Alabama at Birmingham, Birmingham, AL, USA
e-mail: marc.passman@ccc.uab.edu

Abstract

Coordinated treatment of superficial venous insufficiency involves comprehensive patient evaluation, appropriate venous testing usually with venous ultrasound as the cornerstone of diagnostic evaluation, and sound clinical decision making based on current evidence-based guidelines. While nonoperative measures focusing on compression are recommended as initial therapy, operative approaches offer additional opportunity for improved outcomes. As treatment options are shifting to less invasive options, traditional open operative approaches directed at both axial saphenous vein reflux and varicose vein problems still have a role in appropriately selected patients with symptomatic superficial venous insufficiency. This chapter discusses surgical techniques for venous disease.

12.1 Introduction

Superficial venous insufficiency involves incompetence of the great saphenous vein (GSV), small saphenous vein (SSV), and associated patterns of secondary varicose veins. Within the superficial venous system, there is also the potential for primary varicose veins without associated axial or segmental reflux, dilated reticular veins, and venous telangiectases. Venous insufficiency can be isolated to the superficial venous system or can include concomitant deep (see Chap. 16) and perforator disease (see Chap. 14).

E. Mowatt-Larssen et al. (eds.), *Phlebology, Vein Surgery and Ultrasonography*,
DOI 10.1007/978-3-319-01812-6_12, © Springer International Publishing Switzerland 2014

The prevalence of all chronic venous insufficiency has varied in reports but may be as high as 40 % in women and 17 % in men. Active venous ulcers are present in up to 0.5 % of individuals, and between 0.6 and 1.4 % have healed ulcers. Estimates for varicose veins are even higher at 73 % in women and 56 % in men. For all patients with chronic venous insufficiency, those with isolated superficial venous reflux may involve up to 35 %. The age-matched distribution of venous insufficiency corresponding to these prevalence estimates has also translated to a financial burden to patients and society with lost productivity, employment issues, and disabilities. Fortunately, superficial venous insufficiency and associated problems are very amenable to surgical correction [1–4].

This chapter will review treatment of superficial venous insufficiency including patient evaluation, clinical decision making, nonoperative measures, traditional open operative approaches directed at axial saphenous vein reflux and thrombosis and varicose vein problems, outcomes, and current evidence-based guidelines.

12.2 Patient Evaluation

12.2.1 Indications

The most common complaints associated with superficial venous insufficiency and varicose veins are pain, aching, throbbing, heaviness, tingling, burning, cramping, itching, unsightliness, discoloration, tiredness, restlessness, and swelling of the extremity. Complaints are usually pronounced after prolonged limb dependency and relieved with rest or elevation, with further progression of symptoms more notable towards the end of the day. More severe symptoms and advanced venous problems, including chronic venous skin changes and progression to venous stasis ulcers, can occur with both isolated superficial venous insufficiency and deep or perforator venous incompetence. Other pertinent history should include prior personal or family history of venous thromboembolism, superficial thrombophlebitis, established thrombophilia, medication history (particularly oral contraceptives), smoking, pregnancies, family history of varicose veins, spontaneous rupture of varicosity, venous ulceration, and previous venous interventions. It is important to differentiate symptoms due to venous disease from other concomitant musculoskeletal, arterial, neuropathic, dermatologic, pelvic, or lymphatic etiologies.

12.2.2 Diagnostic Evaluation

Physical examination should be performed with the patient standing. On inspection, general position of telangiectases, dilated reticular veins, and varicose veins should be noted, with identification of location, anatomic pattern, size, and presence of inflammation. Documentation can be greatly assisted with handwritten diagrams, electronic drawing systems, or digital photography. Palpation is performed assessing for palpable cord, tenderness, induration, pulses, thrill, and groin or abdominal masses. Auscultation should identify any associated bruits. Evaluation of swelling components should include unilateral vs. bilateral, standardized limb measurements, distribution of edema across the entire extremity, and whether it is pitting or non-pitting, to differentiate lymphedema and other non-venous causes. Additional venous stigmata may include inframalleolar ankle flare, corona phlebectatica, and atrophie blanche. More advanced venous skin findings include hyperpigmentation, venous eczema, stasis dermatitis and other inflammatory changes, induration, lipodermatosclerosis, and healed or active venous ulcerations.

Bedside venous examinations such as Trendelenburg, Ochsner-Mahorner, or Perthes' tests, although occasionally useful, are often unreliable and have been largely replaced by diagnostic imaging. Venous duplex ultrasound is critically important to differentiate obstructive components, presence or absence of venous thrombosis, and competency of deep, superficial,

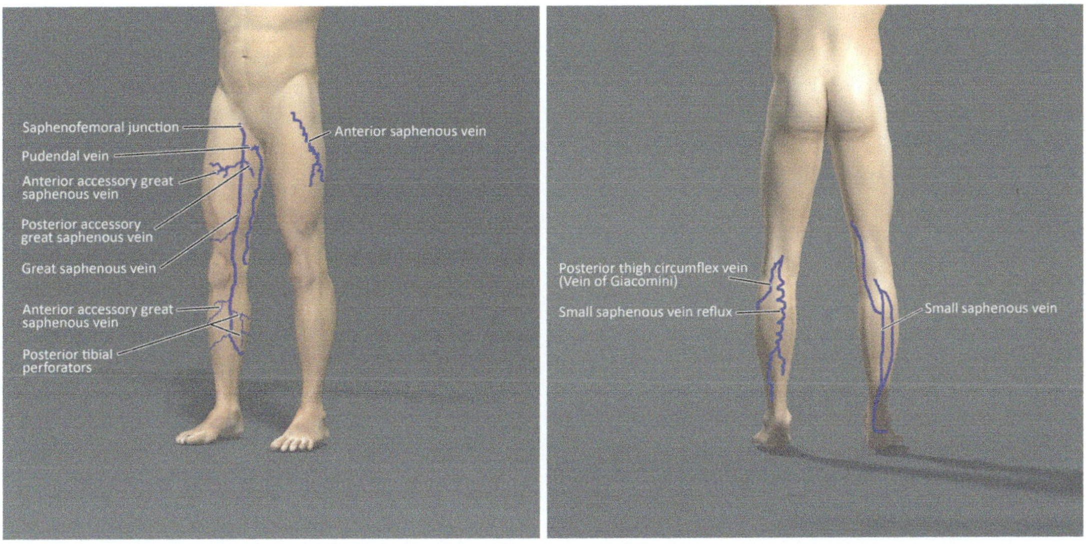

Fig. 12.1 Anatomic distribution of varicose veins and their relationship to documented source of superficial venous reflux, including the great saphenous vein, anterior saphenous vein, pudendal vein, small saphenous vein, and posterior thigh circumflex vein (vein of Giacomini)

and perforator venous systems (see Chap. 6). Identifying sources of reflux and association to clinical patterns of venous findings will help determine the best operative option (Fig. 12.1). Venous physiologic testing (see Chap. 8) and other imaging such as computed tomography (CT) venography, magnetic resonance (MR) venography, ascending and descending contrast venography, and intravascular ultrasound (see Chaps. 9 and 16) can be useful in selected cases when other venous problems beyond superficial venous insufficiency are a consideration, such as post-thrombotic syndrome, thrombotic or non-thrombotic iliac vein obstruction (May-Thurner syndrome), pelvic congestion syndrome, nutcracker syndrome, vascular malformations, venous trauma, or tumors.

12.3 Classification

Venous outcome assessment tools have been used to evaluate severity of venous disease, provide standardized evaluation of treatment effectiveness over time, and are important in objectively assessing effectiveness of superficial venous operations. Clinical, etiologic, anatomic, pathophysiologic (CEAP) classification system (Table 12.1) for chronic venous disease is widely accepted and allows patient comparison among different centers and studies but has been recognized to be relatively static and insensitive for determining changes in venous disease severity over time. Venous Severity Scoring (VSS) which includes Venous Disability Score (VDS), Venous Segmental Disease Score (VSDS), and Venous Clinical Severity Score (VCSS) has been shown to be more useful for comparing patient groups with similar degrees of severity in regard to outcome over time and following different therapies. The VCSS system includes 10 clinical descriptors (pain, varicose veins, venous edema, skin pigmentation, inflammation, induration, number of active ulcers, duration of active ulceration, size of ulcer, and compressive therapy use), scored from 0 to 3 (total possible score, 30) that may be used to assess changes in response to therapy (Table 12.2). VCSS, revised in 2010, has been shown to have minimal intraobserver and interobserver variability,

Table 12.1 Clinical, etiologic, anatomic, pathophysiologic (CEAP) classification system for chronic venous disease

Clinical classification	
C0	No visible or palpable signs of venous disease
C1	Telangiectases or reticular veins
C2	Varicose veins
C3	Edema
C4a	Pigmentation and/or eczema
C4b	Lipodermatosclerosis and/or atrophie blanche
C5	Healed venous ulcer
C6	Active venous ulcer
CS	Symptoms, including ache, pain, tightness, skin irritation, heaviness, muscle cramps, as well as other complaints attributable to venous dysfunction
CA	Asymptomatic
Etiologic classification	
Ec	Congenital
Ep	Primary
Es	Secondary (post-thrombotic)
En	No venous etiology identified
Anatomic classification	
As	Superficial veins
Ap	Perforator veins
Ad	Deep veins
An	No venous location identified
Pathophysiologic classification	
Pr	Reflux
Po	Obstruction
Pro	Reflux and obstruction
Pn	No venous pathophysiology identifiable

Adapted from: Eklöf et al. [2]

and there has been general acceptance and wide dissemination of VCSS for clinical and research purposes. Subjective and functional parameters are tested using venous quality-of-life disease-specific instruments such as the Chronic Venous Insufficiency Quality of Life (CIVIQ), the Venous Insufficiency Epidemiological and Economic Study (VEINES), the Aberdeen Varicose Vein Questionnaire, and the Charing Cross Venous Ulceration Questionnaire. Collectively, integration of all of these venous assessment tools in their appropriate clinical settings as a global venous screening instrument is important to use in all patients undergoing superficial venous operations both before and after treatment to assess effectiveness over time [1–8].

12.4 Clinical Decision Making

12.4.1 Failure of Nonoperative Measures

Lifestyle modifications including weight loss, leg elevation, elastic compression therapy, and exercise are generally recommended for patients with venous insufficiency, but compliance and effectiveness are difficult. Venoactive medications have also been used for the treatment of chronic venous insufficiency. While many medications have been tried, most success has been noted with horse chestnut seed extract (aescin), micronized purified flavonoid fraction (rutosides, diosmin, hesperidin), pine bark extract, and pentoxifylline. While most of these medications have been shown to improve venous tone and decrease capillary permeability leading to diminished symptoms from varicose veins, decreased inflammation and swelling, and improved ulcer healing, overall effectiveness has been variable. However, a recent Cochrane meta-analysis failed to show sufficient evidence to support global use of the venoactive medications in the treatment of chronic venous insufficiency. Compression is standard treatment for all patients with chronic venous insufficiency ranging from spider veins, varicose veins, venous edema, skin changes, and venous ulcerations, with most effectiveness seen in the later more advanced clinical classes. The goal of compression is to decrease venous reflux and improve calf muscle pump function, which has the net effect of decreasing ambulatory venous hypertension. Methods of compression include elastic graduated compression stockings for most patients with C1–3 disease, reserving paste gauze boots (Unna's boot), multilayered compression dressings, elastic and nonelastic bandages, and pneumatic compression devices for advanced C4–6 venous disease that is not controlled with standard compression stockings. While implementation of these nonoperative measures prior to surgical intervention for superficial venous disease is important, the requirement of failure of these measures by third-party payers is not supported by scientific evidence. Unfortunately, most insurance plans require a trial of nonoperative

Table 12.2 Revised Venous Clinical Severity Score (VCSS)

	None: 0	Mild: 1	Moderate: 2	Severe: 3
Pain or other discomfort (i.e., aching, heaviness, fatigue, soreness, burning); presumes venous origin	None	Occasional pain or other discomfort (i.e., not restricting regular daily activity)	Daily pain or other discomfort (i.e., interfering with but not preventing regular daily activities)	Daily pain or discomfort (i.e., limits most regular daily activities)
Varicose veins				
"Varicose" veins must be ≥3 mm in diameter to qualify m the standing position	None	Few: scattered (i.e., isolated branch variosities or clusters); also includes corona phlebectatica (ankle flare)	Confined to calf or thigh	Involves calf and thigh
Venous edema				
Presumes venous origin	None	Limited to foot and ankle area	Extends above ankle but below knee	Extends to knee and above
Skin pigmentation				
Presumes venous origin; does not include focal pigmentation over varicose veins or pigmentation due to other chronic diseases (i.e., vasculitis purpura)	None or focal	Limited to perimalleolar area	Diffuse over lower third of calf	Wider distribution above lower third of calf
Inflammation				
More than just recent pigmentation (i.e., erythema, cellulitis, venous eczema, dermatitis)	None	Limited to perimalleolar area	Diffuse over lower third of calf	Wider distribution above lower third of calf
Induration				
Presumes venous origin of secondary skin and subcutaneous changes (i.e., chronic edema with fibrosis, hypodermitis); includes white atrophy and lipodermatosclerosis	None	Limited to perimalleolar area	Diffuse over Lower third of calf	Wider distribution above lower third of calf
No. of active ulcers	0	1	2	≥3
Active ulcer duration (longest active)	NA	<3 months	>3 months but <1 year	Not healed for >1 year
Active ulcer size (largest active)	NA	Diameter <2 cm	Diameter 2–6 cm	Diameter >6 cm
Use of compression therapy	None: 0	Occasional: 1	Frequent: 2	Always: 3
	Not used	Intermittent use of stockings	Wears stockings most days	Full compliance; stockings

measures, including compression therapy, prior to providing coverage for superficial venous operations, and providers should work with patients and insurance carriers to most accurately represent medical justification for operative planning.

12.4.2 Clinical Severity

Based on clinical severity, there are several considerations that should be factored into the decision to perform superficial venous operations: (1) Patients with more symptoms, higher clinical CEAP (C4/5/6), or higher VCSS will have a higher potential symptomatic benefit; (2) larger varicose vein size and extensive varicose vein burden are less likely to resolve with isolated treatment of superficial axial venous reflux and may need additional therapy with either phlebectomy or sclerotherapy depending on the size, number, and distribution of residual varicosities; (3) patients with recurrent varicose veins after prior venous intervention may represent a more severe group in which more extensive treatment is required; (4) based on venous duplex ultrasound and additional plethysmography testing, patients who have more severe documented physiologic venous impairment would have expected higher margin of benefit and improvement in objective parameters; (5) stratifying patients with isolated superficial venous reflux vs. multilevel disease including deep and/or perforator venous insufficiency may have bearing on outcome, with extended venous treatment more often needed in the latter group; (6) patients with symptoms out of proportion to visualized infra-inguinal reflux, or obstruction, varicosities in the inguinal or peroneal areas, presence of venous stasis ulcer, or history of deep venous thrombosis extending to iliac veins may merit evaluation of the supra-inguinal system.

12.4.3 Patient Risk Factors

Preoperative risk assessment should include standard age stratification and associated medical issues, especially cardiac or pulmonary problems, neurologic status, and overall functional status. Venous risk factors such as personal or family history of venous thrombosis and pulmonary embolism may need to be balanced in terms of anticoagulation prophylaxis and risk of bleeding with planned intervention.

12.4.4 Anatomic Varicose Vein Distribution and Pattern

An important factor in preoperative planning is anatomic distribution of varicose veins and their relationship to documented source of superficial venous reflux: GSV reflux with medial thigh and calf varicosities, anterior accessory GSV reflux with anterior lateral thigh varicosities, pudendal vein reflux with medial posterior thigh varicosities, small saphenous vein reflux with posterior calf varicosities, and reflux in posterior thigh circumflex vein or the thigh extension of the SSV to the posterior accessory GSV, with posterior thigh varicosities (Fig. 12.1). If a direct source of superficial reflux can be identified, then initial treatment of the axial source of reflux may result in increased potential for regression or complete resolution of associated varicosities. However, if noted pattern of varicose vein distribution does not match source reflux, then improvement of varicosities after treatment of superficial axial reflux is less likely and further directed treatment of the varicosities will be required.

12.4.5 Staged vs. Combined Approaches

Based on review of evidence supporting combined or staged approaches for treatment of superficial venous insufficiency and associated varicose veins, definitive recommendations are difficult. A fundamental principle for approaches to superficial venous insufficiency, whether using a combined or staged approach, is elimination of all sources of venous reflux. While saphenous vein-based therapy is important in reducing venous hypertension, patient symptoms, and progression, proponents of combined approaches note that as a sole therapy, there is insufficient elimination of all varicose veins, incomplete reduction of all venous symptoms, higher potential for varicose vein recurrence, and additional frequent need for subsequent procedures. Proponents of a staged approach with saphenous-based treatment first followed by selected phlebectomy, only in those with persistent varicose vein problems, argue that most varicose veins will improve or regress with direct isolated treatment of the underlying saphenous venous reflux and that unnecessary extra surgery is being performed on a significant number of patients undergoing combined approaches. Furthermore, by selectively reserving additional phlebectomy only for those with persistent varicose veins, less invasive techniques like sclerotherapy or microphlebectomy may be used later on since prior varicosities may regress leaving less that may require subsequent treatment. While the global overview of evidence supports either approach as being acceptable, there are various factors that may make one approach preferred over the other in selected clinical scenarios based on clinical severity, risk profile, anatomic pattern, and patient preference, and providers should exercise best judgment in selection of either staged or combined approach on a case-by-case basis.

12.5 Operative Setting

While most thermal (see Chap. 10) and chemical (see Chap. 11) venous ablation procedures and ambulatory phlebectomy can be performed with local and tumescent anesthesia in an outpatient setting, saphenous division, traditional ligation and stripping, and transilluminated powered phlebectomy approaches require general or regional anesthesia in a standard operating room setting. If closer hemodynamic monitoring, airway protection, or bleeding control is needed, the capacity of operating room to handle higher-risk patients may also become a consideration. Furthermore, if general or regional anesthesia is required, then, from an anesthetic risk standpoint, it may be better to perform a more extensive superficial venous operation to avoid the need for multiple trips to the operating room. Ultimately, performing superficial venous operations in an outpatient ambulatory setting or operating room should be most importantly determined by the setting that is most appropriate and safest for the patient.

12.6 Patient Expectations

Patient preferences are important to factor into any decision to proceed with superficial venous operations. Engaging patients in a discussion regarding treatment alternatives, expected symptomatic improvement, postoperative recovery, compression, time off from work, potential complications, recurrence, cosmetic concerns, and potential financial burden should be done in an informed fashion and in an effort to realistically manage patient expectations. Helping patients make a balanced decision prior to superficial venous operations is critical to preventing dissatisfaction after operative intervention in what is sometimes considered a high maintenance patient group [1–8].

12.7 Operative Techniques

12.7.1 Great Saphenous Vein

High ligation and division refers to detachment of the GSV through a small oblique groin incision at its confluence with the saphenofemoral junction and common femoral vein. Incision is usually located along or just above the groin crease. Duplex ultrasound guidance can be used to limit incision size while still allowing appropriate visualization of the saphenofemoral junction and its tributaries. Through the groin incision, the subcutaneous plane over the GSV and saphenofemoral junction is developed. Understanding anatomic relationships and branch anatomy of the GSV at this location is important for most effective ligation technique (see Chap. 1). Most commonly, branch tributary veins at the saphenofemoral junction include inferior epigastric vein, superficial circumflex iliac vein, superficial external pudendal vein, deep external pudendal vein, lateral accessory saphenous vein, and medial accessory saphenous vein. While there may be some variability in branch anatomy, it is important to identify and ligate all tributaries at the saphenofemoral junction to prevent persistent superficial venous flow directly into femoral vein and potential for recurrent reflux and varicosities. Additional exposure of the femoral vein above and below the saphenofemoral confluence and of the proximal GSV below the junction may be required. Flush ligation of the GSV at the saphenofemoral junction without narrowing of the femoral vein is performed to avoid a residual GSV stump as a potential source for thrombus formation and pulmonary embolism. Resection of the proximal 5–10 cm of GSV is performed through the exposed surgical field with distal ligation. The incision is closed in a layered fashion with absorbable sutures in the subcutaneous layers and at the skin level with either absorbable subcuticular closure, interrupted nylon suture, or skin adhesive sealant.

For superficial thrombophlebitis involving the great saphenous vein, if clot is already present up to the saphenofemoral junction, saphenofemoral disconnection may also be required to prevent propagation of clot into the femoral vein (see Chap. 19). Operative approach is similar as described above with extra care taken to avoid dislodgement during exposure. If clot is protruding into the femoral vein, local thrombectomy may also be required prior to flush ligation at the saphenofemoral junction.

Stripping refers to removal of extended segment of the GSV either with external stripper, intraluminal stripper (such as Codman or Myer), or perforation-invagination (PIN) stripper (such as Oesch). Understanding the segmental reflux pattern of the GSV and using a targeted approach directed at incompetent segment are important for most effective treatment. Most GSV reflux patterns will include thigh segment which is most routinely included in stripping. However, if thigh segment is competent, it should not be stripped as it may worsen secondary varicosities by removing a competent and dependent superficial collateral draining vein. Similarly, normal atretic parallel accessory GSV segments should be left intact, while incompetent accessory saphenous veins should be stripped. GSV stripping below the knee is rarely performed today to avoid possible saphenous nerve injury, unless it is obviously incompetent with clinically significant reflux or in the setting of recurring calf varicosities. Through the groin exposure described for high ligation and stripping and a distal counter incision at the level of intended stripping, typically at the knee or ankle, using the intraluminal technique, the GSV is typically secured to the tip of the stripper with inversion of the vein as the stripper is pulled down through the distal incision (Fig. 12.2). GSV stripping in the downward direction using the largest stripper head possible results in most effective avulsion of branches and decreased potential injury to the adjacent saphenous nerve. A heavy silk suture attached to the GSV prior to stripping then allows recovery of the entire stripped GSV segment and tributaries back through the proximal groin incision, thereby limiting the size of the distal incision. For PIN technique, a rod is used to puncture the vein, and a small exit skin incision is used to retrieve the stripper and disconnected invaginated GSV. Expansion of PIN stripper techniques as well as additional techniques using ultrasound guidance for smaller incisions, tumescent anesthesia, leg elevation during stripping, and immediate compression wraps to decrease blood in the tunnel have led to less invasive options for stripping and more of shift into the outpatient setting than in the past.

12.7.2 Small Saphenous Vein

For patients with SSV-associated patterns of varicose veins or posterior lateral venous insufficiency-associated problems, ligation and division of the SSV in the popliteal fossa at saphenopopliteal junction is recommended. The saphenopopliteal junction can be variable in location in relation to the popliteal fossa. Reflux in a cranial extension of the SSV also needs to be identified and may impact treatment. With the patient in the prone position and knee in slight flexion, the saphenopopliteal junction is identified by ultrasound. A small transverse incision is made in the popliteal crease just distal to the junction with exposure of the SSV as it courses through the subcutaneous fascial planes between the medial and lateral heads of the gastrocnemius muscle and into the popliteal fossa. The saphenopopliteal junction is ligated, and the proximal SSV is transected at this level. If a cranial extension is present, it is also ligated at this level. From this exposure, a 3–5 cm distal SSV segment can be excised. Additional segments of SSV can be avulsed through tiny incisions, or stripping can be performed to the mid-calf level, although potential adjacent sural nerve injury is increased.

12.7.3 Varicose Veins

12.7.3.1 Ambulatory Phlebectomy

Ambulatory phlebectomy techniques fall under various descriptors such as excisional phlebectomy, stab avulsion phlebectomy, hook phlebectomy, and micropuncture phlebectomy. While the terminology can be confusing, the basic

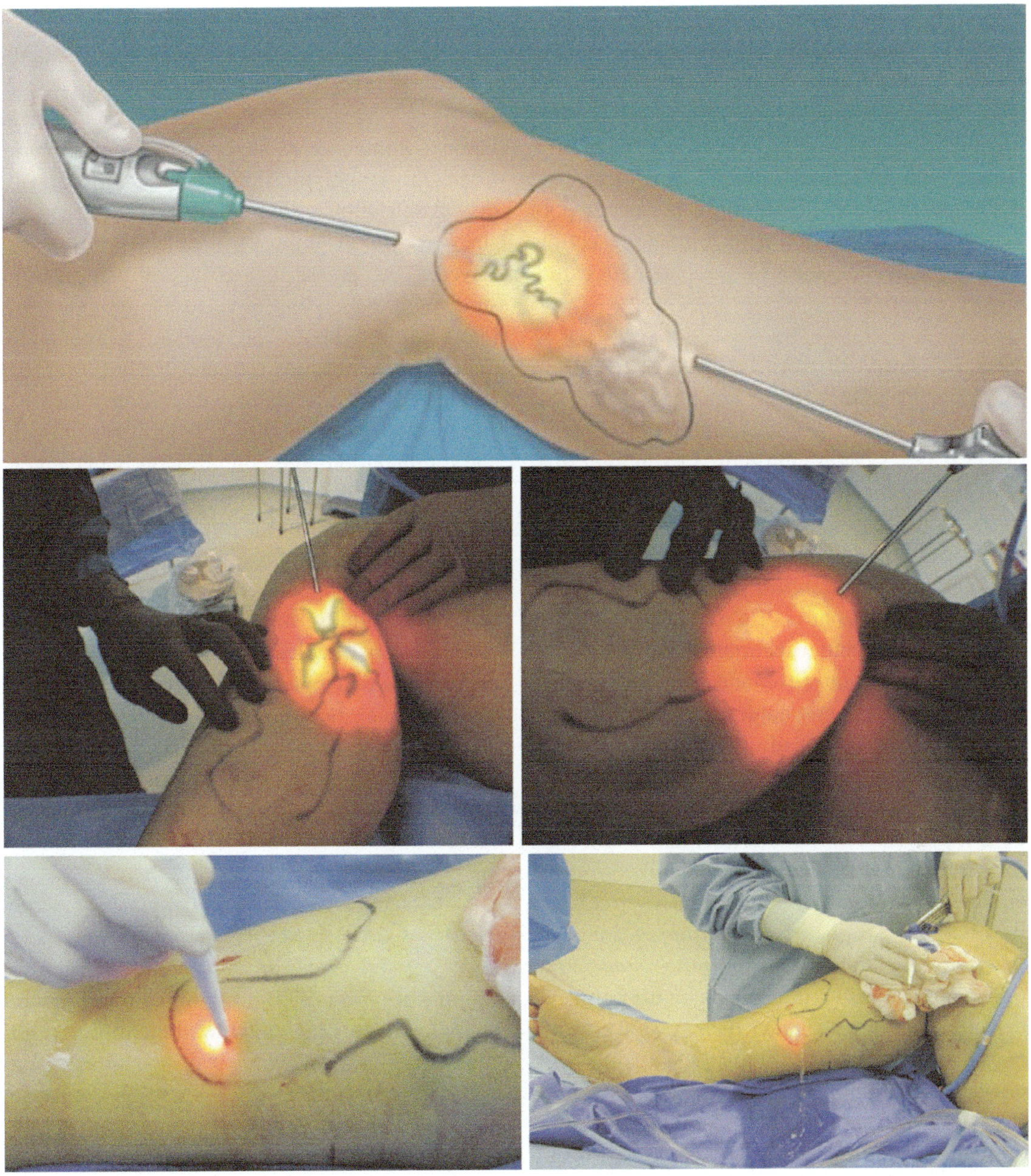

Fig. 12.2 Transilluminated powered phlebectomy technique for removal of varicose veins. Transilluminating instrument allows direct visualization for excision using the powered oscillating resector. Additional tumescence allows flushing of residual blood and tissue from operative field

technique is essentially the same. With advances in tumescent anesthesia, these phlebectomy techniques can be performed in the outpatient setting; are associated with low complications, high patient satisfaction, and excellent cosmesis; and have become a safe and effective method for varicose vein removal. The positions of the varicosities are marked with the patient standing. For phlebectomy in the outpatient setting, tumescent anesthesia is infiltrated along the marked varicosities. Multiple tiny incisions are made with #11 blade, beaver blade, ophthalmic blade, or puncture hole using a large needle. With the use of small profile phlebectomy hooks (such as Muller, Oesch, Tretbar, Ramelet, Varady, or Dortu-Martimbeau), the targeted varicosity is brought up through the small incision and grasped with a hemostat or forceps for further mobilization and avulsion. Incisions are usually too small for suture and are brought together with steri-strips. There are some limitations with ambulatory phlebectomy, however, including the need for multiple incisions, poor visualization, potential for incomplete resection, and technical challenges for patients with extensive varicosities.

12.7.3.2 Transilluminated Powered Phlebectomy

Transilluminated powered phlebectomy (TRIVEX™ system, InaVein, Lexington, MA, USA) combines visualization of varicosities using transillumination and directed resection using endoscopic technology. Instrumentation includes: *System Control Unit* is the central power unit with controls for xenon light source, irrigation pump, and resection oscillation speeds; *Illuminator Handpiece* connects to the control unit with a fiber optic cable and provides high-intensity light for transillumination and tumescence irrigation control; *Resector Handpiece* has both 4.5 and 5.5 mm resector options, control of oscillation direction and rate, and connectors for suction tubing. General, epidural, or spinal anesthesia is required. Through a tiny incision, the illuminator is placed a few millimeters deeper than the target varicosity, and tumescence solution is infiltrated into the area along the course of the vein. Through a counter incision, the resector is positioned directly on the varicosity, and with powered oscillation, varicosities are mobilized free and then suctioned out of the leg. Addition of small dermal punch incisions allows for any blood or tissue debris that collects in the vein tract to be flushed out with further tumescent fluid. Overall, transilluminated powered phlebectomy is the most effective for extensive varicose veins where the improved visualization allows for more complete resection with fewer incisions. However, for patients with fewer varicosities, the margin of benefit of transilluminated powered phlebectomy is less when compared to ambulatory phlebectomy.

12.8 Outcomes

12.8.1 Postoperative Follow-Up

Upon completion of superficial venous operations, most skin incisions can be closed with dissolvable suture, skin adhesives, or even steri-strips for small ambulatory phlebectomy stabs. Layered compression dressing or compression stockings, depending on extent of operative intervention, should be applied immediately upon completion of procedure. Early postoperative instructions should include routine incisional care, initial leg elevation but with transition to early ambulation, and compression management eventually transitioning to compression stockings on a daily basis for a few weeks until pain and swelling have subsided. Pain management with acetaminophen or narcotic pain meds is preferred initially, reserving nonsteroidal anti-inflammatory medications for several days to avoid increased potential bruising. Patients are routinely seen back in outpatient setting within an appropriate time interval. The author prefers an initial postoperative visit within 1 week and then at 6–8 weeks to assess operative results and satisfaction.

12.9 Complications

Complication rates for all superficial venous operations are generally low. Potential complications will vary depending on the treated anatomic venous segment(s), extent of operation, and techniques used. For saphenous-based operations, reported complications include discomfort, bruising, bleeding, wound infection, deep venous thrombosis, and nerve injury (which can range from temporary numb patches to neurapraxia along the saphenous nerve distribution for GSV and sural nerve distribution for SSV-based approaches). Limiting GSV stripping to the knee level and removal of short SSV segments only have decreased potential nerve injury complaints.

Potential complications associated with ambulatory phlebectomy are also low, mostly appearance related, and usually transient. Complaints can include allergic reaction to local anesthetic, skin blistering, subcutaneous dimpling, hypopigmentation, hyperpigmentation, induration, infection, contact dermatitis, skin necrosis, swelling, seroma, telangiectatic matting, numbness, nerve injury, traumatic neuroma, superficial venous thrombosis, and deep venous thrombosis.

Reported complications following transilluminated powered phlebectomy have varied considerably consisting primarily of ecchymosis and/or hematoma formation, paresthesias or nerve injury, skin perforation, superficial phlebitis, swelling, hyperpigmentation, and low potential for deep venous thrombosis. Although most studies reported fewer incisions for transilluminated powered phlebectomy compared to conventional surgery, differences in operating time have varied. With regard to cosmetic scores, outcomes were similar for both groups, and overall patient satisfaction scores were not statistically different. Although there is no published data clearly showing any significant statistical advantage of transilluminated powered phlebectomy except for lower number of incisions, most of the published literature represents earlier generation system and techniques. With a newer generation system, smaller instrumentation, and modification of technique that allow for slower oscillation speed, higher suction, and extensive tumescence irrigation and drainage, most of these earlier problems have been eliminated with decreased potential for complications and improved outcomes over those previously reported.

12.10 Results

Outcomes of open venous surgery have continued to improve and have been shown to be safe and effective with low complication rates and overall excellent outcomes in terms of improved symptoms and quality-of-life parameters compared to nonoperative measures. In the REACTIV trial, results of compression treatment alone were compared to open combined venous surgery including flush ligation, division and stripping of the GSV, and multiple phlebectomies with compression treatment in 246 patients with uncomplicated venous reflux and associated varicose veins. At 2 years, combined open venous surgery provided more symptomatic relief, better cosmetic results, and a significantly improved quality of life over conservative compression management alone. In the ESCHAR study, 500 patients with leg ulcers were randomized to either compression treatment alone or compression in combination with open superficial venous surgery including both saphenous-based approaches and phlebectomy when indicated. In terms of ulcer healing, while compression treatment alone was as effective as compression plus venous surgery, 12-month ulcer recurrence rates were reduced in compression with surgery group (12 %) compared to those with compression alone (28 %) ($P < .0001$).

Reported recurrence rates of varicose veins after surgical treatment have ranged from 6.6 to 37 % at 2 years to 51 % at 5 years. The reasons for varicose vein recurrence have been attributed to technical or judgment errors, neovascularization at the groin, development of new refluxing segments, and residual untreated venous reflux.

12.11 Evidence-Based Guidelines

Clinical practice guidelines of the Society for Vascular Surgery and the American Venous Forum published in 2011 provide a reasonable framework for clinical decision making based on current evidence. Recommendations are based on the Grading of Recommendations Assessment, Development, and Evaluation (GRADE) system. For each guideline, the level of current evidence is documented by letters A, B, and C, and the strength of the recommendation is rated as strong (1) or weak (2). The guidelines specific to treatment of superficial venous reflux including medical therapy, open superficial venous operations, and endovenous ablation (see Chaps. 10 and 11) proposed in this consensus statement are shown in Table 12.3.

Table 12.3 Evidence-based guidelines for treatment of superficial venous insufficiency

Medical therapy
Venoactive drugs (diosmin, hesperidin, rutosides, sulodexide, micronized purified flavonoid fraction, or horse chestnut seed extract [aescin]) in addition to compression for patients with pain and swelling due to chronic venous disease, in countries where these drugs are available (Grade 2B)
Pentoxifylline or micronized purified flavonoid fraction, if available, in combination with compression, to accelerate healing of venous ulcers is suggested (Grade 2B)
Compression therapy
Compression therapy using moderate pressure (20–30 mmHg) for patients with symptomatic varicose veins (Grade 2C)
Against compression therapy as the primary treatment of symptomatic varicose veins in patients who are candidates for saphenous vein ablation (Grade 1B)
Compression as the primary therapeutic modality for healing venous ulcers (Grade 1B)
Compression as an adjuvant treatment to superficial vein ablation for the prevention of ulcer recurrence (Grade 1A)
Open venous surgery
For treatment of the incompetent great saphenous vein, high ligation and inversion stripping of the saphenous vein to the level of the knee (Grade 2B)
To reduce hematoma formation, pain, and swelling, postoperative compression in C2 patients for 1 week (Grade 1B)
For treatment of small saphenous vein incompetence, high ligation of the vein at the knee crease, about 3–5 cm distal to the saphenopopliteal junction, with selective invagination stripping of the incompetent portion of the vein (Grade 1 B)
To decrease recurrence of venous ulcers, ablation of the incompetent superficial veins in addition to compression therapy (Grade 1A)
Ambulatory phlebectomy for treatment of varicose veins, performed with saphenous vein ablation, either during the same procedure or at a later stage. If general anesthesia is required for phlebectomy, we suggest concomitant saphenous ablation (Grade 1B)
Transilluminated powered phlebectomy using lower oscillation speeds and extended tumescence as an alternative to traditional phlebectomy for extensive varicose veins (Grade 2C)
For treatment of recurrent varicose veins, ligation of the saphenous stump, ambulatory phlebectomy, sclerotherapy, or endovenous thermal ablation, depending on the etiology, source, location, and extent of varicosity (Grade 2C)
Endovenous thermal ablation
Endovenous thermal ablations (laser and radio-frequency ablations) are safe and effective for treatment of saphenous incompetence (Grade 1B)
Because of reduced convalescence and less pain and morbidity, endovenous thermal ablation of the incompetent saphenous vein preferred over open surgery (Grade 1B)

Adapted from Gloviczki et al. [3]

12.12 Summary

Coordinated treatment of superficial venous insufficiency involves comprehensive patient evaluation, appropriate venous testing usually with venous ultrasound as the cornerstone of diagnostic evaluation, and sound clinical decision making based on current evidence-based guidelines. While nonoperative measures focusing on compression are recommended as initial therapy, operative approaches offer additional opportunity for improved outcomes. As treatment options are shifting to less invasive options, traditional open operative approaches directed at both axial saphenous vein reflux and varicose vein problems still have a role in appropriately selected patients with symptomatic superficial venous insufficiency.

References

1. Barwell JR, Davies CE, Deacon J, et al. Comparison of surgery and compression with compression alone in chronic venous ulceration (ESCHAR study): randomised controlled trial. Lancet. 2004;363(9424):1854–9.
2. Eklöf B, Rutherford RB, Bergan JJ, et al. American Venous Forum International Ad Hoc Committee for Revision of the CEAP Classification. Revision of the CEAP classification for chronic venous disorders: consensus statement. J Vasc Surg. 2004;40(6):1248–52.
3. Gloviczki P, Comerota AJ, Dalsing MC, et al. The care of patients with varicose veins and associated chronic venous diseases: clinical practice guidelines of the Society for Vascular Surgery and the American Venous Forum. J Vasc Surg. 2011;53:2S–48.
4. Guyatt G, Gutterman D, Baumann MH, et al. Grading strength of recommendations and quality of evidence in clinical guidelines: report from an American College of Chest Physicians Task Force. Chest. 2006; 129:174–81.
5. Michaels JA, Campbell WB, Brazier JE, et al. Randomised clinical trial, observational study and assessment of cost-effectiveness of the treatment of varicose veins (REACTIV trial). Health Technol Assess. 2006;10(13):1–196, iii–iv.
6. Porter JM, Moneta GL. International Consensus Committee on Chronic Venous Disease. Reporting standards in venous disease: an update. J Vasc Surg. 1995;21:635–45.
7. Rutherford RB, Padberg Jr FT, Comerota AJ, et al. Venous severity scoring: an adjunct to venous outcome assessment. J Vasc Surg. 2000;31:1307–12.
8. Vasquez MA, Rabe E, McLafferty RB, Shortell CK, Marston WA, Gillespie D, et al. Revision of the venous clinical severity score: venous outcomes consensus statement: special communication of the American Venous Forum Ad Hoc Outcomes Working Group. J Vasc Surg. 2010;52:1387–96.

13 Transcutaneous Laser Vein Ablation

Joyce Jackson and Craig F. Feied

Contents

J. Jackson, RN, MSN, ANP, BC (✉)
Belmont Aesthetic and Reconstructive Surgery, Chevy Chase, MD, USA

Berman Skin Institute, Palo Alto, CA, USA
e-mail: joycejjackson@msn.com

C.F. Feied, MD, FACEP, FAAEM, FACPh
Department of Emergency Medicine, Georgetown University School of Medicine, Washington, DC, USA
e-mail: craig.feied@gmail.com

Abstract

Patients with vascular lesions may benefit from a combination of different treatment modalities including sclerotherapy, phlebectomy, and intravascular thermoablation of larger vessels. Treatment with lasers and other intense light sources can be an important adjunct to these other modalities, and this is especially true in cases that have proven resistant to sclerotherapy and in patients who have developed telangiectatic matting after sclerotherapy. Surface vascular lesions can be treated effectively with a variety of lasers. There continue to be advances in the treatment of telangiectasias and other undesired veins. In general, lasers with

E. Mowatt-Larssen et al. (eds.), *Phlebology, Vein Surgery and Ultrasonography*,
DOI 10.1007/978-3-319-01812-6_13, © Springer International Publishing Switzerland 2014

shorter wavelengths have been more effective in treating more superficial, red telangiectasias versus those with longer wavelengths for treating deeper blue reticular veins up to 4 mm. Lower extremity telangiectasias can be resistant to laser treatment particularly when other high-pressure vessels have not been eradicated.

13.1 Introduction

Patients with vascular lesions may benefit from a combination of different treatment modalities including sclerotherapy, phlebectomy, and intravascular thermoablation of larger vessels. Treatment with lasers and other intense light sources can be an important adjunct to these other modalities, and this is especially true in cases that have proven resistant to sclerotherapy and in patients who have developed telangiectatic matting after sclerotherapy.

13.2 Underlying Pathology

Although small superficial varicosities and spider veins may cause symptoms such as itching, burning, and soreness, treatment of small superficial vessels most often is performed for cosmetic reasons. Nonetheless, treatment of small superficial vessels is not always a purely cosmetic procedure. The approach to treatment must be guided by a thorough understanding of the underlying pathological venous pathways of the patient being treated. Small visible superficial vessels may be the result of purely local trauma or inflammation, or they may be associated with elevated venous pressures in deeper venous systems. They may arise from small reticular feeder vessels where deeper venous circuits are normal, or from longer venous pathways such as the lateral subdermal plexus, or they may be secondary to significantly elevated venous pressure in larger truncal veins with failed proximal venous valves.

13.3 Treatment of Underlying Causes

When superficial spider veins are actually terminal branches of a deeper reservoir of venous blood with high venous pressures and prolonged recirculation time, therapy directed at the superficial veins alone, whether by sclerotherapy or by laser therapy, will be relatively ineffective. When superficial veins experiencing elevated venous pressure are treated without first addressing the deeper problems, the vessels will be resistant to treatment and prone to early recurrence. In this situation the patient also has an elevated risk for complications such as telangiectatic matting.

13.4 Risks Assessment

A decision to treat superficial or cosmetic vessels must also take into account the patient's overall health and medical situation. Although the treatment of superficial spider veins is often perceived as a benign intervention with very low risk, each patient's situation must be assessed individually. For example, a patient with a hypercoagulable or hypofibrinolytic disorder may develop deep vein thrombosis after treatment of tiny superficial veins by any method because local inflammation can result in pathologic propagation of thrombosis into adjacent vessels, while circulating prothrombotic factors may trigger spontaneous remote thrombosis. There have been many recognized cases of deep vein thrombosis associated with intercurrent treatment of superficial spider veins, and although there is no prospective evidence to prove causality, procoagulant factors are a known component of the physiological response to injury of superficial vessels.

For all these reasons, even when a patient has apparently isolated superficial spider veins, it is important that a careful history and physical examination should be performed and that venous ultrasound should be used to identify and map any associated reflux pathways. Any identified source of elevated venous pressure feeding superficial veins should be ablated before treatment of the more superficial vessels is undertaken.

13.5 Choice of Therapeutic Modality

Once the decision has been made that the patient has superficial small vessel disease with cosmetic implications, the choice of therapeutic modality becomes important. The standard treatment for many years has been chemical ablation of even the smallest vessels, and it is true that a skilled practitioner can successfully introduce sclerosant into vessels much smaller than the diameter of the 30 gauge needles commonly used in treatment. However, the appeal of transcutaneous treatment approaches for small vein ablation is undeniable. Some patients are extremely needle phobic, while others may be allergic to components of sclerosants. Some vessels are highly resistant to chemical sclerosis, and some patients have an aggressive telangiectatic response to sclerosant injection. From the viewpoint of the practitioner, a bloodless field with no sharps is a tremendous convenience in the treatment room. For all these reasons, a wide variety of techniques have been used in attempts to ablate superficial vessels through the delivery of energy in the form of heat, electrical fields, or light. Of these approaches, lasers and noncoherent intense light sources have proven most useful to date.

13.6 Biophysics of Vascular Photoablation

As laser light interacts with the skin, it is either reflected, transmitted, scattered, or absorbed. Absorbed energy causes heating of the intended target and also of surrounding tissues. Although laser light has many interesting characteristics, it is this tissue heating that is responsible for important biological effects: thermal injury is the fundamental mechanism by which phototherapy effects venous ablation.

13.7 Selective Photothermolysis

For many years after their initial introduction into the clinical arena, medical lasers could only be used for nonselective tissue vaporization and nonselective photocoagulation. The modern field of laser medicine has its roots in the work of Anderson and Parrish, who in 1983 described the principles of *selective* photothermolysis, in which light sources of specific wavelengths are used in selective targeting of specific chromophores (e.g., water, melanin, and hemoglobin) to achieve differential heating in adjacent tissues [1]. To destroy unwanted vessels without excessive injury to surrounding or overlying tissues, selective photothermolysis attempts to exploit differences in energy absorption in different tissue types to cause selective heating of the vessel or its contents. In general terms, the frequency (or its inverse: the wavelength) of the energy source is tuned to the absorption spectrum of the tissues into which the energy is delivered. In a perfect system, the abnormal vessel would absorb 100 % of the energy delivered and all other tissues would absorb no energy. In reality, all tissues absorb some energy across a wide range of wavelengths, and thermal energy rapidly diffuses from the site of absorption into nearby tissues. In practical terms, it is sufficient if the temperature in the abnormal veins can be elevated enough to destroy the vessel endothelium while the temperature of surrounding tissues remains low enough that no clinical signs of thermal injury are recognized.

Over the past several decades, advances in the design of medical lasers and intense pulsed light (IPL) sources have made it possible to vary many different parameters in order to improve tissue targeting and reduce collateral injury, and the advent of relatively inexpensive systems for delivering energy via laser and other intense light sources has greatly expanded the practical options for treatment of undesirable superficial vascular lesions. Through manipulation of wavelength, fluence, pulse duration, extrinsic cooling, and other parameters, it is now possible to use phototherapy successfully in the treatment of red spider veins, blue reticular veins, port-wine stains, and many other vascular lesions.

A large number of different devices are available in the marketplace, each offering a slightly different range of parameters and different methods for controlling them. A practitioner using such devices must have a thorough understanding of basic laser biophysics, principles of laser safety, and the concepts underlying a choice of wavelengths and treatment parameters.

13.7.1 Laser Light

An ideal laser emits energy in the form of light that is monochromic (single wavelength), perfectly coherent (having temporally and spatially constant interference), and collimated (non-divergent) [2]. Real-world medical lasers emit light that typically contains some mixture of wavelengths with a fairly high degree of temporal coherence and collimation. Although coherence and collimation are important attributes of lasers for many nonmedical purposes, the attribute of primary importance for medical therapy is the wavelength, since this is what allows a laser to deliver energy selectively to one type of biological structure versus another. An equally important feature of medical lasers is the ability to deliver precise amounts of energy over very short periods of time. Noncoherent IPL sources have also proven useful in delivering energy selectively to different tissue structures. A variety of methods are used to create light pulses of proper wavelength, energy, and pulse duration.

13.7.2 Wavelength and Energy Absorption

The energy absorption of a laser, or other intense light source, depends on the wavelengths of light emitted and the characteristics of the tissues through which it passes. The probability that a photon will be absorbed by chromophores in a particular type of tissue per unit path length is referred to as the absorption coefficient (μa). The absorption coefficient depends upon both the particular wavelength of light and the type of light-absorbing molecules (target molecules) that are present in the tissue [3]. A good target molecule absorbs a high proportion of the energy delivered by light at a wavelength where surrounding tissues absorb very little.

Wavelength also determines how deeply light can penetrate into tissues before being absorbed; near-infrared wavelengths of 755 and 810 nm (e.g., alexandrite and diode lasers) may penetrate deeply enough to target the chromophores of vessels up to 2 mm, among the largest that may be treated primarily with transcutaneous phototherapy. Near-infrared wavelengths of 940 nm and above allow for even deeper penetration and potentially for larger vein treatment, but the longer wavelengths also lead to some loss of selectivity, with increased absorption in tissue water and fat.

Wavelength is the most important determinant of differential light energy absorption in different tissues, but wavelength is not the only parameter to consider when evaluating the suitability of a particular laser device for a specific task. Other important factors include heat diffusion and thermal relaxation time, pulse duration, fluence, power density, epidermal cooling, and selective photothermolysis.

13.7.3 Molecular Targets

The degree of absorption and its thermal effects on the skin vary with the relative number and type of chromophores present in the skin, the vessel to be treated, and surrounding tissues. Each type of vessel absorbs a different fraction of the total tissue energy, based on its color, size, and depth [17]. It is therefore important when choosing a laser to identify a wavelength that will target the lesion to be treated while minimizing the energy delivered to surrounding tissues. The primary molecular targets for the treatment of superficial vascular structures are oxygenated and deoxygenated hemoglobin within the red blood cell, and the primary competitors for energy absorption include skin melanin, water, and tissue fat. The absorption curves for hemoglobin, melanin, water, and fat are shown in Figs. 13.1, 13.2, 13.3, and 13.4.

In the arterial system, hemoglobin saturation is generally above 93 %, whereas in the venous system, it may be 60–80 % in ordinary circulation (mixed venous blood) and lower in the setting of venous stasis with prolonged local recirculation times. Both oxyhemoglobin and deoxyhemoglobin molecules absorb laser energy over a broad range of wavelengths with differential peaks in the visible (blue/green/yellow) portion of the electromagnetic spectrum between 418 and 577 nm [3]. Examples of devices that produce wavelengths in this range include pulsed dye lasers (PDL), potassium titanyl phosphate lasers

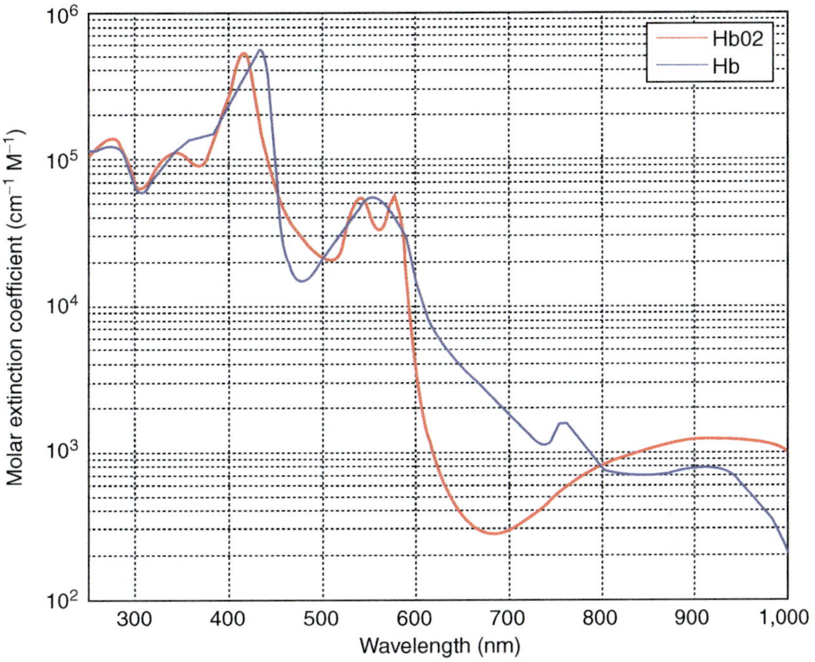

Fig. 13.1 Absorption spectrum of hemoglobin and deoxyhemoglobin (Prahl [27])

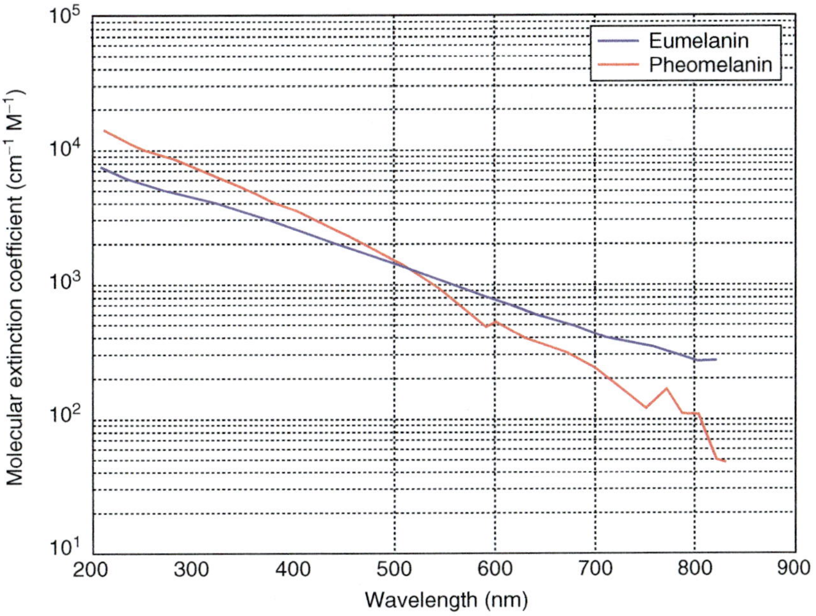

Fig. 13.2 Absorption spectrum of melanin (Jacques [28])

(KTP), and IPL sources used with the appropriate filters [19]. There is also a broad hemoglobin absorption peak from 800 to 1,000 nm, which is of special interest because longer wavelengths can penetrate more deeply into the dermis and thus offer the potential to reach deeper vessels.

13.7.4 Thermal Relaxation

Thermal relaxation time is defined as the time required for a given chromophore to lose 50 % of its heat through diffusion. If a laser pulse is longer than the thermal relaxation time, the

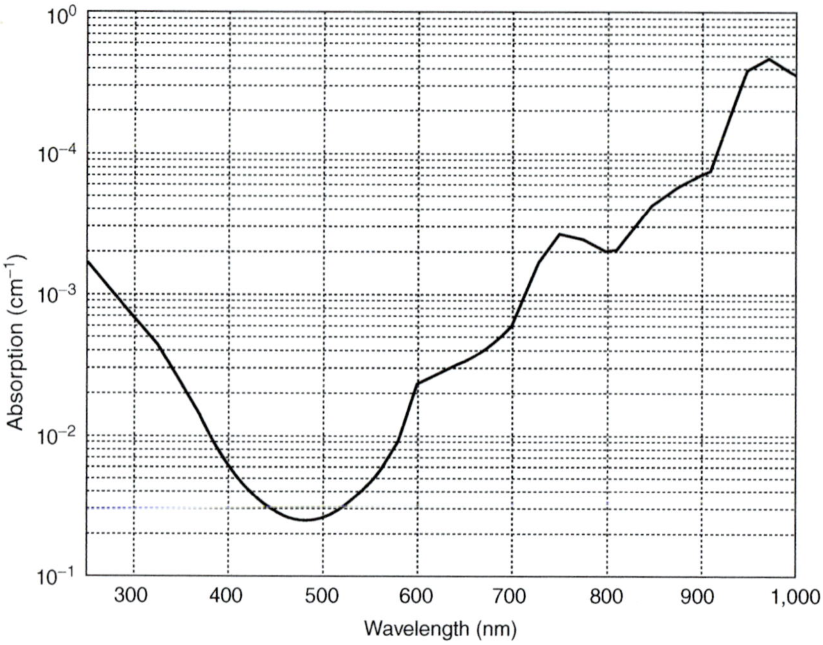

Fig. 13.3 Absorption spectrum of water (Hale and Querry [29])

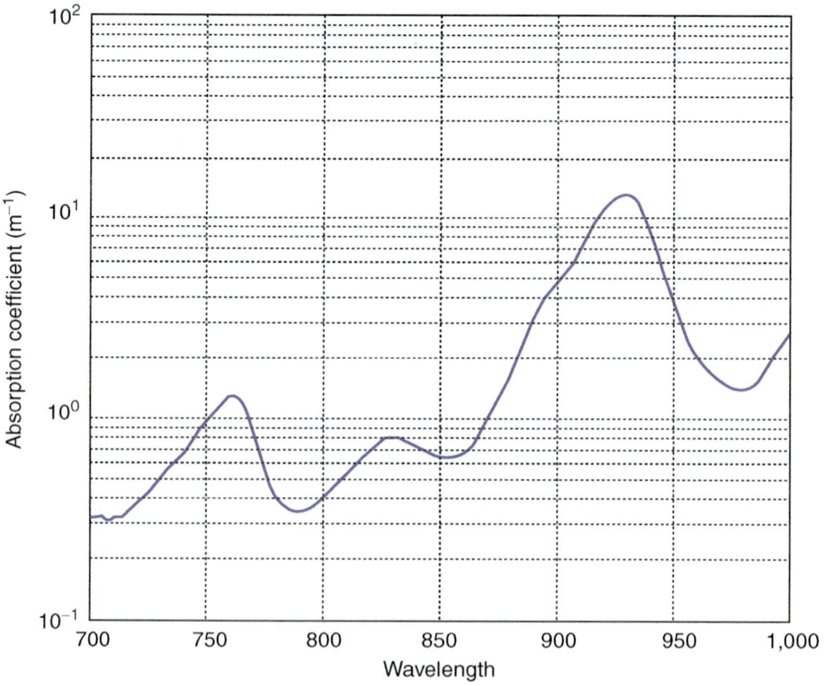

Fig. 13.4 Absorption spectrum of fat (van Veen et al. [30])

chromophore will have absorbed all the energy it can for that pulse, and the remaining energy will be delivered to other tissues, reducing the tissue selectivity of the treatment. In contrast, if the desired energy can be delivered using a pulse of shorter duration than the thermal relaxation time of the target, the largest possible proportion of the light energy can be delivered directly to the desired target, with minimal heating of surrounding tissues.

13.7.5 Pulse Duration/Repetition

Pulse duration, often referred to as pulse width, is the time at which the laser power remains above half its maximum value. Pulse repetition is the number of pulses delivered per second, reported as *Hz*. In general, pulse duration should not exceed the practical thermal relaxation time. The size of the target is also a factor when considering thermal relaxation times: the larger the vessel the greater the amount of total thermal energy that must be delivered to raise its temperature, the greater the amount of energy available to injure adjacent tissues, and the longer it takes to cool down by thermal diffusion.

Delivering the same amount of energy over longer pulse durations (or delivering energy with repetition using multiple pulses) may exploit differential thermal relaxation times in different tissue types, potentially allowing delivery of greater amounts of energy to deeper tissues. Reducing the energy per unit time can also help to reduce epidermal heating. However, when vessels are small and superficial, the more selective thermal targeting of shorter pulse durations offers many advantages.

13.7.6 Fluence

Fluence, sometimes referred to as "radiant exposure," is a measure of the number of photons delivered per unit area. For a fixed set of wavelengths, this is also a measure of the total energy delivered per unit area (usually measured in joules per square centimeter [J/cm^2]). At a fixed power output and pulse width, the fluence will decrease if the spot size increases (the same energy is delivered over a larger area). Given the same laser power and the same spot size, a shorter pulse will deliver a lower fluence than a longer pulse.

13.7.7 Power Density (PD)

The power density or intensity of the laser beam is defined as the beam power per unit of cross-sectional area. If the same amount of energy is delivered over the same amount of time in a smaller spot size, the power density will be increased.

13.7.8 Epidermal Cooling

Absorption of laser light by epidermal melanin causes epidermal heating. In general, the shorter the wavelength, the greater the superficial absorption of energy and the greater the likelihood of epidermal injury. Surface cooling may help to protect the dermis, allowing the delivery of higher fluences to the targeted vessels. Epidermal cooling can also help with analgesia [12]. Epidermal cooling may be particularly useful when longer pulse durations are needed, because heat accumulates in the epidermis more quickly than it accumulates in the blood vessels being treated, increasing the risk of epidermal injury [13]. Commonly used methods for extrinsic cooling of the epidermis include cryogen spray, air cooling, and contact cooling with ice, cold gel, or sapphire or quartz crystals.

13.7.9 Summary

Selective photothermolysis leverages differences in laser power density, pulse width, and wavelength, along with differences in tissue chromophores, thermal relaxation time, and other ambient factors to produce targeted, selective damage to specific tissues while minimizing the effects on surrounding tissue. Selective treatment of a targeted chromophore occurs when a laser system is chosen with a wavelength matching the absorption spectrum of the target, using an appropriate energy level to sufficiently heat the tissue through energy absorption by the targeted chromophore, with a pulse duration shorter than the thermal relaxation time of the target.

13.8 Lasers Commonly Used in Treatment of Vascular Lesions

Lasers can produce light energy in several different modes, including continuous wave (CW), pulsed wave, and Q-switched. Continuous wave lasers deliver energy continuously, which makes them unable to exploit differential thermal relaxation times and reduces the selectivity of energy

Table 13.1 Summary of some laser applications

1,064 nm Nd:YAG	125–150 J/cm²	6 mm spot	25 ms pulse duration
			75–100 ms pulse duration (reticular veins)
	120–170 J/cm²	3 mm spot	5–40 ms pulses
PDL	6.5–7.5 J/cm²	3–5–7–10 mm spot	Pulse duration 20–40 ms
	5–8 J/cm²		
532 nm KTP	16–22.5 J/cm²	500–700 μm spot	Pulse duration 10–30 ms
	17 J/cm²	2 mm spot	
Long-pulsed 532 nm Nd:YAG	12–14 J/cm²		
IPL	35–20 J/cm²		10 ms delay through a 550 nm cutoff filter

delivery, thus increasing the likelihood of thermal damage to surrounding tissue [2]. Pulsed lasers can deliver large amounts of energy over pulse durations measured in milliseconds. The term "Q-switching" refers to a process whereby the laser is first placed in a mode where it is unable to emit light yet is pre-saturated with energetic photons and then is suddenly allowed to emit light, resulting in a very fast emission of all the pre-stored energy in a very short pulse in the range of 10–250 ns. Lasers commonly used in the treatment of cutaneous vascular lesions are mostly pulsed or Q-switched lasers. A variety of suggested treatment parameters have been published for each class of laser. However, in practice, each patient is unique and each device performs differently, thus suggested parameters can be taken only as a rough guide to clinical therapy (Table 13.1).

13.8.1 Neodymium: Yttrium Aluminum Garnet (Nd:YAG)

The long-pulsed 1,064 nm Nd:YAG laser is most effective when treating facial telangiectasias and blue reticular vessels on the face. It has also been used to treat leg veins up to 4 mm in diameter, spider angioma, and cherry angiomas. The principal advantage of the 1,064 nm Nd:YAG is the fact that the longer wavelength allows for deeper penetration and weaker melanin absorption. The longer pulse duration at lower fluences translates into slower heating of the vessels. It has been claimed that this can cause photocoagulation without vessel rupture, minimizing the risk of purpura. This wavelength is well absorbed by both methemoglobin and deoxyhemoglobin and thus can deliver energy to darker blue veins [4].

Published recommendations include: for superficial vessels less than 1 mm in diameter, small spot size (2 mm), short pulse durations (15–30 ms), and high fluences (350–600 J/cm²) and for reticular veins of 1–4 mm in diameter, increased spot size (2–8 mm), longer pulse durations (25–60 ms), and fluences (90–370 J/cm²) [3].

In a study of 20 patients with size-matched superficial telangiectasias of the lower extremities, Lupton et al. compared sclerotherapy treatments to vein irradiation with the 1,064 nm Nd:YAG laser [5]. The telangiectasias responded best to the sclerotherapy, with fewer treatment sessions required, and similar adverse sequelae occurred in both groups. The conclusions were that lower extremity telangiectasias can be effectively treated with both modalities and that laser treatment may be more effective for patients with contraindications to sclerotherapy, including those with needle phobias, telangiectatic matting, or allergies to sclerosant solutions.

Sadick demonstrated longer term (12 months) successful photosclerosis of blue venulectasias and reticular feeder veins in 25 patients treated with the 1,064 nm Nd:YAG laser using a spot size of 6 mm [6]. Treatment parameters for vessels 0.2–2.0 mm: double pulse of 7 ms at 120 J/cm²; vessels 2.0–4.0 mm were treated with a single pulse of 14 ms and fluences of 130 J/cm².

When using the 1,064 nm Nd:YAG laser with the proper settings, effective treatment of many cutaneous vascular lesions can be obtained, especially if epidermal cooling is available. However, complications are not uncommon and can include crusting, hyperpigmentation, hypopigmentation, scarring, transient erythema, bruising, edema, and telangiectatic matting.

13.8.2 Potassium Titanyl Phosphate (KTP) Laser

The potassium titanyl phosphate (KTP) laser, a quasi-CW system, uses an Nd:YAG source passed through a KTP crystal to double the frequency (halve the wavelength), producing a laser with 532 nm wavelength. The system has been further modified to produce millisecond (ms) pulse durations [7]. The resulting KTP laser system delivers high-energy pulses in spot sizes ranging from 0.25 to 4.0 mm and pulse durations of 1–50 ms.

The wavelength of 532 nm allows for some selective absorption by the hemoglobin chromophore, but epidermal melanin is also a target. Compared to the Nd:YAG laser, the shorter wavelength decreases the potential for deep tissue penetration, but this can be offset by extending the pulse duration up to 50 ms [4]. The KTP laser has been used in the treatment of telangiectasias on the face and legs, rosacea, spider angioma, and cherry angiomas. Weiss and Goldman [8] suggest the KTP laser system as one of the useful near-infrared pulsed lasers for the treatment of bright red vessels. Their most encouraging results were achieved with using a spot size of 3–5 mm, longer pulse durations of 10–50 ms, and fluences of 14–20 J/cm^2, with a train of pulses delivered over the vessel until spasm occurs.

To evaluate the efficacy of the 532 nm KTP laser in the treatment of superficial leg telangiectasias, Fournier et al. [9] treated 14 patients with leg vessels, 0.5–1.0 mm in size. Using a nonuniform stacked pulse sequence, veins were treated with a total fluence of 60 J/cm^2, 0.75 mm collimated spot size, with a pulse delay of 250 ms between pulses. The stacked pulses were 100, 30, and 30 ms delivering 38, 11, and 11 J/cm^2, respectively. They demonstrated safe and effective treatment with minimum adverse effects. Side effects seen were transient and included erythema, edema, scabbing, hypopigmentation, and telangiectatic matting.

In addition, Woo et al. [13] compared treatment of telangiectatic leg veins in ten patients using a 532 nm Nd:YAG and a 595 nm PDL using ultra long pulse durations. Leg veins treated measured up to 1.0 mm in diameter. Both lasers showed improvement and some vessel clearance after one treatment with minimum side effects. Treatment parameters used with the Nd:YAG were a fluence of 20 J/cm^2 and a pulse duration of 50 ms using a contact cooling device. The PDL laser used a fluence of 25 J/cm^2, a pulse duration of 40 ms, and cryogen spray precooling.

13.8.3 Intense Pulsed Noncoherent Light (IPL)

The IPL is a noncoherent light source emitting light as a continuous spectrum within the 500–1,200 nm portion of the electromagnetic spectrum. It is used primarily in the treatment of facial telangiectasias and rosacea but is also indicated in the treatment of a variety of vascular lesions, including larger diameter vessels, spider angioma, and cherry angiomas. Light is delivered in a train of pulses, single, double, or triple, with varying time intervals between pulses. The IPL system uses a filtered flashlamp with filters used to remove lower wavelengths of visible light, while pulse durations can be adjusted to match desired thermal relaxation times [8, 19]. Using a light source longer than 600 nm potentiates deeper penetration of thermal energy, targeting the chromophore of deoxyhemoglobin.

Schroeter et al. [10] demonstrated successful treatment of rosacea using IPL. In a study of 60 patients treated with an IPL spectrum ranging from 515 to 1,200 nm with different pulse durations between 4.3 and 6.5 ms and energy densities of 25–35 J/cm^2, there was a reported 77.8 % clearance of lesions. Published treatment parameters include [3]: for smaller vessels, single pulse, 2.5–5 ms, fluence 25–45 J/cm^2, and filters 515–550 nm, and for larger vessels, double or triple pulses, with longer wavelength filters for deeper tissue penetration, higher energy densities of 50–75 J/cm^2, and longer pulse delays between pulses of 40–60 ms.

13.8.4 755 nm Alexandrite Laser

The long-pulsed alexandrite laser operates in the infrared spectrum of the electromagnetic scale. It has been used for the treatment of telangiectasias, but recent studies also show that it may be effective for treatment of larger vessels and for congenital vascular malformations (e.g., port-wine stains) that are resistant to treatment with the pulsed dye laser [18]. Recent device modifications include longer pulse durations of up to 20 ms or longer. The long-pulsed alexandrite laser penetrates to a depth of 2–3 mm, allowing energy delivery to larger and deeper vascular lesions. Published treatment parameters were 20 J/cm^2, double pulsed at a repetition rate of 1 Hz [11].

13.8.5 Flashlamp-Pumped Pulsed Dye Lasers

Pulsed dye lasers (PDL) are used to treat a variety of vascular lesions including port-wine stains, spider angioma, facial telangiectasias, and the superficial components of hemangiomas and rosacea. The original PDL with a wavelength of 585 nm was well suited to the treatment of vascular lesions targeting hemoglobin. However a high fluence with a short pulse duration of 450 μs often resulted in visible bruising that is cosmetically unappealing to patients. The very short pulse duration also resulted in poor results with vessels larger than 0.1 mm.

The PDL has since been modified to deliver a longer wavelength of 595 nm while adding variable pulse width, longer pulse durations, and epidermal cooling. These modifications allow higher fluences over longer pulse durations, thus increasing the size and depth of potential targets while decreasing the likelihood of posttreatment purpura. Alam et al. [14] treated 11 patients with facial telangiectasias to determine whether treatment parameters that did not produce purpura would be as effective as treatment parameters that did produce purpura. Although the longer pulse durations did produce improvement in telangiectasias, larger and darker telangiectasias benefited more from shorter pulse widths that caused purpura.

Ivey and Fitzpatrick [15] showed that making multiple passes, with lower fluencies in each pass, produced cumulative thermal ablation with less postoperative purpura. However, their conclusions were also that this approach was effective for smaller vessels but that larger caliber vessels benefited more from treatment with short pulse widths that did produce purpura.

13.9 Clinical Considerations

13.9.1 Skin Type

Because of differences in skin type, tissue density, pigmentation, and hemoglobin, each patient has a slightly different absorption spectrum for the skin and other tissues surrounding small superficial vessels. Some patients may be safely treated with a wide range of light wavelengths, intensities, and energy fluxes, while others may tolerate only a narrow range of wavelengths with carefully selected intensities and delivery times. Patients with fair skin may pass a larger

Table 13.2 Fitzpatrick skin type classification

Skin type	Skin color	Response to sun exposure
I	White, very fair, red or blond hair, blue eyes, freckles	Always burns, never tans
II	White, fair, red or blond hair, blue, hazel or green eyes	Usually burns, tans with difficulty
III	Cream white, fair with any eye or hair color	Sometimes mild burn, gradually tans
IV	Brown, typical Mediterranean Caucasian skin	Rarely burns, tans with ease
V	Dark brown, Middle Eastern skin types	Very rarely burns, tans very easily
VI	Very dark brown/black	Never burns, tans very easily

Table 13.3 Different fluence and pulse duration settings for different skin types

Skin type	Fluence (J/cm^2)	Pulse duration (ms)
I	40	20
II	30–40	15–30
III	25–35	30
IV	20–30	30
V	15–25	30

amount of energy through to deeper tissues, while those with darker skin will absorb more energy in the skin itself and may be more likely to develop hyperpigmentation or hypopigmentation in response to laser injury.

The Fitzpatrick skin type classification (Table 13.2) is most frequently used to guide treatment selection and predict response to phototherapy [26]. Table 13.3 lists the ways in which recommended influence and pulse duration can differ across the different skin types for a particular wavelength and type of laser.

13.10 Practical Applications for Specific Lesions

13.10.1 Facial Telangiectasias

Facial telangiectasias are visible cutaneous vascular lesions usually 0.1–1 mm in diameter. They are not caused by high venous pressures but are related to a variety of other factors, including but not limited to estrogen, familial influences, trauma, and infection. It is believed that facial telangiectasias result from the action of vasoactive substances leading to venule neogenesis [20]. Facial telangiectasias may present as linear or arborizing vascular patterns or may be papular in clinical appearance. They are primarily seen on the nose, cheeks, and chin.

13.10.2 Leg Telangiectasias

Although lasers can be effective in the treatment of leg telangiectasias, sclerotherapy continues to be the preferred treatment for this class of lesion. Lupton et al. [5] compared sclerotherapy to laser therapy (using a long-pulsed Nd:YAG laser) for lower extremity telangiectasias and found that both were effective in ablating the vessels but that sclerotherapy required fewer treatment sessions. Nonetheless, laser may be of particular interest for patients who have needle phobia or are allergic to sclerosing agents and to those who have proven resistant or who have developed telangiectatic matting after sclerotherapy. Bernstein [25] examined the clinical characteristics of 500 patients presenting with a specific request for laser treatment for ablation of lower extremity spider veins. Half of those patients had previously undergone sclerotherapy and had either persistent vessels, spontaneous new vessels, or sclerotherapy-induced vessels. The remaining patients had not previously undergone any treatment for venous disease but viewed laser therapy as "less painful" and "less risky" when compared to sclerotherapy.

13.10.3 Port-Wine Stains

Port-wine stain (PWS) is a congenital malformation resulting in a large number of confluent superficial dermal ectatic capillaries. Port-wine stains may be associated with other medical conditions, such as Sturge-Weber syndrome. Left untreated, the natural progression of port-wine lesions is one of gradual darkening, thickening, and nodularity.

The pulsed dye laser has become the mainstay in the treatment of port-wine stains and similar vascular lesions [22]. In the past, treatment of port-wine stains was often unsatisfactory, as many lesions proved refractory to treatment. Mariwalla and Dover [22] report success with treatment of pediatric patients using PDL (585 nm or 595 nm), generally starting with a 10 mm spot size and fluences of 7.5 J/cm^2. Depending on results, subsequent treatments may require a decrease in spot size to 7 mm and adjustments in fluence to 9–14 J/cm^2 or 6–8.5 J/cm^2. Several treatments are necessary, usually with treatment intervals of 4–8 weeks. Bernstein [24] evaluated the effectiveness of a high energy 595 nm, variable pulse PDL for treating PWS that had failed to respond to treatment with the 585 nm PDL. Twenty patients were treated with fluences ranging from 7.5 to 9.5 J/cm^2, a 1.5 ms pulse duration, and a 10 mm spot size. Seventy-six percent showed improvement after an average of 3.1 sessions.

In another study, Pence et al. [23] presented the 532 nm frequency-doubled Nd:YAG as an alternative to the PDL, particularly for refractory

Table 13.4 Treatment of rosacea and red facial veins

595 nm PDL	6 ms		7–9 J/cm^2	7 mm spot
	1.5 ms pulse duration		10 J/cm^2	
IPL	550–560 nm cutoff filter	Double pulse: 2.4 ms; 4.0 ms	10 ms delay	30 J/cm^2
532 nm KPT	20 ms		0.7 W	4 mm spot
	20 ms	0.1–0.3 mm/diameter vessels	0.12 W	0.25 mm spot

PWS. A study group of 89 patients with PWS on the face and/or neck were treated with the Nd:YAG laser using a 2–6 mm spot size, 15–50 ms pulse width, and 9.5–20 J/cm^2. Fifty-one percent of the patients showed good to excellent improvement, with pink-red lesions responding more favorably than other colors.

13.10.4 Rosacea

Rosacea is an inflammatory vascular disorder affecting the face and involving a combination of telangiectasia, papules, pustules, and rhinophyma [21]. The KTP laser, IPL, and pulse dye laser with wavelength of 595 nm (Table 13.4) have all been found efficacious in treatment of both the diffuse erythema of rosacea and the linear telangiectasias often seen on the face of these patients [3, 8, 10, 24].

13.11 Adverse Outcomes

Although the physical parameters of lasers and intense pulsed light sources often can be exploited to deliver energy selectively to a vascular lesion while minimizing the effects on adjacent tissues, there is always some degree of collateral injury due to thermal energy absorbed into adjacent or overlying tissues [16]. When the energy delivered to surrounding tissues is sufficient to cause thermal injury, complications or adverse effects can occur [16]. Despite the advances in knowledge and in device capabilities over the last 15 years, blisters or burns still may occur in even the most experienced hands. Most such injuries heal without visible sequelae, but permanent sequelae do still occur with some frequency.

13.11.1 Ocular Injury

Laser wavelengths in the red and infrared spectrum pass with little attenuation through the cornea and lens and may directly damage the retinal vasculature or retinal pigment; thus it is essential that both the patient and the practitioner use eye protection when laser therapy is underway.

13.11.2 Hyperpigmentation/Hypopigmentation

One form of hyperpigmentation is hemosiderin staining, resulting from the rupture of vessel walls and extravasation of red blood cells into the surrounding tissue. This may be visualized with any laser or pulsed light device. It is more likely to occur in patients with darker skin tones or tanned skin. Utilizing longer pulse durations could theoretically result in less pigmentation. Hypopigmentation most often occurs after multiple treatments and with lasers that are targeting melanin, such as those used with laser hair or tattoo removal. As with hyperpigmentation it usually resolves within a few months, but it can be persistent.

13.11.3 Blistering

Blistering is due to epidermal disruption from high temperatures. If deeper dermal structures are involved, blistering may be associated with tissue necrosis and scarring. Treatment measures focus on prevention by lowering the fluence, using external epidermal cooling, or delivering energy more slowly (by prolonging the pulse width for a given fluence) in order to reduce the temperature reached in the skin itself.

Perforator Veins

14

Elna M. Masuda and Darcy M. Kessler

Contents

E.M. Masuda, MD (✉) • D.M. Kessler, RVT
Division of Vascular Surgery,
Straub Clinic and Hospital,
John A. Burns School of Medicine,
Honolulu, HI, USA
e-mail: emasuda@straub.net; dkessler@straub.net

Abstract

Perforator veins (PVs) are one of three major venous systems in the leg directly linked to serious manifestations of chronic venous disease (CVD) including venous ulceration. Although its anatomical details are clearly defined, the physiology and clinical importance of PVs continue to remain less explicit. This chapter will review the evidence to support the diagnosis, indication for treatment, noninvasive and invasive options for management of PVs.

14.1 Introduction

Nearly 100 years ago, Homans presented a comprehensive description of the relationship between perforator veins and leg ulceration [1]. Despite its long history and the fact that perforator veins are frequently identified in the "gaiter area" beneath ulcers and areas of venous stasis dermatitis, controversy still prevails over its clinical significance and role in producing the pathologic state. Additionally, choices for treatment are highly variable and range from invasive eradication by long calf incisions to simple ablation by direct injections. This chapter will attempt to clarify the role of PVs in CVI and discuss the optimal diagnostic and therapeutic strategies.

E. Mowatt-Larssen et al. (eds.), *Phlebology, Vein Surgery and Ultrasonography*,
DOI 10.1007/978-3-319-01812-6_14, © Springer International Publishing Switzerland 2014

14.2 History

Perforator veins were first identified by Russian anatomist von Loder in 1803 then linked to skin changes by John Gay in 1868 who discussed the varicose disease of the leg and its "allied disorders" consisting of skin discoloration, induration and ulcers [2, 3]. In 1917, John Homans published a landmark paper describing the anatomic and pathophysiologic relationship of PVs to venous ulceration and proposed treatment, based solely on his astute clinical skills and careful physical examination [1, 4].

In 1938, Linton followed with a method of treating perforator veins to correct venous ulceration using extensive calf incisions, often through compromised skin, a technique associated with a high rate (up to 58%) of wound complications, which led to other proposed treatment approaches including limited incisions directly over the perforator [5–7]. Cockett and Jones, like Homans and Linton, reported in 1953 their findings that non-healing ulcers were associated with the post-thrombotic syndrome, PV's were important in the production of ulcers in the "gaiter" area or the "ankle blow out syndrome", and that ligation of the perforators promoted healing [8].

The high incidence of wound complications associated with the Linton procedure gave way to less invasive methods with multiple parallel incisions made along the natural skin lines plus skin grafting popularized by Ralph De Palma [9]. Hauer from Germany in 1985 [10] introduced and promulgated the use of endoscope and hence the emergence of SEPS (subfascial endoscopic perforator surgery) in reducing post op wound complications and decreased hospital length of stay. SEPS was the mainstay of therapy for PVs from 1985 to the mid-2000's and has proven to be less invasive than open surgery, and equally effective in eliminating PV's with lower wound complication rates. More recently, other less invasive techniques such as endovenous radiofrequency ablation, laser ablation, and ultrasound guided sclerotherapy have evolved, many of which can be performed under local anesthesia in an office setting, although outcomes have not been validated by controlled studies.

14.3 Anatomy

Perforator veins connect the superficial veins with the deep system and penetrate the deep fascia. There are more than 60–150 perforating veins in the normal leg, 20 of which are most commonly involved with pathology [11, 12]. In normal limbs, the direction of flow is unidirectional from the superficial to the deep system through one to two bicuspid valves, although outward flow has been found in up to 21 % of normal limbs [13]. When associated with chronic venous disease (CVD), the reflux can be outward from the deep to superficial alone (unidirectional) or both deep to superficial and superficial to deep (bidirectional).

New terms have been suggested to replace numerous eponyms and are detailed in Table 14.1 [14]. The majority of clinically important perforators are found along the mid to distal medial calf (Fig. 14.1). The posterior tibial perforators connect the posterior accessory great saphenous vein of the leg (formerly called posterior arch or

Table 14.1 Suggested changes in anatomic terms for leg veins

Previous terms and eponyms	Replaced by newer terms
Superficial femoral vein	Femoral vein
Greater or long saphenous vein	Great saphenous vein (GSV)
Lesser or short saphenous vein	Small saphenous vein (SSV)
Saphenofemoral junction	Confluence of the superficial inguinal veins
Giacomini vein	Intersaphenous vein
Posterior arch vein or Leonardo's vein	Posterior accessory great saphenous vein of the leg
Cockett perforators (I, II, III)	Posterior tibial perforators (lower, middle, upper)
Boyd's perforator	Paratibial perforator (proximal)
Sherman's perforators	Paratibial perforators
"24 cm" perforators	Paratibial perforators
Hunter's and Dodd's perforators	Perforators of the femoral canal
May's or Kuster's perforators	Ankle perforators

Reproduced with permission from Gloviczki and Mozes [14]

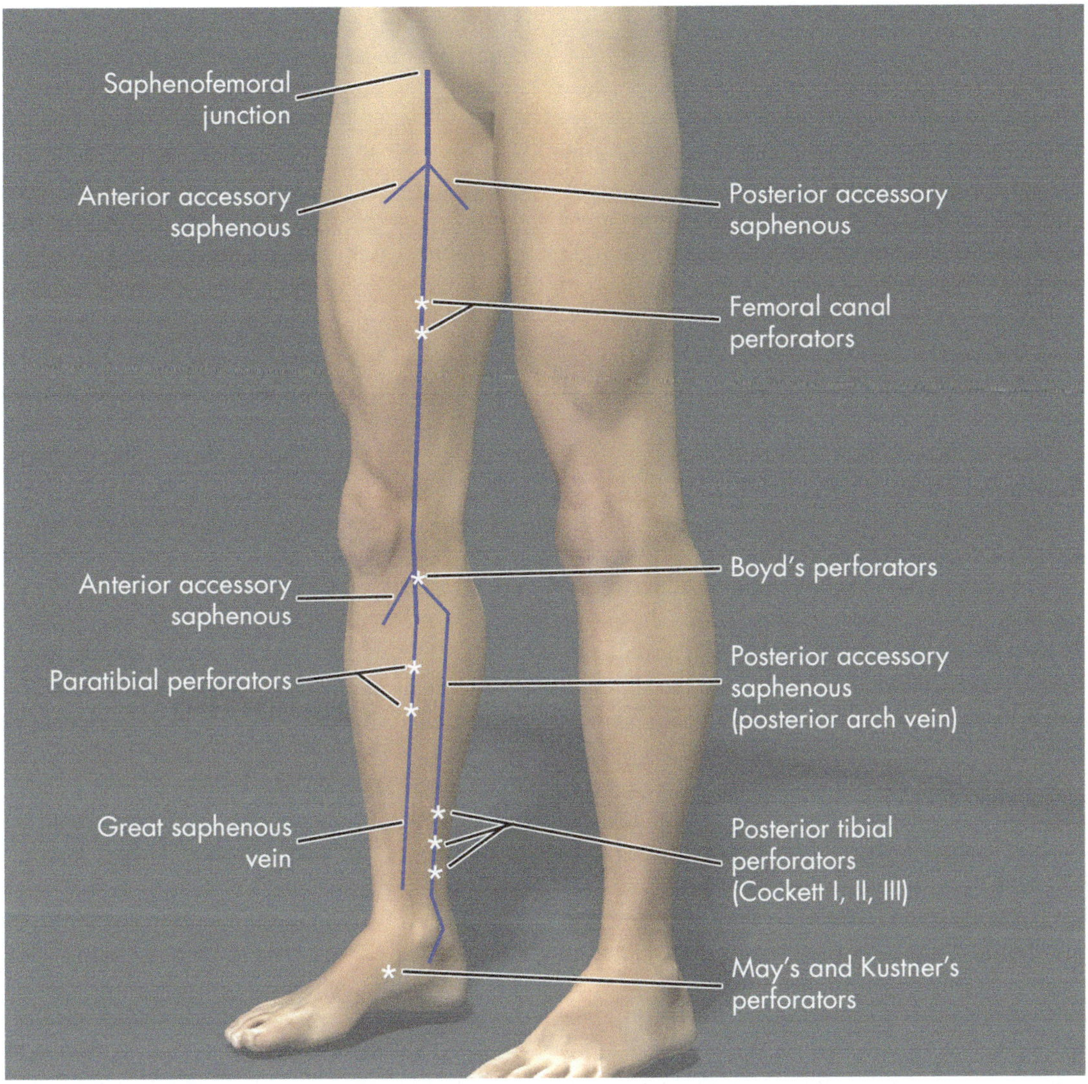

Fig. 14.1 Anatomy of the major perforator veins in the lower limb

Leonardo's vein) to the paired deeper posterior tibial veins. The posterior tibial perforators lower, middle, and upper were previously referred to as Cockett veins I, II, and III. The lower posterior tibial perforator is usually found posterior to the medial malleolus and is not usually accessible by SEPS.

The paratibial perforators connect the great saphenous vein to the posterior tibial veins. Multiple paratibial perforators are found 2–4 cm posterior to the medial edge of the tibia or "Linton's Lane" and are particularly important for conducting a proper SEPS procedure. The perforators of the femoral canal (previously referred to as Dodd and Hunterian perforators) connect the great saphenous and femoral veins.

Ankle perforators include the former May's or Kuster's perforators. In the foot, there are dorsal plantar, medial, and lateral foot perforators where the normal direction of flow is outward, distinctly opposite from PVs in the calf. The large perforator in the foot arises between the first and second metatarsal bones and connects the pedal vein to the superficial dorsal venous arch.

14.4 Pathophysiology

PVs alone do not appear to be the primary cause of venous ulcers. Instead, they are almost always accompanied by local or axial superficial and/or deep venous reflux or obstructive disease. Although PVs are frequently found in areas of intense inflammation, pre-ulcerative skin changes or in the vicinity of ulcers, they are not found as isolated abnormalities in venous ulcers [15]. Frequently, the most recalcitrant ulcers are associated with reflux in all three systems (deep, superficial and PVs). Neither isolated perforator nor isolated deep venous reflux is commonly found associated with severe CVD [16].

Usually two or more venous systems are abnormal in advanced CVD. PVs appear to act as reentry points between two axial systems allowing blood to flow from incompetent superficial to deep or vise versa [17]. If the primary problem is deep venous obstruction or reflux, the elevated venous pressure produced by deep venous obstruction or reflux during calf muscle contraction is transmitted to the connecting perforators and into the superficial veins. The blood under the calf muscle pump is forced to escape via the PVs and "yo-yos" up and down the deep system [17]. This may result in enlargement of the dermal capillary bed and release of proteins into the interstitial space including fibrinogen, which may eventually result in ulceration [18, 19].

In primary venous insufficiency with no prior DVT, the pathology is likely a refluxing saphenous system causing dilatation of the PVs, rendering the valves incompetent and often referred to as a "reentry perforator". This is supported by the findings of Stuart and Campbell who found that in cases of combined PVs and saphenous reflux, by abolishing the superficial saphenous vein alone PVs were no longer detectable or became competent [20, 21]. In a prospective study by Labropoulos and colleagues, new perforator incompetence always occurred with reflux in the superficial veins [22]. If the clinical state worsened, outcomes could not be attributed to development of PVS alone because of the inevitable presence of superficial disease [22].

Increasing size and numbers of PVs are associated with increasing severity of CVD [23, 24]. Size of PVs play an important role since larger diameters of PVs are more likely to be incompetent [25]. Diameters of >3.5mm are associated with reflux in 90% of cases [26]. PVs with diameters >3.9mm possess a high specificity of 96%, but lower sensitivity of 73% for incompetence with the lower sensitivity attributable to one third of incompetent PVs possessing diameters of <3.9mm [22]. The observation that increasing numbers of PVs lead to increasing severity of CVD is supported by the fact that higher numbers of PVs produce higher venous filling indices [23, 24].

14.5 Evidence in Favor of Importance of PVs

The clinical importance of PVs is supported by the fact that ulceration and skin stasis changes inevitably occur in the "gaiter area" between the distal point of the soleus muscle to the ankle where most large incompetent PVs are found. In ulcer disease, 50–60% of patients have incompetent perforators, and as the limb becomes more severely symptomatic , the association of PVs with either superficial or deep vein reflux or obstruction increases [24, 28]. The prevalence of PVs increases with clinical severity stratified by the CEAP classification, and they increase with the prevalence of deep vein reflux [16, 29].

Clinical evidence supporting the importance of PVs are found in studies treating the more severely symptomatic groups of C4–C6. Although there are no RCT's proving its importance, the best data at the time of this publication consists of one large multicenter registry and several observational studies.

The North American Subfascial Endoscopic Perforator Surgery registry (NASEPS) consisted of 155 limbs, collected from 17 US centers, in which 85% were C5–6 [30]. When treated with SEPS, median time to ulcer healing was 54 days; 88% healed at 1 year and 72% remained healed by 2 years. However 71% had concomitant saphenous stripping with SEPS and benefit of SEPS could not be attributed to treating perforators alone. SEPS was appealing since it was associated with low wound complication rate of 6%, much improved over the more invasive Linton procedure. Since most interventions including treatment of superficial reflux, the direct impact of treating PVs alone could not be clearly distinguished from the important effect of treating the superficial axial system.

Several observational studies suggest long term benefit of PV treatment for venous ulceration. Iafrati reported the long term outcome of C5–C6 disease in 35 cases of saphenous or variceal surgery plus SEPS, and 16 cases of SEPS alone in which early ulcer healing rate of 74% at 6 months [31]. Ulcer recurrence was only 13% at 5 years, and best results were associated with GSV stripping, primary venous insufficiency and ulcer <2 cm.

In another long-term follow up study of 9 years, Tawes reported on their retrospective multicenter experience of 832 patients with C4–6 disease undergoing SEPS [32]. Although 55% had stripping plus SEPS, 92% healed their ulcer with a recurrence rate of 4%. Finally, in a study of SEPS and saphenous stripping, healing of C6 cases occurred in 91% by mean of 2.9 months, with an ulcer recurrence of 6% at 30 months [33].

A meta-analysis of SEPS by Luebke found that for severe CVD, SEPs showed early benefit with rapid ulcer healing and decreased ulcer recurrence [34]. They concluded that SEPS in contrast to the Linton procedure was safer, with fewer complications. In another systematic review of 20 studies (one RCT comparing endoscopic to open perforator interruption and 19 case series), Tenbrook and colleagues report early ulcer healing in 88% and recurrence in 13% at 21 months. [35]. But again, this report included studies with both saphenous intervention and SEPS.

In an attempt to isolate the effect of sclerotherapy on perforators alone from treatment of superficial disease, the study from Straub Clinic & Hospital excluded those who had received treatment of the superficial system up to 2 years prior to ultrasound-guided sclerotherapy (UGS) of perforators [36]. The intent was to remove the concomitant confounding effects of treating the GSV and superficial veins. In all 80 limbs in which only the perforators were treated, successful ablation was achieved in 75% at 20.1 month follow-up. Eighteen percent had preexisting deep or superficial axial reflux. In C4–C6 patients, Venous Clincal Severity Score (VCSS) and Venous Disability Score (VDS) significantly improved. Of 37 limbs with ulcers, 86.5% showed rapid healing of ulcers by mean of 35.6 days, Ulcer recurrence was noted in 32.4% after single treatment, which was reduced to 13.5% after a second treatment despite low compliance stocking use of 15%. Recurrence appeared to be related to new or recurrent perforators and post-thrombotic disease [36].

Proof of importance of PV is supported by hemodynamic abnormality in the pathologic state. Leg perforators are associated with abnormal ambulatory venous pressures well above 100 mm Hg during calf muscle contractions. The pressure is released through the PVs from deep to superficial veins with calf contraction analogous to the "broken bellows" described by Negus and Friedgood [37]. Zukowski and Nicolaides showed that 70% of those with ulcerations have moderated to severe hemodynamically significant perforators by ambulatory venous pressure testing [38].

Correction of hemodynamic abnormality has been observed with correction of PVs and is supported by several small studies. Padberg showed ablation of superficial and PVs in 11 cases resulted in improved expulsion fraction and half refill times with no ulcer recurrence when examined by air plethysmograph, foot volumetry and duplex scanning at a mean of 66 months [39]. Rhodes et al. reported significant improvement in calf muscle pump function and vein competence assessed by strain gauge plethysmograhy in 31 limbs following SEPS. Seven underwent SEPS alone and the remaining underwent SEPS plus stripping [40].

14.6 Evidence Against the Importance of IPVs

Isolated incompetent PVs are rare (reported in 3–8 % of CVI patients) [41, 42]. Therefore, separating the effects of isolated IPVs from the effects of superficial or deep venous pathology with respect to pathophysiology and response to treatment has been challenging [43]. To address this important issue, randomized controlled trials (RCTs) have been conducted to measure the effect of IPV treatment on superficial venous treatment by randomizing the groups with or without SEPS.

In mild CVD, abnormalities of the superficial venous system appear to be of greater clinical significance than perforator disease. Two RCTs have shown that with non-ulcer patients, the addition of surgical treatment of IPVs did not impact the clinical results of treating the superficial system alone [44, 45]. Kianiford and colleagues compared stripping of the GSV with or without SEPS and showed no benefit to adding perforator surgery to the GSV treatment [44]. These results were supported by the findings of Fitridge et al. who randomized stripping of the GSV with or without open interruption of previously marked IPVs and found no physiologic benefit (as assessed by air plethysmography) of adding IPV treatment [45]. Superficial axial reflux appeared to show a greater independent contribution toward venous symptoms in uncomplicated disease than IPVs. This is also supported by findings that in cases of both superficial and perforator disease, stripping of the saphenous system from the groin to the knee led to either reversal incompetence in PVs or complete “elimination” of the PVs in 50–80% probably by removing the venous outflow tract. Not only did number of PVs diminish but size of PVs was also reduced [20, 21, 46, 47].

In contrast to mild CVD, evidence for IPV surgery is less clear with clinical, etiologic, anatomic, pathophysiological (CEAP) classes C4–6. With regards to ulceration, a RCT published by the Swedish SEPS group summarized by Nelzen et al., the early results of their trial comparing saphenous surgery with or without SEPS and demonstrating that at 1-year follow-up adding SEPS did not make a difference in mean time to ulcer healing or recurrence [48]. However, the study was limited by the investigators’ inability to accrue the targeted number of patients and was therefore underpowered. It was further limited by the short duration of follow-up. Longer follow-up is needed to establish the effect, if any, that SEPS may have had on healing and ulcer recurrence.

There are two RCTs that did not control for the presence of concomitant GSV surgery and suggested perforator vein surgery had no advantage over compression therapy for ulcers [49, 50]. Stacey et al. examined the effect of IPV ligation on ulcer recurrence in CEAP class C5 patients [49]. They compared IPV ligation combined with saphenous vein surgery with external compression alone and found no hemodynamic advantage in either group, except that those with primary valvular insufficiency (not postthrombotic) had better improvement in calf muscle pump function. The second RCT, by van Gent et al., also suggested no benefit from IPV surgery over compression, although 54 % had concomitant GSV surgery [50]. Despite the limitation that both studies included concomitant GSV surgery, one would have anticipated that adding GSV surgery should have benefitted the IPV surgical group since we know that superficial surgery is superior to compression alone with respect at least in regard to reducing ulcer recurrence [51, 52, 53].

Lastly, hemodynamic studies cannot differentiate the contribution of isolated PVs from those with associated deep or superficial axial reflux which is further confounded by the fact that isolated PVs are rare [22]. Another point to be made against the importance of IPVs is that normal limbs have outward flow in the perforator veins up to 21 % and not all ulcers are associated with incompetent perforator veins [13]. Up to 40 % of venous ulcers have no perforator involvement at all. When IPV is present it is almost always associated with incompetent superficial and/or deep veins [41]. Published evidence that hemodynamic parameters do not improve after IPV ligation have supported the lack of importance of IPVs [49, 54].

14.7 Fate of IPV's After Surgery

PVs will regress afer surgery but increase again with time, thought to be the result of redistribution of venous flow [44]. In a report by van Rij, the majority (76%) of patients developed a new or recurrent PVs after GSV stripping to the knee and direct perforator ligation at 3 years, in stark contrast to the 21% reported after SEPS [55, 56]. The small Dutch group led by Sybrandy reported that after open Linton procedure or SEPS, perforator recurrence rate was 40% at 48 months [57]. Although PV's are associated with recurrence, what remains unclear is whether they are the cause of recurrence. The REVAS group (recurrent varices after surgery) published the experience of eight countries with superficial reflux and previous superficial surgery, and although 55% were associated with incompetent perforators, cause of recurrent symptoms could not be clearly attributed to the perforators [58].

14.8 Diagnosis

Duplex scanning of PVs is best accomplished with the patient in either the reverse Trendelenburg position or standing with the weight placed on the opposite limb. Perforator vein incompetence is defined as the presence of outward or bidirectional flow which can be elicited by manual proximal and distal compression with rapid release, with active dorsiflexion and/or standard rapid cuff release in the standing position with the weight on the opposite limb [59]. Flow lasting greater than 0.5 s in either outward or bidirectional flow is considered abnormal. Pathologic perforator veins must be 3.5 mm or more in diameter based on correlation with clinical severity in the previously mentioned trials [25, 23]. Diameter of the perforator vein is best measured at the level of the fascia. In the case of dividing perforator veins, the measurement is taken away from the division above the fascia to avoid overestimation of the width of the vein.

The optimal method to identify PVs is to scan the GSV first, followed by the posterior accessory GSV of the calf, and then any major tributaries in the calf. Attention should be paid to the presence of skin changes: large tributaries may be clustered in the area that could represent a termination point into the perforator vein. The presence of an ulcer or dressing should not be a deterrent to scanning, as this may be the site of a clinically important perforator. If reflux is detected in the deep vein or superficial vein below a competent valve, it is important to localize the perforator of the femoral canal, which usually connects with a distal incompetent GSV. If reflux is seen in the popliteal vein only, the usual source and point of retrograde outflow is the SSV. The most common IPVs are the posterior tibial perforators middle and upper, which communicate with the posterior accessory GSV of the calf, and the paratibial perforators in the proximal calf, which communicate with the GSV.

Venography is an uncommon method of interrogating perforator veins and has largely been replaced by duplex scanning. Historically, venography was the only method of examining perforators during a time when perforators were being associated with ulcers and treatment by open surgical elimination was widely practiced. The details are well described by Kamida et al. [60]. In brief, to examine perforator veins venographically, a small 22 gauge butterfly needle is inserted into a dorsal foot superficial vein. The exam is best performed in the upright, non-weight-bearing position by having the patient stand with the contralateral leg on a box. Ankle tourniquets are essential to drive the contrast into the deep system and evaluate for perforating veins. The tourniquets are placed at various levels in the leg to identify points of communication between the deep and superficial veins. Fluoroscopic examination of the pattern of venous filling is essential part of identifying the presumably pathologic perforators.

14.9 Treatment Options and Techniques

Current options for treatment are SEPS, direct open surgical division of individual perforators, thermal ablation with either radiofrequency ablation (RFA) or endovenous laser ablation (EVLA), or ultrasound-guided sclerotherapy (UGS).

14.9.1 SEPS

After Hauer described the endoscopic procedure for IPV, O'Donnell introduced the application of the laparoscope to facilitate its technical needs [61]. Gloviczki and colleagues and Conrad are to be credited for introducing the CO_2 inflation method of creating the dissecting space [62, 63]. Standard laparoscopic equipment is required and either the single or double port technique could be used. If the double port method is selected, the 5 mm distal port to pass the 5 mm harmonic scalpel, scissors, or dissecting instruments and a 10 mm proximal port with 10 mm camera are set up. The leg is exsanguinated with an Esmarch bandage and proximal thigh tourniquet inflated to 300 mmHg. Balloon dissection is performed with pressures of 30 mmHg. The proximal port is placed 10 cm distal to tibial tuberosity; distal port is placed 10–12 cm further down but above the medial ankle or diseased gaiter area.

For best results, Rhodes and colleagues recommend paratibial fasciotomy to ligate the middle and upper posterior tibial perforators in the intermuscular septum [64]. Care is taken to place the fasciotomy close to the tibia to avoid injury to the posterior tibial vessels and nerve. The retromalleolar lower posterior tibial perforator is best treated by small incision directly over it or ultrasound-guided foam or liquid sclerotherapy. If treatment of the superficial axial system is required, the ablation or stripping and phlebectomy are performed following the SEPS procedure.

14.9.2 Percutaneous Ablation

Percutaneous ablation techniques include radiofrequency ablation (RFA), endovenous laser ablation (EVLA), and ultrasound-guided sclerotherapy (UGS). Percutaneous ablation allows precise identification and localization of each perforator vein that can provide treatment without disruptive incisions or tissue dissections. It can be done in the outpatient setting; local (RFA, EVLA) or no (UGS) anesthesia is necessary, and it can be used as an adjunct procedure during surgery for CVD. It is beneficial in cases where the overlying skin is severely sclerotic or with the presence of an active ulcer. Percutaneous ablation is also helpful in patients who are obese or poor candidates for SEPS due to anesthesia risks. These procedures can be repeated without sequelae.

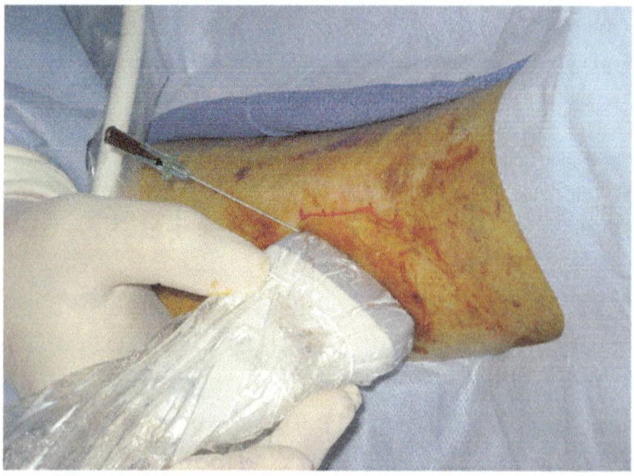

Fig. 14.2 Importance of identifying the perforator artery begins with confirming Doppler data with image. Initially perforator is identified with typical to and fro flow

With percutaneous ablation, it is imperative to identify the perforator artery (Figs. 14.2, 14.3, 14.4, 14.5, and 14.6). "Blind sticks" are discouraged due to the significant risk of inadvertently ablating the perforator artery, which could lead to skin necrosis. While injecting the vein under duplex guidance, occasionally, resistance is encountered which could indicate the needle is now outside the vein or the vein is maximally filled, at which time the flow can appear stagnant during the injection. At that point, ablation must be stopped and the duplex used to check access for PV patency and color flow. Alternatively, some advocate injecting or ablating the superficial vein into which the incompetent perforator vein drains. Finally, good results have been obtained with UGS by injecting the microvasculature associated with IPV skin changes.

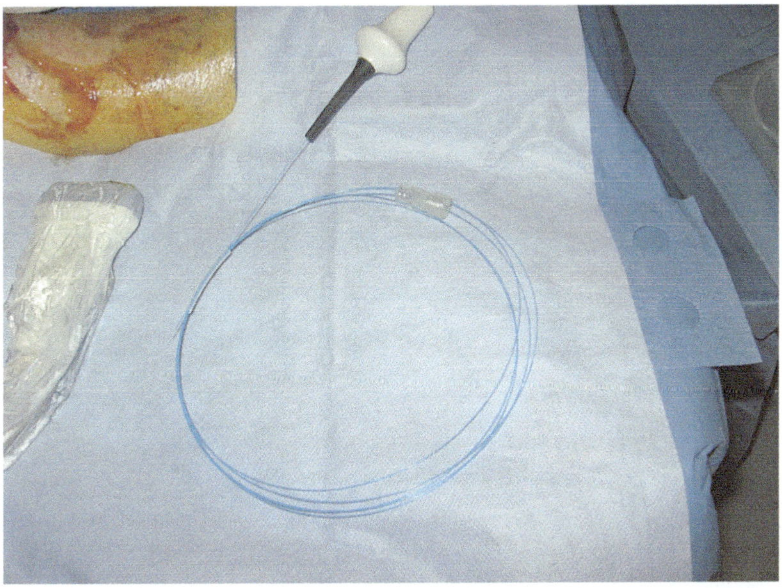

Fig. 14.3 Perforator artery adjacent to vein is clearly identified by arterial signal

Percutaneous ablation is generally confirmed when there is no spontaneous flow and no flow with proximal and distal compression and release. If there is persistent flow through the PV, reinjection with the same technique can be done either at the same site or through a superficial vein communicating with the PV since often times reaccessing a previously treated PV can be difficult. Inadvertent infiltration of the perivascular tissue during UGS at standard volumes usually results in no major consequences unless the perforator artery is injected.

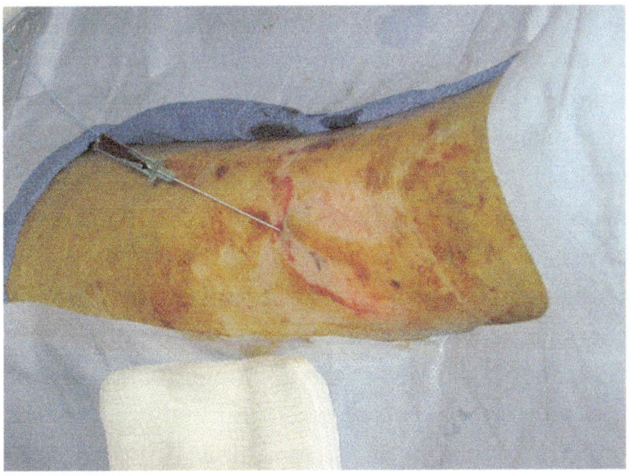

Fig. 14.4 Perforator artery is avoided and not in the path of the needle while access of vein is achieved

14.9.3 Thermal Ablation Techniques

The application of RFA energy to treat PVs was first described and presented by Whiteley et al. and was referred to as "TRLOP," for *transluminal occlusion of perforator* [65]. Others have referred to all transcutaneous methods of treatment including RFA, EVLA, and UGS as "PAPS," for *percutaneous ablation of perforators* [66]. Whichever term is applied, the RFA results by Bacon et al. showed the surrogate outcome of successful perforator ablation by RFA was 81 % at 5 years [67]. Clinical outcomes, particularly in patients with advanced CVD, however, are still lacking.

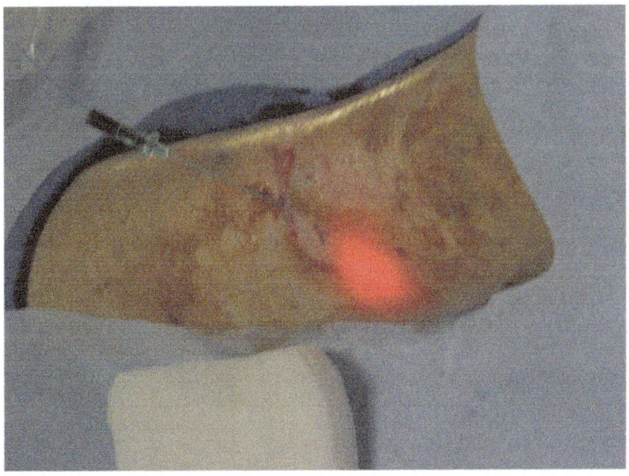

Fig. 14.5 Successful ablation of perforator vein

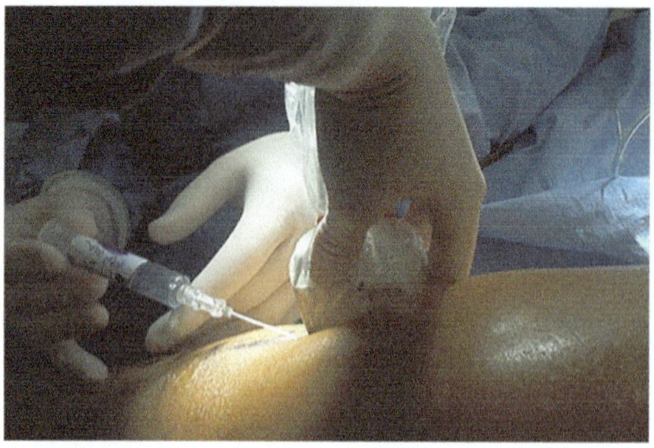

Fig. 14.6 Confirmation that perforator artery is left undisturbed posttreatment

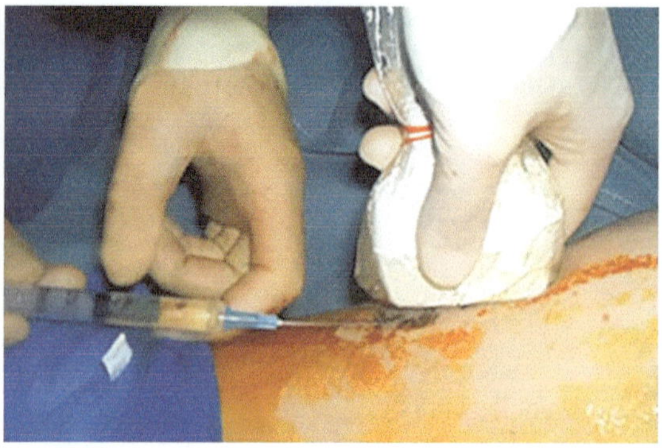

Fig. 14.7 Laser ablation with duplex ultrasound isolation of perforator and needle access (Courtesy of Dr. Lowell Kabnick)

RFA access is achieved by ultrasound guidance with the patient in the reverse Trendelenburg position and the ultrasound transducer longitudinal and parallel to the PV. In order to avoid injury to the deep vessels and nerve, the tip is placed at the level of the fascia. The stylet is placed under ultrasound guidance into the PV to the fascia and confirmed by measuring impedance goal of 150–350Ω. Prior to treatment in the Trendelenburg position, tumescent with local anesthetic is infiltrated around the stylet to create a "halo" around the catheter or laser fiber to achieve optimal contact between treating element and vein, to avoid thermal skin injury, to provide anesthesia during the ablation, and to provide a heat sink for the delivered thermal energy. The stylet is heated to 85°C and allowed to treat four quadrants each for 1 min; a second treatment is done after withdrawing the stylet 2 mm or in the same location if completion duplex shows persistent flow. Posttreatment, the PV is examined by duplex for success as indicated by lack of flow by proximal and distal compression and release, and adjacent deep veins are examined for DVT.

Endovenous laser treatment is a technically simpler method than the current RFA procedure and is shown to be safe and feasible [68] (Figs. 14.7, 14.8, 14.9, and 14.10). Access is identical to RFA, but the ablation is performed through a needle, depending on size of laser fiber. For the 600 μm fiber, a 16 gauge angiocatheter is needed; for a 400 μm fiber, a 21 gauge needle is required. Tumescent anesthesia is applied after the tip of the laser is at or just below the fascia. Elias et al. recommend 120 J per segment treated with the 810 nm laser, with power set at 15 W at 4-s pulse intervals and two treatment pulses per segment [66]. A total of three segments per vein are treated if possible. Proebstle and Herdemann also suggest treating three segments or levels, below the fascia, at the fascia, and above the fascia, with each segment receiving 60–100 J [68]. Treating three segments is sometimes not possible due to the tortuosity and short length of many perforators. Posttreatment, the PV is examined by duplex for success as indicated by lack of flow by proximal and distal compression and release, and adjacent deep veins are examined for DVT.

14.9.4 Ultrasound-Guided Sclerotherapy Techniques

Injection of varicose veins and, hence, perforator veins has been performed for decades. Fegan described his method of injecting "control points" or perforator veins based on clinical exam localizing the PV by palpation followed by injection into an adjacent varix while the limb was elevated [69]. With the guidance of duplex imaging, Thibault and Lewis reported their prospective experience in 1992, where they found the surrogate endpoint of successful perforator ablation of 83.7 % at 6 months [70]. Likewise, Guex reported a 90 % success rate of obliterating PVs with one to three injection sessions using Sotradecol® 3 % or polidocanol 3 % for veins >4 mm, and a more

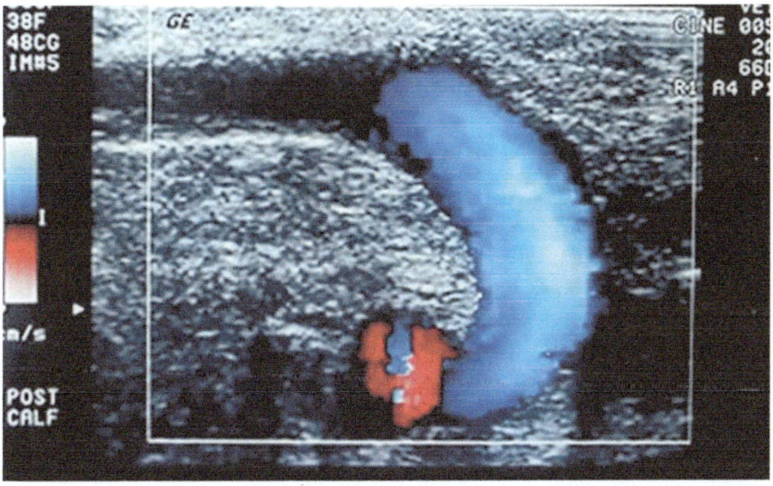

Fig. 14.8 Laser fiber for ablation (Courtesy of Dr. Lowell Kabnick)

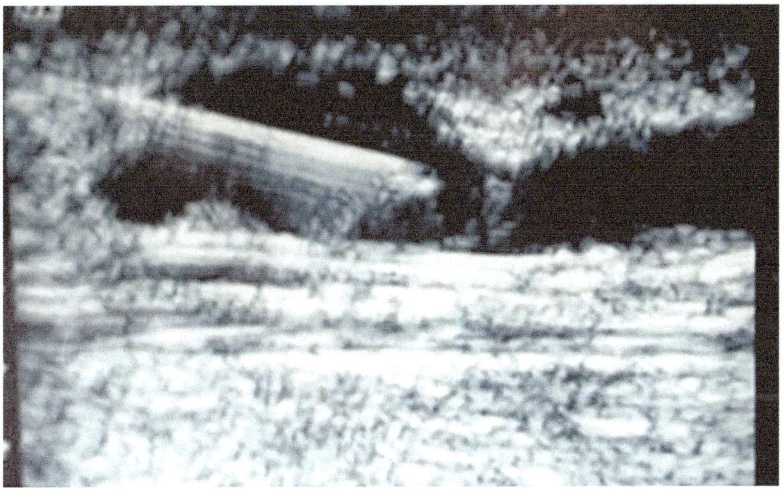

Fig. 14.9 Laser fiber inserted into existing needle (Courtesy of Dr. Lowell Kabnick)

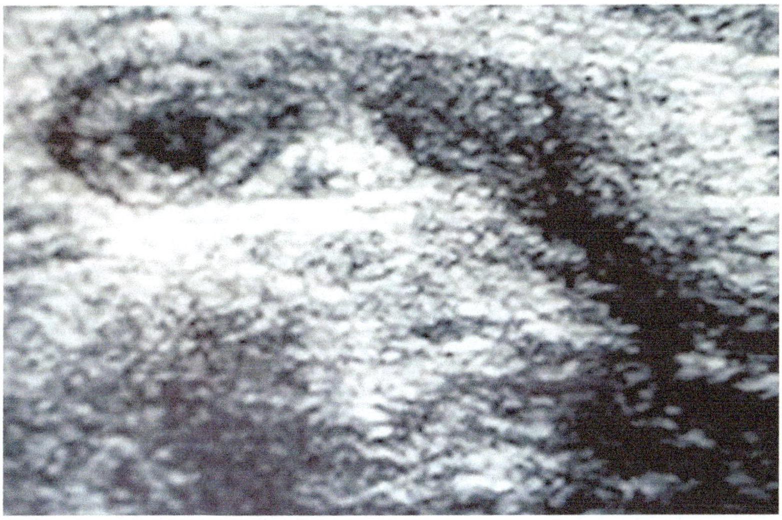

Fig. 14.10 Laser fiber with visible transmission (Courtesy of Dr. Lowell Kabnick)

dilute solution for veins <4 mm [71]. In the clinical series at Straub, 75 % remained successfully ablated at 20.1 months, and 86.5 % showed rapid healing of ulcers at a mean time of 35.6 days [36].

The initial localization and marking of the perforator vein is achieved with a linear pulsed wave transducer 4–12 MHz. For injection in the office setting or operating room, using the "hockey-stick" probe (10–12 MHz) is technically easier, but the same can be achieved with the standard diagnostic transducer. In our institution, the procedure is performed by a vascular surgeon with the assistance of a registered vascular technologist both in the outpatient clinic and in the operating room.

All planned injection sites are marked prior to procedure, and the patient is kept warm to avoid vasoconstriction. One may apply nitropaste if necessary to counteract vasoconstriction especially in the colder operating room. If vasospasm is encountered, position the patient in the reverse Trendelenburg position to maximally fill the IPV. Under duplex guidance, the 25 or 27 gauge needle is inserted into the skin close to the transducer, either parallel or in cross section to the probe. The target is the perforator vein or the communicating varicosity just above the perforator vein. By ultrasound guidance, if the artery is in the path of the needle, it is best to access a varix 5–10 mm from the PV that communicates with the perforator vein as opposed to accessing the PV directly.

Venous blood is withdrawn, and then 1.0–1.5 cc of sclerosant (sodium morrhuate 5 %, polidocanol 1 % or sodium tetradecyl sulfate 3 %) is injected. Depending on the size of the PV, larger ones may take up to 2.0 cc to completely obliterate. It is imperative to avoid the perforator artery that is usually a single vessel but can occasionally be paired. The perforator artery will have a low Doppler resistance waveform prior to injection. After successful UGS, the Doppler waveform of the perforator artery will typically convert to a high-resistance waveform with a lower end-diastolic velocity suggestive of vasospasm or previous shunting of blood through the perforator vein.

The needle is withdrawn and local pressure is applied. At completion, final duplex scan of the area confirms no flow in the PV and elastic compression wraps or stockings are applied for 4–7 days. At our institution, both liquid and foam sclerotherapy is utilized: liquid sclerosant is used for small PVs less than 3.5 mm, and for larger PVs, foam is preferred.

Serious complications of UGS are rare but include risk of anaphylaxis, pulmonary emboli, and death in <0.01 %. With foam, there is increased risk of bubbles passing through a patent foramen ovale into the ocular and cerebral circulation, where they can produce transient ischemic attacks, temporary blindness or scotoma, or stroke [71–75]. Visual disorders can occur with liquid sclerotherapy but are more common with foam, at 0.5–1 per 100 sessions, and may occur more frequently in patients with migraines and visual aura, possibly through a patent foramen ovale (PFO) [72]. Others can have vasovagal fainting, not specific to UGS, but which can result in traumatic injury. Deep vein thrombosis or skin ulceration is rare.

Foam has a theoretical advantage over liquid because the detergent sclerosant class works by a mechanism of protein theft denaturation. Aggregates of detergent molecules form a lipid bilayer in the form of a micelle, cylinder, or sheet which disrupts the cell surface membrane. The surface area of the lipid bilayer is maximized when shaken as foam, hence potentially increasing its effectiveness. The foam displaces blood and increases the contact time between sclerosant and endothelium, resulting in a more effective treatment than liquid sclerotherapy.

Foam can be made using a technique initially described by Tessari [76]. We use two 5 cc syringes and either a three-way stopcock or a two-way female-to-female Luer-Lok connector to create foam using a detergent sclerosant. Options include polidocanol, sodium tetradecyl sulfate, or sodium morrhuate. We use 1 mL of sclerosant drawn up into one 5 cc syringe and 3 mL of air into the other syringe. The air can be filtered and made sterile. The three-way stopcock is used to attach the two syringes, and with 15–20 alternating movements from one syringe to the next through the stopcock, a foam of about 4 mL will be created. Since the stability of the foam is only 2–3 min, the solution is prepared just before planned injection and after the perforator is already identified by duplex ultrasound.

14.10 Influence of Postthrombotic Syndrome on Outcomes

Outcomes after treating PVs appear more favorable with primary disease as opposed to secondary or post-thrombotic disease. Eliminating PVs in the presence of PTS needs to be carefully considered, since they may serve as important alternative drainage routes for the deep system in the presence of deep obstruction. In the presence of deep vein obstruction, Burnand concluded surgery on superficial or perforating veins did not effectively control recurrence [77]. The NASEPS registry showed that PTS had a negative impact on outcomes, with increased recurrent ulcers [30]. Likewise PTS was found to represent an adverse factor associated with ulcer recurrence following ultrasound guided sclerotherapy [36].

14.11 Suggested Indications for PV Treatment

Selective PV intervention particularly for those with primary valvular disease is recommended for advanced CVD for venous ulceration, healed or active. For C5–6, American Venous Forum (AVF) guidelines suggest that PV treatment be considered when outward flow duration is >500ms (0.5 sec), PV diameter of 3.5 mm or more, and PV under a healed or active ulcer [78]. In more advanced levels of CVD, correction of PVs is likely warranted particularly when combined with correction of other axial reflux segments.

PV intervention is not recommended as sole treatment in the presence of correctable axial superficial reflux for milder clinical classes of CVD. In mild CVD, the superficial system appears to play a more important role than PV and probably serve as extensions of axial superficial, deep reflux and/or superficial varices. AVF guidelines recommend against selective treatment of incompetent perforator veins in mild C2 disease [78].

It is unclear as to what role PVs play in patients with postthrombotic disease. PV ablation in the presence of deep venous obstruction from DVT must be approached with caution since ablation of a potentially critical outflow vessel may worsen the venous hypertension and clinical state.

Future studies should be directed towards examining the role of PVs in the development of recurrent varicose veins and in the presence of deep venous reflux and obstruction. Indications for intervention will continue to evolve and need to be clarified by carefully designed studies, void of concomitant intervention of the superficial and deep systems, in order to determine the primary effect of PVs in CVD.

References

1. Homans J. The etiology and treatment of varicose ulcer of the leg. Surg Gynecol Obstet. 1917;24:300–11.
2. Von Loder JC. AnatomischeTafeln. Landes-Industrie-Comptoir, Text, vol. 2. Weimar; 1803 (Tab. 127).
3. Gay J. Lettsonian lectures 1867. Varicose disease of the lower extremities. London: Churchill; 1868.
4. Kistner RL. Etiology and treatment of varicose ulcer of the leg. J Am Coll Surg. 2005;200:646–7.
5. Linton RR. The communicating veins of the lower leg and the operative technique of their ligation. Ann Surg. 1938;107:582–93.
6. Field P, van Boxel P. The role of the Linton flap procedure in the management of stasis, dermatitis and ulceration in the lower limb. Surgery. 1971;70:920–6.
7. Puts JP, Gruwez JA. Surgical treatment of the post-thrombotic syndrome: improvement of the Linton operation by use of piracetam. Br J Surg. 1993; 80(Suppl):115.
8. Cockett FB, Elgan Jones DE. The ankle blow-out syndrome. A new approach to the varicose ulcer problem. Lancet. 1953;i:17–23.
9. DePalma RG. Surgical therapy for venous stasis: results of a modified Linton operation. Am J Surg. 1979;137:810–3.
10. Hauer G. The endoscopic subfascial division of the perforating veins—preliminary report. Vasa. 1985;14:59–61.
11. Thomson H. The surgical anatomy of the superficial and perforating veins of the lower limb. Ann R Coll Surg Engl. 1979;61:198–205.
12. Van Limborgh J. L'anatomie du systemeveineux de l'extremiteinferieure en relation avec la pathologievariqueuse. Folia Angiol. 1961;8:240–57.

13. Sarin S, Scurr JG, Coleridge Smith PD. Calf perforating veins in venous disease. In: Raymond-Martimbeau P, Prescott R, Zummo M, editors. Phlebology 92. Paris: John LibbeyEurotext; 1992. p. 102–3.
14. Gloviczki P, Mozes G. Development and anatomy of the venous system. In: Gloviczki P, editor. Handbook of venous disorders: guidelines of the American venous forum. 3rd ed. London: Edward Arnold Ltd; 2009. p. 12–24.
15. Labropoulos N, Giannoukas AD, Nicolaides AN, Ramaswami G, Leon M, Burke P. New insights into the pathophysiologic condition of venous ulceration with color-flow duplex imaging: implications for treatment? J Vasc Surg. 1995;22:45–50.
16. Myers KA, Ziegenbein RW, Zeng G, Matthews PG. Duplex ultrasonography scanning for chronic venous disease: patterns of venous reflux. J Vasc Surg. 1995;21:605–12.
17. Burnand KG, Wadoodi A. The physiology and hemodynamics of chronic venous insufficiency of the lower limb. In: Handbook of venous disorders. 3rd ed. London: Edward Arnold Ltd; 2009. p. 47–55.
18. Burnand KG, Whimster I, Clemenson G, et al. The relationship between the number of capillaries in the skin of the venous ulcer bearing area of the lower leg and the fall in foot vein pressure during exercise. Br J Surg. 1981;68:297–300.
19. Burnand KG, Whimster I, Naidoo A, Browse NL. Pericapillary fibrin in the ulcer bearing skin of the leg. Br Med J. 1982;285:1071–2.
20. Stuart WP, Adam DJ, Allan PL, Ruckley CV, Bradbury AW. Saphenous surgery does not correct perforator incompetence in the presence of deep venous reflux. J Vasc Surg. 1998;28:834–8.
21. Campbell WA, West A. Duplex ultrasound audit of operative treatment of primary varicose veins. Phlebology. 1995;10(Suppl):407–9.
22. Labropoulos N, Tassiopoulos AK, Bhatti AF, Leon L. Development of reflux in the perforator veins in limbs with primary venous disease. J Vasc Surg. 2006;43:558–62.
23. Labropoulos N, Mansour MA, Kang SS, et al. New insights into perforator vein incompetence. Eur J Vasc Endovasc Surg. 1999;18:228–34.
24. Stuart WP, Adam DJ, Allan PL, Ruckley V, Bradbury AW. The relationship between the number, competence, and diameter of medial calf perforating veins and the clinical status in healthy subjects and patients with lower-limb venous disease. J Vasc Surg. 2000;32:138–43.
25. Delis KT, Husmann M, Kalodiki E, Wolfe JH, Nicolaides AN. In situ hemodynamics of perforating veins in chronic venous insufficiency. J Vasc Surg. 2001;33:773–82.
26. Sandri JL, Barros FS, Pontes S, et al. Diameter-reflux relationship in perforating veins of patients with varicose veins. J Vasc Surg. 1999;30:867–74.
27. Ibegbuna V, Delis KT, Nicolaides AN. Haemodynamic and clinical impact of superficial, deep and perforator vein incompetence. Eur J Vasc Endovasc Surg. 2006;31:535–41.
28. Lees TA, Lambert D. Patterns of venous reflux in limbs with skin changes associated with chronic venous insufficiency. Br J Surg. 1993;80:725–8.
29. Delis KT, Ibegbuna V, Nicolaides AN, Lauro A, Hafez H. Prevalence and distribution of incompetent perforating veins in chronic venous insufficiency. J Vasc Surg. 1998;28:815–25.
30. Gloviczki P, Bergan JJ, Rhodes JM, Canton LG, Harmsen S, Ilstrup DM, The North American Study Group. Mid-term results of endoscopic perforator vein interruption for chronic venous insufficiency: lessons learned from the North American subfascial endoscopic perforator surgery registry. J Vasc Surg. 1999;29:489–502.
31. Iafrati MD, Pare GJ, O'Donnell TF, Estes J. Is the nihilistic approach to surgical reduction of superficial and perforator vein incompetence for veous ulcer justified? J Vasc Surg. 2002;36:1167–74.
32. Tawes RL, Barron ML, Coello AA, Joyce DH, Kolvenbach R. Optimal therapy for advanced chronic venous insufficiency. J Vasc Surg. 2003;37:545–51.
33. Bianchi C, Ballard JL, Abou-Zamzam AM, Teruya TH. Subfascial endoscopic perforator vein surgery combined with saphenous vein ablation: results and critical analysis. J Vasc Surg. 2003;38:67–71.
34. Luebke T, Brunkwall J. Meta-analysis of subfascial endoscopic perforator vein surgery (SEPS) for chronic venous insufficiency. Phlebology. 2009;24:8–16.
35. Tenbrook Jr JA, Iafrati MD, O'Donnell Jr TF, Wolf MP, Hoffman SN, Pauker SG, et al. Systematic review of outcomes after surgical management of venous disease incorporating subfascial endoscopic perforator surgery. J Vasc Surg. 2004;39:583–9.
36. Masuda EM, Kessler DM, Lurie F, Puggioni A, Kistner RL, Eklof B. The effect of ultrasound-guided sclerotherapy of incompetent perforator veins on venous clinical severity and disability scores. J Vasc Surg. 2006;43:551–7.
37. Negus D, Friedgood A. The effective management of venous ulceration. Br J Surg. 1983;70:623–7.
38. Zukowski AJ, Nicolaides AN, Szendro G, Irvine A, Lewis R, Malouf GM, Hobbs JT, Dudley HAF. Haemodynamic significance of incompetent calf perforating veins. Br J Surg. 1991;78:625–9.
39. Padberg Jr FT, Pappas PJ, Araki CT, Back TL, Hobson 2nd RW. Hemodynamic and clinical improvement after superficial vein ablation in primary combined venous insufficiency with ulceration. J Vasc Surg. 1996;24:711–8.
40. Rhodes JM, Gloviczki P, Canton L, Heaser TV, Rooke TW. Endoscopic perforator vein division with ablation of superficial reflux improves venous hemodynamics. J Vasc Surg. 1998;28:839–47.
41. Labropoulos N, Leon M, Geroulakos G, Volteas N, Chan P, Nicolaides AN. Venous hemodynamic abnormalities in patients with leg ulceration. Am J Surg. 1995;169:572–4.
42. Hanrahan LM, Araki CT, Rodriguez AA, Kechejian GJ, LaMorte WW, Menzoian JO. Distribution of

valvular incompetence in patients with venous stasis ulceration. J Vasc Surg. 1991;13:805–12.
43. O'Donnell TF. The role of perforators in chronic venous insufficiency. Phlebology. 2010;25:3–10.
44. Kianifard B, Holdstock J, Allen C, Smith C, Price B, Whiteley MS. Randomized clinical trial of the effect of adding subfascial endoscopic perforator surgery to standard great saphenous vein stripping. Br J Surg. 2007;94:1075–80.
45. Fitridge RA, Dunlop C, Raptis S, Thompson MM, Leppard P, Quigley F. A prospective randomized trial evaluating the haemodynamic role of incompetent calf perforating veins. Aust N Z J Surg. 1999;69:214–6.
46. Mendes RR, Marston WA, Farber MA, Keagy BA. Treatment of superficial and perforator venous incompetence without deep venous insufficiency: is routine perforator ligation necessary? J Vasc Surg. 2003; 38:891–5.
47. Al-Mulhim AS, El-Hoseiny H, Al-Mulhim FM, Bayameen O, Sami MM, Abdulaziz K, Raslan M, Al-Shewy A, Al-Malt M. Surgical correction of main stem reflux in the superficial venous system: does it improve the blood flow of incompetent perforating veins? World J Surg. 2003;27:793–6.
48. Nelzen O, Fransson I, The Swedish SEPS Study Group. Early results from a randomized trial of saphenous surgery with or without subfascial endoscopic perforator surgery in patients with a venous ulcer. Br J Surg. 2011;98:495–500.
49. Stacey MC, Burnand KG, Layer GT, Pattison M. Calf pump function in patients with healed venous ulcers is not improved by surgery to the communicating veins or by elastic stockings. Br J Surg. 1988;75:436–9.
50. van Gent WB, Hop WC, van Pragg MC, MacKaay AJ, Wittens CH. Conservative versus surgical treatment of venous leg ulcers: a prospective, randomized, multicenter trial. J Vasc Surg. 2006;44:563–71.
51. Barwell JR, Davies CE, Deacon J, Harvey K, Minor J, Sassano A, Taylor M, et al. Comparison of surgery and compression with compression alone in chronic venous ulceration (ESCHAR study): randomized controlled trial. Lancet. 2004;363:1854–9.
52. Gohel MS, Barwell JR, Taylor M, Chant T, Foy C, Earnshaw JJ, Heather BP, Mitchell DC, Whyman MR, Poskitt KR. Long term results of compression therapy alone versus compression plus surgery in chronic venous ulceration (ESCHAR): randomized controlled trial. BMJ. 2007;335:83.
53. Zamboni P, Cisno C, Marchetti F, Mazza P, Fogato L, Carandina S, De Palma M, Liboni A. Minimally invasive surgical management of primary venous ulcers vs. compression treatment: a randomized clinical trial. Eur J Vasc Endovasc Surg. 2003;25:313–8.
54. Akesson H, Brudin L, Cwikiel W, Ohlin P, Plate G. Does the correction of insufficient superficial and perforating veins improve venous function in patients with deep venous insufficiency? Phlebology. 1990;5: 113–23.
55. Van Rij AM, Hill G, Gray C, Christie R, Macfarlane J, Thomson I. A prospective study of the fate of venous leg perforators after varicose vein surgery. J Vasc Surg. 2005;42:1156–62.
56. Roka F, Binder M, Bohler-Sommeregger K. Mid-term recurrence of incompetent perforating veins after combined superficial endoscopic perforating vein surgery. J Vasc Surg. 2006;44:359–63.
57. Sybrandy JE, van Gent WB, Pierik EG, Wittens CH. Endoscopic versus open subfascial division of incompetent perforating veins in the treatment of venous leg ulceration: long-term follow-up. J Vasc Surg. 2001;33:1028–32.
58. Perrin MR, Labropoulos N, Leon LR. Presentation of the patient with recurrent varices after surgery (REVAS). J Vasc Surg. 2006;43:327–34.
59. Van Bemmelen PS, Bedford G, Beach K, Strandness Jr DE. Quantitative segmental evaluation of venous valvular reflux with duplex ultrasound scanning. J Vasc Surg. 1989;10:425–31.
60. Kamida CB, Kistner RL, Eklof B, Masuda EM. Lower extremity ascending and descending phlebography. In: Gloviczki P, editor. Handbook of venous disorders: guidelines of the American Venous Forum. 3rd ed. London: Edward Arnold Ltd; 2009. p. 160–8.
61. O'Donnell Jr TJ. Surgical treatment of incompetent perforating veins. In: Bergan JJ, Kistner RL, editors. Atlas of venous surgery. Philadelphia: W.B. Saunders Company; 1992. p. 111–24.
62. Gloviczki P, Cambria RA, Rhee RY, Canton LG, McKusick MA. Surgical technique and preliminary results of endoscopic subfascial division of perforating veins. J Vasc Surg. 1996;23:517–23.
63. Conrad P. Endoscopic exploration of the subfascial space of the lower leg with perforator interruption using laparoscopic equipment: a preliminary report. Phlebology. 1994;9:154–7.
64. Rhodes JM, Kalra M, Gloviczki P. The management of incompetent perforating veins with open and endoscopic surgery. In: Gloviczki P, editor. Handbook of venous disorders: guidelines of the American Venous Forum. 3rd ed. London: Edward Arnold Ltd; 2009. p. 523–35.
65. Whiteley MS, Holdstock J. Percutaneous radiofrequency ablations of varicose veins (VNUS closure). In: Greenhalgh RM, editor. Vascular and endovascular challenges. London: Biba Publishing; 2004. p. 361–81.
66. Elias S, Peden E. Ultrasound-guided percutaneous ablation for the treatment of perforating vein incompetence. Vascular. 2007;15:281–9.
67. Bacon JL, Dinneen AJ, Marsh P, Holdstock JM, Price BA, Whiteley MS. Five-year results of incompetent perforator vein closure using trans-luminal occlusion of perforator. Phlebology. 2009;24:74–8.
68. Proebstle TM, Herdemann S. Early results and feasibility of incompetent perforator vein ablation by endovenous laser treatment. Dermatol Surg. 2007;33:162–8.
69. Fegan WG. Injection with compression as a treatment for varicose veins. Proc R Soc Med. 1965;58:874–6.
70. Thibault PK, Lewis WA. Recurrent varicose veins. Part 2: injection of incompetent perforating veins

using ultrasound guidance. J Dermatol Surg Oncol. 1992;18:895–900.
71. Guex JJ. Ultrasound guided sclerotherapy (UGS) for perforating veins (PV). Hawaii Med J. 2000;59:261–2.
72. Guex JJ. Complications and side-effects of foam sclerotherapy. Phlebology. 2009;24:270–4.
73. Guex JJ, Allaert FA, Gillet JL, Chleir F. Immediate and midterm complications of sclerotherapy: report of a prospective multicenter registry of 12,173 sclerotherapy sessions. Dermatol Surg. 2005;31:123–8.
74. Coleridge Smith P. Saphenous ablation: sclerosant or sclerofoam? Semin Vasc Surg. 2005;18:19–24.
75. Hanisch F, Muller T, Krivokuca M, Winterholler M. Stroke following variceal sclerotherapy. Eur J Med Res. 2004;9:282–4.
76. Tessari L. Nouvelle technique d'obtention de la sclero-mousse. Phlebologie. 2000;53:129.
77. Burnand KG, O'Donnell TF, Thomas LM, et al. The relationship between post-phlebetic changes in the deep veins and the result of surgical treatment of venous ulcers. Lancet. 1976;1:936.
78. Gloviczki P, Comerota AJ, Dalsing MC, Eklof BG, Gillespie DL, Gloviczki ML, Lohr JM, McLafferty RB, Meissner MH, Murad MH, Padberg FT, Pappas PJ, Passman MA, Raffetto JD, Vasquez MA, Wakefield TW. The care of patients with varicose veins and associated chronic venous diseases: clinical practice guidelines of the Society for Vascular Surgery and the American Venous Forum. J Vasc Surg. 2011; 53:2S–48.

Upper Deep Vein Disease

15

Sapan S. Desai, Eric Mowatt-Larssen, and Mitchell Cox

Contents

S.S. Desai, MD, PhD, MBA (✉)
Department of Surgery,
Duke University Medical Center,
Durham, NC, USA

Department of Cardiothoracic and Vascular Surgery,
University of Texas at Houston Medical School,
Houston, TX, USA
e-mail: sapan.desai@surgisphere.com

E. Mowatt-Larssen, MD, FACPh, RPhS
757 Pacific Street, Suite C-2, Monterey,
CA 93940, USA
e-mail: eric.mowatt.larssen@gmail.com

M. Cox, MD
Department of Surgery,
Duke University Medical Center,
Durham, NC, USA
e-mail: mitchell.cox2@duke.edu

Abstract

Chronic cerebrospinal insufficiency, venous thoracic outlet syndrome, and superior vena cava syndrome are disease processes that are considered pathology of the deep upper venous system. The incidence, pathophysiology, diagnosis, and management are discussed in this chapter.

15.1 Chronic Cerebrospinal Insufficiency

15.1.1 Definition

Chronic cerebrospinal insufficiency (CCSVI) is a syndrome of stenosis of the cerebrospinal venous system, especially the internal jugular and azygos systems [1]. There is collateralization around these stenotic obstructions, and blood flow mean transit time is increased. On venography, these lesions consist of primarily intraluminal defects. CCSVI was recently incorporated into the International Union of Phlebology consensus document as a truncular venous malformation [2].

E. Mowatt-Larssen et al. (eds.), *Phlebology, Vein Surgery and Ultrasonography*,
DOI 10.1007/978-3-319-01812-6_15,

15.1.2 Symptoms

A strong association between CCSVI and multiple sclerosis (MS) has been proposed by Dr. Paolo Zamboni [3], corroborated by some, and challenged by others [4]. Common symptoms of MS are listed in Fig. 15.1. MS symptoms often improve or resolve (remit) and then recur (relapse) but can progress without remission.

Other vascular problems of the cerebrospinal system produce different symptoms. Acute dural sinus or jugular vein obstruction, such as that caused by hypercoagulability, catheterization complication, or compression (tumor or lymphadenopathy), can cause acute symptoms of mental confusion, severe headaches, and visual disturbances. Treatment with angioplasty, with or without stenting, is often clinically successful [5]. Transient global amnesia has been hypothesized to be caused by internal jugular vein reflux [6]. CCSVI has not been found in association with other neurodegenerative diseases like Alzheimer's disease, Parkinson's disease, or amyotrophic lateral sclerosis [1].

- Blurry or double vision
- Numbness
- Tingling
- Limb weakness
- Loss of balance

Fig. 15.1 Some common symptoms of multiple sclerosis

CCSVI is distinct from venous sinus thrombosis, which is a well-established cause of acute mental status change, headache, and stroke. Venous sinus thrombosis may be caused by hypercoagulability, catheterization complications, or compression by tumor. The mainstay of treatment is systemic anticoagulation, but interventional techniques including catheter-directed lysis, mechanical thrombectomy, and angioplasty have been sporadically reported.

15.1.3 Anatomy and Physiology

Intracranial blood passes through the dural sinuses into the extracranial system of the internal jugular and (IJV) vertebral veins (Fig. 15.2). Most blood volume drains anteriorly through the IJV in the supine position and posteriorly through the vertebral veins in the standing position. The vertebral system also communicates with deep thoracic and lumbar and hemiazygos veins. The vertebral, deep thoracic and lumbar, and hemiazygos veins all drain into the final collecting azygos vein (AV).

The IJV and AV drain into the superior vena cava (SVC). Most CCSVI abnormalities occur

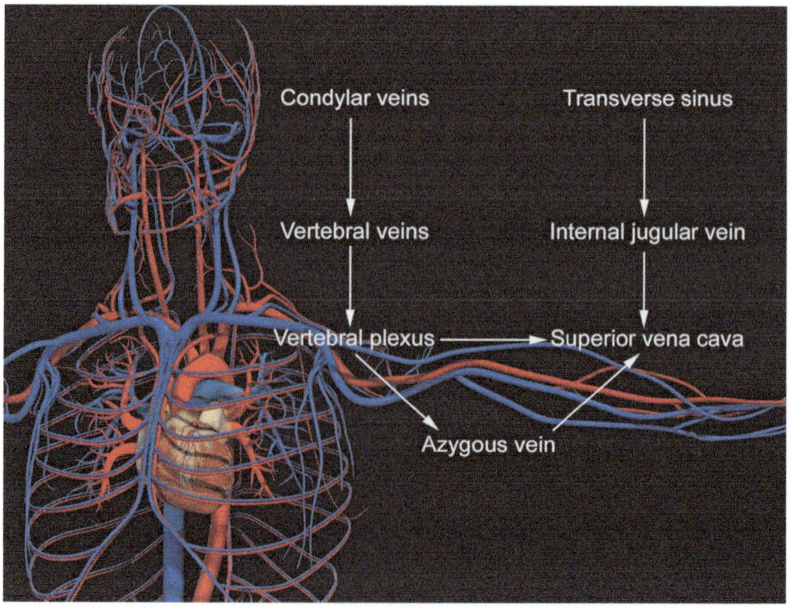

Fig. 15.2 Anatomy

near the junction at either the IJV or AV with the SVC and usually near at or near a valve. Physiologic obstructions also occur, such as at the skull base, adjacent to the carotid bulb, and where the strap muscles compress the vein [5]. Physiologic obstructions must be separated from pathologic obstructions, since the former should not be treated.

15.1.4 Pathophysiology

The classic pathophysiologic model of multiple sclerosis is that of an autoimmune disorder [7]. CCSVI advocates largely do not challenge the importance of this model in understanding the disease. MS plaques, however, also show impressive pathophysiologic similarities to chronic venous insufficiency of the lower extremities. Both show perivenous iron deposition and pericapillary fibrin cuffs. Activated macrophages show hemosiderin deposits and ferritin-like structures. There is hyperactivation of metalloproteinases and hypoactivation of tissue inhibitors of metalloproteinases [8].

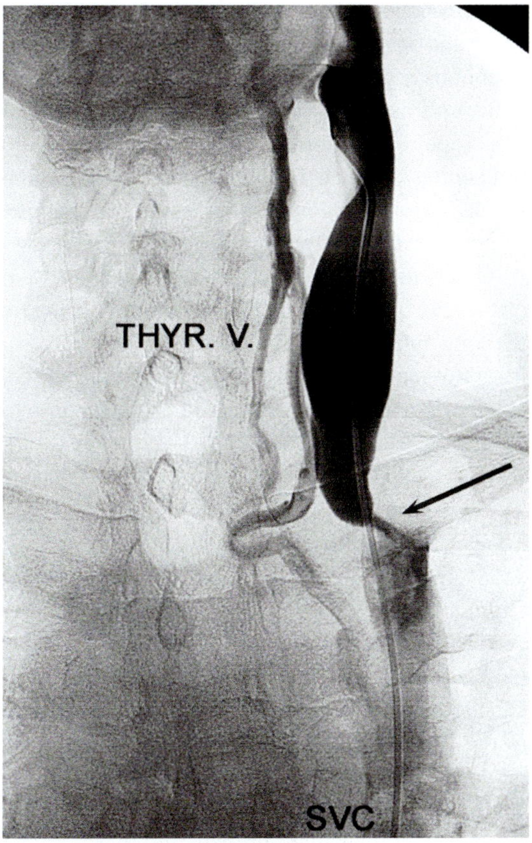

Fig. 15.3 Venogram showing venous obstruction (*arrow*) (Courtesy of Roberto Galleoti, University of Ferrara, Italy)

15.1.5 Diagnosis

Duplex ultrasound has been proposed as a screening test for CCSVI. Key ultrasound findings are summarized in Fig. 15.3. Zamboni and colleagues have defined the details of the protocol. In this protocol, two or more of the five ultrasound criteria in Fig. 15.1 are considered positive for CCSVI [3]. The use of a different ultrasound protocol was ineffective in differentiating MS patients from controls [9]. The use of ultrasound to screen for CCSVI is training and protocol dependent [1].

Venography is currently the primary test used to confirm CCSVI (Fig. 15.4) [10]. Common findings include, among others, annulus, septum malformation, or membranous obstruction. Magnetic resonance and computerized tomography venography as well as intravascular ultrasound have also been considered [1, 5].

15.1.6 Treatment

Angioplasty and stenting have been proposed as treatments for CCSVI. Treatment with angioplasty is being performed at specialized centers with good technical success. Stenosis recurrence is a problem, especially in the internal

- Reflux in the internal jugular or vertebral veins
- Reflux in the deep cerebral veins
- Evidence of a proximal internal jugular vein stenosis in high–resolution B-mode
- Undetectable flow in the internal jugular or vertebral vein,
- Absence of the normal decrease in cross-sectional area of the internal jugular vein when moving from a supine to an upright position

Fig. 15.4 CCSVI ultrasound findings (Adapted from Melby et al. [3])

jugular veins [10]. Deep venous thrombosis and vein rupture have been rare complications [11]. Stent placement has also been performed, but there has been a case of stent migration reported [11, 12].

15.1.7 Conclusions

It is presently highly controversial whether CCSVI plays a clinically significant role in MS and whether fixing these venous obstructions will help MS patients. Clinical outcomes are currently the subject of an ongoing randomized controlled trial in Italy. The Society of Interventional Radiology Foundation recommends further study [13]. It is an important area of research, because it carries the potential to help a significant number of patients with a severely disabling disease at minimal risk.

15.2 Venous Thoracic Outlet Syndrome

15.2.1 Etiology

The etiology of subclavian vein obstruction may be primary, when there is no known reason for the obstruction, or secondary, in which there is a known reason for the obstruction to occur. In both primary and secondary subclavian venous obstructions, extrinsic pressure or intrinsic trauma can produce either a thrombotic or nonthrombotic occlusion secondary to stenosis of the subclavian vein.

A thrombus must be treated separately prior to further intervention to relieve the cause of the obstruction. The majority of patients have secondary subclavian vein obstruction from intimal damage due to the insertion of catheters or pacemaker wires.

Other known secondary causes are thrombosis from underlying coagulopathies, extrinsic pressure on the subclavian vein due to cancer, and from irradiation (which can cause intimal damage from ongoing vasculitis or extrinsic compression from scarring and fibrosis).

15.2.2 Pathophysiology

Primary subclavian vein obstruction is also known as effort thrombosis or Paget-Schrötter syndrome, which was first described by Paget in 1875 and von Schrötter in 1884. The underlying cause of primary subclavian vein occlusion is often due to a congenitally narrowed costoclavicular space (also termed the *thoracic outlet*) for passage of the subclavian vein as it joins the innominate vein. In the costoclavicular space, the costoclavicular ligament and subclavius muscle surround the subclavian vein as it passes between the first rib and the clavicle to enter the mediastinum.

The possible causes for primary obstruction of the subclavian vein are (1) enlargement of either the ligament or the muscle, (2) a narrow angle between the clavicle and the first rib, or (3) the position of the subclavian vein that is too medial compared to normal. In any of these possibilities, the vein lies too close to the costoclavicular ligament and is subject to trauma, particularly from strenuous arm motion, hence the rise of the term "effort thrombosis" to describe this condition. The repetitive trauma leads to intimal injury, thickening, or web formation, and stenosis can result. Thrombosis is the final event, and it may be acute or chronic or never occur.

Other more rare causes of subclavian vein obstruction are (1) an anterior-lying phrenic nerve, (2) congenital bands and ligaments, (3) the pectoralis minor tendon, and (4) thickened venous valves, either congenitally hypertrophied or in response to extrinsic pressure and trauma [13–39].

15.2.3 Symptoms

Clinically, two-thirds of reported cases of subclavian vein thrombosis occur on the right side. This may be due to the acute angle between the right subclavian and innominate veins when compared to the left, which is almost straight, resulting in hemodynamically more turbulent flow on the right. Another proposed explanation is that more people are right-hand dominant and therefore the right arm is more likely to be used for strenuous activities. Men are more likely than women to develop subclavian vein obstruction, and the exact reason for this is still unknown. Paget-Schrötter syndrome is most often a disease of young, active, healthy patients.

Symptoms are the same for both thrombotic and non-thrombotic occlusions, and these include sudden swelling of the hand and arm, a pressure sensation of the arm, and pain, all of which are aggravated by physical activity. Some patients may describe the arm as having a "bursting" feeling. The majority of patients with non-thrombotic occlusions will have had a gradual onset of symptoms, while patients with thrombotic occlusions may have had an acute or gradual onset. In retrospect, many people with an acute thrombotic presentation often had earlier milder symptoms of pain and swelling but did not initially seek medical attention until more severe symptoms suddenly appeared. Patients who present after the initial venous thrombosis has resolved may only demonstrate symptoms with physical activity.

15.2.4 Diagnosis

On physical exam, in addition to the swelling of the hand and arm, there may be cyanosis or rubor and distended veins around the shoulder or lateral chest, indicating the development of collateral circulation ("first rib collaterals"). In patients with effort thrombosis, pallor, sweating, and fatigue may also accompany their hand and arm symptoms. Workup often starts with noninvasive duplex scanning, but occasionally it may not be possible to visualize the subclavian vein due to the clavicle. A positive duplex scan is followed by diagnostic venogram, which is the gold standard for diagnosis. If there is partial obstruction, dynamic venography is essential, as occlusions may not be seen unless the arm is elevated to 90–180°, hyperabducted, or even adducted [39]. See Chap. 9 for a further discussion of workup and diagnostic imaging.

15.2.5 Treatment

Secondary subclavian venous thrombosis is usually treated conservatively with anticoagulation: heparin initially followed by warfarin for 3–6 months. The offending indwelling catheters or wires should be removed. In dialysis patients, where their functioning arteriovenous fistula (AVF) is in the offending arm, removal of the AVF will often relieve the symptoms. However, if retention of the AVF is necessary, transluminal angioplasty (with stent placement if absolutely required) or surgical bypass via axillary, brachial-internal jugular bypass, or central vein bypass may be performed to decompress the arm.

Primary subclavian vein obstruction is usually symptomatic when presented and must be treated aggressively in the following order: (1) remove the acute thrombus if present and reestablish axillosubclavian venous patency, (2) relieve the extrinsic pressure by decompression of the costoclavicular space, and (3) eliminate the intrinsic defect. The acute thrombus is treated by catheter-directed thrombolysis with tissue plasminogen activator (tPA), urokinase (UK), or potentially, in some cases, by pharmacomechanical thrombolysis, followed by systemic anticoagulation to maintain venous patency with heparin followed by warfarin. Lytic management of acute venous thoracic outlet syndrome (TOS) is demonstrated in Fig. 15.5. Although thrombolysis is most successful in thrombus less than a few days old, it can dissolve clot several weeks to (in some cases) several months old. Indications for surgical thrombectomy are failure of lysis to reestablish venous outflow, patients who have contraindications to fibrinolytic therapy, or technical inability to deliver the agent directly into the thrombus of patients who experience persistence of severe symptoms (Fig. 15.6).

Once venous patency is established, the underlying cause of the occlusion should be repaired, and in most cases, this is due to the extrinsic compression of the subclavian vein at the costoclavicular ligament. The relief of extrinsic compression is by first rib resection, either by a transaxillary, supraclavicular, or infraclavicular approach. The supra- or infraclavicular approach may be optimal if concomitant exploration or reconstruction of the subclavian vein is anticipated. In any case, it is necessary that the anterior portion of the first rib be removed along with

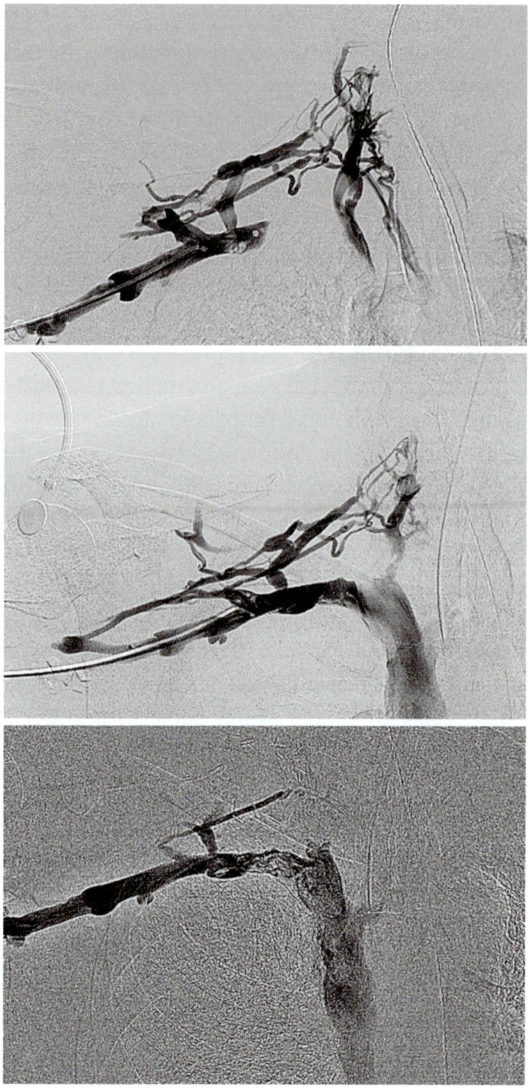

Fig. 15.5 Venous thoracic outlet syndrome

sufficient costal cartilage to totally free the subclavian vein.

The timing of resection of the first rib remains controversial. Traditional protocols advocated systemic anticoagulation for 3 months prior to surgical intervention, due to potential coagulation issues in the patient following lysis. Most surgeons believe there is no difference in rethrombosis of the vein despite a 3-month delay in surgery for extrinsic compression. However, currently in many centers, first rib resection is performed either during the same hospitalization or at the time of thrombectomy [39]. Rethrombosis of the vein following lysis or decompression should be treated with repeat lysis. If the subclavian vein cannot ultimately be opened by lysis or other techniques, some would omit first rib resection since there is no reason to decompress an already occluded vein, perhaps with the exception of an open proximal subclavian vein from a cephalic vein collateral. However, some argue that there is a potential role for first rib resection or other TOS surgery even in those with an occluded subclavian vein [28].

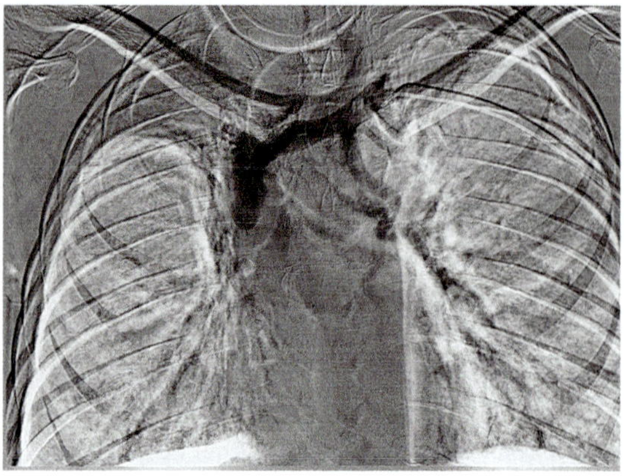

Fig. 15.6 Subclavian venous thrombosis

Complications of decompression include violation of the pleural space and postoperative pneumothorax, injury to the subclavian vein and artery (rare), injury to the brachial plexus due to excessive retraction, and injury to other nerves such as the long thoracic and phrenic. Other rare complications include postoperative causalgia, Horner's syndrome, thoracic duct injuries, and injury to the laryngeal nerve, although these are more common in the reoperative setting [40, 41].

Finally, if the vein is opened and extrinsic pressure relieved, efforts turn to the intrinsic defect of the vein; venography and symptom assessment determine the next step. If there is significant stenosis, but symptoms are relieved, no further intervention is necessary. If symptoms are present, or develop later, percutaneous balloon angioplasty can be performed. However, balloon angioplasty treats the intrinsic defect only, and therefore first rib resection and lysis must be performed first before any percutaneous angioplasty is attempted.

If balloon angioplasty fails, then vein patch angioplasty with or without endovenectomy can be considered. This is indicated if the subclavian vein has flow into the innominate, but it is narrowed by webbing, scarring, or old thrombus. This is done through an infraclavicular approach, with or without a modified mediastinotomy for adequate exposure. If the subclavian vein is totally occluded or patch angioplasty is not desired, then jugulosubclavian bypass can be used to restore outflow from the arm. There must be adequate inflow into the axillary vein for successful bypass.

It may be essential to perform axillary thrombectomy, even in chronic occlusion, to obtain good inflow. If inflow cannot be established, jugulosubclavian bypass should not be performed. If both the axillary and subclavian veins are occluded, other venous bypasses can be attempted by using saphenous vein, crossover cephalic vein, or a long prosthesis, anticipating more limited expectations for the results of such compromised reconstructions.

Any of these venous repair or bypass procedures may have improved patency if supported by a temporary AVF in the ipsilateral arm. These AVFs can be created by anastomosis of a nearby vein to the axillary artery, sewing a section of saphenous vein to the axillary artery and using the distal end as an onlay vein patch during endovenectomy or similar maneuver. Closure of the fistula, which is usually done approximately 3 months later, can be done under local anesthesia if the AVF is just under the skin, or it can be coiled percutaneously via endovascular methods.

Results of treatment of venous TOS were also addressed in the recent series demonstrating satisfactory return to work and symptom improvement previously discussed under neurogenic TOS [32]. Most TOS surgeons obtain good to very good immediate results with surgery for venous TOS on a routine basis. However, recurrence rates following first rib resection via the transaxillary or supraclavicular route have been documented to be in the 15–20 % range, and if recurrence occurs, it will tend to be in the first 2 years. Subjective improvement is noted to be >80 % immediately postoperatively, falling to 59 % at 2 years and 69 % at 5 years. Reoperation may improve the overall improvement back to greater than 80 % when patients have late recurrence of their symptoms [28, 36, 40–42].

15.3 Superior Vena Cava Syndrome

15.3.1 Definition

Superior vena cava (SVC) syndrome is the development of clinically significant congestion in the head, neck, and upper extremities due to severe stenosis or occlusion of the SVC. The most common cause is from lung cancer and mediastinal tumors leading to compression of the SVC [1]. Benign causes tend to be iatrogenic injuries in general, such as following the placement of a pacemaker, central line placement, or other instrumentation of the major veins [2].

15.3.2 Symptoms

SVC syndrome typically presents with venous congestion of the head, neck, and upper extremities leading to a feeling of fullness. This fullness is often relieved by increasing the number of pillows while the patient sleeps in an attempt to use gravity to improve venous outflow. Very severe symptoms may lead to difficulty breathing, headache, and visual changes. Dramatic jugular venous distention is often present, along with a characteristic swelling of the face. Prominent collateral veins may develop if enough time elapses from the time of onset [3, 4].

15.3.3 Diagnosis

Following a thorough history and physical examination, diagnosis proceeds with imaging of the affected regions. Ultrasound is a good early test to identify aberrant venous outflow and to confirm the presence of collateral circulation. Computerized tomography (CT) scanning is particularly useful to determine the potential etiology of the SVC syndrome and can help identify hilar masses or mediastinal tumors. With appropriate timing of the contrast bolus, CT can also help identify aberrant venous circulation [5, 6]. See Chap. 9 for a further review of imaging of SVC syndrome.

Venography is typically performed before endovascular or surgical intervention. Real-time visualization of the venous system with contrast allows the clinician to determine the point of obstruction, map collaterals, and potentially complete an endovenous intervention [7]. Four patterns of SVC syndrome have been described based on the extent of stenosis or obstruction [8]. Type I disease presents with up to 90 % stenosis of the SVC and normal outflow of the azygos system; this type of disease is relatively uncommon. Type II disease presents with subtotal stenosis of the SVC with normal anterograde outflow of the azygos system. Type III disease, the most common of the four types, presents with subtotal stenosis of the SVC and retrograde flow within the azygos system. Type IV disease presents with occlusion of the SVC and adjacent major veins.

15.3.4 Treatment

The preferred management of SVC syndrome is through various endovascular interventions. Balloon angioplasty with possible stent placement can be beneficial for patients and typically provides immediate improvement in their symptoms [9]. Between 90 and 100 % of patients typically respond well to endovascular techniques, with about 70 % of patients reporting continuing relief at 1 year [10–12] (Fig. 15.7).

Open management of SVC syndrome has largely fallen out of favor due to the need for median sternotomy in most cases. In selected patients, such as those undergoing median sternotomy to remove mediastinal masses, treatment involves resection of the affected segment and anastomosis with either reversed femoral or saphenous vein or the use of polytetrafluoroethylene (PTFE) graft. Outcomes vary between 70 and 100 % patency at 1 year [13, 14].

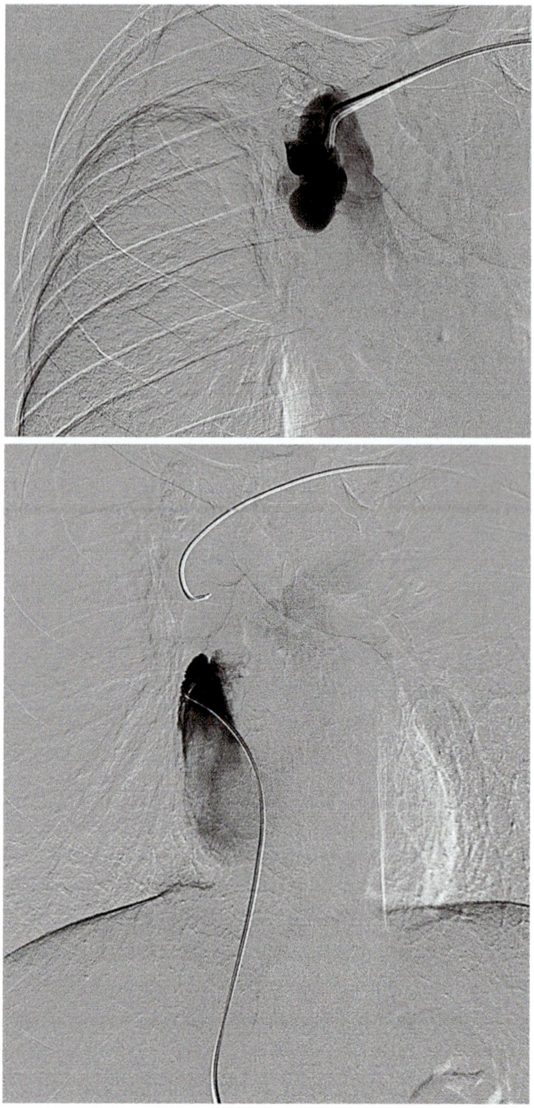

Fig. 15.7 Superior vena cava syndrome

15.3.5 Conclusions

SVC syndrome affects approximately 15,000 patients per year and is a relatively common complication of lung cancer [15]. The effective management of clinically significant presentations of SVC syndrome should involve diagnosis and classification of the type of disease via venography, followed by endovascular repair of the defect.

References

1. de León RA, Chang DC, Hassoun HT, Black JH, Roseborough GS, Perler BA, Rotellini-Coltvet L, Call D, Busse C, Freischlag JA. Multiple treatment algorithms for successful outcomes in venous thoracic outlet syndrome. Surgery. 2009;145(5):500–7.
2. Doyle A, Wolford HY, Davies MG, Adams JT, Singh MJ, Saad WE, Waldman DL, Deweese JA, Illig KA. Management of effort thrombosis of the subclavian vein: today's treatment. Ann Vasc Surg. 2007;21(6):723–9.
3. Melby SJ, Vedantham S, Narra VR, Paletta Jr GA, Khoo-Summers L, Driskill M, Thompson RW. Comprehensive surgical management of the competitive athlete with effort thrombosis of the subclavian vein (Paget-Schroetter syndrome). J Vasc Surg. 2008;47(4):809–20.
4. Fugate MW, Rotellini-Coltvet L, Freischlag JA. Current management of thoracic outlet syndrome. Curr Treat Options Cardiovasc Med. 2009;11(2):176–83.
5. Chang DC, Rotellini-Coltvet LA, Mukherjee D, De Leon R, Freischlag JA. Surgical intervention for thoracic outlet syndrome improves patient's quality of life. J Vasc Surg. 2009;49(3):630–5.
6. Caparrelli DJ, Freischlag JA. Thoracic outlet syndromes. In: Cameron JC, editor. Current surgical therapy. 9th ed. Philadelphia: Elsevier Mosby; 2007. p. 878–84.
7. Huang JH, Zager EL. Thoracic outlet syndrome. Neurosurgery. 2004;55(4):897–902.
8. Hasanadka R, Towne JB, Seabrook GR, Brown KR, Lewis BD, Foley WD. Computed tomography angiography to evaluate thoracic outlet neurovascular compression. Vasc Endovascular Surg. 2007;41(4):316–21.
9. Mackinnon SE, Novak CB. Thoracic outlet syndrome. Curr Probl Surg. 2002;39(11):1070–145.
10. Demondion X, Herbinet P, Van Sint Jan S, Boutry N, Chantelot C, Cotten A. Imaging assessment of thoracic outlet syndrome. Radiographics. 2006;26(6):1735–50.
11. Sanders RJ, Hammond SL, Rao NM. Diagnosis of thoracic outlet syndrome. J Vasc Surg. 2007;46(3):601–4.
12. Caparrelli DJ, Freischlag J. A unified approach to axillosubclavian venous thrombosis in a single hospital admission. Semin Vasc Surg. 2005;18(3):153–7.
13. Rigberg D, Freischlag J. Complications of thoracic outlet surgery. In: Towne JB, Hollier LH, editors. Complications in vascular surgery. 2nd ed. New York: Marcel Decker, Inc; 2004. p. 429–38.
14. Chang DC, Lidor AO, Matsen SL, Freischlag JA. Reported in-hospital complications following rib resections for neurogenic thoracic outlet syndrome. Ann Vasc Surg. 2007;21(5):564–70.
15. Caparrelli DJ, Tabulov DM, Freischlag JA. Image of the month. Subclavian artery aneurysm secondary to cervical rib. Arch Surg. 2006;141(5):513.
16. Sanders RJ, Cooper MA. Thoracic outlet syndrome. In: Dean RH, Yao JST, Brewster DC, editors. Current diagnosis and treatment in vascular surgery. Norwalk: Appleton & Lange; 1995. p. 133–52.
17. Rice TW, Rodriguez RM, Light RW. The superior vena cava syndrome: clinical characteristics and evolving etiology. Medicine (Baltimore). 2006;85:37.
18. Parish JM, Marschke Jr RF, Dines DE, Lee RE. Etiologic considerations in superior vena cava syndrome. Mayo Clin Proc. 1981;56:407.
19. Laguna Del Estal P, Gazapo Navarro T, MurillasAngoitti J, et al. Superior vena cava syndrome: a study based on 81 cases. An Med Interna. 1998;15:470.
20. Rizvi AZ, Kalra M, Bjarnason H, et al. Benign superior vena cava syndrome: stenting is now the first line of treatment. J Vasc Surg. 2008;47:372.
21. Yedlicka JW, Schultz K, Moncada R, Flisak M. CT findings in superior vena cava obstruction. Semin Roentgenol. 1989;24:84.
22. Bashist B, Parisi A, Frager DH, Suster B. Abdominal CT findings when the superior vena cava, brachiocephalic vein, or subclavian vein is obstructed. AJR Am J Roentgenol. 1996;167:1457.
23. Stanford W, Doty DB. The role of venography and surgery in the management of patients with superior vena cava obstruction. Ann Thorac Surg. 1986;41:158.
24. Bierdrager E, Lampmann LEH, Lohle PNM, et al. Endovascular stenting in neoplastic superior vena cava syndrome prior to chemotherapy or radiotherapy. Neth J Med. 2005;63:20.
25. Kim YI, Kim KS, Ko YC, et al. Endovascular stenting as a first choice for the palliation of superior vena cava syndrome. J Korean Med Sci. 2004;19:519.
26. Dyet JF, Cook A, Nicholson A. Use of the Wallstent in the treatment of malignant superior vena caval obstruction. J Vasc Interv Radiol. 1994;5:2.
27. Barshes NR, Annambhotla S, El Sayed HF, et al. Percutaneous stenting of superior vena cava syndrome: treatment outcome in patients with benign and malignant etiology. Vascular. 2007;15:314.
28. Magnan PE, Thomas P, Giudicelli R, et al. Surgical reconstruction of the superior vena cava. Cardiovasc Surg. 1994;2:598.
29. Wisselink W, Money SR, Becker MO, et al. Comparison of operative reconstruction and percutaneous balloon dilatation for central venous obstruction. Am J Surg. 1993;166:200.
30. Wilson LD, Detterbeck FC, Yahalom J. Superior vena cava syndrome with malignant causes. N Engl J Med. 2007;356:1862.
31. Zamboni P. Galleoti: the chronic cerebrospinal insufficiency syndrome. Phlebology. 2010;25:269–79.
32. Lee BB, Bergan JB, Gloviczki P, et al. Diagnosis and treatment of venous malformations. Consensus Document of the International Union the International Union of Phlebology. Int Angiol. 2009;28:434–51.
33. Zamboni P, Galleoti R, Menegatti E, et al. Chronic cerebrospinal venous insufficiency in patients with multiple sclerosis. J Neurol Neurosurg Psychiatry. 2009;80:392–9.
34. Khan O, Filippi M, Freedman MS, et al. Chronic cerebrospinal insufficiency and multiple sclerosis. J Neurol Neurosurg Psychiatry. 2009;80:392–9.

35. Sclafani JA. Chronic cerebrospinal insufficiency: a new paradigm and therapy for multiple sclerosis. Endovasc Today. 2010.
36. Gonzalez MM, Rivera MM. Transient global amnesia. Arch Neurol. 2006;63:1334–6.
37. Frohman EM, Racke MK, Raine CS. Multiple sclerosis – the plaque and its pathogenesis. N Engl J Med. 2006;354:942–55.
38. Zamboni P. The big idea: iron-dependent inflammation in venous disease and proposed parallels in multiple sclerosis. J R Soc Med. 2006;99:589–93.
39. Doepp F, Friedemann P, Valdueza PM, Schmierer K, Schreiber SJ. No cerebrocervical venous congestion in patients with multiple sclerosis. Ann Neurol. 2010;68:173–83.
40. Zamboni P, Galleoti R, Menegatti E, et al. A prospective open-label study of endovascular treatment of chronic cerebrospinal venous insufficiency. J Vasc Surg. 2009;50:1348–58.
41. Ludyga T, Kazibudzki M, Simka M, et al. Endovascular treatment for chronic cerebrospinal venous insufficiency: is the procedure safe? Phlebology. 2010;25:286–95.
42. Burton TM. MS program halted amid controversy. Wall Street J. 2010.

Lower Deep Vein Disease

16

Jovan N. Markovic and Mitchell Cox

Contents

J.N. Markovic, MD (✉) • M. Cox, MD
Department of Surgery,
Duke University Medical Center, Durham, NC, USA
e-mail: jovan.markovic@duke.edu
mitchell.cox2@duke.edu

Abstract

Deep venous insufficiency may manifest as limb edema, chronic leg pain, stasis dermatitis, or ulceration, and the symptoms may be chronically disabling. Initial therapy is directed at ulcer healing and control of symptoms with wound care and compression. Once conservative measures have been instituted, the next step may be evaluation for any surgically correctable contributors to the symptomatology. Although valvular dysfunction and consequent venous reflux are a major cause of the venous hypertension that underlies the clinical manifestations of chronic venous insufficiency (CVI), recent studies suggest that iliac venous outflow obstruction plays a more important role in the pathogenesis of CVI than previously estimated. Any combination of superficial, perforator, and/or deep venous reflux can result in various stages of CVI, but when multiple segments of venous system are affected, the manifestations of CVI increase in severity. The combination of reflux and obstruction produces the highest levels of venous hypertension and the most severe clinical symptoms. This chapter discusses iliocaval vein obstructions and pelvic venous congestion.

16.1 Overview

Management of deep venous insufficiency can be a uniquely frustrating endeavor for both patient and physician. While minimally invasive ablative

E. Mowatt-Larssen et al. (eds.), *Phlebology, Vein Surgery and Ultrasonography*,
DOI 10.1007/978-3-319-01812-6_16, © Springer International Publishing Switzerland 2014

therapy for superficial venous reflux can represent definitive treatment and a symptomatic cure, there are only rarely surgical or endovascular solutions for incompetence of the deep veins. For the phlebologist, the challenge in management is to select the few patients who are candidates for a surgical or endovascular approach and avoid an invasive and expensive workup or a morbid surgical procedure in patients that would be better served by conservative management with wound care and compression.

In the past, the only options for surgical treatment of deep venous insufficiency were valve repair or valve transposition for insufficiency and venous bypass for obstruction. These procedures are both relatively morbid and have had marginal results and therefore have been performed at only a relative handful of tertiary referral centers by a few enthusiastic and persistent surgeons. Over the past decade, there has been a boom in endovascular approaches which are less technically demanding and significantly less invasive while achieving similar or better results than these classic surgical procedures. Given the obvious early technical success and surprising durability of venous angioplasty and stenting, a somewhat more aggressive approach to evaluation and surgical referral may be justified.

As discussed in previous chapters, deep venous insufficiency may manifest as limb edema, chronic leg pain, stasis dermatitis, or ulceration, and the symptoms may be chronically disabling. Initial therapy is directed at ulcer healing and control of symptoms with wound care and compression. Once conservative measures have been instituted, the next step may be evaluation for any surgically correctable contributors to the symptomatology.

Although valvular dysfunction and consequent venous reflux are a major cause of the venous hypertension that underlies the clinical manifestations of chronic venous insufficiency (CVI), recent studies suggest that iliac venous outflow obstruction plays a more important role in the pathogenesis of CVI than previously estimated [1]. Any combination of superficial, perforator, and/or deep venous reflux can result in various stages of CVI, but when multiple segments of venous system are affected, the manifestations of CVI increase in severity. The combination of reflux and obstruction produces the highest levels of venous hypertension and the most severe clinical symptoms. Fortunately, both reflux and obstruction can be surgically addressed, resulting in significant symptomatic improvement. Therefore, a more complete characterization of the underlying pathophysiology can be critical in a subset of patients.

16.2 Clinical Presentation of Iliocaval Obstruction

Iliac vein obstruction in the setting of superficial reflux disease should be suspected and evaluated in CVI patients with symptoms that are out of proportion to detectable infrainguinal pathology, in patients lacking another explanation for their CVI symptoms, and in patients with a history of deep venous thrombosis (DVT). Patients with isolated left leg symptoms and minimal infrainguinal venous abnormalities on duplex might be suspected to have May-Thurner syndrome and represent another high-risk group. In a study from 1953, May and Thurner examined pelvic venous anatomy in 430 cadavers and found that in approximately 22 % of cases, the left iliac vein was compressed against the fifth lumbar vertebra by the right iliac artery [2]. Authors of the same study reported that thrombosis of the pelvic veins was found about eight times more frequently on the left than the right. Although compression of the vein by the overlying artery was not necessarily proven to be causative for DVT, the association was highly suggestive, and in fact, symptoms of CVI may result from this compression even without a clear history of thrombosis.

Although perimalleolar edema is common in patients with superficial reflux disease, prominent edema that involves calf and thigh suggests iliac vein obstruction. Central venous imaging of a patient presenting with severe chronic lower extremity edema, but minimal abnormalities on duplex, is illustrated in Fig. 16.1. In this case, a stricture of the inferior vena cava (IVC) was identified by venogram, confirmed by intravascular

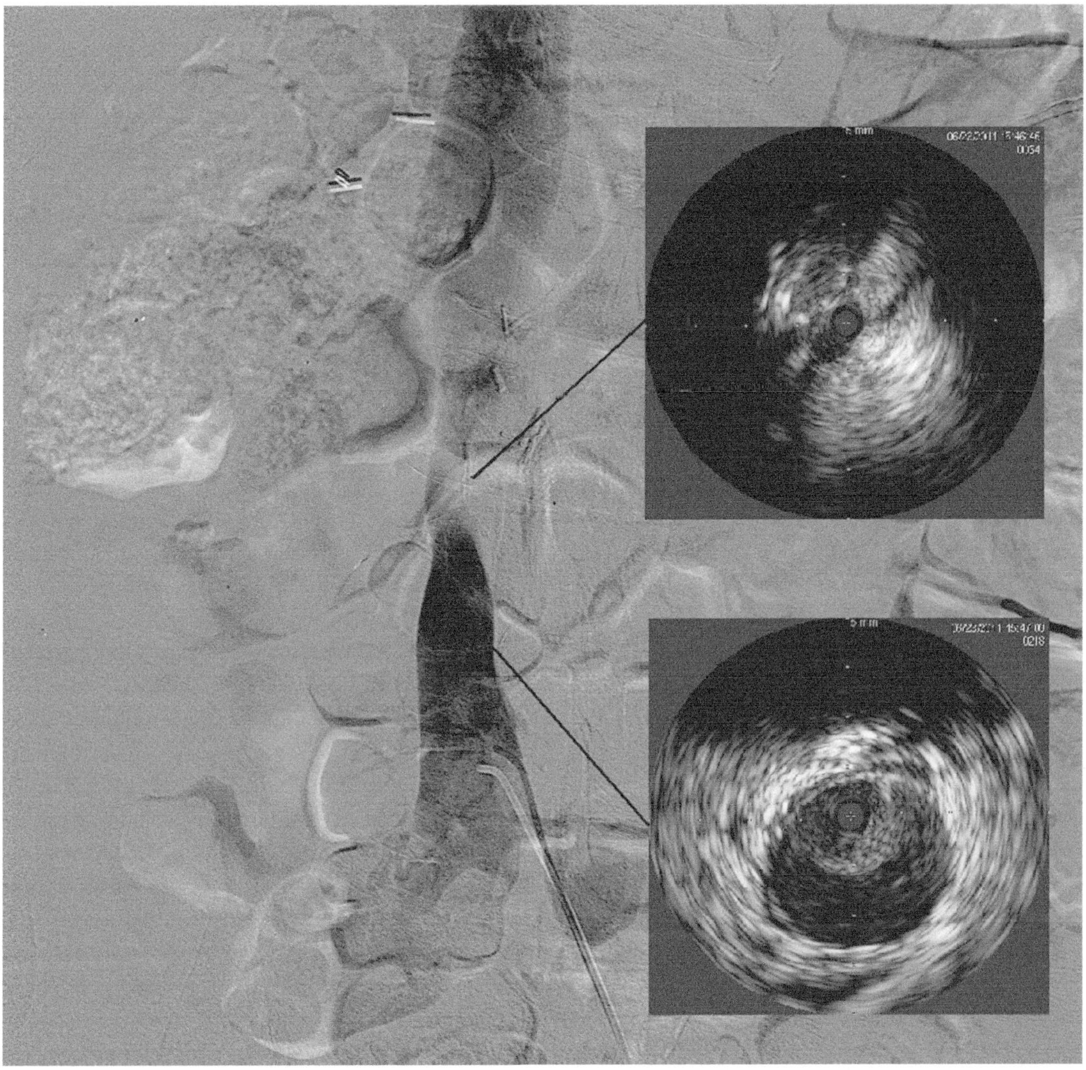

Fig. 16.1 This 68-year-old man presented with gradual onset of massive bilateral lower extremity edema several years after a course of radiation therapy to the abdomen for an ampullary carcinoma. Duplex ultrasound showed no evidence of reflux; however, venogram and IVUS demonstrated a clear stenosis of the IVC. This was treated with angioplasty and stenting and there was near-complete resolution of the leg edema. IVUS images through the stenotic portion of the IVC and the more normal distal IVC are shown in the insets

ultrasound (IVUS), and successfully treated with venous angioplasty and stenting. Similarly, patients who present with lower extremity pain that is not located near varicosities and patients who present with exercise-induced pain in the thigh and the calf muscles ("venous claudication") should be evaluated for venous outflow obstruction. Some degree of suspicion for iliac obstruction should also be present in patients with advanced CVI (C4–C6 stage) [3]. Collateral venous circulation will develop in most patients with a history of long-standing venous disease, and the pattern of visible collaterals may be a clue to the anatomy of a deep venous obstruction. Suprapubic and abdominal wall collaterals are not typically present in patients with isolated infrainguinal disease and may be indicative of central stenosis. The incidence of hemorrhage from high-pressure varicosities is also higher in CVI patients with coexisting iliac obstruction, since venous outflow obstruction may lead to a particularly significant elevation of pressure in veins distal to an obstruction.

Patients with a known history of iliofemoral DVT represent a uniquely high-risk group for iliac or caval obstruction. Previous longitudinal studies have demonstrated that only 20–30 % of iliac vein thrombi completely recanalize with anticoagulation alone, while the remaining veins develop persistent obstruction with variable collateral formation [4, 5]. Thus, pelvic imaging should be obtained in patients with a history of DVT and/or thrombophilic disorders and coexisting CVI. Although frequently clinically silent, the importance of primary, non-thrombotic iliac vein obstruction (May-Thurner syndrome or iliac vein compression syndrome) can play an important role in the pathogenesis of iliac vein obstruction. As reported by Meissner et al., among approximately 1,000 limbs that were treated for iliocaval obstruction, approximately 40 % had non-thrombotic occlusion [6].

16.3 Diagnostic Imaging

The absence of a "gold standard" imaging modality represents an obstacle in the systematic study of patients with iliac vein obstruction. There are now multiple imaging studies that are complementary, however, and together can provide a clear view of the underlying pathophysiology. With judicious application of these available tests, the savvy practitioner can amass enough information to reliably diagnose and treat nearly all patients with deep venous reflux.

The evaluation of both valvular incompetence and obstruction almost always begins with duplex ultrasonography (US). Unfortunately, duplex US is unreliable for assessment of the iliac veins, especially in obese patients. Duplex US is, however, the starting point for a comprehensive evaluation and will yield the first clues that there may be an issue above the level of the inguinal ligament. Loss of respiratory variation in the femoral tracing or poor signal augmentation with distal limb compression during duplex US examination of the femoral vein may be indicative of venous outflow obstruction. Data from a large retrospective study by Lin et al. that included 2,963 limbs scanned with duplex US documented abnormal monophasic waveforms in the common femoral veins in 124 patients [7]. Just under 50 % of these patients with abnormal waveforms had evidence of prior DVT or iliac vein stenosis on computerized tomography (CT) scan. Based on this and other similar studies, it is reasonable to pursue central imaging in all CVI patients with abnormal Doppler waveforms in the common femoral vein. But while specific criteria for duplex detection of central venous stenosis have been described, the most significant finding is usually what the duplex does not show. That is, if there are severe symptoms of chronic venous insufficiency, but minimal infrainguinal reflux or occlusion, a more proximal cause must be suspected.

Ascending venography provides greater detail than simple duplex US, detects extensive iliac vein stenosis, and images collateral flow. It is an essential study when surgical intervention is planned [6]. The Achilles heel of venography is that it often does not provide adequate visualization of focal obstructions with a post-thrombotic or non-thrombotic cause [9]. For instance, a post-thrombotic iliac vein may still appear to have flow with multiple small recanalized channels while still representing a major physiologic obstruction (Fig. 16.2a). In addition, anterior-posterior (AP) compression, as might be present in a May-Thurner syndrome, will be completely missed by a standard venogram in an AP projection. CT and magnetic resonance venography (MRV) appear to be more sensitive for detection of spatially complex and focal lesions (Fig. 16.3). Unfortunately, significant technical expertise in MRV or CT is required to produce consistently reliable images and may not be widely available in all locales. Significant obstructions are also not uncommon in asymptomatic patients [10]. IVUS is increasingly viewed as the superior imaging modality in estimating the extent of iliac vein stenosis since it allows real-time visualization of the details and morphology of intraluminal obstruction [11, 12]. In addition, IVUS allows definitive

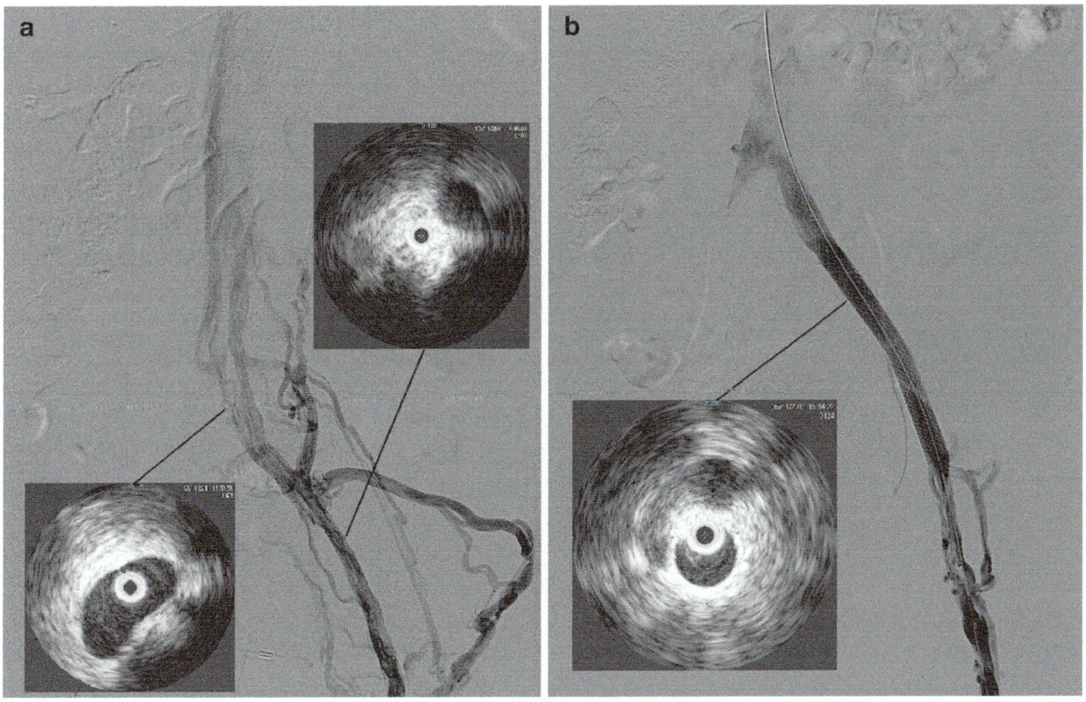

Fig. 16.2 This 44-year-old woman presented with a history of approximately 20 years of left leg edema, beginning with a DVT during pregnancy. Duplex findings were notable only for GSV incompetence; however, after an ablation of the great saphenous vein, she developed worsening symptoms with chronic, severe pain and worsening edema. Venogram shows what appears to be a patent left iliac system, but with extensive collaterals (**a**), and IVUS shows near occlusion of the common and external iliac veins (*inset*). After angioplasty and stenting, there is free flow through the iliac veins with minimal collateral flow (**b**) and IVUS shows a patent, re-expanded lumen (*inset*)

identification of focal lesions and can be used as a guide during angioplasty and stenting. When performed in conjunction with direct pressure measurement, many practitioners feel that it is the most sensitive and specific method of identifying hemodynamically significant stenoses in the iliocaval system. While IVUS is an invasive procedure, high-quality images are easily obtained, and interpretation is straightforward. Figure 16.2 demonstrates a situation in which a post-thrombotic iliac vein appeared patent on venogram but was near occluded as demonstrated by IVUS. In this case, the post-thrombotic vein was treated successfully with angioplasty and stenting, resulting in near-complete resolution of the symptoms. In current practice, while purists may debate which imaging modality is the gold standard, the simple fact is that a combination of venogram and IVUS will identify nearly all significant obstructive lesions.

The only real concern is that IVUS might be oversensitive to physiologic compression and the degree of stenosis which merits intervention is a matter of discussion and debate. The point at which stenosis should be considered hemodynamically significant in the venous system remains controversial, but stenosis of greater than 50 % is probably considered the minimum indication for intervention [6, 8]. In practice however, the decision to intervene is based on multiple factors including the degree of stenosis, the clinical presentation, and the perceived odds of success. One might be hard pressed to recommend intervention on an older patient with mild lower leg edema and a 70 % compression of the iliac vein by the overlying iliac artery. In contrast, a 70 % stenosis of the iliac vein may well-merit treatment in a post-thrombotic 35-year-old with symptomatic thigh and lower leg edema accompanied by venous claudication.

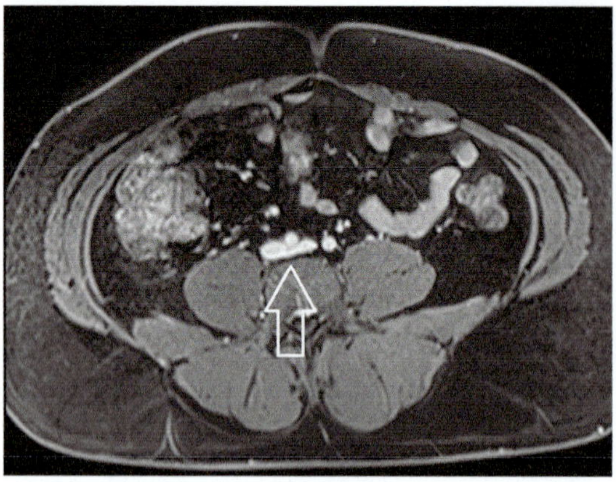

Fig. 16.3 A 65-year-old man presented with severe, recurrent varicosities of the left leg extending up to the inguinal area and buttocks. Given some suspicion of proximal obstruction, an MRV was ordered which showed only mild compression of the left common iliac vein by the left common iliac artery. This was deemed not to be physiologically significant and was not treated

16.4 Venous Angioplasty and Stenting

Currently available treatment modalities for the management of iliac vein obstruction are large vein bypass and percutaneous stenting. In the past, the only available option for patients with iliac vein or IVC obstruction was surgical bypass. These procedures are, however, maximally invasive and technically challenging and have been associated with poor long-term results in all but the most experienced hands. Over the last decade, the success associated with percutaneous angioplasty and stenting for venous obstruction on an outpatient basis has largely relegated surgical procedures to a handful of the most intractable cases which have failed multiple attempts with an endovascular approach.

Data from several studies has demonstrated that venous stenting is associated with low morbidity and strikingly high long-term patency rates. In a case series including 982 lower extremities, Neglen et al. reported cumulative patency rates of 86 and 100 % at 5 years in patients treated for post-thrombotic and non-thrombotic iliac vein occlusion, respectively [13, 14]. The same authors reported complete pain relief in 64 % of patients, resolution of leg swelling in 34 %, and ulcer healing in 58 % of treated patients, despite the presence of untreated infrainguinal reflux in many limbs [13, 14]. Hartung et al. demonstrated that stenting of iliac obstruction was associated with significant improvement of the venous clinical severity scores (VCSS). In their study, which included 44 patients followed for an average of 27 months, VCSS were 8.5 and 2.0 before and after the procedure, respectively [15]. These excellent patency rates, and documented symptomatic improvement with a minimally invasive procedure, have revolutionized the management of deep venous obstruction. A typical case of iliac venous obstruction due to May-Thurner syndrome which was treated with venous angioplasty and stenting is presented in Fig. 16.4.

Even very extensive iliocaval obstructions can be addressed effectively with endovascular approaches. As recently documented by Neglen and Raju, long-standing caval obstructions due to an IVC filter can be successfully and durably addressed with angioplasty and stenting [16]. Figure 16.5 illustrates a case of extensive iliac and IVC obstruction in the presence of an IVC filter which was not retrievable. This patient presented with recurrent right leg stasis ulceration that was refractory to conservative management with compression and wound care. In this case, the occluded iliac segment and IVC were recanalized and stented with almost immediate symptomatic improvement and eventual ulcer healing.

The technical approach to venous angioplasty and stenting begins with percutaneous access of the popliteal, femoral, or greater saphenous vein. Our preference is to access the femoral vein in the mid-thigh under ultrasound guidance, since the patient can be positioned supine while still allowing visualization of the entire iliac and proximal femoral drainage. A venogram is obtained which will often diagnose obvious long-segment occlusions and document collateral flow. If the venogram is relatively normal or equivocal, the IVUS catheter is passed up over a wire and the entire iliocaval system is interrogated. If there is an occlusion, we attempt to cross the

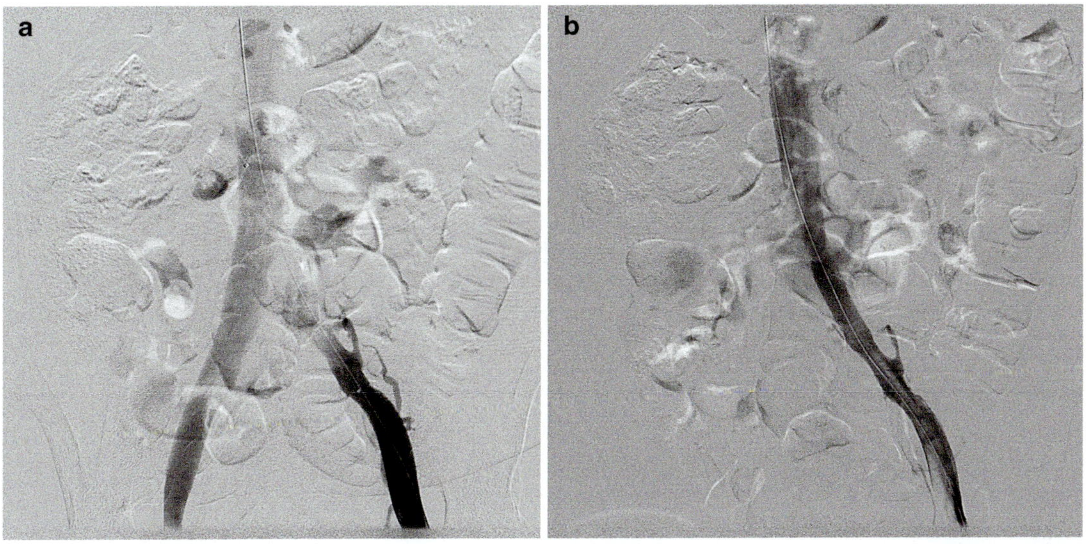

Fig. 16.4 A classic presentation of May-Thurner syndrome is illustrated by this 35-year-old woman with sudden onset of massive left leg swelling. After thrombolysis of an occluded iliac vein, there is a residual iliac stenosis (**a**), which was addressed successfully with angioplasty and stenting (**b**). The leg returned to a normal diameter within 48 h

lesion with a guidewire/catheter combination and then obtain imaging proximal to the occlusion, as well as IVUS of the affected segment. Pullback pressures across a stenosis or occlusion may be obtained; however, venous pressure differentials may be quite small and difficult to interpret and are not typically a major part of our decision-making process.

If the stenosis or occlusion is deemed to be clinically significant, the next step is serial predilation to near the normal expected diameter of the vein segment. Balloon dilation alone will almost never be sufficient for venous obstructions of the lower extremities, and a self-expanding stent, sized to a diameter 10–20 % greater than the expected vein diameter, is nearly always placed. The Wallstent® (Boston Scientific, Natick, MA) and SmartStent (Cordis, Bridgewater, NJ) are the most frequently used devices in this setting. After post-dilation, a completion venogram and IVUS are obtained. In our practice, patients requiring long-term warfarin are restarted on enoxaparin and warfarin immediately post-procedure, while those not on long-term systemic anticoagulation are begun on aspirin and Plavix. Presence of a stent in the iliac system alone does not necessarily mandate long-term anticoagulation with warfarin.

16.5 Venous Bypass

For a patient with the most severe and intractable symptoms of CVI, a documented central venous occlusion, and multiple failed attempts at endovascular recanalization, one of the traditional venous bypass procedures might still be considered. The first and most famous large vein bypass procedure, described by Dr. Palma ("Palma procedure"), uses contralateral great saphenous vein as a bypass conduit [17]. This procedure is designed to bypass a chronically obstructed iliac vein by mobilizing the contralateral greater saphenous vein and turning it over onto the ipsilateral femoral vein (Fig. 16.6). The largest available series, with data from an analysis of 412 procedures, demonstrated clinical improvement in 63–89 % of patients and long-term patency rates of up to 80 % [6]. A particularly optimistic review from the Mayo Clinic documented patency rates for the Palma procedure as

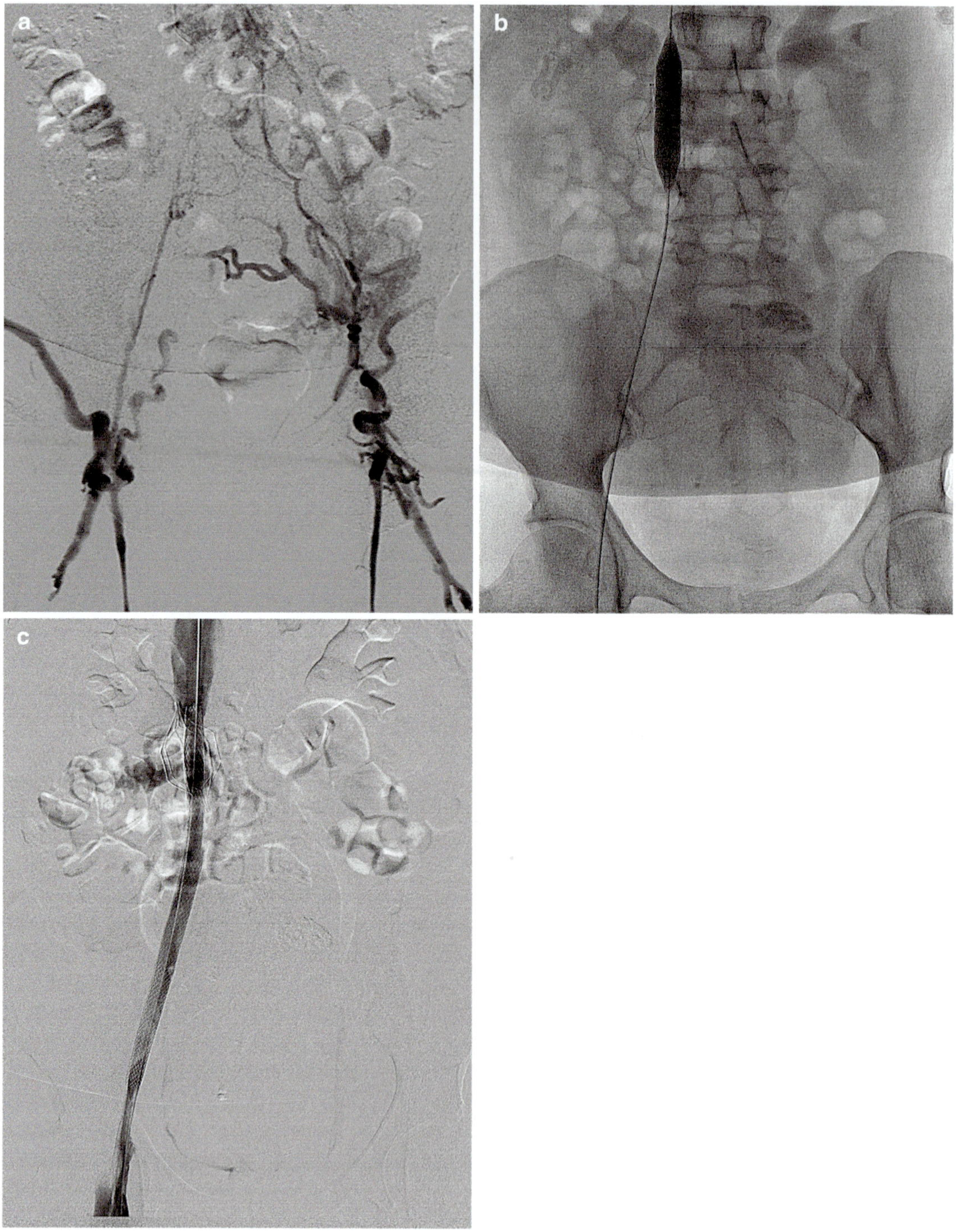

Fig. 16.5 This 55-year-old woman had a history of multiple bilateral DVTs as well as prior placement of an IVC filter and presented with recurrent right leg stasis ulcers. Complete iliocaval occlusion is demonstrated by venogram (**a**); however, the right iliac veins were easily crossed with a wire and the entire segment, including the occluded filter, was balloon dilated and stented (**b**). Completion venogram shows brisk flow across the treated segment (**c**)

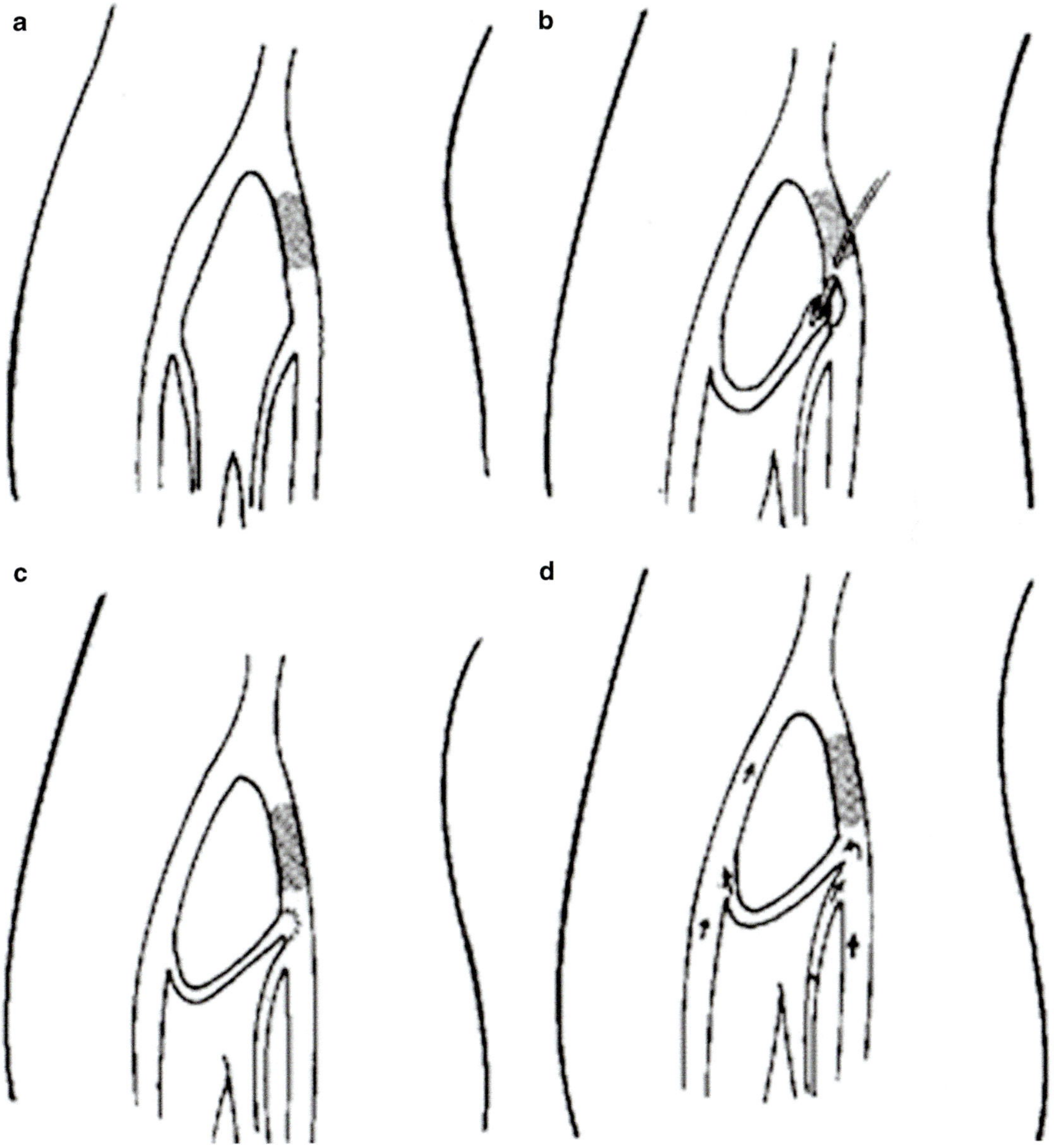

Fig. 16.6 The Palma procedure is designed to address unilateral iliac occlusion (**a**) by mobilization and anastomosis of the contralateral great saphenous vein to the ipsilateral common femoral vein (**b**, **c**). Drainage of the affected leg then flows through the saphenous vein and the contralateral iliac system (**d**) [30]

high as 83 %, at 4 years [18]. Unfortunately, clinical success hinges on long-term patency of a fairly small conduit with relatively low flow, and the procedure is technically challenging, so real-world results may not be as advertised. Nevertheless, the morbidity of the procedure is limited, and it may be worthwhile in a small subset of patients.

The Palma procedure is not, however, appropriate for patients with bilateral iliac occlusions or patients with complex iliocaval stenosis or occlusion. In such cases, an in-line bypass with polytetrafluoroethylene (PTFE) may be considered. In-line bypass (femorocaval, iliocaval, or even ilioatrial) may be indicated

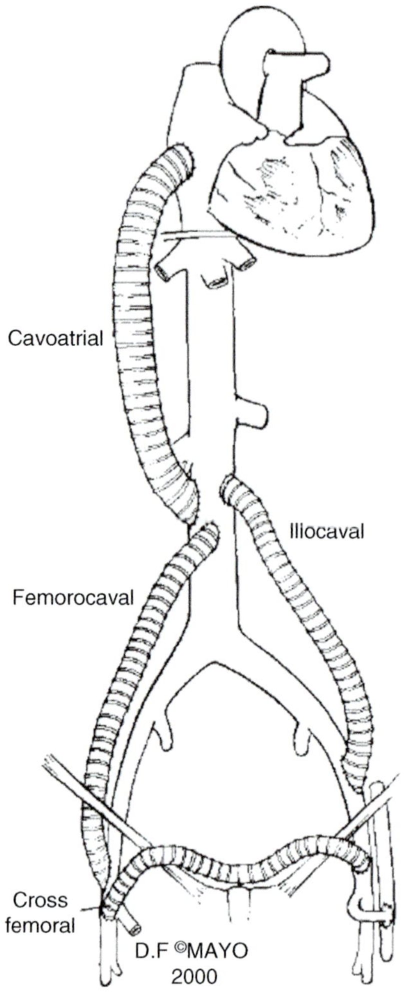

Fig. 16.7 Various configurations of PTFE bypass for chronic venous occlusion are illustrated in this diagram based on the Mayo Clinic experience [18]

in patients with bilateral iliac occlusions, isolated caval occlusion, or very extensive iliocaval obstructions who also have relatively non-diseased venous segments proximally and distally to provide adequate inflow and outflow for the graft. In-line bypass may also be considered in cases of unilateral iliac obstruction where autologous conduit for a suprapubic graft (Palma procedure) is not available. Some typical graft configurations are seen in Fig. 16.7 [18]. One-year primary patency rates associated with in-line venous bypass have been reported to be as high as 93 % [6]. However, somewhat lower patency rates are documented in a series from the Mayo Clinic, the best realistically achievable results (Fig. 16.8) [18].

Excellent results can only be achieved with the most judicious patient selection, and venous bypass is not to be offered to all comers with extensive iliac occlusion. To be candidates for a major surgical procedure, the patient must report pain in a pattern which is clearly referable to the underlying venous disease, have minimally diseased veins proximal and distal to the planned graft, and should not be obese. Long-term anticoagulation with warfarin is mandatory, and patients must be compliant with their medical regimen, consistently present for follow-up, and have no contraindications to anticoagulation. As alluded to earlier, venous bypass is typically reserved for relatively young patients who are excellent surgical candidates and have failed multiple aggressive attempts at endovascular recanalization and stenting.

16.6 Valve Repair

For patients without proximal venous obstruction, but with isolated lower extremity valvular incompetence, one option in addition to conservative measures might be valve repair or transposition. While operative repair of the diaphanous lower extremity venous valves may seem to be an exercise in futility, a very few dedicated and persistent practitioners have demonstrated that these procedures are technically feasible.

For patients with primary valvular incompetence in the absence of chronic thrombus, direct valve repair is a possibility. Valvular incompetence may result from dilation of the involved vein segment or prolapse of elongated valve cusps. Primary repair may be performed with a variety of techniques, all of which aim to resuspend the prolapsing valve cusps and restore the normal contour of the involved vein segment. Figure 16.9 demonstrates an external valvuloplasty, one variant of these difficult-to-conceptualize techniques.

In cases where the valve is too damaged for repair, one may consider valve transposition.

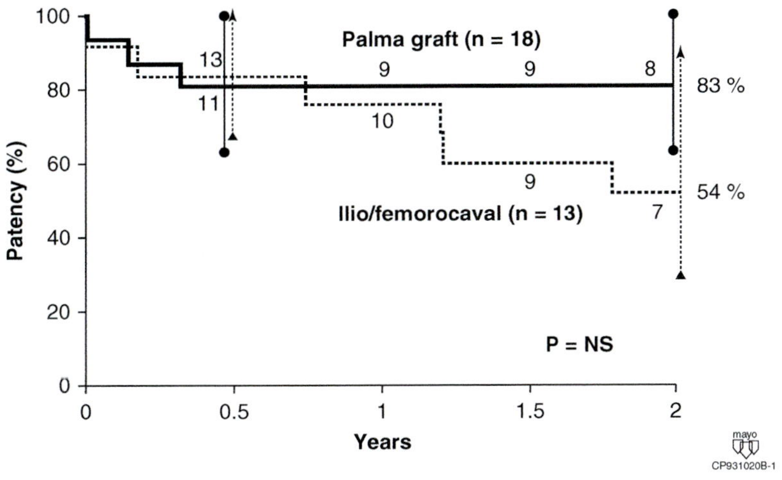

Fig. 16.8 Long-term patency of bypass procedures for chronic venous occlusion is represented by this figure from the large Mayo Clinic experience. The Palma procedure is noted to be superior to in-line bypass with PTFE [18]

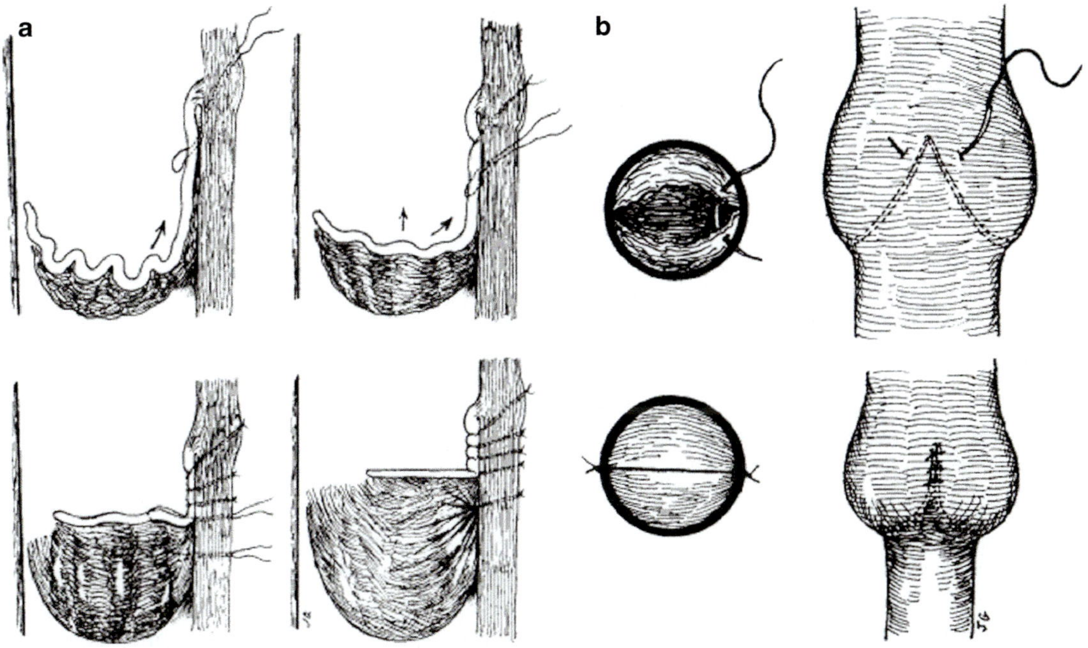

Fig. 16.9 Valve repair is difficult to conceptualize; however, this diagram from Neglen and Raju illustrates the technique of external valvuloplasty, which aims to resuspend the prolapsing valve cusps. (A-D) Demonstrates that each suture, following initial through-and-through oblique transluminal suture, is placed deeper and less oblique than the suture above to pull the valve in cephalic direction and to assure good valve apposition. A lateral cut-away view of the vein (**a**) shows the redundant valves tightened against the vein wall by the externally placed sutures (**b**) [19]

Most commonly, the axillary vein is exposed, and a segment with a competent valve is excised. The harvested vein can be used to replace a vein segment in the lower extremity, often the proximal femoral vein, with an incompetent valve. Another technique, the Kistner Transfer, involves transposition of an incompetent femoral vein onto a competent profunda vein (Fig. 16.10). As mentioned earlier, these tend to be niche procedures performed in significant volume at only a few centers of excellence; however, reported success rates in highly selected patients are reasonably good. In a large series from Raju and Neglen, patency with a competent valve after valve repair has been documented in 59 % of cases at 30 months [19].

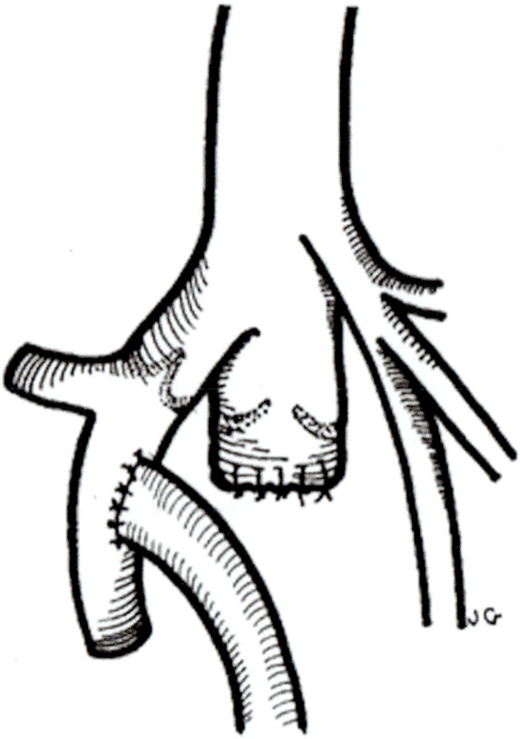

Fig. 16.10 The Kistner transfer involves dividing a proximal incompetent femoral vein and anastomosis to a competent profunda femoral vein [31]

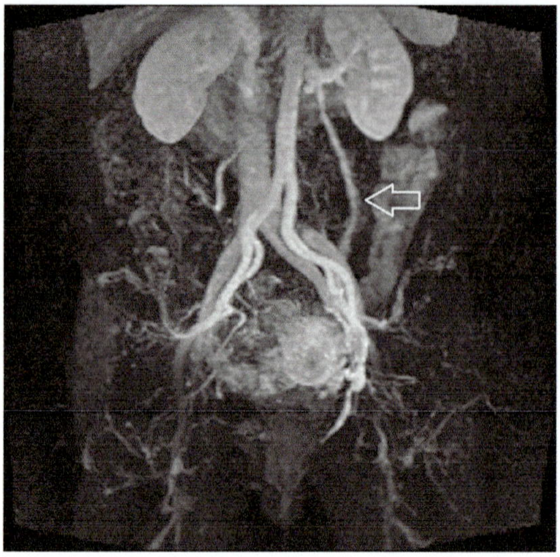

Fig. 16.11 MRV of a patient with symptoms of pelvic venous congestion demonstrates a markedly dilated left ovarian vein filling parauterine varicosities

16.7 Pelvic Venous Congestion

Valvular incompetence of the infrainguinal veins and the accompanying sequelae of venous insufficiency have been appreciated for decades, and obstruction of the iliac veins has recently been widely recognized as a significant issue in many patients with venous stasis. Pelvic venous incompetence should be considered in female patients with varicosities in an atypical distribution, namely, over the labia, perineum, or buttocks. Varicosities at the very proximal thigh should be followed proximally on exam or ultrasound to see if the supra-inguinal area is involved. Patients can also have chronic pelvic pain.

Imaging of the pelvic veins should be considered in patients with a suggestive history, including symptoms of dyspareunia, chronic pelvic pain, or dysuria. Noninvasive imaging with CT or MR will usually be the first choice for evaluation, and suggested diagnostic criteria for pelvic venous congestion include four or more tortuous parauterine veins, parauterine veins >4 mm in diameter, or an ovarian vein diameter >8 mm. While exact diagnostic criteria are not clear-cut, a recent consensus statement from the Society for Vascular Surgery (SVS) suggests that at venography, an ovarian vein diameter greater than 6 mm, contrast retention for more than 20 s, and filling of vulvar or thigh varicosities are all indicative of pelvic venous congestion [20]. Figure 16.11 shows an MRV which would be considered highly suggestive of pelvic venous congestion.

Treatment modalities may include medical ovarian suppression, hysterectomy, operative ligation of the ovarian vein, or percutaneous transcatheter embolization. While surgical approaches have been advocated in the past, currently, most patients failing medical management are offered transcatheter therapy as the preferred option. Endovascular treatment begins with a diagnostic venogram via a jugular or femoral approach, and in most cases contrast injection into the left ovarian vein will demonstrate reflux into pelvic varicosities (Fig. 16.12). Once reflux is confirmed, the most complete approach to endovascular treatment includes both coiling of the main ovarian vein as well as embolization or transcatheter

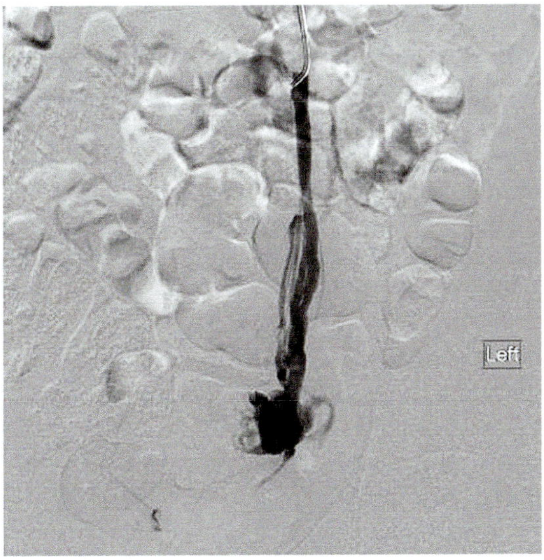

Fig. 16.12 Direct contrast injection of the ovarian vein demonstrates reflux into the pelvis, supporting the diagnosis of pelvic venous congestion

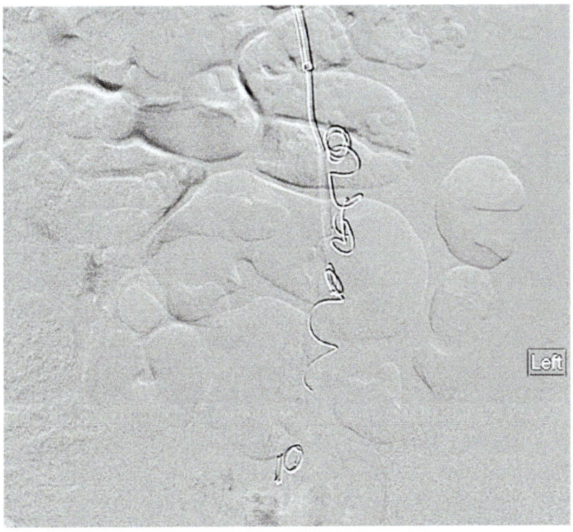

Fig. 16.13 Coiling of the ovarian vein will eliminate the main source of reflux and usually improve the symptoms of pelvic venous congestion

sclerotherapy of the pelvic varicosities [21]. Figure 16.13 demonstrates coiling of the ovarian vein in a patient undergoing treatment for pelvic venous congestion.

16.8 Nutcracker Syndrome

Nutcracker syndrome (NCS) is a rare clinical entity characterized by obstructed outflow from the left renal vein into the inferior vena cava due to extrinsic compression of the renal vein between the aorta and the overlying superior mesenteric artery (SMA). Although the first patient with NCS was described in 1950s [22], the problem is still only rarely recognized, and definitive diagnosis is difficult. Some degree of renal vein compression by the superior mesenteric artery may be physiologic, and surgical ligation of the left renal vein during aortic procedures is usually well tolerated, so even the existence of a true clinical syndrome may be disputed by some practitioners.

The most commonly reported symptoms associated with NCS include chronic left flank pain, gross or microscopic hematuria, and scrotal or vulvar varices [23]. More severe symptoms may include dysuria, proteinuria, dyspareunia, dysmenorrhea, and chronic pelvic pain. NCS may be suspected based on history and physical examination; however in most cases, patients present with vague complaints of abdominal pain and have seen multiple practitioners without a specific diagnosis. Often a CT scan is ordered to evaluate the vague abdominal complaints or hematuria, and renal vein compression is incidentally noted. Further evaluation may be pursued with either computed tomographic angiography (CTA) or magnetic resonance angiography (MRA), and either study will demonstrate the classic findings of left renal vein compression by the SMA and pelvic varicosities fed by gonadal vein reflux (Fig. 16.14).

Although multiple imaging studies are often ordered during the evaluation of a patient with suspected NCS, venography is typically pursued as the confirmatory test since it allows for measurement of a renocaval pressure gradient and documents reflux into gonadal and pelvic collaterals in real time. Existing literature suggests that a pressure gradient >3 mmHg is consistent with NCS [24–26]. However, there is probably not a true gold standard diagnostic test, and a decision to intervene surgically is based on a combination of imaging findings, clinical presentation, and patient preference.

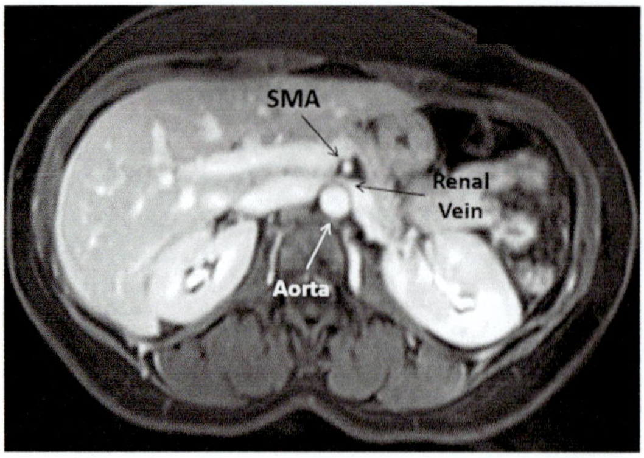

Fig. 16.14 This MRA demonstrates typical findings in a case of nutcracker syndrome with the left renal vein compressed between the SMA and the aorta

The major goal of NCS treatment is the reduction of the left renal vein hypertension, and current treatment options include observation, surgical decompression, and endovascular stenting. Observation alone is certainly appropriate for patients with mild symptoms or in cases of an incidental finding of renal vein compression in the absence of classic symptoms. Most operative and endovascular procedures are performed in NCS patients with hematuria and/or significant flank pain.

A panoply of surgical procedures have been reported in the literature including transposition of the SMA, excision of fibrous compressive tissue, and external stenting of the left renal vein, but currently, the most commonly used surgical techniques are transposition of the left renal vein and autotransplantation. Transposition of the left renal vein onto a more distal segment of the inferior vena cava should alleviate compression from the overlying SMA and restore normal flow [27]. In cases where it may be technically difficult to transpose the renal vein, autotransplantation of the kidney into the pelvis may be the only option. Given the potential morbidity of these operative approaches, the diagnosis and therapeutic goals should be very clear-cut preoperatively.

Over the last couple of decades, as central venous stenting in other locations has been shown to be durable, stenting of the left renal vein in the treatment of patients with NCS has been described. One large retrospective experience was reported in 2011 by Chen et al. and noted that 33 % of patients had symptomatic improvement at 6 months [28]. Despite some isolated pockets of enthusiasm, however, there is still concern about the short-term efficacy and long-term durability of angioplasty and stenting, and traditional surgical approaches are typically considered optimal for the average good-risk patient.

16.9 Popliteal Vein Compression

Another entity which may result in lower extremity deep venous obstruction is popliteal vein compression. Popliteal artery compression is well recognized as a distinct clinical phenomenon, but isolated popliteal venous compression is very infrequently recognized and treated. The clinical setting to consider popliteal venous entrapment is a patient with significant CVI symptoms isolated below the knee and no evidence of more proximal reflux. These patients may have significant edema below the knee or recurrent varicosities in the small saphenous distribution.

Some degree of intermittent compression of the popliteal vein with hyperextension of the knee joint is a normal component of the calf muscle pump, but in certain cases the compression may be pathologic. Abnormal fibrous bands, anomalous insertion of the gastrocnemius, or the popliteus muscle may create a fixed or dynamic compression. The unusual patient with symptoms of clear-cut, severe venous hypertension and no reflux above the level of the knee probably merits investigation for popliteal vein entrapment.

The diagnostic test of choice will be venography, optimally with contrast injected via one of the tibial veins to maximally opacify the popliteal vein. The study should include multiple views with provocative maneuvers including plantar and dorsiflexion against resistance. Patients with a suggestive history and fixed or dynamic obstruction on venogram may be candidates for a surgical popliteal vein release. As described by Neglen and Ragu, this is optimally performed via a medial approach, exposing the length of the popliteal vein and dividing any constricting fibrous bands or anomalous slips of muscle. Results with this approach are variable, but experienced practitioners report reasonably good results in very highly selected patients [29–31].

16.10 Summary

The thorough phlebologist should consider pelvic venous abnormalities as an important part of the differential in patients presenting with lower extremity venous insufficiency. One should have a low threshold for extending investigation beyond duplex US evaluation of the lower extremity in CVI patients with a clinical severity beyond the demonstrated hemodynamic abnormalities, patients lacking another explanation for their symptoms, and patients with a history of DVT. MRV or CT may be good noninvasive screening tests if the appropriate technical expertise is available, while venography with the adjunctive use of IVUS is the optimal technique for evaluation of iliac and caval pathology. Percutaneous endovenous stenting has emerged during the last decade as the method of choice to treat venous outflow obstruction, but traditional surgical reconstruction may be indicated in select patients who fail endovascular approaches. For patients with perineal varicosities, pelvic venous congestion should be considered as a diagnosis, and it can be treated very effectively with coil embolization of the ovarian vein and transcatheter sclerotherapy or embolization of pelvic varicosities. Nutcracker syndrome and popliteal venous entrapment are rare diagnoses but should be considered in the differential of certain atypical presentations of CVI. Both conditions may be treated surgically in certain circumstances.

While the majority of patients with chronic deep venous insufficiency of the lower extremities will not have a surgically remediable cause, there is a small subset of patients, often with the most severe and disabling symptoms, that merit consideration for an interventional approach. Iliocaval vein obstructions and pelvic venous congestion in particular are maladies which are very effectively addressed with minimally invasive procedures. These approaches are documented to provide significant symptomatic improvement in most patients.

References

1. Neglen P, Thrasher TL, Raju S. Venous outflow obstruction: an underestimated contributor to chronic venous disease. J Vasc Surg. 2003;38:879–85.
2. May R, Thurner J. The cause of the predominantly sinistral occurrence of thrombosis of the pelvic veins. Angiology. 1957;8:419–27.
3. Eklöf B, Rutherford RB, Bergan JJ, et al. Revision of the CEAP classification for chronic venous disorders: consensus statement. J Vasc Surg. 2004;40:1248–52.
4. Johnson BF, Manzo RA, Bergelin RO, Strandness DE. Relationship between changes in the deep venous system and the development of the postthrombotic syndrome after an acute episode of lower limb deep vein thrombosis: a one- to six- year follow-up. J Vasc Surg. 1995;21:307–13.
5. Akesson H, Brudin L, Dahlstrom JA, Eklof B, Ohlin P, Plate G. Venous function assessed during a 5-year period after acute iliofemoral venous thrombosis treated with anticoagulation. Eur J Vasc Surg. 1990;4:43–8.
6. Meissner MH, et al. Secondary chronic venous disorders. J Vasc Surg. 2007;46(Suppl 6):S68–83.
7. Lin EP, Bhatt S, Rubens D, Dogra VS. The importance of monophasic Doppler waveforms in the common femoral vein: a retrospective study. J Ultrasound Med. 2007;26:885–91.
8. Labropoulos N, Borge M, Pierce K, Pappas PJ. Criteria for defining significant central vein stenosis with duplex ultrasound. J Vasc Surg. 2007;46(1):101–7.
9. Neglen P, Thrasher TL, Raju S. Chronic venous insufficiency and varicose veins. N Engl J Med. 2006;360:22.
10. Kibbe MR, Ujiki M, Goodwin AL, Eskandari M, Yao J, Matsumura J. Iliac vein compression in an asymptomatic patient population. J Vasc Surg. 2004;39:937–43.
11. Hartung O, Benmiloud F, Barthelemy P, Dubuc M, Boufi M, Alimi YS. Late results of surgical venous thrombectomy with iliocaval stenting. J Vasc Surg. 2008;47:381–7.
12. Neglén P, Raju S. Intravascular ultrasound scan evaluation of the obstructed vein. J Vasc Surg. 2002; 35:694–700.
13. Neglén P, Hollis KC, Olivier J, Raju S. Stenting of the venous outflow in chronic venous disease: long-term stent-related outcome, clinical, and hemodynamic result. J Vasc Surg. 2007;46:979–90.
14. Raju S. Endovenous treatment of patients with iliac-caval venous obstruction. J Cardiovasc Surg (Torino). 2008;49:27–33.
15. Hartung O, Otero A, Boufi M, Decaridi G, Barthelemy P, Juhan C, et al. Mid-term results of endovascular treatment for symptomatic chronic nonmalignant iliocaval venous occlusive disease. J Vasc Surg. 2005;42: 1138–44; discussion 44.

16. Neglén P, Oglesbee M, Olivier J, Raju SJ. Stenting of chronically obstructed inferior vena cava filters. Vasc Surg. 2011;54(1):153–61.
17. Palma EC, Esperon R. Vein transplants and grafts in the surgical treatment of the postphlebitic syndrome. J Cardiovasc Surg. 1960;1:94–107.
18. Jost CJ, Gloviczki P, Cherry Jr KJ, McKusick MA, Harmsen WS, Jenkins GD, et al. Surgical reconstruction of iliofemoral veins and the inferior vena cava for nonmalignant occlusive disease. J Vasc Surg. 2001;33:320–7; discussion 7-8.
19. Raju S, Berry MA, Neglen P. Transcommisural valvuloplasty: technique and results. J Vasc Surg. 2000; 32(5):969–76.
20. Gloviczki P, Comerota AJ, Dalsing MC, et al. The care of patients with varicose veins and associated chronic venous diseases: clinical practice guidelines of the Society for Vascular Surgery and the American Venous Forum. J Vasc Surg. 2011;53(5 Suppl):2S–48.
21. Kim HS, Malhotra AD, Rowe PC, Lee JM, Venbrux AC. Embolotherapy for pelvic congestion syndrome: long-term results. J Vasc Interv Radiol. 2006;17(2 Pt 1): 289–97.
22. El-Sadr A, Mina E. Anatomical and surgical aspects in the operative management of varicocele. Urol Cutaneous Rev. 1950;54:257–62.
23. Rudloff U, Holmes RJ, Prem JT, Faust GR, Moldwin R, Seigel D. Mesoaortic compression of the left renal vein (nutcracker syndrome): case reports and review of the literature. Ann Vasc Surg. 2006;20:120–9.
24. Zerhouni EA, Siegelman SS, Walsh PC, White RI. Elevated pressure in the left renal vein in patients with varicocele: preliminary observations. J Urol. 1980;123:512–3.
25. Beinart C, Sniderman KW, Tamura S, Vaughan ED, Sos TA. Left renal vein to inferior vena cava pressure relationship in humans. J Urol. 1982;127:1070–1.
26. Hohenfellner M, Steinbach F, Schultz-Lampel W, et al. The nutcracker syndrome: new aspects of pathophysiology, diagnosis and treatment. J Urol. 1991;146:685–8.
27. Reed NR, Kalra M, Bower TC, Vrtiska TJ, Ricotta 2nd JJ, Gloviczki P. Left renal vein transposition for nutcracker syndrome. J Vasc Surg. 2009;49:386–93.
28. Chen S, Zhang H, Shi H, et al. Endovascular stenting for treatment of Nutcracker syndrome: report of 61 cases with long-term followup. J Urol. 2011;186(2):570–5.
29. Raju S, Neglen P. Popliteal vein entrapment: a benign venographic feature or a pathologic entity? J Vasc Surg. 2000;31(4):631–41.
30. Lalka S. Management of chronic obstructive venous disease of the lower extremity. In: Rutherford RB, Johnson KW, et al., editors. Vascular surgery. Philadelphia: WB Saunders Company; 1995. p. 1869.
31. Raju S. Operative management of chronic venous insufficiency. In: Rutherford RB, Johnson KW, et al., editors. Vascular surgery. Philadelphia: WB Saunders Company; 1995. p. 1858.

Low-Flow Vascular Malformations 17

Jovan N. Markovic and Cynthia K. Shortell

Contents

Abstract

Congenital vascular malformations (CVM) are a group of unique vascular disorders that can be defined as "diffuse or localized embryologically developed errors of vascular morphogenesis leading to true structural anomalies". The presence of CVM in the general population is estimated to be around 1.5 %, with no known sex predilection. Venous malformations are the most common type of CVM, and they comprise approximately two-thirds of all CVMs. The diagnosis and treatment of CVM can be complex and challenging. Patients with CVM can easily be misdiagnosed and also mismanaged. Consequently, many patients have been discouraged by the lack of correct diagnosis and proper treatment despite numerous visits to different clinics (from primary care physicians to subspecialists). Moreover, patients with CVM have frequently been left untreated, due to the mistaken presumption that these types of lesions can spontaneously regress, while others were considered too high risk to treat. This chapter discusses CVM: classification, multidisciplinary approach diagnosis, and management.

17.1 Introduction

Congenital vascular malformations (CVM) are a group of unique vascular disorders that can be defined as "diffuse or localized embryologically developed errors of vascular morphogenesis

J.N. Markovic, MD (✉)
Department of Surgery,
Duke University Medical Center, Durham, NC, USA
e-mail: jovan.markovic@duke.edu

C.K. Shortell, MD, FACS
Department of Vascular Surgery,
Duke University Medical Center, Durham, NC, USA
e-mail: cynthia.shortell@duke.edu

E. Mowatt-Larssen et al. (eds.), *Phlebology, Vein Surgery and Ultrasonography*,
DOI 10.1007/978-3-319-01812-6_17,

leading to true structural anomalies" [1]. The presence of CVM in the general population is estimated to be around 1.5 %, with no known sex predilection [2]. Venous malformations are the most common type of CVM, and they comprise approximately two-thirds of all CVM [3, 4]. The estimated incidence of predominantly venous malformations is approximately 0.8–1 % [5]. The majority of CVM arise sporadically, but in rare cases (1–2 %), they are familial and characterized by an autosomal dominant pattern of inheritance [6–8]. Although genetic mutations are suspected to be the underlying etiology, the exact mechanism responsible for development of CVM still remains to be elucidated [9–14].

The diagnosis and treatment of CVM can be complex and challenging since it exceeds the level of expertise of any single medical specialty. Patients with CVM can easily be misdiagnosed and also mismanaged. Consequently, many patients have been discouraged by the lack of correct diagnosis and proper treatment despite numerous visits to different clinics (from primary care physicians to subspecialists). Moreover, patients with CVM have frequently been left untreated, due to the mistaken presumption that these types of lesions can spontaneously regress, while others were considered too high risk to treat.

17.2 Classification

Historically, numerous attempts have been made to classify CVM [15–19]. Early classification published by Virchow divided all vascular lesions into angiomas and lymphangiomas [20]. This classification was based on the vessels' histopathologic appearance and did not consider biological behavior and natural history of the lesion. Thus, there was a tendency to classify any type of vascular anomaly as a hemangioma. This tendency still persists among practitioners. Based on endothelial characteristics and on a biologic classification of vascular birthmarks, initially proposed by Mullikin and Glowicki in 1982, the International Society for the Study of Vascular Anomalies (ISSVA) approved in 1996 a classification system

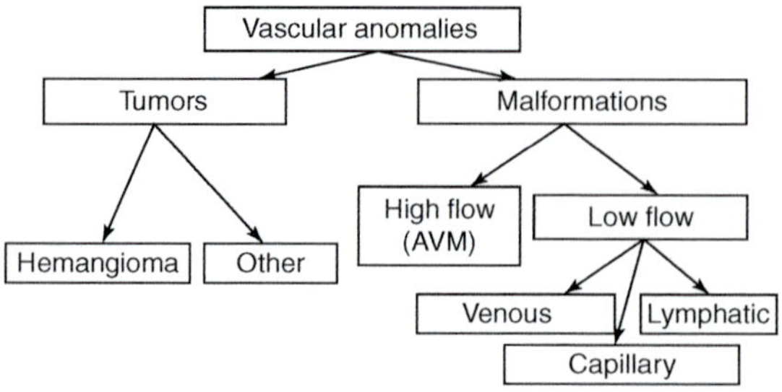

Fig. 17.1 The International Society for the Study of Vascular Anomalies classification system. Vascular anomalies are divided on the basis of cellular kinetics and clinical behavior into two major categories: vascular tumors and vascular malformations. Vascular malformations are subdivided into high-flow and low-flow vascular malformations (capillary, venous, and lymphatic malformations)

in which all vascular anomalies were divided on the basis of cellular kinetics, anatomy, and clinical behavior into two major categories: vascular tumors and vascular malformations [21, 22]. Depending on the type of vessel involved, vascular malformations were subdivided into high-flow vascular malformations (HFVM), such as arteriovenous malformation, and low-flow vascular malformations (LFVM), such as capillary, venous, and lymphatic malformations (Fig. 17.1). Based on their embryonic stage of developmental arrest, there are two different types of venous malformations: extratruncular and truncular as emphasized in the Modified Hamburg's Classification [23]. Extratruncular venous malformations are the outcome of developmental arrest in the early stages, whereas truncular venous malformations are a result of developmental arrest in the late stages of embryogenesis. Extratruncular malformations are associated with a higher rate of recurrence and resistance to therapy, presumably because they possess mesenchymal characteristics of independent growth potential [24]. There are also complex-combined vascular malformations that are typically associated with osteomuscular hypertrophy and various internal organ anomalies.

The separation of vascular anomalies into tumors and malformations permits more effective communication between different medical specialists, since, as previously mentioned, the management of CVM has been characterized by confusing and contradictory nomenclature and classification that was present in the majority of the medical literature discussing these lesions. Unfortunately, despite the ISSVA classification, the use of confusing nomenclature persists in the literature, and archaic terms such as "cavernous hemangioma," "port wine stains," "salmon patch," "angel's kiss," and "nevus simplex" are still frequently used by some specialists.

17.3 Pathophysiology

Congenital vascular malformations arise by vascular dysmorphogenesis, between the fourth and tenth weeks of intrauterine life, without increased endothelial proliferation affecting a limited number of vessels in a restricted area of the body [3]. Recent data suggest that the pathophysiologic mechanism underlying the formation of CVM is caused by dysfunctions in the signaling process responsible for regulation of proliferation, differentiation, maturation, adhesion, and apoptosis of vascular cells [25–27]. A genetic TIE2 mutation has been described in certain hereditary cutaneomucosal venous malformations [28]. A number of genes have also been identified in the process of lymphangiogenesis including VEGFR3, VEGFC, Ang2, Lyve1, Nrp2, and podoplanin [29]. It is postulated that genetic aberrations of these genes and their regulatory mechanisms underline developmental defects during embryonic lymphangiogenesis, resulting in lymphatic malformations. In contrast to CVM, vascular tumors are true neoplastic disorders, and pathohistologically they demonstrate increased endothelial cell turnover rate [26, 30]. Hemangiomas represent the most common type of vascular tumor. Less common vascular tumors include Kaposiform hemangioendothelioma, angiolipoma, angiosarcoma, and hemangiopericytoma. Although hemangiomas and CVM have distinct histopathologic characteristics and clinical courses, occasionally, they coexist in the same settings, suggesting a possible overlap in the pathogenesis of the vascular tumors and malformations in certain cases [31].

17.4 Clinical Presentation

The differential diagnosis of vascular tumors and vascular malformations can be made by clinical assessment in the majority of cases. Vascular malformations are present at birth and do not spontaneously regress. Often they grow proportionately with the child's growth with many becoming more prominent later in life. Their rapid growth and appearance may be stimulated by trauma, infection, and the effects of hormones (during puberty or pregnancy), or they may occur spontaneously in the absence of any identified triggering factors [32]. By contrast, infantile hemangiomas are characterized by a rapid proliferative phase in the first several months of life, followed by an involutional phase of slow, spontaneous regression in the majority of cases, frequently leaving adipofibrotic overlying dermis and telangiectasias that can remain visible at the location of the initial hemangioma [33]. In challenging and complex cases, histopathologic evaluation, immunohistopathologic markers, and radiologic studies are needed to help distinguish vascular tumors from vascular malformations.

The morphology, clinical presentation, and course of vascular malformations are variable in their extent and severity, depending upon location, proximity to vital structures, size or organ involved, and the type of vessel affected. Congenital vascular malformations are rarely asymptomatic. Usually they cause discomfort, pain, hemorrhage, and negatively affect the patient's appearance as well as emotional well-being. In addition, these patients often have a significant reduction in daily functional capacity and quality of life. As discussed previously, if the malformation has an arterial component, it is classified as HFVM. The absence of arterial blood flow is the characteristic used to differentiate HFVM from LFVM. Some authors use the term fast-flow or arteriovenous malformation to describe HFVM. Low-flow vascular malformations are subdivided into venous malformations, lymphatic malformations, capillary malformations, and lesions that combine two or more of these elements.

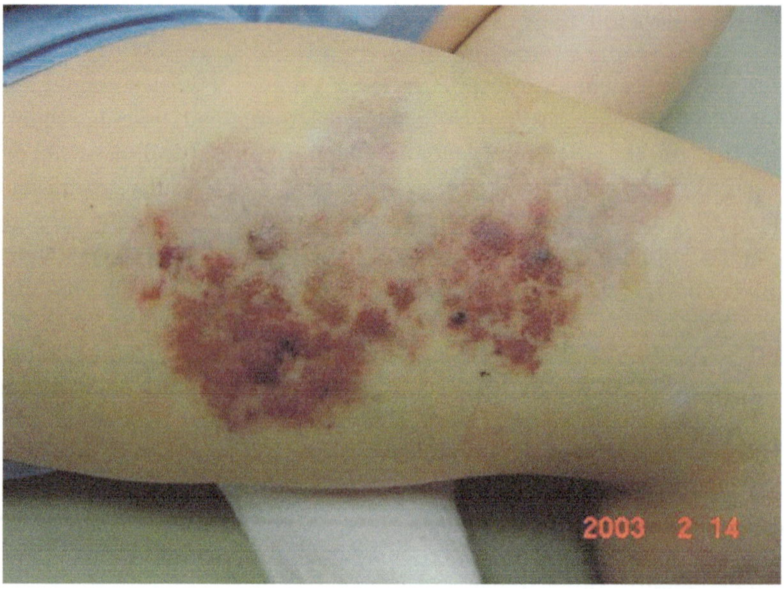

Fig. 17.2 Capillary malformation affecting the latero-medial aspect of the right thigh in the patient with Klippel-Trenaunay syndrome. Capillary malformations frequently occur in association with venous malformations and other structural abnormalities such as osteomuscular hypertrophy

Capillary malformations usually appear as localized pink or red lesions. They are present at birth and grow in proportion to the growth of the child. They appear darker immediately after the birth and lighten slightly in the first several weeks of life. This is believed to be secondary to the higher hemoglobin concentration that characterize the immediate newborn period [34]. Capillary malformations can occur as isolated cutaneous lesions or in association with other vascular malformations or other structural abnormalities such as bony or soft tissue hyperplasia or atrophy and neurological defect. In the limbs, capillary malformations are usually associated with osteomuscular hypertrophy (Fig. 17.2). When located on the head, they may extend to the gingiva, lips, and oral mucosa. Midline occipital capillary malformations can herald the presence of an encephalocele or ectopic meninges. Capillary malformations over the spine can be associated with occult spinal dysraphism [35]. In a retrospective review, Guggisberg et al. suggested that the combination of two or more midline capillary malformations is highly suggestive of spinal dysraphism [36]. However, the significance of capillary malformations as a marker for underlying spinal abnormalities is still unclear, and currently there are no evidence-based guidelines regarding screening of patients with capillary malformations for spinal defects. The most common syndrome associated with capillary malformations is Sturge-Weber syndrome. This neuroectodermal syndrome is characterized by an overabundance of capillaries around the ophthalmic branch (V_1) of the trigeminal nerve, ipsilateral leptomeningeal angiomatosis, glaucoma (in approximately 50 % of patients), and seizures. Seizures are frequently present within the first year of life and tend to worsen over time.

Venous malformations are the most common peripheral LFVM encountered clinically. They are composed of anomalous dilated venous channels. They affect males and females equally with a reported prevalence of approximately 1 % [37]. On physical examination they appear as bluish, soft, and easily compressible, non-pulsatile masses that usually enlarge with activity, Valsalva maneuver (crying in children) or dependent posture, and empty with elevation. There is no increase in local skin temperature or thrill when the malformation is palpated, and there is no bruit present on auscultation (in contrast to HFVMs) (Fig. 17.3). Venous malformations are associated with swelling and episodes of pain as well as functional difficulties secondary to the involvement of muscles and joints. Although most venous malformations are solitary and occur in the skin and subcutaneous tissues, they

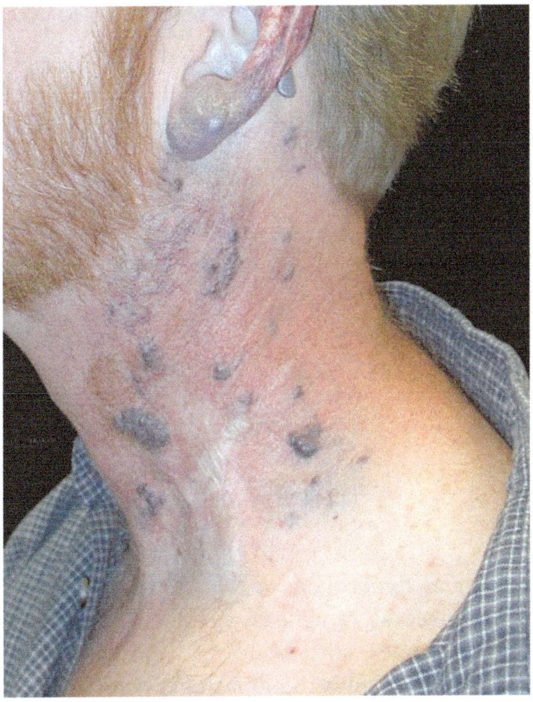

Fig. 17.3 Venous malformations appear as bluish, soft, and easily compressible, non-pulsatile masses that usually enlarge with activity. In contrast to high-flow vascular malformations, there is no increase in local skin temperature or thrill when the malformation is palpated, and there is no bruit present on auscultation

can also occur as multiple, infiltrating lesions that can involve multiple soft tissue planes including muscles, abdominal viscera, and the central nervous system [38]. In terms of connection to the conducting veins, venous malformations are characterized as sequestered or communicating. In contrast to sequestered venous malformations, communicating malformations have direct connection to deep venous system. It is important to determine whether malformation is communicating since treatment of this type of malformation carries an increased risk of distal venous thromboembolic events. Venous malformations can also occur as part of syndromes. Klippel-Trenaunay syndrome (KTS) is a complex capillary-lymphatic-venous malformation which is associated with pathognomonic osteomuscular hypertrophy of the affected extremities in association with mixed venous and lymphatic and capillary lesions [39, 40]. In addition to obvious concerns about cosmesis, these patients often present with pain, swelling, orthostatic hypotension, or in severe cases pulmonary embolism secondary to insufficiency of the anomalous vein structures or repeated occult pulmonary emboli from intralesional thrombus. Blue rubber bleb nevus syndrome (BRBNS) is another rare syndrome associated with venous malformations. This sporadic disorder is characterized by multifocal venous malformations of the skin, soft tissues, and gastrointestinal tract [41, 42]. In addition to the risk of bleeding and subsequent anemia, gastrointestinal involvement makes these patients susceptible to intussusception and volvulus [43].

Lymphatic malformations are usually noted at birth or before the patient reaches the age of 2 years. Prenatal ultrasonography (US) can detect macrocystic lymphatic malformations during the late first trimester. The skin overlying these sponge-like lesions is usually normal or of bluish hue (Fig. 17.4). Lymphatic malformations can be characterized as microcystic, macrocystic, or combined. Macrocystic lymphatic malformations are generally defined as lesions that contain cyst spaces greater than 2 cm and microcystic as cysts smaller than 2 cm in diameter. Bleeding, bacterial infection, and swelling are the most common complications associated with lymphatic malformations. These complications can lead to the compression of surrounding structures, including the airway (if the malformation is located in the head or neck), or the optic nerve in the case of orbital lesions. In these patients, prompt management and urgent decompression are required to decompress the lesion and subsequently restore the normal function of the affected vital structures. Infection is a common complication of lymphatic malformations, and prompt recognition and treatment with systemic antibiotics that cover skin pathogens is imperative.

17.5 Diagnosis

Despite distinct clinical, radiologic, and histological findings, LFVM are often confused with vascular tumors (most frequently with infantile

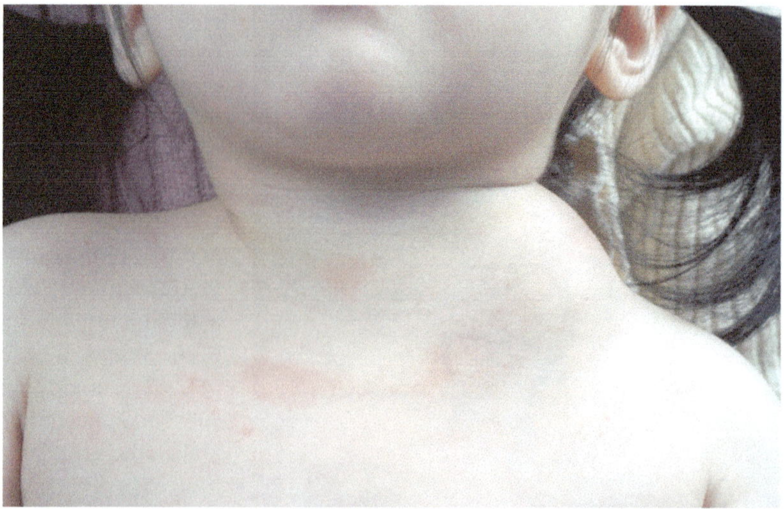

Fig. 17.4 A large lymphatic malformation extending from the left side of the neck. Lymphatic malformations are usually noted at birth (or before the patient reaches the age of 2 years). Macrocystic lymphatic malformations are defined as lesions that contain cyst spaces greater than 2 cm in diameter (*Courtesy of Dr. B.B. Lee)

hemangiomas) and many physicians do not understand the difference between these two vastly different lesions. Moreover, the complexity of many CVM contributes to the diagnostic challenge of differentiating LFVM from HFVM and differentiating LFVM from other congenital vascular anomalies. Since the prognosis, morbidity, and treatment significantly differ between vascular tumors, HFVM, and LFVM, proper diagnosis and accurate classification are critical for the successful management of these lesions [44]. A meticulous medical history and a detailed physical examination are essential initial steps in the management of CVM. However, clinical evaluation often underestimates the involvement of deep structures such as muscles, bones, joints, or abdominal viscera and is not sufficient to differentiate HFVM from LFVM and malformations from tumors in some of the more complicated lesions. Therefore, evaluation by advanced imaging modalities (color flow duplex ultrasound, magnetic resonance imaging) is of paramount importance for the correct diagnosis and management of CVM [45–47]. Ultrasonography of HFVMs is characterized by multidirectional blood flow and high-amplitude arterial waveform with spectral broadening. Ultrasonography of venous and lymphatic malformations reveals mixed venous waveform and complete absence of signal, respectively. On gray scale ultrasound, venous malformations appear as hypoechoic or heterogeneous lesions with anechoic structures visible in <50 % of cases. Duplex ultrasound of venous malformations generally demonstrates monophasic low-velocity flow. In some cases flow is only detectible with compression and release of the malformation. Macrocystic lymphatic malformations appear as anechoic cavities, often with internal septa and debris. Microcystic lymphatic malformations are hyperechoic, giving a more solid appearance.

In the evaluation of CVM, duplex ultrasound is useful to confirm the diagnosis, as it is rapid, readily available, and shows the flow velocity and vascularization [48]. It is also useful for initial assessment of superficial malformations; however it is frequently inadequate to demonstrate the extent of larger lesions. Therefore, magnetic resonance imaging (MRI) is the imaging modality of choice in the evaluation of CVM [49, 50]. It gives a bright hypersignal on T2-weighted spin-echo sequences that delineates the extent of the malformation throughout the involved tissues [51, 52]. In addition, MRI shows the lesion's flow characteristics, relation to normal vascular and nonvascular structures, and provides good soft tissue definition (Fig. 17.5). In inconclusive cases, when suspicion of arterial flow is present based on MRI findings, an appropriate diagnostic workup includes an arteriogram, but only if treatment is deemed necessary. Every

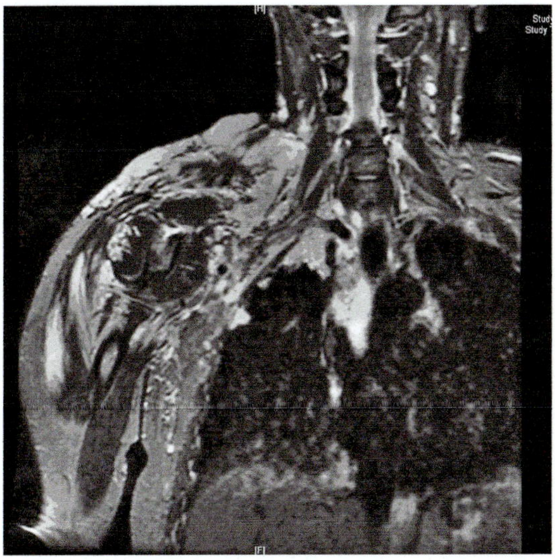

Fig. 17.5 Coronal T2-weighted image of the right upper extremity venous malformation. MRI gives a bright hypersignal on T2-weighted spin-echo sequences that delineates the extent of the malformation throughout the involved tissues

effort should be exerted to rule out a high-flow arterial component. It is worth emphasizing that this differentiation is of critical value in the management of CVM as treatment options for high-flow and low-flow lesions are different and the presence of an arterial component represents an absolute contraindication to transcutaneous sclerotherapy (due to the risk of arterial thrombosis and extensive tissue necrosis) which can be effectively used in the treatment of LFVM. In T2-weighted MRI, venous malformations demonstrate high-signal intensity, and this sequence is the best sequence to determine the full extent of the lesion and its relationship to adjacent tissues (Fig. 17.6a, b). Lymphatic malformations demonstrate predominantly fluid-type characteristics on all MRI sequences (low signal on T1 and high signal on T2 sequences). Macrocystic and microcystic components are easily differentiated since microcystic malformations demonstrate intermediate signal intensity on T1 and T2 spin-echo sequences.

From a diagnostic standpoint, evaluation of the deep venous system deserves special consideration. In a study of 392 patients with CVM, Eifert et al. documented aplasia or hypoplasia of deep

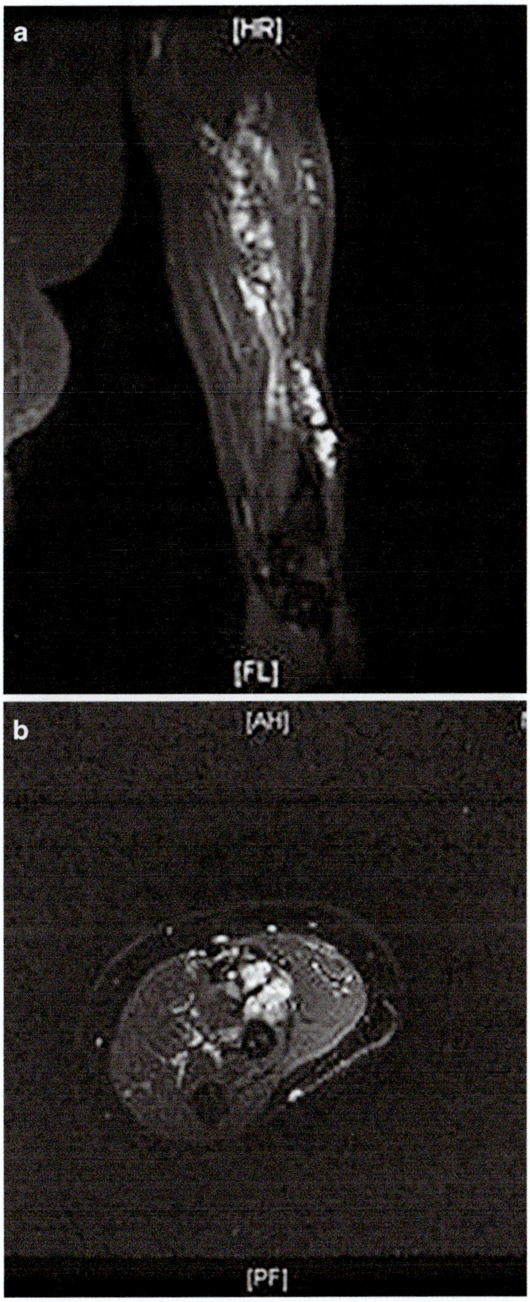

Fig. 17.6 MRI of the patient with venous malformation affecting the left upper extremity. A and B: coronal and axial (respectively) T2-weighted images of left upper extremity demonstrates multiple dilated venous channels in the subcutaneous and deeper soft tissues in the antero-lateral aspect of the left upper extremity

venous trunks in 8 % of patients (with venous predominance) [2]. In these patients venous blood

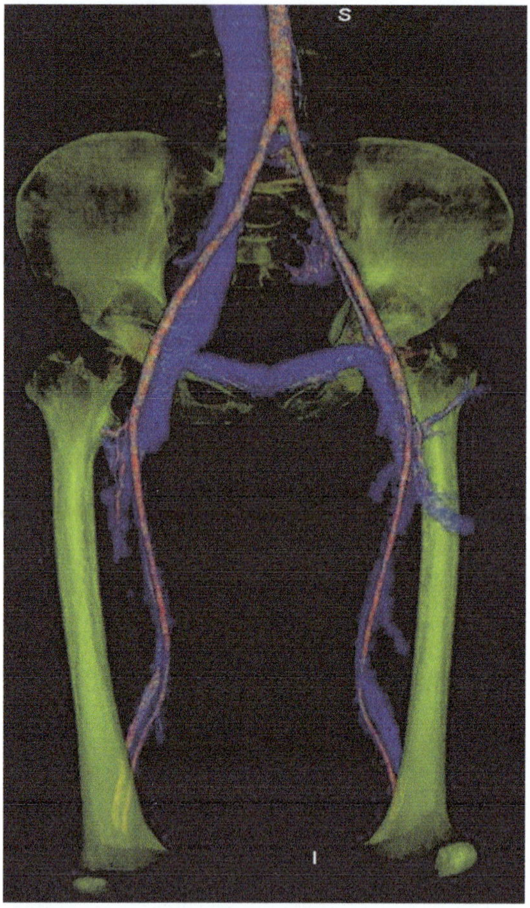

Fig. 17.7 MRI reconstruction of patient with Klippel-Trenaunay Syndrome (KTS) demonstrates absence of the left iliofemoral vein segment. The prevalence of deep venous anomalies is high (18 %) in patients with KTS. Evaluation of patency and anatomic variations of the deep venous system is important in patients with vascular malformations

flow from the affected limbs depends on superficial and abnormal vessels. Obliteration of these venous structures would compromise the venous circulation of the affected limb. Evaluation of patency and anatomic variations of the entire venous system (deep and superficial) is vital in these patients (Fig. 17.7). It has been reported that the prevalence of deep venous anomalies is even higher (18 %) in patients with KTS [53]. Based on the venous drainage channels and their response to treatment and rates of complications, Puig et al. divided venous malformations into four types: isolated malformations without discernible venous drainage (type I), lesions draining into normal veins (type II), lesions draining into dysplastic veins (type III), and lesions consisting primarily of venous ectasia (type IV). According to the same authors, types I and II respond best to sclerotherapy and higher rates of complications are attributed to types III and IV [17].

In addition to being at increased risk of having deep venous anomalies, patients with extensive LFVMs may develop an intralesional consumptive coagulopathy [54, 55]. In a study of 118 patients, Mazoyer et al. demonstrated that localized intravascular coagulopathy (LIC) was present in 58 % of venous malformation patients [56]. In the literature, this coagulopathy is often erroneously labeled as Kasabach-Merritt syndrome (a distinct clinical entity characterized by disseminated intravascular coagulation and profound thrombocytopenia associated with vascular tumors) [57]. The platelet count in LIC is minimally diminished (in the $100–150 \times 10^3$/mL range). This distinction is important because, in contrast to patients with Kasabach-Merritt syndrome, LIC can be treated with heparin. Localized intravascular coagulopathy can be asymptomatic, but it may, rarely, be associated with painful intralesional thrombotic episodes and can progress to disseminated intravascular coagulation with life-threatening hemorrhage [58–60]. Although controversial, some authors advocate the use of aspirin or low molecular weight heparin (depending on the severity of symptoms) to be administered in patients with painful thrombotic episodes [58]. The increased risk of bleeding in some of these patients can be attributed to the increased consumption of coagulation factors. This is especially concerning in patients undergoing surgical resection of the lesion. A hypercoagulability profile should be considered in LFVM patients prior to undergoing imaging studies, surgical intervention, or sclerotherapy. An elevated D-dimer level and variable fibrinogen level is the hallmark of LIC. This finding is so common that some authors use D-dimer to differentiate venous malformations from lymphatic malformations (which do not show elevated D-dimer levels). Although LIC is usually latent and asymptomatic, it is worth emphasizing that these patients can become severely coagulopathic even during diagnostic procedures (US, MRI, angiography).

17.6 Treatment

Since the management of CVM falls in the range of several medical and surgical specialties, it is critical to establish a multidisciplinary approach for their diagnosis and treatment [61–64]. This was first discussed and introduced at the International Symposium for Congenital Vascular Malformations held in Seoul in 1996 [65]. In the past several years, several medical centers have developed multidisciplinary CVM teams [66]. Ideally, to achieve a consensus view of management, representatives from different medical specialties should be involved in the management of CVM patients and all treatments should be based on team assessments and decisions. This also affords the opportunity to streamline the evaluation process for patients with vascular anomalies, to coordinate the care of these patients, and to treat them comprehensively by reducing the need for multiple visits to different clinics. Given the heterogeneous nature and complexity of CVM, every patient and every lesion should be individually discussed. Multidisciplinary preoperative evaluation is of paramount importance, especially to rule out vascular tumors and to differentiate LFVM from HFVM and to identify lesions most amenable to resection. The decision for intervention has to take into account the size, location, proximity to vital structures and the natural history of the lesion, the risk of complications, and the relative risk of surgical or endovascular intervention. Low-flow vascular malformations can be treated with laser therapy, sclerotherapy, surgical excision, or combination therapy.

The flashlamp-pumped pulsed dye laser (FPDL) is the most frequently used as a treatment of choice for capillary malformations especially in areas in which there are concerns about ulcerations or hyperpigmentation from sclerotherapy. The most commonly used wavelengths are 577, 585, and 595 nm since they selectively target oxyhemoglobin. Pulse duration is used to concentrate and limit heat distribution (and subsequent collagen contraction and obliteration) to the capillary malformation while preserving surrounding structures in epidermis and dermis. Efficacy rates of the FPDL in the treatment of capillary malformations are variable. Reyes et al. reported good response in as many as 80 % of treated patients [67]. In a retrospective study of 259 adults and children, Renfro et al. demonstrated that responsiveness of the capillary malformations depends on the anatomical location of the lesion [68]. Lesions located on the central face or limbs were less responsive to FPDL than lesions located on the neck and trunk. It must be noted that multiple treatments are needed to achieve acceptable results. Treatments are usually scheduled every 6–8 weeks over the course of several months to a year depending upon the size, location, and responsiveness of the malformation to the therapy.

Despite the high rates of recurrence (25–52 %), surgical excision has been historically used as the treatment of choice for vascular malformations [69]. Traditionally, surgical resection was effectively used for encapsulated and small lesions. When a malformation is diffuse and multifocal, the surgical approach is relatively contraindicated as damage to major vital structures and massive hemorrhage may ensue. For larger lesions, complete surgical resection might not be possible and multiple partial surgical resections may be required. Partial surgical resections are associated with higher recurrence rates. Encapsulated, circumscribed, localized lesions and lesions composed of numerous small venous channels are the most amenable to surgical resection.

Since its introduction, sclerotherapy has been used as an effective alternative to surgery in the treatment of LFVM. Currently there are numerous agents available for sclerotherapy including ethanol, sodium tetradecyl sulfate (STS), polidocanol, ethibloc, and bleomycin. The most commonly used agents are ethanol and STS (in the United States) and polidocanol (in Europe), although the use of polidocanol in the United States has been increasing since its approval by the Food and Drug Administration (FDA) in March of 2010. Although proven to be effective

[70, 71], ethanol sclerotherapy (ES) is associated with limitations and major side effects (local and systemic), including severe pain requiring general anesthesia, ethanol toxicity, and local tissue damage, and its use in pediatric patients remains controversial. In a study of 71 patients, Mason et al. demonstrated that patients who received up to 1 mL/kg of ethanol during ethanol embolization or sclerotherapy may have elevated serum ethanol levels that could be associated with increased risk of respiratory depression, cardiac arrhythmias, seizures, rhabdomyolysis, and hypoglycemia [72]. In a study of 98 sessions of ES in 30 CVM patients, Lee et al. documented complications in 26.7 % of patients which ranged from mild to severe and acute to delayed [73]. Authors reported nine cases with ischemic bullae, two with tissue fibrosis, two with tissue necrosis, one with deep venous thrombosis (DVT), one with pulmonary embolism, five with nerve palsy, and four cases of transient pulmonary pressure elevation. Of the five nerve palsies, one (affecting the peroneal nerve) was permanent. Other studies reported episodes of transient bradycardia and cardiac arrest during the treatment with ES [74]. Ethanol sclerotherapy can also result in transmural vessel necrosis, massive swelling (sometimes resulting in compartment syndrome), central nervous system (CNS) depression, hypertension, and pulmonary vasospasm [75, 76]. Some practitioners recommend continuous pulmonary pressure monitoring during ES and avoiding ethanol in regions adjacent to nerves such as the facial nerve or the sympathetic plexus in cervical lesions [76].

Since liquid sclerosants become diluted and inactivated by intralesional blood, the use of sclerosants in microfoam form significantly improves the procedure for LFVM [77–79]. The foam bubbles displace intralesional blood (preventing the sclerosant from becoming diluted) and achieve maximal effective exposure between the sclerosing agent and the endothelial lining. In addition, the echogenicity of the bubbles makes them visible on US surveillance making the procedure easier to perform (Figs. 17.8a, b). Foam treatments, in contrast to ES, can be given on a strictly ambulatory basis as they are minimally painful.

The use of foam sclerosants was initially described by Orbach in 1944 [80], and foam sclerotherapy gained popularity in the last decade. Foam can be produced with different techniques that result in differences in bubble size, foam stability, and reabsorption rates [81–83]. In 2000, Tessari reported a new method for microfoam production, using two syringes connected with a three-way stopcock (Fig. 17.9) [84]. Since then, this technique has been widely accepted in producing stable foam for the treatment of vein disorders. STS is a synthetic, detergent-based sclerosant, first described by Reiner in 1946 [85]. The mechanism of action is the creation of irreversible chemical damage to the vascular endothelial lining by the disruption of cell membranes. The response to the subendothelial collagen exposure is vasospasm, platelet aggregation, and subsequent endofibrosis that obliterates the vessel. Different concentrations of STS solution have been commonly used in the treatment of telangiectasias and reticular veins [86–89]. However, larger veins (greater than 10 mm in diameter) have also been effectively treated with STS [90]. In a double-blind prospective comparative trial that included 129 patients with varicose veins and telangiectasias, Goldman demonstrated that STS and polidocanol had approximately the same effectiveness and that there was no significant difference in adverse effects between these two sclerosants [91]. The properties of sclerosant in the form of microfoam made it possible to use smaller doses, decreasing the risk of side effects and toxicity. The echogenicity of microfoam bubbles made them visible on US surveillance, ensuring that the injection of STS was intraluminal and preventing extravasation necrosis.

Adverse events described with STS are skin hyperpigmentation and allergic reactions (ranging from urticaria to anaphylaxis). Patients susceptible to allergic reactions should be treated with precaution regarding prophylaxis. Skin hyperpigmentation depends on skin type, and its incidence parallels that of other sclerosing agents. Recently, some authors have voiced concern that

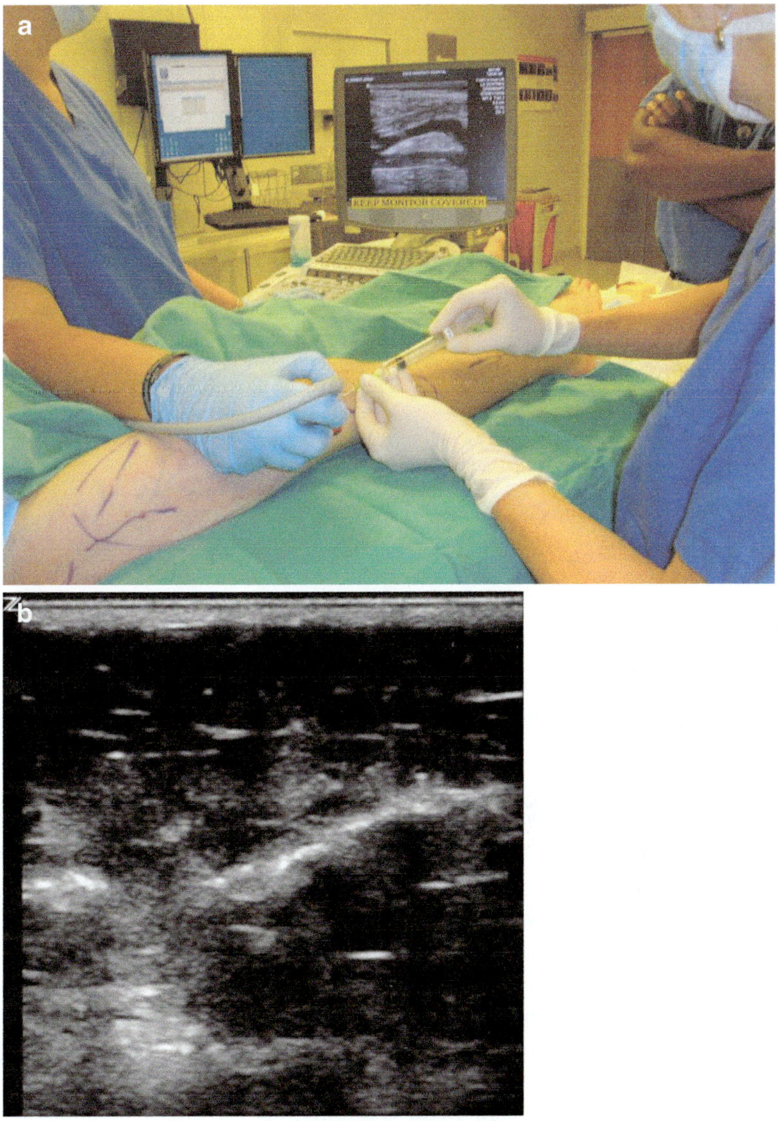

Fig. 17.8 Foam sclerotherapy. (**a**) Foam sclerotherapy is performed by percutaneous injection of the sclerosant under the ultrasound (US) guidance. (**b**) Echogenicity of the bubbles makes them visible on US surveillance ensuring that the injection of sclerosant is intraluminal and preventing extravasation necrosis

foam-induced microembolism is a common phenomenon during foam sclerotherapy and that caution should be utilized in using foam sclerotherapy, especially in patients with a patent foramen ovale [92]. To minimize the possibility of distal embolic events, all malformations with arterial flow should be excluded prior to starting the treatment using the diagnostic methodologies discussed above.

Cabrera et al. published the first study of a large group of patients treated by foam sclerotherapy [93]. The report included 50 patients (35 with venous malformations and 15 with KTS). Sclerotherapy was performed by US-guided injection of 0.25–4 % polidocanol microfoam. The treatment was beneficial in 46 (92 %) patients. Eighteen showed total disappearance of treated malformation, 15 had a reduction in malformation size of more than 50 %, and 13 showed a reduction in malformation size of 50 % or less. Out of the 39 patients who presented with pain, 25 experienced total relief, and in the

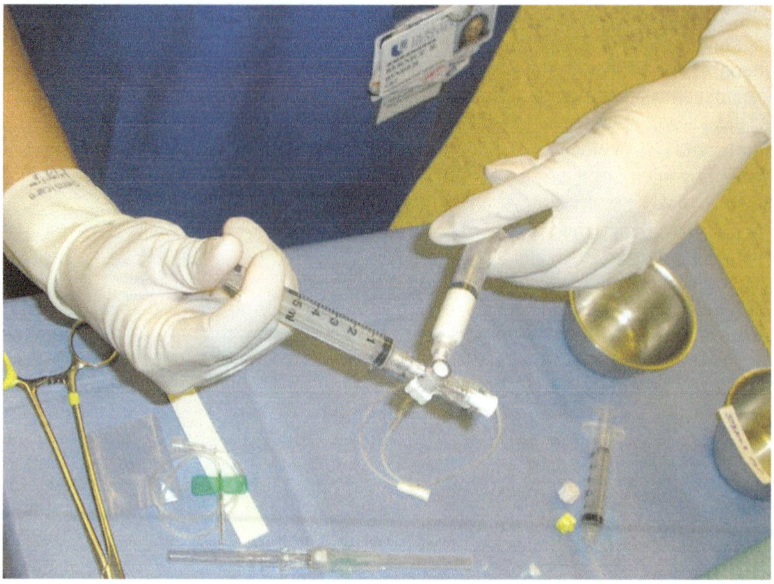

Fig. 17.9 Sodium tetradecyl sulfate (STS) foam produced by Tessari method of mixing using two syringes connected with a three-way stopcock. Optimal foam consistency is achieved with 20 passes between syringes and with the STS to air ratio of 1:2

remaining 14 patients, the pain was significantly reduced. There were no major adverse events. Skin necrosis developed in three patients, and four patients developed transient skin hyperpigmentation. Another study that confirmed the efficacy of foam sclerotherapy was that of Bergan's group [94]. Dr. Bergan reported a retrospective study on the efficiency and safety of outpatient treatment of LFVM based on 14 patients (eight with KTS) who were treated with polidocanol foam sclerotherapy. Foam was produced by the Tessari technique using 1 or 2 % polidocanol, specific for each patient. This study demonstrated that the use of polidocanol foam sclerotherapy was effective and was associated with no major complications, no recovery time, and no anesthetic requirements. The most recent data from a prospective study evaluating 135 patients with CVM (77.2 % were LFVM) treated at our institution demonstrate that symptoms in 93.5 % of patients significantly improved or resolved following US-guided foam sclerotherapy with STS or polidocanol. There were no complications. In a subgroup of LFVM patients treated with ES, symptoms significantly improved in 42.9 % of cases, and complication rate was 57.1 % (DVT, ulceration at the site of injection, bradycardia, and oxygen desaturation during the procedure). Consistent with these findings, we previously reported similar STS efficacy rates. 91.7 % of patients treated at our institution with STS had significant symptom improvement, and STS foam sclerotherapy was associated with no complications [95].

Conclusion

Vascular malformations are complex lesions that still pose a serious diagnostic and therapeutic challenge. During the last two decades, numerous efforts have been made to improve the management of patients with LFVM. Proper classification, MRI, US-guided sclerotherapy, and introduction of the multidisciplinary team concept all represent advancements in the management of this traditionally underserved population. However, further research is warranted to provide insights into the genetics and pathogenesis of vascular malformations. In addition, level 1 data from prospective, double-blind, controlled, randomized clinical trials are needed to compare therapeutic efficacy and safety of different sclerosing agents and surgical approach in the treatment of this challenging patient population.

References

1. Mulliken JB, Glowacki J. Hemangiomas and vascular malformations in infants and children. A classification based on endothelial characteristics. Plast Reconstr Surg. 1982;69:412–22.
2. Eifert S, Villavicencio JL, Kao TC, Taute BM, Rich NM. Prevalence of deep venous anomalies in congenital vascular malformations of venous predominance. J Vasc Surg. 2000;31:462–71.
3. Young AE. Pathogenesis of vascular malformations. In: Mulliken JB, Young AE, editors. Vascular birthmarks: hemangiomas and malformations. Philadelphia: W.B. Saunders Co; 1988. p. 107–13.
4. Villavicencio JL, Scultetus A, Lee BB. Congenital vascular malformations: when and how to treat them. Semin Vasc Surg. 2002;15(1):65–71.
5. Tasnadi G. Epidemiology and etiology of congenital vascular malformations. Semin Vasc Surg. 1993;6:200–3.
6. Boon LM, Mulliken JB, Enjolras O, Vikkula M. Glomuvenous malformation (glomangioma) and venous malformation: distinct clinicopathologic and genetic entities. Arch Dermatol. 2004;140(8):971–6.
7. Blei F, Walter J, Orlow SJ, Marchuk DA. Familial segregation of hemangiomas and vascular malformations as an autosomal dominant trait. Arch Dermatol. 1998;134:718–22.
8. Gallione CJ, et al. A gene for familial venous malformations maps to chromosome 9p in a second large kindred. J Med Genet. 1995;32(3):197–9.
9. Boon LM, Mulliken JB, Vikkula M, et al. Assignment of a locus for dominantly inherited venous malformations to chromosome 9p. Hum Mol Genet. 1994;3:1583–7.
10. Calvert JT, et al. Allelic and locus heterogeneity in inherited venous malformations. Hum Mol Genet. 1999;8(7):1279–89.
11. Irrthum A, Brouillard P, Boon LM, Warman ML, Olsen BR, Mulliken JB, Enjolras O, Vikkula M. Linkage disequilibrium narrows locus for venous malformations with glomus cells (VMGLOM) to a single 1.48-Mbp YAC. Eur J Hum Genet. 2001;9:34–8.
12. Cohen Jr MM. Vasculogenesis, angiogenesis, hemangiomas, and vascular malformations. Am J Med Genet. 2002;108(4):265–74.
13. Brouillard P, Olsen BR, Vikkula M. High-resolution physical and transcript map of the locus for venous malformations with glomus cells (VMGLOM) on chromosome 1p21-p22. Genomics. 2000;67(1):96–101.
14. Diehl S, et al. Altered expression patterns of EphrinB2 and EphB2 in human umbilical vessels and congenital venous malformations. Pediatr Res. 2005;57(4):537–44.
15. Degni M, Gerson L, Ishikava K, et al. Classification of the vascular diseases of the limbs. J Cardiovasc Surg. 1973;14:109–16.
16. Belov S. Anatomopathological classification of congenital vascular defects. Semin Vasc Surg. 1993; 6:219–24.
17. Puig S, Aref H, Chigot V, Bonin B, Brunelle F. Classification of venous malformations in children and implications for sclerotherapy. Pediatr Radiol. 2003;33:99–103.
18. Marler JJ, Mulliken JB. Vascular anomalies: classification, diagnosis, and natural history. Facial Plast Surg Clin North Am. 2001;9(4):495–504.
19. Bartels C, Horsch S. Classification of congenital arterial and venous vascular malformations. Angiology. 1995;46(3):191–200.
20. Virchow R, editor. Die krankhaftenGeschwu¨ lste. Berlin: A. Hirschwald; 1863. p. 456–61.
21. Enjolras O, Mulliken JB. Vascular tumors and vascular malformations, new issues. Adv Dermatol. 1997; 13:375–423.
22. Chiller KG, Frieden IJ, Arbiser JL. Molecular pathogenesis of vascular anomalies: classification into three categories based upon clinical and biochemical characteristics. Lymphat Res Biol. 2003;1(4):267–81.
23. Belov S. Classification of congenital vascular defects. Int Angiol. 1990;9(3):141–6.
24. Lee BB. Critical issues in management of congenital vascular malformation. Ann Vasc Surg. 2004;18(3):380–92.
25. Vikkula M, Boon LM, Mulliken JB, Olsen BR. Molecular basis of vascular anomalies. Trends Cardiovasc Med. 1998;8:281.
26. Lawley LP, Cerimele F, Weiss SW, North P, Cohen C, Kozakewich HPW, Mulliken JB, Arbiser JL. Expression of wilms tumor 1 gene distinguishes vascular malformations from proliferative endothelial lesions. Arch Dermatol. 2005;141:1297–300.
27. Morris PN, et al. Functional analysis of a mutant form of the receptor tyrosine kinase Tie2 causing venous malformations. J Mol Med. 2005;83(1):58–63.
28. Wouters V, Limaye N, Uebelhoer M, et al. Hereditary cutaneomucosal venous malformations are caused by TIE2 mutations with widely variable hyper-phosphorylating effects. Eur J Hum Genet. 2010;18:414–20.
29. Puig S, Casati B, Staudenherz A, Paya K. Vascular low-flow malformations in children: current concepts for classification, diagnosis and therapy. Eur J Radiol. 2005;53:35–45.
30. Mulliken JB, Fishman SJ, Burrows PE. Vascular anomalies. Curr Probl Surg. 2000;37:517.
31. Frieden IJ, Garzon M, Enjolras O. Vascular tumors and vascular malformations: does overlap occur? In: Program and abstracts of the 12th International Workshop on Vascular Anomalies, Berlin; June 27–28, 1998.
32. Enjolras O, Wassef M, Chapot R. A color atlas of vascular tumors and vascular malformations. New York: Cambridge University Press; 2007.
33. Boon LM, Enjolras O, Mulliken JB. Congenital hemangioma: evidence of accelerated involution. J Pediatr. 1996;128:329–35.
34. Cordoro KM, Speetzen LS, Koerper MA, et al. Physiologic changes in vascular birthmarks during

early infancy: mechanisms and clinical implications. J Am Acad Dermatol. 2009;60(4):669–75.
35. Boyvat A, et al. Lumbosacral vascular malformation: a hallmark for occult spinal dysraphism. Dermatology. 2000;201(4):374–6.
36. Guggisberg D, Hadj-Rabia S, Vinet C, et al. Skin markers of occult spinal dysraphism in children: a review of 54 cases. Arch Dermatol. 2004;140(9):1109–15.
37. Legiehn GM, Heran MK. Venous malformations: classification, development, diagnosis, and interventional radiologic management. Radiol Clin North Am. 2008;46:545–97.
38. Hein KD, et al. Venous malformations of skeletal muscle. Plast Reconstr Surg. 2002;110(7):1625–35.
39. Gloviczki P, et al. Klippel-Trenaunay syndrome: the risks and benefits of vascular interventions. Surgery. 1991;110(3):469–79.
40. Lee A, et al. Evaluation and management of pain in patients with Klippel-Trenaunay syndrome: a review. Pediatrics. 2005;115(3):744–9.
41. Nahm WK, et al. Venous malformations in blue rubber bleb nevus syndrome: variable onset of presentation. J Am Acad Dermatol. 2004;50(5 Suppl):S101–6.
42. Andersen JM. Blue rubber bleb nevus syndrome. Curr Treat Options Gastroenterol. 2001;4(5):433–40.
43. Rossler L, Lamesch A. The blue rubber bleb nevus or the cellular blue nevus or Bean syndrome. A rare case of iron-deficiency anemia. Phlebologie. 1992;45(4):471–5.
44. Lee BB, et al. Congenital vascular malformations: general diagnostic principles. Phlebology. 2007;22(6):253–7.
45. Dubois J, Garel L, Grignon A, et al. Imaging of hemangiomas and vascular malformations in children. Acad Radiol. 1998;5(5):390–400.
46. Paltiel HJ, Burrows PE, Kozakewich HP, Zurakowski D, Mulliken JB. Soft-tissue vascular anomalies: utility of US for diagnosis. Radiology. 2000;214(3):747–54.
47. Dubois J, et al. Soft-tissue venous malformations in adult patients: imaging and therapeutic issues. Radiographics. 2001;21(6):1519–31.
48. Trop I, et al. Soft-tissue venous malformations in pediatric and young adult patients: diagnosis with Doppler US. Radiology. 1999;212(3):841–5.
49. Burrows PE, Laor T, Paltiel H, Robertson RL. Diagnostic imaging in the evaluation of vascular birthmarks. Dermatol Clin. 1998;16(3):455–88.
50. Wilms G, et al. MRI of non-ischemic vascular disease: aneurysms and vascular malformations. Eur Radiol. 1999;9(6):1055–60.
51. Herborn CU, et al. Comprehensive time-resolved MRI of peripheral vascular malformations. AJR Am J Roentgenol. 2003;181(3):729–35.
52. Dubois J, Garel L. Imaging and therapeutic approach of hemangiomas and vascular malformations in the pediatric age group. Pediatr Radiol. 1999;29(12):879–93.
53. Browse NL, Burnand KG, Lea TM. The Klippel-Trenaunay syndrome. In: Browse NL, Burnand KG, Thomas ML, editors. Diseases of the veins: pathology, diagnosis and treatment. London: Edward Arnold; 1988. p. 609–25.
54. Enjolras O, Ciabrini D, Mazoyer E, Laurian C, Herbreteau D. Extensive pure venous malformations in the upper or lower limb: a review of 27 cases. J Am Acad Dermatol. 1997;36(2, pt 1):219–25.
55. Mazoyer E, Enjolras O, Laurian C, Houdart E, Drouet L. Coagulation abnormalities associated with extensive venous malformations of the limbs: differentiation from Kasabach-Merritt syndrome. Clin Lab Haematol. 2002;24(4):243–51.
56. Mazoyer E, et al. Coagulation disorders in patients with venous malformation of the limbs and trunk: a case series of 118 patients. Arch Dermatol. 2008;144(7):861–7.
57. Enjolras O, Mulliken JB, Wassef M, et al. Residual lesions after Kasabach-Merritt phenomenon in 41 patients. J Am Acad Dermatol. 2000;42(2, pt 1): 225–35.
58. Dompmartin A, et al. Association of localized intravascular coagulopathy with venous malformations. Arch Dermatol. 2008;144(7):873–7.
59. Hermans C, et al. Venous malformations and coagulopathy. Ann Chir Plast Esthet. 2006;51(4–5):388–93.
60. Mazereeuw-Hautier J, et al. Extensive venous/lymphatic malformations causing life-threatening haematological complications. Br J Dermatol. 2007;157(3):558–63.
61. Lee BB, Bergan JJ. Advanced management of congenital vascular malformations: a multidisciplinary approach. Cardiovasc Surg. 2002;10(6):523–33.
62. Donnelly LF, Adams DM, Bisset 3rd GS. Vascular malformations and hemangiomas: a practical approach in a multidisciplinary clinic. AJR Am J Roentgenol. 2000;174(3):597–608.
63. Nagy M, Brodsky L. Multidisciplinary approach to management of hemangiomas and vascular malformations. Facial Plast Surg Clin North Am. 2001;9(4):551–9.
64. Redondo P. The hidden face of venous malformations: a multidisciplinary therapeutic approach. Arch Dermatol. 2008;144(7):922–6.
65. Lee BB. What is new in venous disease: new approach to old problem of venous disease: congenital vascular malformation. In: Angelides NS, editor. Advances in phlebology. Limassol: Hadjigeogiou Printing & Co; 1998. p. 59–64.
66. Erin FDM, et al. Clinical characteristics and management of vascular anomalies: findings of a multidisciplinary vascular anomalies clinic. Arch Dermatol. 2004;140(8):979–83.
67. Reyes BA, Geronemus R. Treatment of port-wine stains during childhood with the flashlamp-pumped pulsed dye laser. J Am Acad Dermatol. 1990;23(6 Pt 1):1142–8.
68. Renfro L, Geronemus RG. Anatomical differences of port-wine stains in response to treatment with the pulsed dye laser. Arch Dermatol. 1993;129(2):182–8.
69. Mathur NN, Rana I, Bothra R, Dhawan R, Kathuria G, Pradhan T. Bleomycin sclerotherapy in congenital lymphatic and vascular malformations of head and neck. Int J Pediatr Otorhinolaryngol. 2005;69:75–80.

70. Svendsen P, Wikholm G, Fogdestam I, Naredi S, Edén E. Instillation of alcohol into venous malformations of the head and neck. Scand J Reconstr Hand Surg. 1994;28:279–84.
71. Yakes WF, Luethke JM, Parker SH, Stavros AT, Rak KM, Hopper KD, et al. Ethanol embolization of vascular malformations. Radiographics. 1990; 10:787–96.
72. Mason KP, Michna E, Zurakowski D, Koka BV, Burrows PE. Serum ethanol levels in children and adults after ethanol embolization or sclerotherapy for vascular anomalies. Radiology. 2000;217:127–32.
73. Lee BB, Kim DI, et al. New experiences with absolute ethanol sclerotherapy in the management of a complex form of congenital venous malformation. J Vasc Surg. 2001;33(4):764–72.
74. Yakes WF, Baker R. Cardiopulmonary collapse: sequelae of alcohol embolotherapy. Radiology. 1993; 189:145.
75. Yakes WF, et al. Symptomatic vascular malformations: ethanol embolotherapy. Radiology. 1989;170 (3 Pt 2):1059–66.
76. Burrows PE, Mason KP. Percutaneous treatment of low flow vascular malformations. J Vasc Interv Radiol. 2004;15(5):431–45.
77. Yamaki T, et al. Prospective randomized efficacy of ultrasound-guided foam sclerotherapy compared with ultrasound-guided liquid sclerotherapy in the treatment of symptomatic venous malformations. J Vasc Surg. 2008;47(3):578–84.
78. Bergan J, Cheng V. Foam sclerotherapy of venous malformations. Phlebology. 2007;22(6):299–302.
79. Yamaki T, Nozaki M, Iwasaka S. Comparative study of duplex-guided foam sclerotherapy and duplex-guided liquid sclerotherapy for the treatment of superficial venous insufficiency. Dermatol Surg. 2004; 30(5):718–22. discussion 722.
80. Orbach EJ. Sclerotherapy of varicose veins—utilization of an intravenous air block. Am J Surg. 1944; 66:362–6.
81. Eckmann DM, Kobayashi S, Li M. Microvascular embolization following polidocanol microfoam sclerosant administration. Dermatol Surg. 2005;31:636–43.
82. Frullini A. New technique in producing sclerosing foam in a disposable syringe. Dermatol Surg. 2000; 26:705–6.
83. Rao J, Goldman MP. Stability of foam in sclerotherapy: differences between sodium tetradecyl sulfate and polidocanol and the type of connector used in the double-syringe system technique. Dermatol Surg. 2005;31(1):19–22.
84. Tessari L, Cavezzi A, Frullini A. Preliminary experience with a new sclerosing foam in the treatment of varicose veins. Dermatol Surg. 2001;27:58–60.
85. Reiner L. The activity of anionic surface active compounds in producing vascular obliteration. Proc Soc Exp Biol Med. 1946;62:49.
86. Lucchi M, Bilancini S, Tucci S. Sclerosis with foam of the great saphenous vein—short term results. Phlebologie. 2003;4:389–94.
87. Rao J, Wildemore JK, Goldman MP. Double-blind prospective comparative trial between foamed and liquid polidocanol and sodium tetradecyl sulfate in the treatment of varicose and telangiectatic leg veins. Dermatol Surg. 2005;31(6):631–5. discussion 635.
88. Stirling M, Shortell CK. Endovascular treatment of varicose veins. Semin Vasc Surg. 2006;19(2):109–15.
89. Bergan J, Cheng V. Foam sclerotherapy for the treatment of varicose veins. Vascular. 2007;15(5):269–72.
90. Barrett J, Allen B, Ockelford A, Goldman MP. Microfoam ultrasound- guided sclerotherapy for varicose veins in a subgroup with diameter at the junction of > 10 mm compared with a subgroup < 10 mm. Dermatol Surg. 2004;30:1386–90.
91. Goldman MP. Treatment of varicose and telangiectatic leg veins. Double-blind prospective comparative trial between aethoxyskerol and sotradecol. Dermatol Surg. 2002;28:52–5.
92. Ceulen RP, Sommer A, Vernooy K. Microembolism during foam sclerotherapy of varicose veins. N Engl J Med. 2008;358(14):1525–6.
93. Cabrera J, Cabrera J, Garcia-Olmedo MA, Redondo P. Treatment of venous malformations with sclerosant in microfoam form. Arch Dermatol. 2003;139:1494–6.
94. Pascarella L, Bergan JJ, Yamada C, Mekenas L. Venous angiomata: treatment with sclerosant foam. Ann Vasc Surg. 2005;19:457–64.
95. Markovic JN, Shortell CK. Initial experience in the treatment of low flow vascular malformations with sodium tetradecyl sulfate foam sclerotherapy. Presented at the 62nd Vascular Annual Meeting of the Society for Vascular Surgery. San Diego; June 2008.

Part V

Thrombosis

Ultrasound for Thrombosis 18

Jennifer Heller

Contents

J. Heller, MD
Department of Surgery, Johns Hopkins Vein Centers, Johns Hopkins University, Baltimore, MA, USA
e-mail: jheller6@jhmi.edu

Abstract
This chapter discusses the technique, advantages, and limitations of duplex examination for evaluation of the venous system in the lower extremities. It will also discuss additional clinical considerations including the use of ultrasound in recurrent thrombosis, surveillance, and its role in endovenous therapy.

18.1 Introduction

Since its description by Rudolf Virchow in the mid-nineteenth century, deep venous thrombosis (DVT) has continued to challenge clinicians. Although risk factors for development of a thromboembolic event have been well described, the actual diagnosis by physical examination has yet to be so firmly established. Clinical findings of a DVT are variable at best, and there are no pathognomonic features upon which we can base a diagnosis. Further, the natural history of DVT can be fraught with recurrent morbidity, namely, recurrent deep venous thrombosis and post-thrombotic syndrome. To add more complexity to the problem, with each subsequent episode of a DVT, the risk of a pulmonary embolism is increased.

Because of these issues, the diagnosis of a DVT is dependent upon imaging techniques. Ascending phlebography was initially utilized as the primary imaging modality. Contrast venography provides superior images, and anatomic detail

E. Mowatt-Larssen et al. (eds.), *Phlebology, Vein Surgery and Ultrasonography*,
DOI 10.1007/978-3-319-01812-6_18,

of the venous anatomy is unparalleled. However, the technique is invasive, expensive, and requires intravenous contrast. Post-procedural complications include pain, thrombophlebitis, extravasation of contrast, and venous thrombosis.

In the 1980s, the ultrasound supplanted venography as the primary diagnostic tool upon which to base a diagnosis of venous thrombus. The ultrasound eradicated the risk of vessel injury and contrast-associated complications. There was no radiation exposure. Further, the examination could be performed without patient preparation or sedation. The medical community has embraced the duplex examination as the new gold standard imaging modality. Certainly, this method has improved our ability to diagnose what can be an elusive and potentially fatal disorder.

In this chapter, we will discuss the technique, advantages, and limitations of duplex examination for evaluation of the venous system in the lower extremities. Further, we will discuss additional clinical considerations including the use of ultrasound in recurrent thrombosis, surveillance and its role in endovenous therapy.

18.2 Technique

18.2.1 Lower Extremity

The quality and accuracy of a venous duplex examination is dependent upon a thorough knowledge of the venous anatomy of the lower extremity. Although this is described in detail in a separate chapter, a brief review is provided. There are three venous systems in the lower extremity: deep, superficial, and perforating. The deep system parallels the main bony structures of the lower extremity: femur and tibia. The saphenous system resides within a fascial compartment; tracking the fascial lines facilitates visualization of the great saphenous vein during venous mapping. The perforator system connects the superficial to deep veins by penetrating the investing fascial layer.

In brief, the two main superficial axial veins of the lower extremity are the great saphenous and the small saphenous. The great saphenous vein (GSV) originates near the medial malleolus, courses in a medial fashion, and terminates at the saphenofemoral junction. The small saphenous vein travels from near the lateral malleolus, courses cephalad along the posterior mid-calf, and terminates variably at the saphenopopliteal junction or further cephalad along the posterior thigh.

The deep veins of the foot empty into a network of metatarsal veins that comprises the deep plantar arch. These coalesce into plantar veins that drain into the posterior tibial veins, posterior to the tibia and adjacent to the medial malleolus. The posterior tibial veins run under the deep posterior compartment fascia and with the posterior tibial artery. The dorsalis pedis veins on the dorsum of the foot form the paired anterior tibial veins at the ankle. The anterior tibial veins run in parallel with the anterior tibial artery and cross along the anterior calf compartment. The third pair of calf veins is the peroneal veins, which run medial to the posterior aspect of the fibula. These three pairs of calf veins course cephalad and join to form the popliteal vein. Smaller, more variable veins also can drain into these calf veins. They include the soleal sinuses and the gastrocnemius veins. The gastrocnemius veins tend to empty into the popliteal vein distal to the point of entry of the small saphenous vein.

The popliteal vein enters the adductor magnus, or Hunter's canal, at which point it becomes the femoral vein (previously called the superficial femoral vein). The femoral vein ascends and receives venous drainage from the profunda femoris, or deep femoral vein, and after this confluence, it is termed the common femoral vein. As the common femoral vein crosses the inguinal ligament, it becomes the external iliac vein. The external and internal iliac veins, with multiple pelvic venous tributaries, coalesce to form the common iliac veins, which combine to form the inferior vena cava.

18.2.1.1 Technique

The venous ultrasonographic exam consists of sequential compression, color-flow duplex, and spectral Doppler sonography. Transducer compression provides information on luminal

Table 18.1 Normal Doppler findings

Complete compression of the vein
Vein walls completely apposed with less compression than required to compress adjacent artery
Spontaneous phasic flow signals in all veins

irregularity and can precisely locate a region of thrombus. The color-flow portion of the examination presents a global image of venous flow. Anatomic anomalies are easily demonstrated. The color-flow improves interpretation of recanalization and collateralization. The spectral Doppler portion of the exam is essential because these signals will allow the examiner to evaluate augmentation and phasicity of flow, corresponding with normal flow, partial occlusion, or total occlusion. These signals incorporate phasicity with respiration, augmentation, and pulsatility. All of these components are evaluated during the examination (Table 18.1).

The examination is performed with the patient supine. The head of the bed is elevated 30° to facilitate venous pooling of the lower extremity. The extremity is externally rotated. Duplex or color-flow scanning is performed utilizing a linear transducer in the 5–7.5 mHz range. In patients with an elevated body mass index, a lower frequency transducer such as a 2.5–3.5 mHz is used to facilitate visualization of deeper structures. The transducer is placed in the groin, inferior to the inguinal ligament, to identify the common femoral vein. This structure lies medial to the common femoral artery. Transverse plane compressions using the transducer are performed at 1–2 cm intervals along the vein and images are obtained. Compression images should reveal complete compression of the vein being interrogated. Further, the vein lumen should completely compress, and the walls should coapt. Adequate compression is being applied if the adjacent artery diameter is reduced. If proximal compression cannot be performed, the Valsalva maneuver can be utilized to observe if there is respiratory phasicity or augmentation. With Valsalva, a normal vein expands to more than 50 % of its baseline diameter. Further if there is a proximal deep venous thrombus, the Valsalva maneuver will decrease vein dilatation.

The transducer is oriented so that a longitudinal image can be obtained. This view will afford comprehensive images of flow characteristics of the vein being interrogated. Normal venous flow characteristics include spontaneous flow and phasic flow. Additionally, during compression, augmentation of the Doppler signal is demonstrated. Color imaging is used with distal compression to obtain augmentation measurement.

The examination begins with complete interrogation of the common femoral vein and saphenofemoral junction, as well as the proximal deep femoral vein. This sequential compression is performed along the common femoral vein, with continuation into the femoral vein and popliteal vein. At Hunter's canal, patient positioning may need to be changed, by either placing the patient in the lateral decubitus or prone position to aid in visualization of the infrapopliteal venous system. Incidental findings may be evident at the popliteal fossa. These include Baker's cyst, hematoma, abscess, or edema. Attention is now turned towards the calf veins. As previously described, the infrapopliteal venous system consists of three paired sets of veins, (anterior tibial, posterior tibial, and peroneal) as well as the soleal sinuses and the gastrocnemius veins.

Evaluation of the infrapopliteal veins is performed in most centers from the foot and then traveling proximally with the transducer. Alternatively, sequential venous segmental compression should be performed as one travels distal towards the foot. Spectral analysis is performed with plantar flexion or squeezing the calf to assess veins with sluggish flow. Further, these maneuvers can facilitate patency of the iliac venous system. If possible, repositioning of the patient with the lower extremity in a dependent position may facilitate imaging. Despite these additional maneuvers, it is still quite common to inadequately compress and/or visualize the entirety of the calf veins. This is due to the small caliber of the calf veins, patient edema, body habitus, and inexperience of the examiner.

The great and small saphenous veins are interrogated throughout their course, imaged, and sequentially compressed in utilizing the techniques previously described.

18.3 Acute Deep Vein Thrombus

The pathognomonic ultrasonographic findings for acute deep venous thrombosis on ultrasound are non-compressibility of the vein and the presence of a thrombus. Acute thrombus also is characterized by clot mobility that is evident for the first 7–10 days after thrombus formation. After this period, thrombus begins to adhere to the vein wall. An acutely thrombosed vein may actually be partially compressible because for the first 24 h of thrombus formation, the thrombus is still soft. Acute thrombi may have smooth edges because of continued partial flow. Acute thrombus tends to be hypoechogenic. Echogenicity refers to the brightness of the clot compared to surrounding structures. However, echogenicity can be variable and is therefore not indicative of age of thrombus (Table 18.2).

18.4 Chronic Deep Vein Thrombus

Although it can be challenging to determine the precise age of a chronic thrombus and, further, more challenging to determine if a thrombus is recurrent, there are certain ultrasonographic identifiers that distinguish a chronic thrombus from an acute process. Over time, the thrombus resorbs, and complete occlusion will evolve to become partial recanalization. With this process, vein collateralization takes place. Further, the echogenicity of a chronic thrombus tends to be hyperechoic, due to flow resorption surround the aging thrombus. Over time, the vein walls intimately involved with the thrombus become thickened and demonstrate decreased compressibility compared to their normal vein wall counterparts. Over time, the dilated vein visualized with acute thrombus tends to decrease, affording a diminutive, attenuated vein, with thickened walls and decreased compressibility. It is this sonographic picture that best describes the chronic thrombus state (Table 18.3).

Table 18.2 Abnormal ultrasonographic findings. Doppler findings in acute DVT

Inability to compress the vein/complete occlusion, partially
Visualization of thrombus
Absence of spontaneous flow
Absence of phasic flow with respiration, no flow signal with vein occluded
Hypoechogenicity
Mobile thrombus, poor attachment to the vein wall
Dilated vein

Table 18.3 Doppler findings in chronic DVT

Thrombus retraction
Increasing echogenicity
Vein wall characteristics in chronic thrombus: walls thickened, decreased compressibility
Formation of venous collaterals
Recanalization
Partial occlusion
Immobile thrombus
Continuous or minimally phasic flow signals
Additional incidental findings
Baker's cyst
Calf hematoma
Abscess
Lymph nodes
Arteriovenous malformation (AVM)

18.5 Discussion

18.5.1 Limitations of Ultrasound for Deep Venous Thrombosis

Although the basis for a normal venous duplex is complete easy compression, there are some locations in the lower extremity that may be difficult to compress and thereby limit the results. The distal femoral and popliteal veins may be too deep, and despite patient repositioning, the depth of these structures may limit visualization. The posterior tibial vein at the ankle may be obscured by the adjacent medial malleolus.

A variety of clinical conditions can limit the information obtained by venous ultrasonography of the lower extremities. An elevated body mass index may limit visualization of the deeper lying veins, despite use of a lower frequency transducer. Extensive edema of the lower extremity can also impede image accrual. Further, patients

Table 18.4 Advantages of duplex ultrasonography

Noninvasive
Extremely sensitive
Cost effective
Reproducible
Excellent modality for assessment of chronic thrombus over time

Table 18.5 Disadvantages/limitations of duplex ultrasonography

Technologist Skill
Body habitus
Venous duplication
Misidentification of veins
Soft tissue edema
Orthopedic devices, casts, external fixations etc.

may report severe pain that will therefore restrict the ability of compression. If extensive dressings or orthopedic devices are in place, inadequate imaging will ensue.

Alternative pathology may confound ultrasound images. Inguinal adenopathy, soft tissue edema, or arterial aneurysmal disease can confound interpretation of venous flow and luminal characteristics. At the popliteal fossa, edema, a Baker's cyst, or a popliteal aneurysm may cause decreased popliteal venous compression, inaccurately suggesting intraluminal venous disease. The calf veins, as discussed in the next section, are of small caliber and can be extremely difficult to visualize, thereby limiting definitive conclusions. Despite these limitations, sensitivity and specificity of ultrasound for diagnosis of the proximal veins of the lower extremities exceeds 97 % (Tables 18.4 and 18.5).

18.5.2 What About the Calf Veins?

Ultrasonographic evaluation of the calf veins has variable accuracy. Investigators have documented complete visualization of all three pairs of calf veins in only 60–90 % of studies. As previously discussed, ultrasonographic imaging of the proximal lower extremity veins is outstanding; sensitivity and specificities are consistently greater than 95 %. However, a significant reduction is demonstrated in the calf vein system: sensitivities range from 11 to 100 % and specificity from 90 to 100 %. This discrepancy is due to many factors. First, the small caliber of the calf veins, especially in a dehydrated patient, impedes visualization. Calf vein anatomy is quite variable, and inaccuracy of anatomy, particularly the gastrocnemius branches, can occur. Lower extremity edema, when present, usually is focused in the calf, which also negatively impacts imaging.

With these limitations, the importance of accurate, comprehensive imaging of the calf veins cannot be overemphasized as, currently, controversy still exists over the clinical significance of calf vein thrombus. Some centers do not consider isolated calf thrombus a true deep venous thrombus and do not treat, whereas other clinicians cite studies that demonstrate a significant proportion of calf thrombi that propagate and cause venous thromboembolic manifestations. Further research will be required to determine the best method to either improve ultrasonographic sensitivity and specificity or another superior diagnostic modality.

18.5.3 Recurrent Deep Venous Thrombosis

The diagnosis of a recurrent deep venous thrombus is the one of the most challenging ultrasonographic diagnoses to make. The reason is that chronic changes of a DVT may still be present in a vein, and it can be difficult to distinguish chronic changes from recurrent thrombus. Certainly, incompressibility in a previously compressible segment is consistent with recurrence. Color duplex can be an essential component of the exam in these cases as collateralization of flow channels will help distinguish acute recurrence from chronic processes. Prandoni and colleagues reported that thrombus thickness of greater than 2 mm in the common femoral or popliteal veins correlates with recurrent thrombosis, with sensitivity and specificity of 100 %.

Standardized protocols for ultrasound surveillance do not exist. There is a tendency to reexamine in settings that are not based on strong clinical evidence. Groups that would warrant serial examinations include patients who have completed anticoagulation and require a baseline study, patients who exhibit high risk factors for recurrent DVT, and potentially patients in whom free-floating thrombus is identified. Further investigation is required to further understand the natural history of chronic thrombus and recurrent thrombotic disease.

18.6 Special Considerations

18.6.1 Endovenous Therapy

Endovenous ablation has revolutionized treatment of superficial venous insufficiency. The technique has brought with it many significant advantages over high ligation and stripping of the axial veins: faster return to activity of daily living, decreased rate of neovascularization, decreased saphenous nerve injury, improved quality of life, and rapid recovery, to name a few. However, endovenous therapy harbors its own significant risk: deep venous thrombosis. Interestingly, venous thrombosis is evaluated at several points in time during the treatment course of endovenous ablation.

First, preoperative duplex imaging is an essential element of the patient pre-procedural evaluation. Acute occlusive deep venous thrombosis is an absolute contraindication to the procedure. Further, chronic thrombosis of deep veins is a relative contraindication to axial ablation. If adequate recanalization is demonstrated, and the patient has advanced symptomatic superficial disease, endovenous ablation may be indicated. However, it is important to ensure that adequate deep venous drainage will be sufficient after superficial ablation is performed. Obviously, this is an issue that must be comprehensively addressed prior to ablation and not realized afterwards.

The superficial veins must be interrogated, not only for reflux, but also for acute and chronic thrombus. This author ablates areas proximal and distal to foci of chronic superficial thrombus in a saphenous vein but ensures that the catheter does not abut the thrombosed region.

Endovenous technique requires ultrasonography at various steps during the procedure. First, the axial vein to be treated must be mapped and access point confirmed. Occasionally, patients will harbor a new area of superficial thrombus that was not evident on prior exam, and this alters management. This author either delays treatment or accesses above or below the thrombus site, as long as the thrombus is immobile and the practitioner is assured that he/she can obtain excellent images during these access and compression steps.

Once the catheter is positioned with the patient in Trendelenburg, the ultrasound is utilized to measure distance of the catheter tip from the deep system (femoral vein). Controversy exists as to whether increasing catheter tip distance decreases the incidence of post-procedural thrombotic events. This author places the tip at 2.5 cm distal to the deep system until definitive studies can be performed.

The final step of procedural ultrasound is at the conclusion of ablation. The ultrasound is used to evaluate the deep system patency and to assess flow, including retrograde flow of the epigastric vein. Further, the ultrasound is utilized to assess closure of the ablated segment. Usually, thrombus is not visualized at this time, but decreased compressibility of the treated vein can be evident.

The final component of ultrasonography in the percutaneous endovenous patient is the post-procedural duplex. This exam is generally performed within 1 week of the procedure, although definitive data on timing is not available. There is an early study that reported 16 % incidence of deep venous thrombosis after ablation; however, many subsequent investigators have reported significantly lower incidences, which range from 0 to 2.2 %.

Although absence of a classic deep venous thrombosis is typical, practitioners have identified an iatrogenic phenomenon that occurs after endovenous ablation, the endovenous heat induced thrombus (EHIT). Many investigators believe that this process is due to direct thermal damage of the endothelium. This process occurs in both laser and radiofrequency ablation techniques. There are four stages of EHIT: Class I

EHIT extends to the saphenofemoral junction or saphenopopliteal junction, but not into the deep system; Class II extends into deep system of a cross sectional area less than 50 %; Class III extends into the deep venous system cross sectional area of greater than 50 %; and Class IV is occlusive deep venous thrombus of the common femoral or popliteal vein. Although controversy exists on the precise management of the first two stages, many phlebologists anticoagulate stage III and IV EHIT. Further research is required to determine best practices for each of the classifications as well the best timing for follow-up ultrasound examination in each of the stages.

Superficial Venous Thrombophlebitis

19

Marlin W. Schul

Contents

M.W. Schul, MD, MBA, RVT, FACPh
Venous and Lymphatic Medicine,
Lafayette Regional Vein and Laser Center,
A division of Unity Healthcare, LLC, Lafayette, IN, USA
e-mail: mschul@lafayetteveincenter.com

Abstract

Superficial thrombophlebitis offers an array of presentations. Yet despite the knowledge that has emerged over the past 20 years, the curricula in medical schools and residencies fail to acknowledge STP as anything more than a self-limiting disease. The gap in venous education in the USA leads many unknowing providers to prescribe a recipe for thrombus extension, based upon established yet inaccurate dogma associated with STP. Although clinical trials are emerging, there is far more to be learned about this topic. This chapter discusses the latest in peer-reviewed literature, enabling the reader to optimize outcomes through minimizing the risk of complications related to this common venous condition of the lower extremity.

19.1 Introduction

Evidence pertaining to the diagnosis and management of superficial thrombophlebitis (STP) is controversial and poorly understood. This condition is common, yet largely minimized when compared to its big brother, deep vein thrombosis (DVT) [1]. Existing data suggests this venous

E. Mowatt-Larssen et al. (eds.), *Phlebology, Vein Surgery and Ultrasonography*,
DOI 10.1007/978-3-319-01812-6_19,

condition is more than a trivial concern, yet despite what we know, debate remains on best management strategies [2, 3]. Frequent reports of concomitant deep vein thrombosis with or without pulmonary embolus, align the pathophysiology of STP more closely with DVT [1, 2].

Anatomically, this chapter addresses superficial thrombosis above the level of the muscular fascia, including phlebitis involving saphenous trunks and tributaries (Fig. 19.1). The abbreviation of STP will be utilized throughout the chapter to distinguish this entity from the common cardiac arrhythmia. Discussion of post-ablation superficial thrombosis, both thermal and chemical, is reserved for other sections of this text.

Superficial thrombophlebitis offers an array of presentations. Yet despite the knowledge that has emerged over the past 20 years, the curricula in medical schools and residencies fail to acknowledge STP as anything more than a self-limiting disease. The gap in venous education in the USA leads many unknowing providers to prescribe a recipe for thrombus extension, based upon established yet inaccurate dogma associated with STP. Although clinical trials are emerging, there is far more to be learned about this topic. Mass adoption of present management principles is not likely to occur overnight. The case presentations shared in this chapter will arm providers with the latest in peer-reviewed literature, enabling the reader to optimize outcomes through minimizing the risk of complications related to this common venous condition of the lower extremity.

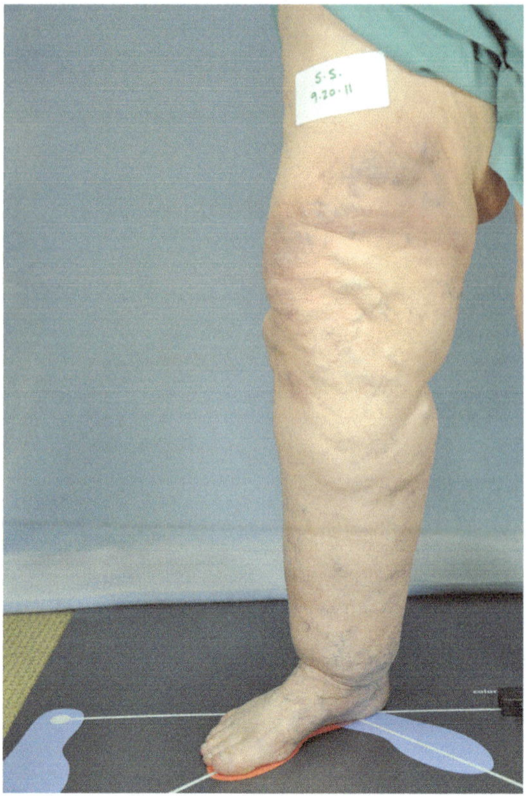

Fig. 19.1 Inflamed bulbous varices above and below the knee with an acute bout of STP

Case 1. JJ

JJ is a 35-year-old Caucasian male with chief complaint of leg pain, aching, and heaviness for 2 weeks. He reports sudden onset of symptoms with "firm knots" over the medial and anterior thigh. JJ has suffered from symptomatic varicosities over the past 5 years. At the time of presentation, no therapy had been instituted.

There is no past medical history except for the presence of varicosities. He takes no medicines and shares no drug allergies. Family history is negative for varicose veins, venous ulcers, or "blood clots." JJ is a business owner of a sports bar and limousine service and works long hours standing or sitting. He does not drink or smoke. Review of systems reveals no further concerns.

Vital signs as follows: Respiratory rate 12, heart rate 82, blood pressure 131/76, oxygen saturation 99 %, and a body mass index (BMI) of 40.4. Physical exam was unremarkable with the exception of left lower extremity cluster of veins with overlying erythema and proximal streaking (Fig. 19.2). No palpable cord is appreciated through the girth of the affected extremity.

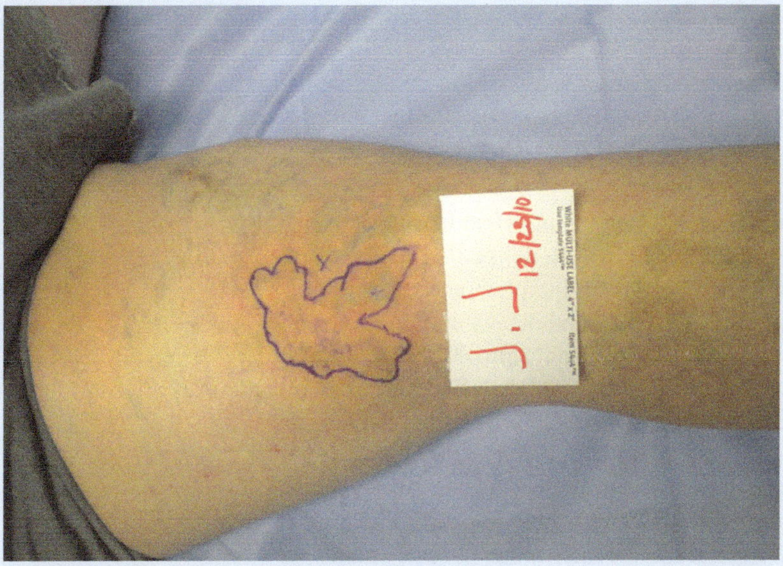

Fig. 19.2 Case #1 – JJ's physical findings. A dramatic inflammatory response is seen corresponding to painful thrombosed superficial varices

Given JJ's history and physical findings:
Does this patient have the working diagnosis of STP?
What are the clinical features of STP?
What is the differential diagnosis of STP?
Does this patient have risk factors for DVT?
What tests are indicated at the initial evaluation of clinically suspected STP?

19.2 Clinical Features

Superficial thrombophlebitis offers a spectrum of presentations, yet the most common is that of sudden onset of leg discomfort with firm, inflamed varicosities. A palpable cord may be present with saphenous or deep venous involvement [1]. Fluctuance is frequently noted over the varicosities involved, and edema may be present. Inflammation over the region may at times be extreme despite the lack of a true infectious etiology [2]. In patients with severe and sustained inflammatory response in a superficial varix, hemorrhage may occur and thrombus may be expelled as the skin weakens [3]. As Sobreira et al. reported, the proximal most point of thrombus extends, on average, 15 cm beyond where clinically evident, rendering the physical exam a limited tool [4].

The inflammatory process that is commonly linear, forces us to consider other potential pathology and a broader differential diagnosis

Table 19.1 Differential diagnosis considerations for STP

Posttraumatic – hematomas adjacent to veins
Venipuncture
Intravenous drug abuse
Allergic reaction to insect bites
Filarial infestation
Lymphangitis
Cellulitis
Erythema nodosum
Erysipelas

Alternative considerations for patients presenting with red streaks and suspicion for superficial thrombophlebitis

(Table 19.1). Historical features of exotic travel, intravenous drug abuse, recent hospitalization with intravenous catheter, insect bites, etc., offer added insight to the potential underlying pathology. The lower extremities are the most commonly involved site, yet STP may occur in superficial veins throughout the body, including upper extremity, breast, and genital veins [5–8]. Although the diagnosis of STP is typically not in question, the true extent and nature of thrombus burden must be verified.

19.3 Epidemiology/ Pathophysiology

The Tecumseh Community Health Study was the first large-scale effort to define the incidence of venous thromboembolic phenomena including superficial thrombophlebitis. Combining sequential history and physical exams, Coon et al. estimated the STP incidence between 3 and 11 % of the population [5]. At the time of the Tecumseh study, it was estimated that 123,000 cases occur each year [6]. The true prevalence is likely much higher. As duplex ultrasonography has emerged, we have learned much more about patterns of STP and complications associated with this disease state.

Nothing has been more important in understanding the patterns and clinical sequelae of superficial thrombophlebitis than the development of duplex ultrasound technology. In Lutter's series of nearly 13,000 lower extremity duplex evaluations for deep vein thrombosis, 1,412 were found to have acute venous thrombosis. Of these, one of every eight was found to involve superficial venous system. The location of thrombus most commonly involved the great saphenous vein (GSV) (69 %), followed by the small saphenous vein (30 %), and isolated to varicose veins (13 %) [7]. Multi-segment involvement is commonly seen as is bilateral involvement (9 %) (Fig. 19.3).

The pathophysiology of STP is thought to be similar to deep vein thrombosis, except STP is clearly associated with varicose veins as the predominant pattern [9]. Histopathology has been suggested to differ with regard to the extent of inflammation involving the vein wall, where STP involves a tremendous amount of inflammation compared to that found with acute deep vein thrombosis [8]. As shown in Fig. 19.4, extensive inflammatory changes are noted throughout the vein wall in a patient with phlebitis isolated to the superficial vessels. Over time the region of thrombus may become more organized and incorporated into the vein wall, may become completely recanalized, or may remain scarred with venous septae in an otherwise refluxing vessel [10] (Fig. 19.5).

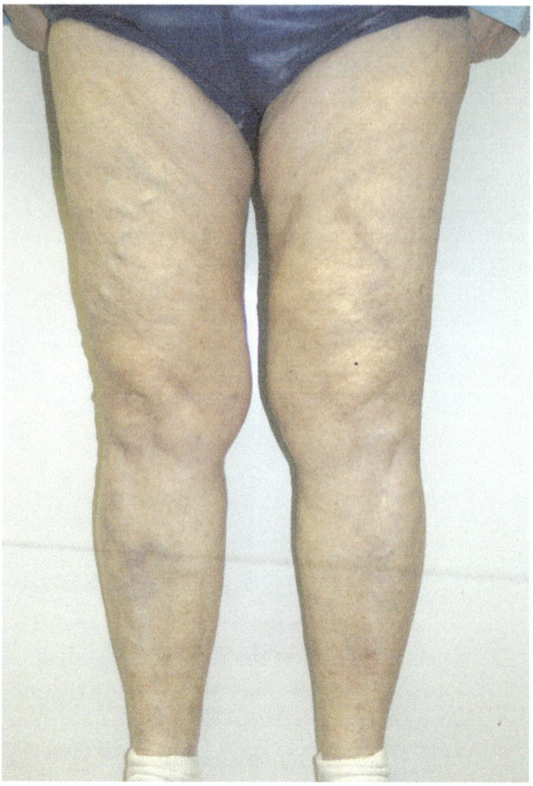

Fig. 19.3 Bilateral STP Image. This image depicts bilateral STP involving varices below the knee on the right leg and the left anterior thigh

19.4 Risk Factors for STP

When considering risks for the development of STP, one must reflect on Virchow's triad including venous stasis (immobilization or reflux), vessel injury or trauma, and thrombophilia states due to hereditary or acquired conditions. The risks for developing superficial thrombophlebitis have been gleaned from numerous studies, many of which, not surprisingly, are well aligned with those of deep vein thrombosis (Table 19.2). The most common predisposing risk includes varicose veins in the lower extremity, occurring in 61–93 %, advancing age ≥60, female/male ratio of 2:1, obesity in 20 %, multiparity, recent

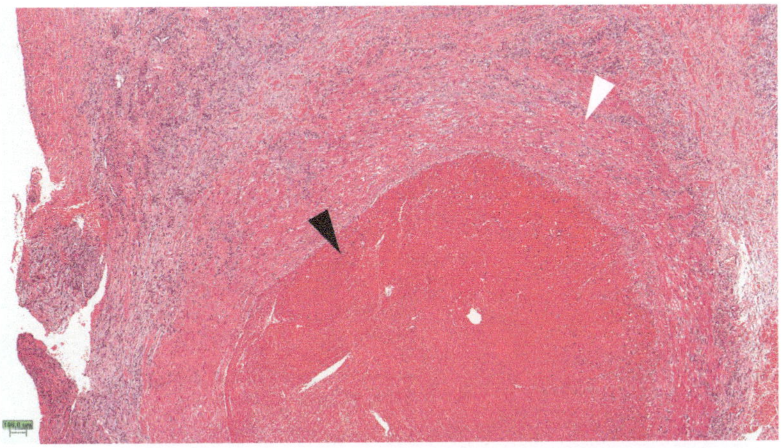

Fig. 19.4 Histopathology seen in acute STP, Case #1. *Black arrow* indicates thrombus within the vein lumen. *White arrow* indicates the transmural inflammation and neutrophil infiltration

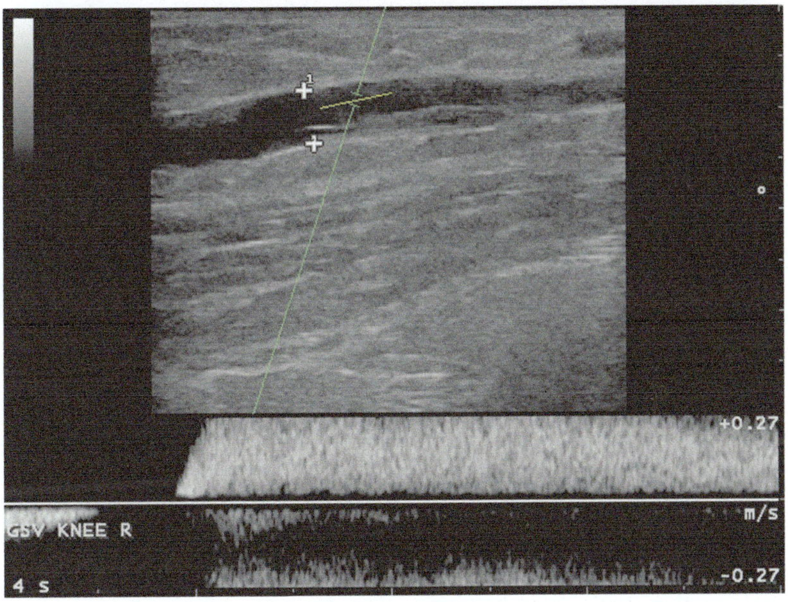

Fig. 19.5 Residual scar from STP in lumen of the great saphenous vein

Table 19.2 Common risk factors for STP and DVT

Shared risk factors for STP or DVT
Varicose veins
Previous DVT/STP
Immobilization
Malignancy
Trauma
OCP/puerperium
Hypercoagulable states

surgery/immobilization, hormonal influences, history of prior venous thromboembolism (VTE), and hypercoagulable states including malignancy [9, 11]. Seasonal variations have also been reported where a peak incidence is seen in warmer summer months [11].

19.5 Risk for VTE Complications/Recurrence

Superficial thrombophlebitis and the association with complications of DVT, with or without pulmonary embolus, have been noted for 7 years. Once thought to be a rare finding, duplex ultrasonography reports have revealed concomitant deep and superficial vein thrombosis at a rate of 8.6–24 % [9, 12–14] This confirms a reality that

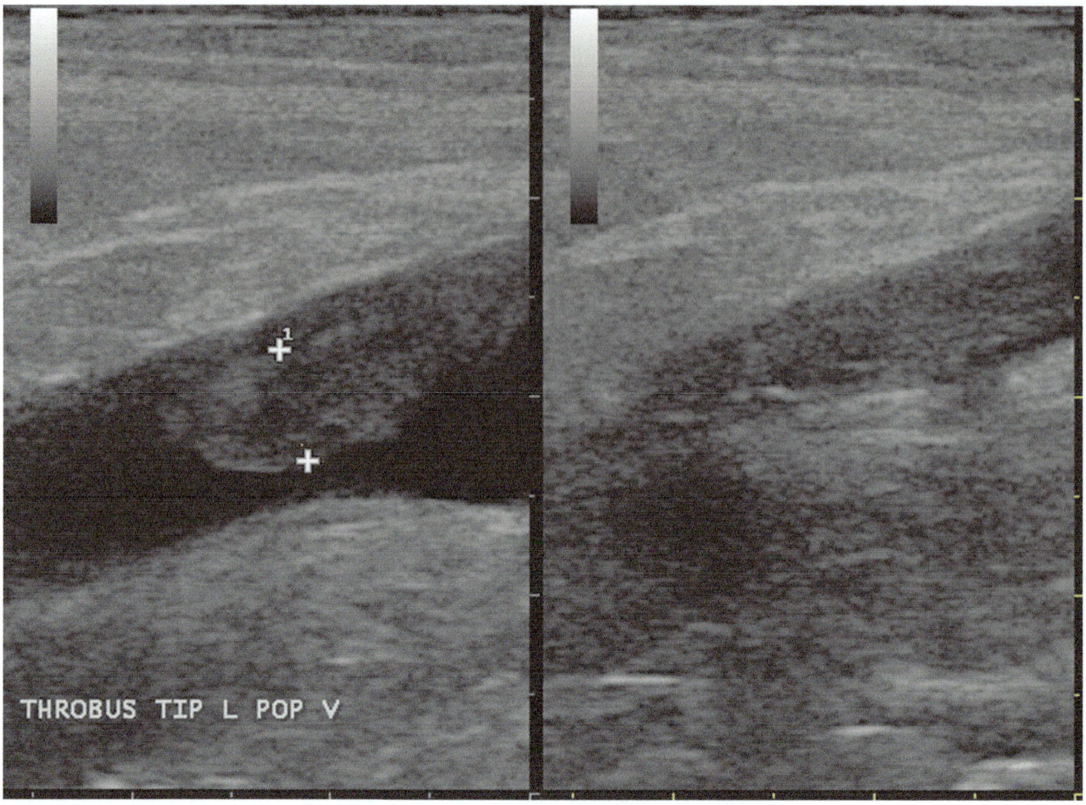

Fig. 19.6 STP at the saphenopopliteal junction with free-floating tongue

the clinical picture of superficial thrombophlebitis may, and often, harbors more serious sequelae than previously suspected.

There are two patient populations at the time of initial presentation, one of isolated STP and another with complications of concomitant DVT or pulmonary embolus. Identifying which patients possess the greatest propensity in developing VTE complications is of paramount importance.

19.6 Deep Vein Thrombosis

Anatomic location of the thrombus (e.g., near the saphenofemoral or saphenopopliteal junctions) has not been proven to yield a higher proclivity for VTE events. Lutter's study compared populations with isolated STP to those with combined disease at initial presentation and found age >60, prior history of DVT, recent immobilization, and systemic infection as statistically significant risk factors for developing concomitant DVT and STP (Fig. 19.6). Quenet identified 427 consecutive hospitalized patients with isolated STP. Over the following 3 months, 4.1 % (17/413) were confirmed to have developed deep vein thrombosis. Univariate and multivariate regression analysis revealed male sex, history of VTE, severe chronic venous insufficiency, and sudden onset of STP as statistically significant risk factors for developing VTE complications [4].

19.7 Pulmonary Embolus

The life-threatening complication of pulmonary embolus (PE) has been largely thought to occur only in the presence of deep vein thrombosis.

STP as a suspected cause of pulmonary embolus was first described by Richter in 1905 [9]. Is it possible that isolated superficial thrombophlebitis may in fact cause pulmonary embolus? Verlato et al. prospectively studied 21 consecutive patients with isolated STP involving the proximal great saphenous vein. Each subject received systemic duplex scanning excluding presence of DVT through the calf veins and underwent chest radiography and pulmonary perfusion scanning. Surprisingly, despite general lack of symptomatology for pulmonary embolus, one-third was found to have high probability scintigraphy studies [12]. Sobreira et al. studied 60 consecutive patients with clinical findings of STP. Each subject received complete duplex scanning of the lower extremities and pulmonary perfusion scanning. Although 13 (21.7 %) patients were found to have concomitant DVT at presentation, 17 (28 %) were found to have high probability scans. Five of the 17 (29 %) found to have pulmonary embolus had concomitant DVT [10].

Although large randomized trials are lacking, the simultaneous occurrence of superficial and deep vein thrombosis suggests that this is more than a benign disease process [13, 14]. Epidemiology studies declaring the relatively high incidence of concomitant DVT and/or PE among STP patients warrant further consideration toward the prevention of further thromboembolic events. If merely 1 % of these cases result in PE or VTE complications, thousands of lives are placed at risk [15].

Case 2. JD (Fig. 19.7)

JD is a 70-year-old Caucasian male presenting with "knots" in the left calf after a 16 h car ride from coastal North Carolina to Chicago. He sat in the back seat of a car with confined space for leg room. He reported to an urgent care facility who made a diagnosis of STP, and he was referred for fitted gradient compression.

Past medical history is significant for degenerative joint disease, hypertension, hypercholesterolemia, and type II diabetes mellitus. He has no prior history of thrombosis yet has had varicose veins in the calf that have not previously been problematic. Family history is negative for varicose veins, venous ulcers, or "blood clots." JD does not drink or smoke. He enjoys golf and church activities. Review of systems was noncontributory.

JD has normal vital signs, oxygen saturation of 98 %, and a BMI of 29.0. He communicates easily and appears in no distress. Physical findings reveal a firm, tender, inflammatory region in the medial proximal calf, corresponding to an intersaphenous branch. A pink hue is present over the firm varicosities. Trace edema is noted at the ankle in addition to high-pressure telangiectasia.

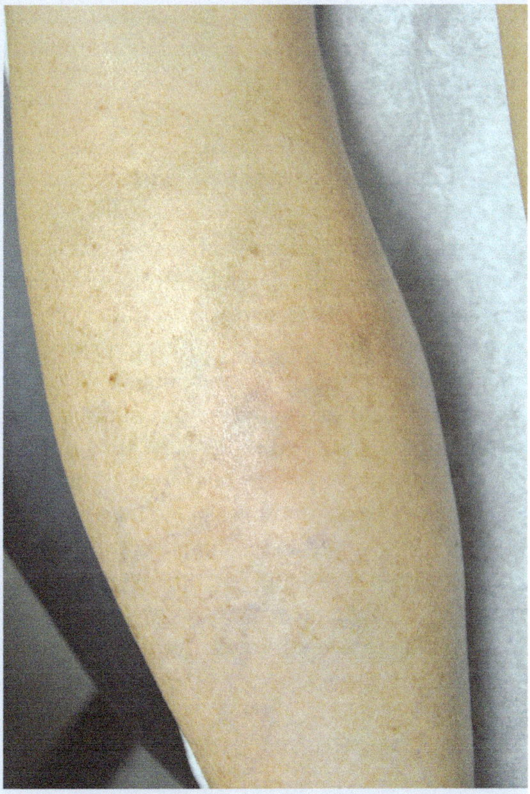

Fig. 19.7 Case #2 – JD's calf image. This patient demonstrates painful bulbous varices of the calf with a *faint pink* hue after long car ride in a confined space

The urgent care advised the use of an anti-inflammatory reported that an antibiotic may be required if there was no improvement. No laboratory tests or imaging tests performed at the time of his initial evaluation.

What risk factors does JD possess that place him at risk for developing STP?

What risk factors does JD possess that place him at risk for VTE?

Describe a practical approach to evaluate JD and guide his treatment.

Do you agree with the urgent care recommendations of anti-inflammatory agents, an antibiotic, and compression therapy? Please explain.

19.8 Diagnostic Approach

Superficial thrombophlebitis most often occurs in patients with varicose veins but may also occur in normal saphenous veins in patients with an underlying thrombophilia. Given the common findings of DVT and/or pulmonary embolus in patients with superficial thrombophlebitis, once the clinical assumption is made, affirmation requires further diagnostic testing.

19.8.1 Duplex Ultrasonography

The prevalence of concomitant venous complications in patients with superficial thrombophlebitis mandate duplex ultrasound for each patient suspected of this condition [13, 14]. Duplex evaluation is valued for proving the diagnosis of STP while accurately assessing the thrombus burden throughout the lower extremity. The results of the duplex study serve to not only declare the presence or absence of thrombus but aid in identifying presence of complications found commonly in patients with STP. Simply put, duplex ultrasonography is the most critical of studies to perform and may indicate a need for more advanced imaging.

19.8.2 Acute Phase Testing

Principles of assessing a lower extremity for thrombosis are well documented. Systematic comprehensive whole-leg assessment of venous anatomy be mapped and for thrombus burden and the extent of venous reflux [13]. Bilateral scanning is indicated when bilateral symptoms are present and when institutional protocols mandate the study. Complete testing of an asymptomatic contralateral limb is debatable beyond assessing the most proximal segments of the limb [14].

As seen in an acute setting, probe compression in the region of thrombosis reveals noncompressible vessels which are hypoechoic (Fig. 19.8). The standard commonly used in clinical studies to define thrombus in the great or small saphenous vein includes a segment at least 5 cm in length (Fig. 19.9). A free-floating thrombus tip may be seen as an extensive STP protrudes into the lumen of the common femoral or popliteal vein (Fig. 19.10a, b). Valsalva testing and spectral waveform patterns are helpful in assessing presence of proximal obstruction (Fig. 19.11). Duplex findings or signs of proximal involvement should trigger algorithms to address pelvic vein pathology and the central circulation.

19.8.3 Follow-Up Duplex Scanning

Although there may be institutional standards, there are generally no accepted principles for serial duplex scans in this patient population [16]. Despite the argument regarding cost effectiveness, periodic surveillance of thrombus burden is strongly recommended for patients at higher risk for thrombus extension (e.g., involving proximity of the saphenous junctions or proximal one-third of the great saphenous vein) [4]. If the patient is not a candidate for anticoagulation,

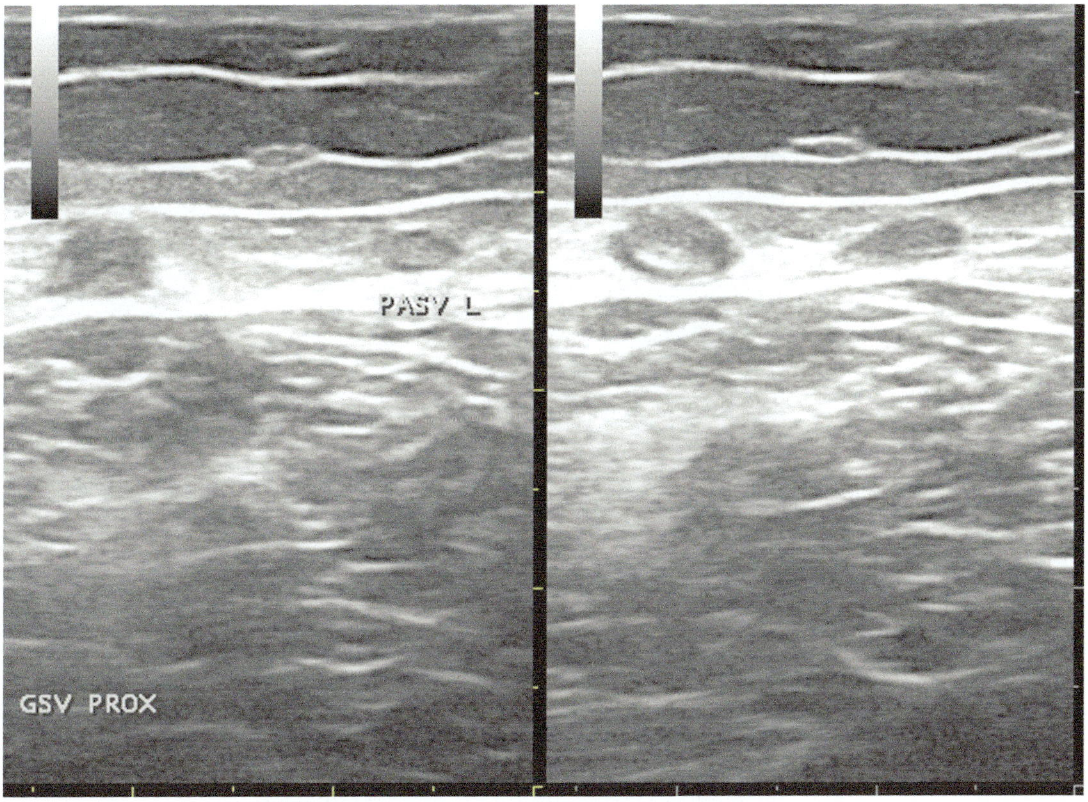

Fig. 19.8 STP of the GSV. Probe compression reveals limited compression of the great saphenous vein of the proximal thigh

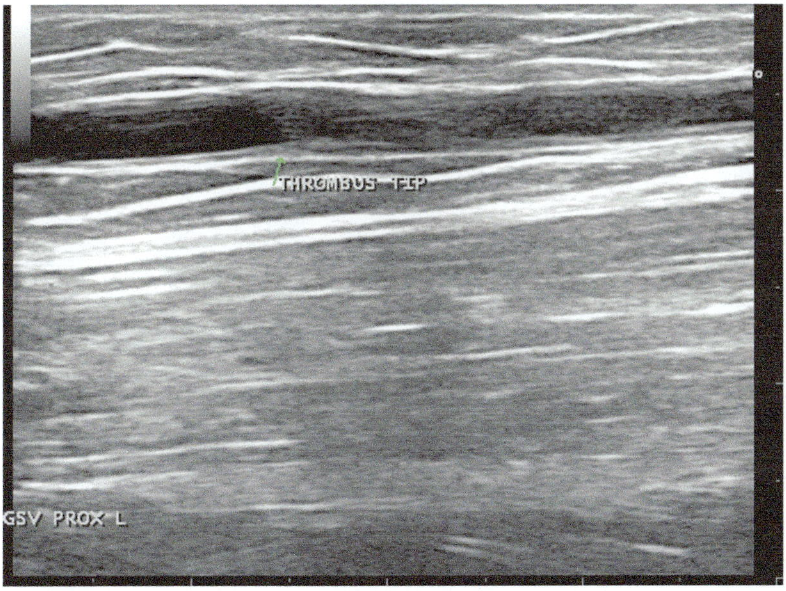

Fig. 19.9 STP and thrombus tip in mid-thigh in a nondilated saphenous vein

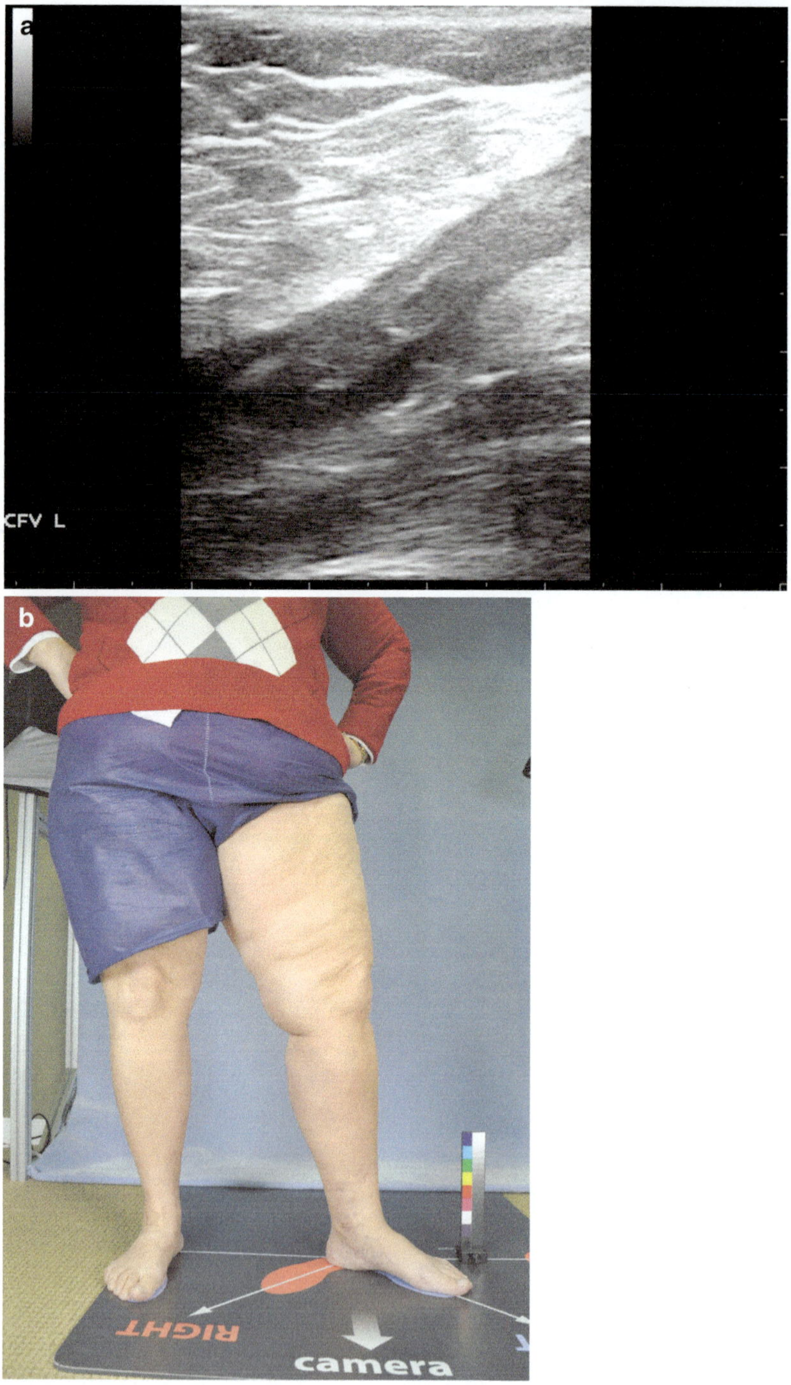

Fig. 19.10 STP at the saphenofemoral junction (duplex and standing photo of limb). (**a**) This image depicts the thrombus extending from the GSV through the SFJ and into the CFV for the patient below. (**b**) This image demonstrates limited findings with focal tenderness at the knee

sequential scanning is imperative. As the majority of thrombus extends during the first week, a general rule of thumb is to reimage patients within 2–10 days [17, 18]. Additional studies are recommended for increasing pain or swelling of the affected limb and near the anticipated end of anticoagulation. This permits not only an assessment of residual thrombus burden

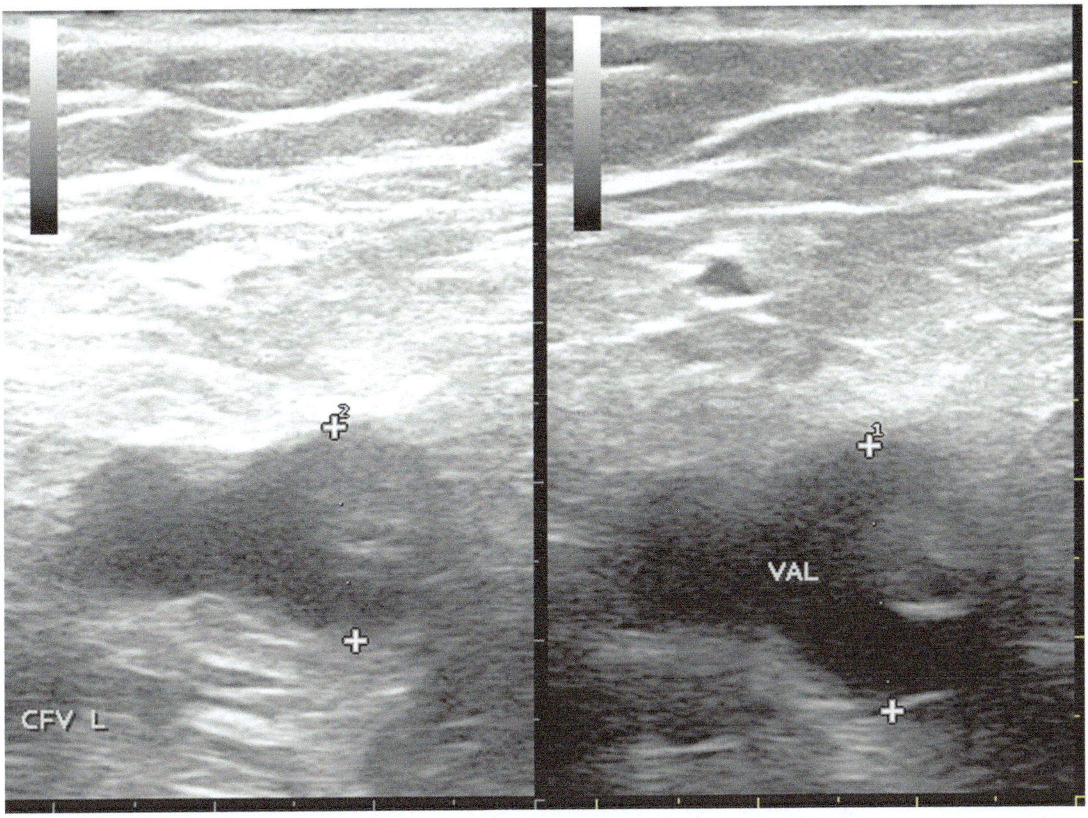

Fig. 19.11 CFV with STP extension with and without Valsalva

but insight to residual reflux and permits a provider to determine the best surgical course of action if indicated.

19.8.4 Laboratory Testing

Patients with their first bout of superficial thrombophlebitis may indeed be manifesting their first event of an as of yet unknown thrombophilia [17]. The incidence of hypercoagulable conditions has been as high as 35 % in a series reported by Hanson et al. [19]. Schonauer prospectively observed 615 patients with first VTE who had completed 3 months anticoagulation therapy. Over an average of two and one-half years, 45 (7.3 %) STP events were reported. When analyzed, elevated factor VIII levels proved to be an independent risk factor for developing STP [20]. Recently, MTHFR C677T polymorphism was found to be significantly higher in patients with superficial thrombophlebitis when compared to patients with DVT [21]. Despite the reality that an underlying thrombophilic state may exist in a substantial percentage of patients with STP, acute phase laboratory testing is best geared toward those commonly performed prior to initiating anticoagulation. In these patients, a complete blood count with differential and platelets, PT/aPTT, and D-dimer generally suffice in the acute phase. Given the features of assessing a patient for inherited thrombophilia, it is not only timing of testing that is important, but rather an assessment whether the findings may change the course of management [21]. A thorough review of thrombophilia and testing may be found in the chapter dedicated to this topic.

Case 3. JA (Fig. 19.12)

JA is a 38-year-old Caucasian male presenting with chief complaint of "firm painful knot" over the right anterior thigh for 1 week. The discomfort is constant and associated with red streaking along the inner thigh and superficial vessels of the anterior thigh and leg. There are no aggravating or relieving factors and no therapy had been instituted. Past medical history is significant for apparent uncomplicated STP 3 years prior, and a remote right ankle injury without loss of function. Family history is negative for "blood clots" or known thrombophilia, yet positive for varicose veins and severe venous insufficiency. JA is married, he is a nonsmoker. He is a successful farm equipment salesman, spending long hours on the road. Review of systems revealed a 1 week history of nonproductive cough and dyspnea.

Vital signs reveal a respiratory rate of 20, heart rate of 72, a blood pressure of 128/70, and oxygen saturation of 98 %. JA is morbidly obese in no apparent distress. Physical exam was unremarkable with the exception of an extensive superficial thrombophlebitis with firm, painful varices with overlying inflammation above and below the knee. A palpable cord was easily noted along the medial thigh from just below the knee to the proximal thigh. Pretibial edema is noted, and pulses are equal bilaterally.

Duplex study revealed a normal deep system from calf veins through the common femoral vein without signs of proximal obstruction.

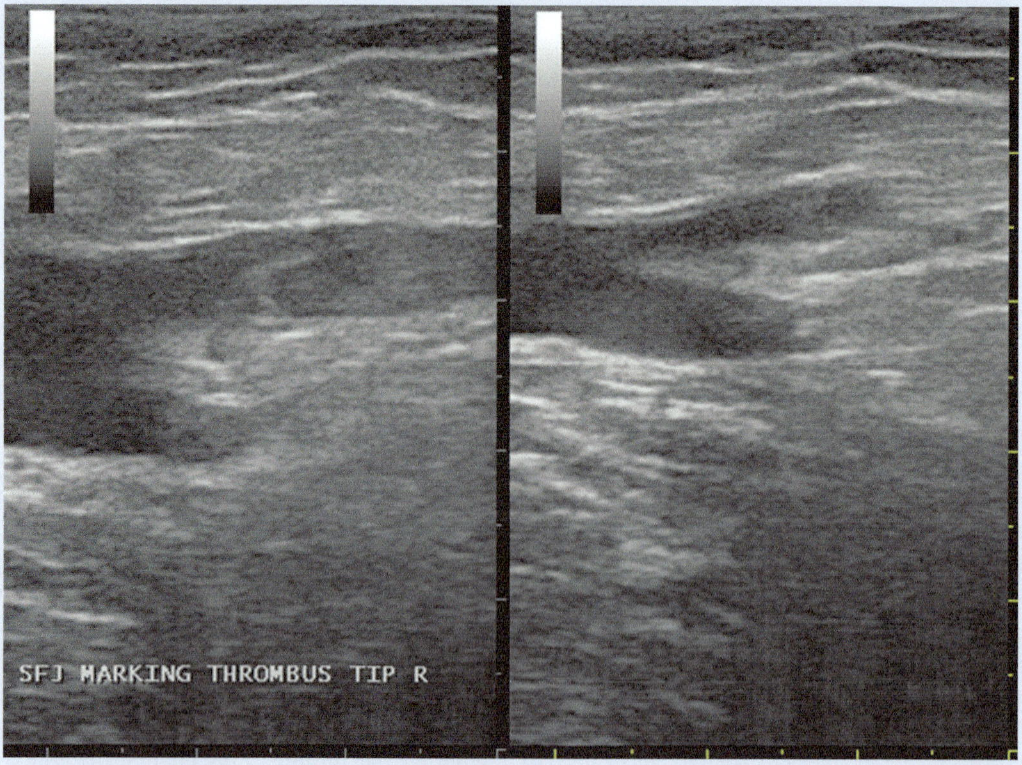

Fig. 19.12 Case #3 – JA SFJ with and without compression

Superficial thrombosis was noted in the GSV from just below the knee proximally to the superficial epigastric vein (Fig. 19.12). Tributaries in the thigh and leg were involved in the thrombotic process and contiguous with the GSV. A thrombosed intersaphenous vein coursed to the popliteal fossa, joining the small saphenous vein near the saphenopopliteal junction (SPJ). The thrombus extended to the SPJ yet the small saphenous was compressible and without reflux in the distal two-thirds.

What is the likelihood that JA has already passed pulmonary emboli to explain his dyspnea?
What risk factors suggest JA is at higher risk of developing VTE complications?
Are any further diagnostic tests indicated?
What management strategies would you consider?

19.9 Treatment Options

Controversies surrounding management of superficial thrombophlebitis are abundant. Best practice guidelines exist for patients with STP and complications of VTE, but data is lacking for all other categories. Existing treatment options are reviewed further on, sharing existing evidence as it pertains to preventing VTE complications in patients with STP.

19.9.1 Ambulation Versus Bed Rest

Many reference texts in vascular surgery and primary care continue to tout bed rest as part of the mainstay of therapy for STP and DVT. Ambulation alone is not suspected to be the sole means to prevent VTE, yet an effective calf pump will effectively reduce venous stasis. The recommendation for bed rest in patients with acute thrombosis is a simply recipe for thrombus extension and potential complications [15]. In a randomized study by Partsch, compression and walking were shown superior to bed rest and elevation in reducing edema, reducing the amount of discomfort, and in minimizing thrombus extension in patients with proximal DVT [22]. Although we may not extrapolate the value of ambulation to encompass all thrombotic events of the lower extremity, one cannot dismiss the potential benefit.

19.9.2 Compression Therapy

There should be little argument that compression offers the most scientific benefit for this condition. Established benefits include symptomatic relief as well as prophylaxis against the development of DVT [18]. In a recent multicenter epidemiologic study involving 844 patients with STP, 99.7 % were prescribed elastic compression stockings or compression bandages until they could be seen by a vascular specialist [18]. Given the series of Decousus studies, we may easily report that compression therapy using gradient compression stockings or leg wraps is recommended for patients with superficial thrombophlebitis.

19.9.3 Pharmacotherapy

19.9.3.1 Anticoagulation

Whether to employ systemic anticoagulation is dependent upon the burden of thrombus, or geographic standards of care. The management of uncomplicated deep vein thrombosis and pulmonary embolus are clear, while the management of STP continues to evolve, incorporating low-molecular-weight heparin, warfarin, and fondaparinux [23, 24]. The prevalence of comorbid pathology and risk of complications with acute superficial thrombosis have led many investigators to favor systemic anticoagulation when the thrombus is near the saphenous junctions

Table 19.3 Summary of current guidelines for duration of anticoagulation

Disease state	Compression	Anticoag	NSAIDs	Ambulation	I and D	Antibiotics	Surgery
Isolated tributaries	++	–	+	++	+++	–	–
Saphenous involvement and VVs	++	+45 days	–	++	++	–	–
Combined STP and DVT, STP without VVs	++	+3 months	–	++	–	–	–
Septic thrombophlebitis	++	+/–	–	++	+	+++	+++++

or over 5 cm of the saphenous trunk in length. Systemic reviews by Wichers et al. demonstrated anticoagulation using low-molecular-weight heparin (LMWH) was beneficial in reducing the risk of thrombosis extension in the near term but failed to provide reduction in VTE events during the longer-term follow-up [23, 24]. The American College of Chest Physician (ACCP) guidelines recommend a recipe and duration of anticoagulation corresponding to thrombus burden [23]. Table 19.3 summarizes the current recommendations and duration of therapy.

Discontinuing anticoagulation presents another dilemma. Two separate studies showed an initial benefit to anticoagulation which was not sustained when anticoagulation was discontinued at 8–12 or 30 days. With duration of 45 days, anticoagulation benefits were sustained. Presence of residual thrombus on duplex scan at 4 weeks is not an indication for ongoing anticoagulation [24]. Extrapolating from the DVT literature, D-dimer could perhaps be useful to distinguish high from low recurrence risk. Although not perfect, if the result is positive at the end of anticoagulation, recommendations would be to maintain systemic anticoagulation and repeat in 1–2 months. If the result is negative, it is recommended that anticoagulation be discontinued with plan to repeat the testing 1 month later. In the PROLONG trial in patients with venous thromboembolism, D-dimer was assessed every 2 months for a year after discontinuing anticoagulation. In patients with persistent elevations of D-dimer after stopping anticoagulation, the recurrence risk was 27 % per year [25]. Patients with isolated superficial phlebitis will present with or without varicose veins. Some may declare their respective thrombophilia risk with persistently elevated D-dimer levels. It is recommended that each patient with STP be assessed carefully for ongoing thrombosis risk and care tailored accordingly [25–41].

19.9.3.2 Anti-inflammatory Agents

Nonsteroidal anti-inflammatory agents (NSAIDS) are effective in reducing the pain and inflammation of STP. In a pilot program conducted by the Enoxaparin Study Group, 427 patients were randomized to placebo, enoxaparin, and tenoxicam. Although there were no significant differences between the active treatment arms, when compared to placebo, each active arm demonstrated a meaningful reduction in the incidence of DVT [42]. At the present time, the role of NSAIDS should be reserved for patients with iatrogenic STP, tributary vein clot with normal saphenous trunks, or who are low risk for significant clot extension.

19.9.3.3 Role of Antibiotics

The acute inflammatory response commonly seen with superficial phlebitis can raise concerns over a potential infectious process (Fig. 19.1). Contrary to general appearance, these painful superficial lesions are almost always sterile [7]. Fever, leukocytosis, and toxicity suggest an infectious process and septicemia. Patients with suppurative thrombophlebitis require open drainage and broad spectrum antibiotics. Unless the phlebitis is of the suppurative type or accompanied by clinical ascending lymphangitis, there is no indication for the use of antibiotics [3, 28].

19.9.4 Surgical Intervention

19.9.4.1 Incision and Drainage

In cases where bulbous varices are acutely inflamed, painful, and fluctuant, symptoms may be rapidly relieved with local incision and drainage. After cleansing the area, local anesthesia may be infiltrated with a small needle allowing for small incisions or punctures to be made over

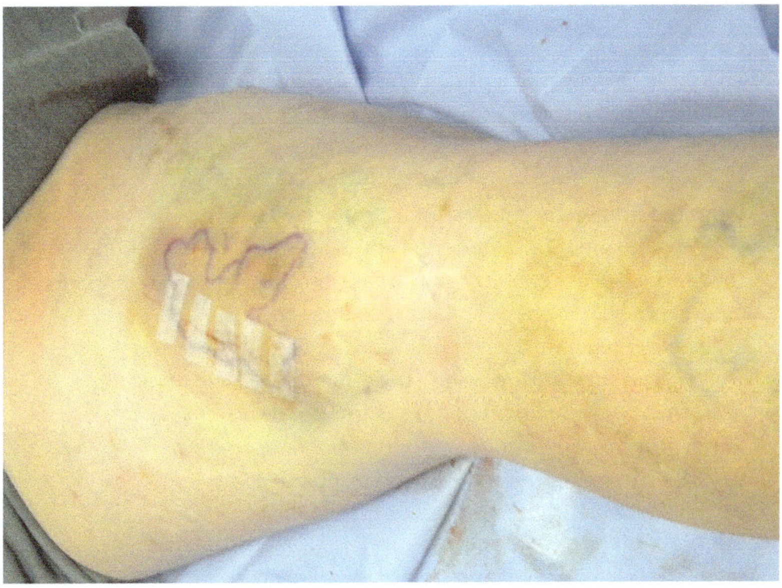

Fig. 19.13 Decreasing inflammation following local surgical removal of STP

the regions of fluctuance. Once the punctures are made, the physician may effectively expel the superficial thrombus [25]. This minor in-office procedure is very well tolerated by patients; it serves to dramatically reduce inflammation and pain, with added benefit if reducing risk of pronounced hyperpigmentation over the affected region (Fig. 19.13).

19.9.4.2 High Ligation and Stripping

Debate exists as to whether surgical intervention versus conservative medical therapy with LMWH or anti-inflammatories offers a better outcome and reduction in VTE events [23]. In reality, the best answer may come down to the combination of patient and physician preference. In the only level I trial, Belcaro et al. compared surgical to medical therapy. Results were comparable, yet the surgical group employing high ligation, stripping, and perforator ligation had the best response with no thrombus extensions at 3 months and a single event at 6 months. Although no VTE events were noted in the medical arms, four (2.7 %) patients in the surgical arm suffered extension of thrombus into the deep venous system, but there were no pulmonary emboli [26].

In a prospective study, 20 consecutive patients with thrombophlebitis within 1 cm of the SFJ were managed nonoperatively. Ascer et al. found a 40 % incidence of concurrent DVT in the sample. Medical therapy included bed rest, leg elevation, and full anticoagulation for 6 months. No pulmonary emboli, no recurrences, and no complications from anticoagulation were noted [27]. In a review by the American College of Chest Physicians, when surgical management is compared to medical management, the surgical therapy (high ligation, surgical stripping, +/− perforator ligation) is more than threefold more costly and carries a higher rate of VTE complications. As a result, present ACCP recommendations favor medical treatment with anticoagulants over surgical treatment (grade 1B) [43–46].

19.9.4.3 Warm Versus Cold Compresses

Warm moist compresses have been recommended to help manage superficial thrombophlebitis for decades, yet there is little evidence besides common practice to support its use [7]. According to present day indications for heat therapy, acute inflammation is a relative contraindication for using warm compresses. There is no mistaking the inflammatory response that is commonly seen. Cold packs or ice are indicated for acute inflammatory processes and for acute injuries, the local tissue effect reduces inflammation and pain. There is little evidence to support benefit from the use of warm compresses. Ultimately the use of warm compresses or ice packs is dependent upon provider choice.

Case 4. DH (Fig. 19.14)

DH is a 28-year-old white, male with chief complaint of left leg pain for 3 weeks. Symptoms include aching, burning, and swelling. He reports he has had repeated flares involving each lower extremity where regions become inflamed and firm to the touch. DH was recently evaluated in the emergency department, where he was prescribed cephalexin. He reports no diagnosis was shared, and no imaging study has been performed. Past medical history is unremarkable with the exception of previous bouts as described above. Family history is positive for varicose veins, but no known thrombophilia or VTE. No previous surgeries. Social history reveals casual alcohol and tobacco use. DH is actively employed in the golf maintenance industry, walking as much as 6 h per day. Review of systems was otherwise negative.

Vital signs reveal a respiratory rate of 14, heart rate of 61, a blood pressure of 139/58, oxygen saturation of 99 %, and a BMI of 31.4. Physical exam was unremarkable with the exception of a faint pink hue along the inseam of the left thigh. There were no visible varicosities or palpable cord. No edema was noted.

Duplex study reveals a noncompressible GSV from the level of the knee to the SFJ. There was no sign of DVT or evidence of deep or saphenous vein reflux. The vessel diameters are within normal limits.

List the risk factors DH possesses for developing VTE?

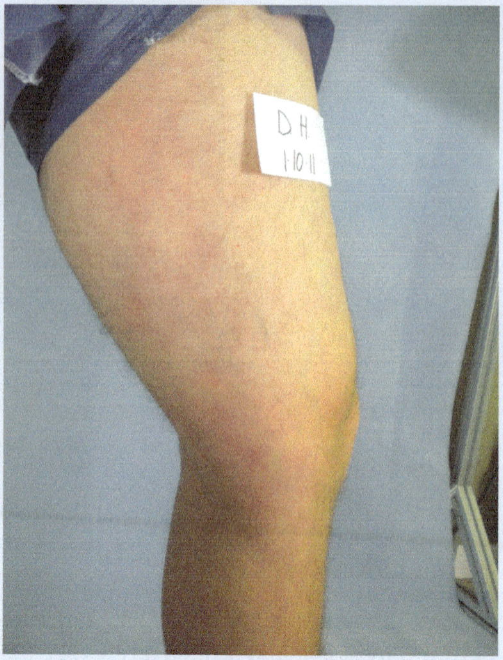

Fig. 19.14 Case #4 – Acute STP with no physical findings of venous pathology

Assuming DH had previously normal saphenous veins, how would your management strategy change?

Which of the following are strongly recommended for this presentation?

Ambulation
Therapeutic compression therapy
Systemic anticoagulation
Surgical ligation of the saphenofemoral junction
Thrombophilia testing
Intravenous antibiotic
Warm compresses

19.10 Management Strategies

Once the diagnosis is made, whether isolated STP or combined STP with or without VTE, patients should be effectively counseled. Many patients may have never been burdened by their veins, and now they are found to have a painful condition that has potential life or limb threatening complications. Increasing leg pain, swelling, sudden chest pain, or dyspnea are all indications for emergent evaluation and potential change in management. This may be a tremendous amount of information for a patient to digest. Building patient expectations and follow-up must be effectively managed. The patient's primary care physician may be unaware of complications associated with STP. In this instance, opportunities exist to bring an elevated awareness to complications of venous stasis.

Not all patients with superficial phlebitis are alike. Differing presentations were shared in the cases above, but there are many other examples. This section summarizes recommendations in three distinct groups of patients and outline proposed best practice guidelines.

19.10.1 Superficial Thrombophlebitis Isolated to Tributaries

These patients often have significant discomfort from inflamed superficial varices, yet they generally possess the lowest risk for potential VTE complications. Therapy in this category of patients should be supportive involving each of the following: ambulation, properly fitted compression stocking or wraps 20–30 mmHg or higher, anti-inflammatories, and local incision and drainage of inflamed varices if symptoms warrant. Time should be taken to educate patients arming them with awareness of warning signs should symptoms worsen. Ideally, these patients should be followed up with repeat duplex study over the following weeks.

19.10.2 Superficial Thrombophlebitis with Saphenous Vein Involvement in the Presence of Varicose Veins

Patients with saphenous vein involvement in the presence of varicose veins are at risk for extension of existing thrombus and VTE complications. For this reason, near-term follow-up with ultrasound within 5–10 days is recommended. At present, the ACCP recommends prophylactic to intermediate dosing of LMWH or fondaparinux for a minimum of 45 days, when thrombus involves the saphenous veins or approximate the saphenofemoral/saphenopopliteal junctions. This author typically anticoagulates patients with acute saphenous thrombosis whether or not it is close or long enough. Additional recommended therapy includes ambulation, properly fitted compression, and local incision and drainage if symptoms warrant.

19.10.3 Superficial Thrombophlebitis with VTE Complications at Presentation/STP Without Varicose Veins

As with the category above, these patients should walk, wear properly fitted compression, and begin anticoagulation according to ACCP guidelines for VTE. Signs and symptoms suggesting a need for prompt reassessment should be shared. What makes this group somewhat unique is the potential to possess an underlying hypercoagulable cause for their present condition. In the interest of preventing future VTE, risk may be mitigated by promoting healthy vein habits and considering thrombophilia work-ups on those with clear indications.

19.10.4 Unusual Sites of Superficial Thrombophlebitis

19.10.4.1 Upper Extremity STP

Superficial thrombophlebitis of upper extremity veins is most commonly encountered as a complication of intravenous infusions and, at times, drugs that lead to inflammation at the infusion site. Rarely associated with VTE, the ACCP guidelines recommend oral or topical anti-inflammatory agents until symptoms resolve (grade 2B). Anticoagulation for this disorder is not recommended (grade 1C).

19.10.4.2 Mondor's Disease

This is classically reported as superficial thrombosis of breast veins along the anterolateral aspect. Symptoms include pain, tenderness, and erythema. On physical exam a cord is commonly felt, and the skin is tensed or dimpled as the ipsilateral arm is elevated. This may occur following surgery, with malignancy (12 %), or hormonal and hereditary thrombophilia. Care is usually supportive with anti-inflammatories, cold compresses, and time.

Superficial thrombophlebitis may also be seen in the superficial dorsal vein of the penis. Although rare, the presentation may be related to prolonged excessive sexual intercourse, hernia operations, as well as other concomitant thrombotic events. Duplex ultrasonography confirms noncompressibility of the vessel and permits assessment of adjacent deep and superficial vessels. Treatment is supportive with anti-inflammatory agents, reserving dorsal penile surgery for refractory cases.

19.10.4.3 Septic Thrombophlebitis

Suppurative thrombophlebitis is a life-threatening condition frequently associated with septicemia [8]. Patients may present with grossly inflamed superficial vein, fever, leukocytosis, and signs of sepsis. The most common source of infection stems from an intravenous puncture, yet soft tissue and solid organ infections have been reported [27]. The mainstay of therapy is urgent surgical excision and broad spectrum antibiotics.

19.11 Conclusion/Summary

Superficial thrombophlebitis is a common condition associated with substantial morbidity, though less than that seen with femoropopliteal deep vein thrombosis. The best practice may be debatable at present, yet principles to protect patients from complications of venous stasis remain of paramount importance. Benign neglect of heat, elevation, and bed rest are no longer acceptable options. In fact, present management strategies largely parallel those used for deep vein thrombosis, varying only in the use and duration of anticoagulation.

Case Study Questions and Considerations

Case 1

Does this patient have the working diagnosis of STP?

The short answer is yes.

What are the clinical features of STP?

This patient possesses acute onset, firm, painful, inflamed varices, along the medial thigh. Other potential findings include red streaking, fluctuance over cluster of varices, a palpable cord, and presence of edema. Of important note, the most proximal point of thrombus by physical exam is on average 15 cm short of most proximal point by duplex ultrasound.

What is the differential diagnosis of STP?

Table 19.1 provides an overview of alternative considerations.

Does this patient have risk factors for DVT?

The risk factors of STP are the same as DVT as shown in Table 19.2.

What tests are indicated at the initial evaluation of clinically suspected STP?

The noninvasive, yet highly accurate duplex exam is indicated for every patient with clinical findings consistent with STP. Only upon duplex testing does it become possible to optimize treatment while reducing the risk for VTE if it has not already occurred.

Case 2

What risk factors does JD possess that place him at risk for developing STP?

Prolonged immobilization and known history of varicose veins.

What risk factors does JD possess that place him at risk for VTE?

If one was to consider both the Lutter and Quenet studies, age >60, male sex, sudden onset, and recent immobilization are JD's risks for VTE.

Describe a practical approach to evaluate JD and guide his treatment.

Everything starts with a systematic assessment of the limb(s) with duplex ultrasonography. If anticipating the implementation of anticoagulation, initial laboratory tests may be ordered.

Do you agree with the urgent care recommendations of anti-inflammatory agents, an antibiotic, and compression therapy? Please explain.

Anti-inflammatories? If there is no indication for anticoagulation, anti-inflammatories may prove quite helpful in reducing symptoms and arguably minimizing the risk of thrombus extension.

Antibiotics? Unless JD is toxic, no antibiotics are indicated as the lesions are sterile by nature.

Compression therapy? Unless a contraindication exists, compression is indicated for nearly any vein-related concern or for the swollen limb pending diagnosis. The reality is that if anticoagulation is to occur, stockings may be applied at the same stage as the initial dose of LMWH.

Case 3 (Fig. 19.12)

What is the likelihood that JA has already passed pulmonary emboli to explain his dyspnea?

According to series by Verlato and Sobreira, the risk approximates 25–33 % simply by possessing STP at the level of the saphenofemoral junction.

What risk factors suggest JA is at higher risk of developing VTE complications?

He is male, obese, and reported an acute onset of symptoms.

Are any further diagnostic tests indicated?

This is debatable, as JA was hemodynamically stable and did not appear grossly ill. The recommended duration of anticoagulation varies significantly however (e.g., 4 weeks for isolated STP of the GSV versus 6 months for patients with pulmonary embolus). If there is any doubt as to the question of PE, perfusion scanning or spiral computed tomography works well in establishing the diagnosis. In this instance, it was the acute onset of symptoms associated with dyspnea that led to spiral computed tomography (CT) scanning to confirm multiple pulmonary emboli.

What management strategies would you consider?

Reimaging in near term (3 months)

Although repeat duplex scanning did not significantly change in the near term, complete recanalization was seen at 3 months. All of the previously affected vessels were now refluxing and thermal ablation was successfully performed. Twelve months later, his GSV is no longer detectable by ultrasound.

Compression therapy/ambulation

JA continues to make compression a routine part of his daily life as a farm machinery salesman. He is losing weight and is making walking a daily part of his exercise regimen.

Anticoagulation

JA was given LMWH and transitioned to warfarin which he continues to take today. He was found to have thrombophilia, and multiple bouts of phlebitis with complication of PE have led him and his hematologist to favor long-term anticoagulation. If he had not been diagnosed with PE, he may not have undergone thrombophilia testing.

Thrombophilia testing

Multiple bouts of phlebitis with complications of pulmonary embolus in a young patient led to the thrombophilia work-up. The patient was incorporated into the decision making and understood the potential ramifications should a significant finding be noted. He also recognized that he could have a yet to be discovered disorder should the work-up have proven negative.

Case 4 (Fig. 19.14)

List the risk factors DH possesses for developing VTE

DH is male, he smokes, he has no physical findings of venous disease, and yet he has had multiple bouts of phlebitis.

Assuming DH had previously normal saphenous veins, how would your management strategy change?

In this instance, DH should be considered at risk for an underlying thrombophilia. He reports multiple bouts of phlebitis and is young. The work-up identified DH as being homozygous for Factor V Leiden.

Which of the following are strongly recommended for this presentation?

Ambulation: every patient should be encouraged to walk.

Therapeutic compression therapy: every patient should be fitted with at minimum calf high compression therapy. It is our practice to compress the areas involved (e.g., thigh-high, panty height, or Capri-style stockings could each be employed in this case).

Systemic anticoagulation: STP approximated the saphenofemoral junction (SFJ) and thus LMWH was initiated acutely with subsequent transition to warfarin.

Surgical ligation of the SFJ: although this may be a regional choice, medical therapy is preferred in this instance. These patients are already hypercoagulable and the VTE risk is higher when compared to medical therapy.

Thrombophilia testing: in this instance, the history and age of the patient led to a candid discussion. The risks were explained and the patient wanted to know if there was a reason for recurrent bouts of phlebitis. In this instance, a rather important thrombophilia was identified in homozygous factor V Leiden (FVL).

Intravenous antibiotics: antibiotics are not indicated unless septic thrombophlebitis is suspected.

Warm compresses: warm or cold compresses are a reasonable option to help provide symptomatic relief.

References

1. Hingorani A, Ascher E. Superficial venous thrombophlebitis. In: Gloviczki P, editor in chief. Handbook of venous disorders. 3rd ed. London: Hodder Arnold; 2009. p. 314–9.
2. Hill S, Hancock D, Webb T. Thrombophlebitis of the great saphenous vein – recommendations for treatment. Phlebology. 2008;23:35–9.
3. DeMaeseneer M. Letter to editor RE: treatment of superficial thrombophlebitis of the great saphenous vein. Phlebology. 2008;23:299.
4. Quenet S, Laporte S, Decousus H, et al. Factors predictive of venous thrombotic complications in patients with isolated superficial vein thrombosis. J Vasc Surg. 2003;38:944–9.
5. Feied C. Venous thrombosis and pulmonary embolism. In: Marx J, Hockberger R, Walls R, editors. Rosen's emergency medicine: concepts and clinical practice. 5th ed. St. Louis: Mosby; 2002. p. 1211–2.
6. DeGowin R. Thrombophlebitis. DeGowin & DeGowin's bedside diagnostic examination. 5th ed. New York: Macmillan Publishing Company; 1987. p. 441–5.
7. Allen E, Barker N, Hines E, et al. Peripheral vascular diseases. Philadelphia: WB Saunders Company; 1946. p. 636–8.
8. DePalma R, Johnson G. Superficial thrombophlebitis: diagnosis and management. In: Rutherford R, editor. Vascular surgery, vol. 143. 5th ed. Philadelphia: W.B. Saunders Company; 2000. p. 1979–81.
9. Decousus H, Leizorovicz A. Superficial thrombophlebitis of the legs: still a lot to learn. J Thromb Haemost. 2005;3:1149–51.
10. Sobreira M, Maffei F, Yoshida W, et al. Prevalence of deep vein thrombosis and pulmonary embolism in superficial thrombophlebitis of the lower limbs: prospective study of 60 cases. Int Angiol. 2009; 28:400–8.
11. Conant E, Wilkes A, Mendelson E, Feig S. Superficial thrombophlebitis of the breast (Mondor's disease): mammographic findings. AJR Am J Roentgenol. 1993;160:1201–3.
12. Coon W, Willis P, Keller J. Venous thromboembolism and other venous disease in the Tecumseh Community Health Study. Circulation. 1973;48:839–46.
13. DeWeese MS. Nonoperative management of acute superficial thrombophlebitis and deep femoral venous thrombosis. In: Ernst CB, Stanley JC, editors. Current therapy in vascular surgery. Philadelphia: BC Decker; 1991. p. 952–60.
14. Lutter K, Kerr T, Roedersheimer R, et al. Superficial thrombophlebitis diagnosed by duplex scanning. Surgery. 1991;110:42–6.

15. Skillman JJ, Kent KC, Porter DH, Kim D. Simultaneous occurrence of superficial and deep thrombophlebitis in the lower extremity. J Vasc Surg. 1990;11:818–24.
16. Blättler W, Schwarzenbach B, Largiadér J. Superficial vein thrombophlebitis-serious concern or much ado about little? Vasa. 2008;37(1):31–8.
17. Cotran R, Kumar V, Robbins S, editors. Robbins pathologic basis of disease. 4th ed. Philadelphia: WB Saunders Company; 1989.
18. Chengelis D, Bendick P, Glover J, et al. Progression of superficial venous thrombosis to deep vein thrombosis. J Vasc Surg. 1996;24:745–9.
19. Hanson J, Ascher E, DePippo P, et al. Saphenous vein thrombophlebitis (SVT): a deceptively benign disease. J Vasc Surg. 1998;27:677–80.
20. Dewar C, Panpher S. Incidence of deep vein thrombosis in patients diagnosed with superficial thrombophlebitis after presenting to an emergency department outpatient deep vein thrombosis service. Emerg Med J. 2010;27:758–61.
21. Kakkos S, Lampropoulos G, Papadoulos S, et al. Seasonal variation in the incidence of superficial thrombophlebitis. Thromb Res. 2010;126(2):98–102.
22. Blumenberg R, Barton E, Gelfand M, et al. Occult deep vein thrombosis complicating superficial thrombophlebitis. J Vasc Surg. 1998;27:338–43.
23. Sullivan V, Denk P, Sonnad S, et al. Ligation versus anticoagulation: treatment of above-knee superficial thrombophlebitis not involving the deep venous system. J Am Coll Surg. 2001; 193(5):556–62.
24. Verlato F, Zucchetta P, Prandoni P, et al. An unexpectedly high rate of pulmonary embolism in patients with superficial thrombophlebitis of the thigh. J Vasc Surg. 1999;30:1113–5.
25. Leon L, Giannoukas AD, Dodd D, et al. Clinical significance of superficial vein thrombosis. Eur J Vasc Endovasc Surg. 2005;29:10–7.
26. Olubaniyi BO, Kumar S, Dimitri S, et al. Superficial thrombophlebitis of lower limb veins – far from a benign condition. Br J Surg. 2009;96(S1):1–15.
27. Decousus H, Epinat M, Guillot K, et al. Superficial vein thrombosis: risk factors, diagnosis, and treatment. Curr Opin Pulm Med. 2003;9:393–7.
28. Cesarone M, Belcaro G, Agus G, et al. Management of superficial vein thrombosis and thrombophlebitis: status and expert opinion document. Angiology. 2007;58(1):7–15.
29. Coleridge-Smith P, Labropoulos N, Partsch H, et al. Duplex ultrasound investigation of the veins in chronic venous disease of the lower limbs – UIP consensus document. Part I: basic principles. Phlebology. 2006;21:158–67.
30. Ascer E, Lorenson E, Pollina R, Gennaro M. Preliminary results of a nonoperative approach to saphenofemoral junction thrombophlebitis. J Vasc Surg. 1995;22:616–21.
31. Wasserman D, Bonner K, et al. Duplex surveillance of superficial thrombophlebitis. Vasc Surg. 1997;31(4):427–31.
32. Chopra A. Thrombophlebitis and occlusive arterial disease. In: Tintinalli J, Kelen G, Stapczynski J, editors. Emergency medicine a comprehensive guide. 6th ed. New York: McGraw-Hill; 2004. p. 409–10.
33. Comerata A. Comment on duplex surveillance of superficial thrombophlebitis. Vasc Surg. 1997;31(4):430–1.
34. Schönauer V, Kyrle P, Weltermann A, et al. Superficial thrombophlebitis and risk for recurrent venous thromboembolism. J Vasc Surg. 2003;37:834–8.
35. Wilmanns C, Casey A, Schinzel H, Walter P. Superficial thrombophlebitis in varicose vein disease: the particular role of methylenetetrahydrofolate reductase. Phlebology. 2011;26:135–9.
36. Nutescu E, Michaud J, Caprini J. Evaluation of hypercoagulable states and molecular markers of acute venous thrombosis. In: Gloviczki P, editor in chief. Handbook of venous disorders. 3rd ed. London: Hodder Arnold; 2009. p. 113–28.
37. Junger M, Diehm C, Storiko H, et al. Mobilization versus immobilization in the treatment of acute proximal deep vein thrombosis: a prospective, randomized, open, multicenter trial. Curr Med Res Opin. 2006;22(3):593–602.
38. Partsch H, Blattler W. Compression and walking versus bed rest in the treatment of proximal deep venous thrombosis with low molecular weight heparin. J Vasc Surg. 2000;32:861.
39. Ramelet A. Compression therapy. Dermatol Surg. 2002;28:6–10.
40. Decousus H, Quere I, Presles E, et al. Superficial venous thrombosis and venous thromboembolism. Ann Intern Med. 2010;152:218–24.
41. Decousus H, Prandoni P, Mismetti P, et al. Fondaparinux for the treatment of superficial-vein thrombosis in the legs. N Engl J Med. 2010;363:1222–32.
42. Decousus H, Bregeault M, Darmon J, et al. A pilot randomized double-blind comparison of a low-molecular weight heparin, a nonsteroidal anti-inflammatory agent, and placebo in the treatment of superficial vein thrombosis. Arch Intern Med. 2003;163:1657–63.
43. Wichers I, DiNisio M, Buller H, Middeldorp S. Treatment of superficial vein thrombosis to prevent deep vein thrombosis and pulmonary embolism: a systematic review. Haematologica. 2005;90:672–7.
44. Di Nisio M, Wichers I, Middeldorp S. Treatment for superficial thrombophlebitis of the leg. Cochrane Database Syst Rev. 2007;(2):CD004982.
45. Kearon C, Kahn S, Agnelli G, et al. Antithrombotic therapy for venous thromboembolic disease: American College of Chest Physicians evidence based clinical practice guidelines (8th Edition). Chest. 2008;133:454S–545.
46. Bauer K. Duration of anticoagulation: applying the guidelines and beyond. Hematology Am Soc Hematol Educ Program. 2010;2010:210–5.

Deep Vein Thrombosis

20

Sapan S. Desai, Eric Mowatt-Larssen, and Ali Azizzadeh

Contents

Abstract

Venous thromboembolism (VTE) is characterized by the acute pathology of deep venous thrombosis (DVT) and/or pulmonary embolus (PE). DVT affects nearly a quarter million people per year in the USA, with an incidence of about one case per 1000 people. In addition to its local effects with inflammation, swelling, and pain, DVT is responsible for the vast majority of pulmonary embolism (PE). This chapter discusses the incidence, pathophysiology, diagnosis, and management of DVT.

20.1 Introduction

The Ebers Papyrus was written about 3,500 years ago, but is based on medical knowledge dating as far back as 3,400 BC. This 110 page scroll is one of the oldest surviving medical records from Egypt. Within this document is one of the earliest descriptions of deep vein thrombosis (DVT) [1]. Hippocrates coined the term "leucophlegmasia" to describe the swelling that occurs in conjunction with DVT formation in the leg [2]. Galen discusses rubor (redness), dolor (pain), calor (heat), and tumor (swelling) as the cardinal

S.S. Desai, MD, PhD, MBA (✉)
Department of Surgery, Duke University Medical Center, Durham, NC, USA

Department of Cardiothoracic and Vascular Surgery, University of Texas at Houston Medical School, Houston, TX, USA
e-mail: sapan.desai@surgisphere.com

E. Mowatt-Larssen, MD, FACPh, RPhS
757 Pacific Street, Suite C-2, Monterey, CA 93940, USA
e-mail: eric.mowatt.larssen@gmail.com

A. Azizzadeh, MD
Department of Cardiothoracic and Vascular Surgery, University of Texas at Houston Medical School, Houston, TX, USA
e-mail: ali.azizzadeh@uth.tmc.edu

E. Mowatt-Larssen et al. (eds.), *Phlebology, Vein Surgery and Ultrasonography*,
DOI 10.1007/978-3-319-01812-6_20, © Springer International Publishing Switzerland 2014

manifestations of DVT formation – a description that still pertains to our clinical practice today[3].

An association between DVT and pregnancy was elucidated in the thirteenth century and gradually became known as an independent risk factor [4]. Yet, as a consequence of the paucity of knowledge about human anatomy until the fourteenth and fifteenth centuries, the association between actual clot formation and physical obstruction of the deep veins leading to swelling, pain, and inflammation would not be recognized until the early eighteenth century [5].

Rudolf Ludwig Karl Virchow advanced the theory that deep vein thrombosis is related to embolism formation, even leading to large and potentially fatal pulmonary emboli. Building upon the work of surgeons and physicians in the late eighteenth and early nineteenth centuries, Virchow synthesized that the presence of venous stasis (i.e., immobility), vessel wall damage (i.e., surgery and trauma), and hypercoagulable states (i.e., pregnancy) were the chief factors that contributed to venous thromboembolism [6]. This codification permitted the first meaningful interventions against DVT formation, including vein stripping in the nineteenth century and the use of heparin as an anticoagulant in 1916 [7, 8].

20.2 Epidemiology

20.2.1 Incidence

Venous thromboembolism (VTE) is characterized by acute pathology of deep venous thrombosis (DVT) and/or pulmonary embolus (PE). DVT affects nearly a quarter million people per year in the USA, with an incidence of about one case per 1000 people [9, 10]. In addition to its local effects with inflammation, swelling, and pain, DVT is responsible for the vast majority of pulmonary embolism (PE). The commonly accepted values for the risk of fatal PE from a DVT are estimated to be about 5 % [11–14]. In addition to PE, DVT formation is associated with recurrent DVT in about 10 % of all patients and postthrombotic syndrome in about 30 % of patients [15, 16]. Venous thromboembolism occurs more often in African-American and Caucasian populations than in Asians and Hispanics. Most VTE events begin in the deep calf veins. Though many calf vein thromboses resolve spontaneously, 15 % will propagate into proximal veins. When untreated, DVT occurring above the knee leads to symptomatic PE in more than 50 % of patients. Venous thromboembolism is the leading cause of preventable in-hospital deaths, and the 30-day mortality for PE and DVT are 12 and 6 %, respectively [13–16].

20.2.2 Risk Factors

The risk factors contributing to DVT are well known. While more than 20 separate risk factors have been described, they can all generally be divided into the three primary categories first described by Virchow. Hypercoagulable states include cancer, nephrotic syndrome, ulcerative colitis, major trauma or surgery, burns, lupus and other autoimmune disorders, antithrombin III deficiency, protein C and S deficiency, factor V Leiden, oral contraceptives and estrogens, pregnancy, heparin-induced thrombocytopenia, and various defects in plasminogen activation. Venous stasis occurs with prolonged immobilization (such as bedridden patients or those taking long trips in planes or cars), spinal cord injury, multiple trauma, potentially in May-Thurner syndrome (discussed later), and in the chronically ill. Venous wall injury occurs in surgical procedures, trauma, instrumentation of the vasculature, and inflammatory responses to injury or infection [17–42]. Without prophylaxis, 40–60 % of orthopedic surgery patients and 60–80 % of spinal cord injured patients will develop DVT.

20.3 Pathophysiology

20.3.1 Overview

A venous thrombus is attached to the venous wall by thrombin, which then attaches to platelets. Venous thrombi are rarely caused by vessel wall injury, unlike arterial thrombi. Coagulation and fibrinolysis are key physiological processes which must be kept in equilibrium. Disturbances favoring coagulation include venous blood stasis, hypercoagulable states, and cancer. Key mechanisms through which these disturbances create thrombus may include endothelial expression of P-selectin (which binds leukocytes), endothelial secretion of von Willebrand Factor (which binds platelets, leukocytes, and erythrocytes), and monocyte synthesis of tissue factor (which often causes thrombus on P-selectin-expressing endothelial or platelet cells).

The cascade model of coagulation is the foundation of modern thinking about hemostasis. This paradigm has proven durable in part because its components can be quantified: prothrombin time (PT) measures the extrinsic pathway and partial thromboplastin time (PTT) measures the intrinsic pathway. Recent work has revealed that the regulation of blood coagulation is far more dynamic and complex than depicted by the cascade model.

The current cell-based model of coagulation combines components of both the intrinsic and extrinsic pathways into a single mechanism occurring on cellular surfaces and involving factors that arise from cellular surfaces and free-flowing blood. This model has multiple steps including initiation, resulting in the deposition of thrombin; priming, resulting in platelet activation; propagation of thrombus leading to fibrin deposition; and stabilization of coagulation through modulation of fibrinolysis. Moreover, endothelial cell repair and death are vital to the subject of thrombophilia and vascular bed-specific thrombotic potential. The ability to promote endothelial integrity (structural and functional) following injury and the prompt regulation of apoptotic cell-mediated prothrombotic activity are key to the biology of hemostasis and thrombosis. The phenotype of thrombosis is the end result of vascular bed-specific responses to endothelial cell injury, environmental prothrombotic triggers (internal, external), and distinct molecular (genetic) thromboregulatory systems.

Upon completion of all the stages in both clot formation and regulation, the endothelial cell returns to the resting state where its surface expresses heparin sulfates and thrombomodulin and it releases molecule such as t-PA, nitric oxide, and prostacyclins, in effect, providing permanent endogenous anticoagulation.

20.3.2 Coagulation Cascade

An exploration of the coagulation cascade and its attendant contributors is important to understand the various pathologies that contribute to DVT. A breakdown in one of several critical steps is all that is necessary to initiate a hypercoagulable state. Normal coagulation relies on three main contributors, including the exposed endothelium, platelets, and circulating proteins in the plasma. Just as important as these three main contributors, fibrinolytic enzymes are also required to help reform the clot and restore vascular patency. This last component is critical for normal wound healing [43–52].

Normal coagulation typically begins with trauma to the vessel wall, exposing thrombogenic proteins under the endothelium such as von Willebrand Factor (vWF). vWF binds to a variety of circulating clotting factors, including collagen and factor VIII. This creates a matrix upon which platelets bind using glycoprotein Ia/IIa and Ib/IX/V receptors. Platelet activation then leads to release of alpha and dense granules (Fig. 20.1). Release of thrombogenic proteins and growth factors occurs, leading to platelet clumping and the formation of fibrinogen cross-links using glycoprotein IIb/IIIa receptors. This process is known as primary hemostasis [52].

Disruption of primary hemostasis such as in disseminated intravascular coagulopathy (DIC); drug-induced reactions with quinidine, quinine, vancomycin, or gold salts; bone marrow suppressed states; cardiopulmonary bypass; and alcohol toxicity leads to the inability to form an enduring clot and presents as mucocutaneous bleeding. Defects in primary hemostasis can be diagnosed with platelet aggregation assays, von Willebrand Factor functional assays, and a platelet function analyzer (PFA) [52].

After formation of the platelet plug, secondary hemostasis is initiated with the coagulation cascade to form a stable fibrin plug. Both an intrinsic and extrinsic pathway are available to initiate secondary hemostasis (Fig. 20.2); this dual pathway ensures that even patients with defects in primary hemostasis eventually develop some form of enduring clot over time (Fig. 20.3) [53]. The most important pathway in secondary hemostasis is

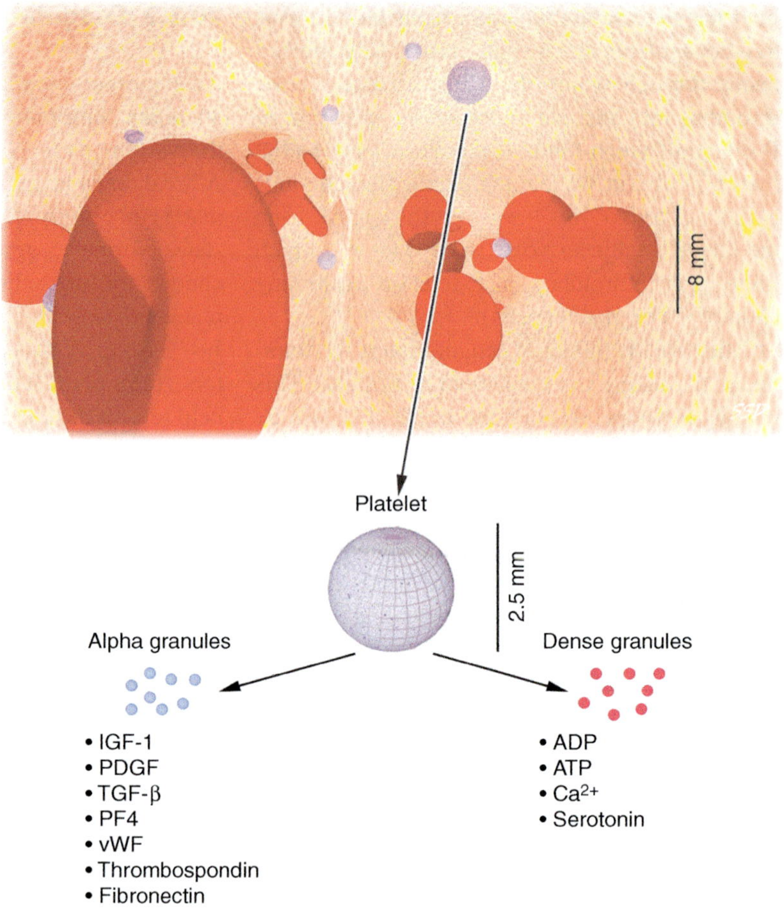

Fig. 20.1 Platelets and the two types of granules they contain. Alpha granules contain insulin-like growth factor 1 (*IGF-1*), platelet-derived growth factor (*PDGF*), transforming growth factor-beta (*TGF-B*), platelet factor 4 (*PF4*), von Willebrand Factor (*vWF*), thrombospondin, and fibronectin. Dense granules contain ADP, ATP, calcium, and serotonin. Both types of granules are necessary for the coagulation cascade to function correctly

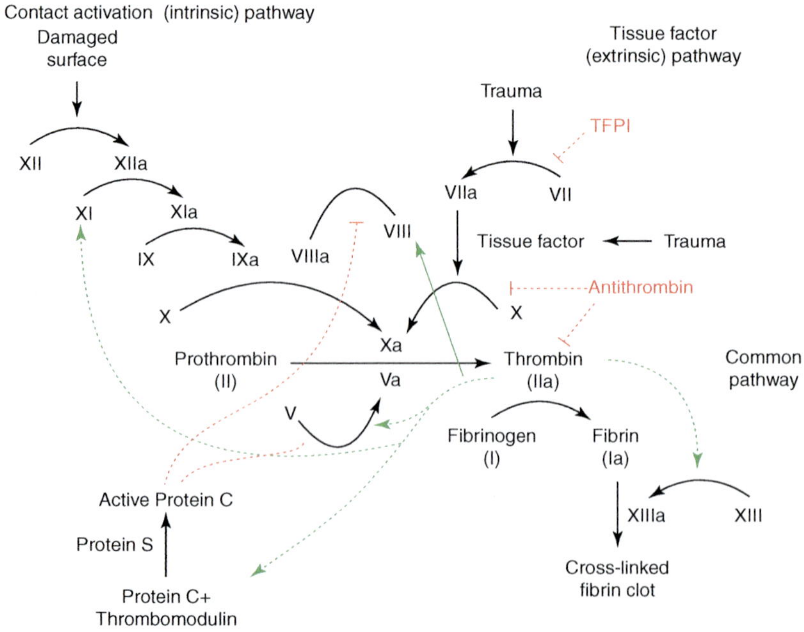

Fig. 20.2 The intrinsic and extrinsic pathway of coagulation with the interplay between the various types of factors demonstrated. Illustration by Joe Dunckley. Used in accordance with the GNU Free Documentation License Version 1.2

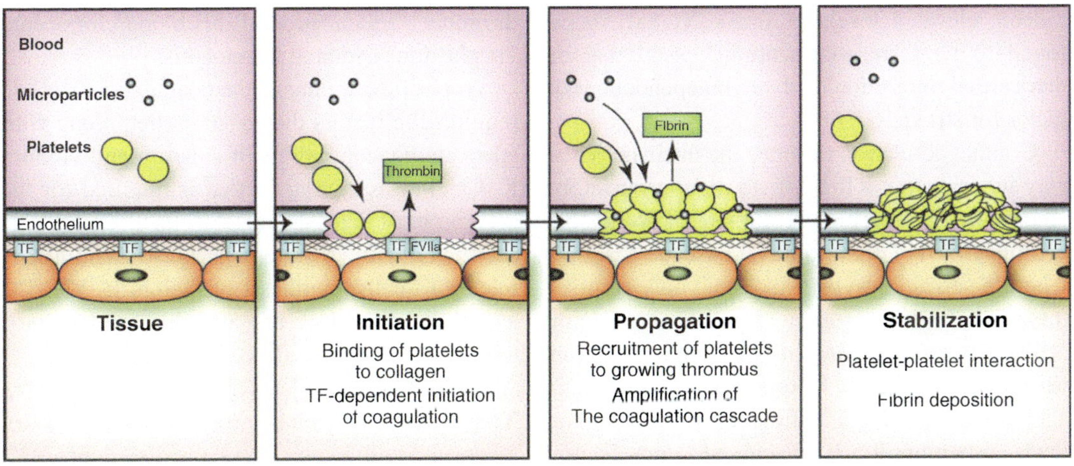

Fig. 20.3 Formation of a clot at the site of blood vessel injury. In a healthy individual, TF expressed by vascular smooth muscle cells, pericytes, and adventitial fibroblasts in the vessel wall is physically separated from its ligand FVII/FVIIa by the endothelium. Vessel injury leads to the rapid binding of platelets to the subendothelium and activation of the coagulation cascade by TF. Propagation of the thrombus involves recruitment of additional platelets and amplification of the coagulation cascade by the intrinsic pathway, and possibly by TF-positive MPs and TF stored in platelets. Finally, fibrin deposition stabilizes the clot. De novo synthesis of TF by platelets may also play a role in stabilization of the clot

the extrinsic pathway, which relies upon the transmembrane receptor tissue factor (TF).

Tissue factor is found within vascular endothelium, adventitia, brain, lung, heart, and placenta [54–61]. While deficiencies in factors VIII and IX (hemophilia A and B, respectively) have been identified, the absence of tissue factor is typically incompatible with life [62]. Constitutively, low production of tissue factor is associated with spontaneous hemorrhage in the heart, lung, and placenta [60].

Tissue factor is normally unmasked from the vascular wall following trauma. However, this factor is expressed by monocytes and possibly neutrophils and may initiate thrombosis in patients with disseminated intravascular coagulation [63–65]. Tissue factor expression upon neutrophils has been implicated as one of the causes of autoimmunity-based hypercoagulable disorders such as antiphospholipid antibody syndrome [65].

20.3.3 Extrinsic Pathway

Trauma initiates a process whereby tissue factor interacts with factor VII, forming an activated complex and beginning the cycle of thrombosis. This activated complex leads to the activation of factor X and the beginning of the final common pathway that both the extrinsic and intrinsic pathways share, discussed below.

The extrinsic pathway has a number of strict controls to prevent runaway thrombosis. This is necessary as factor VII is one of the most common factors in circulation and the lack of strict regulation would lead to rapid propagation of clot [66]. The tissue factor-factor VIIa complex is inhibited by tissue factor pathway inhibitor (TFPI), a single chain polypeptide that also inhibits factors Xa and IIa (thrombin).

20.3.4 Intrinsic Pathway

While the extrinsic pathway seems critical for thrombosis, defects in the intrinsic pathway are associated with delayed clot formation with arterial injury. The primary importance of the intrinsic pathway therefore appears to be with arterial thrombosis; clot formation throughout the veins and much of the rest of the body appears to be controlled by the extrinsic pathway [53, 59–61].

Indeed, elevated levels of factor XI have been found to be associated with increased risk of myocardial infarction and an independent risk factor for stroke [67, 68].

Contact activation initiates the intrinsic pathway when factor XII binds to an appropriately charged surface, typically the site of some sort of injury [69]. This initiates a cascade reaction where a series of trypsin-like enzymes amplify the reaction and promote thrombosis. Factor XII is activated, leading in turn to the activation of factor XI. These factors work together to activate factor IX; a deficiency of this factor leads to hemophilia B (discussed later). Factor IXa binds to activated factor VIII to initiate the activation of factor X and the beginning of the final common pathway; defects in factor VIII lead to hemophilia A. Of note, independent activation of factor XI can also occur, as seen in patients with defects in factor XII (Hageman factor deficiency) [70].

20.3.5 Final Common Pathway

The final common pathway begins with factor Xa and is regulated by factor V. The activation of factor V is inhibited by protein C; the activation of protein C is modulated by protein S. Therefore, protein C and S serve as inhibitory mediators for coagulation and their deficiency leads to a hypercoagulable state; this is seen in warfarin administration without prior anticoagulation with heparin. Protein C and S are vitamin K-dependent factors with short half-lives and are downregulated within the first 24–48 h of warfarin administration. This leads to a transient hypercoagulable state while the other factors are still being downregulated to sufficient levels [71].

Activated factors X and V lead to the conversion of prothrombin (factor II) to thrombin (factor IIa). Thrombin leads to feedback regulation by stimulating the production of protein C and thrombomodulin. Thrombin serves to convert fibrinogen to fibrin, leading to the deposition of the hemostatic plug. Cross-linking of the fibrin clot occurs with the action of factor XIII, the production of which is also upregulated by thrombin. Organization of this blood clot occurs via plasmin-mediated fibrinolysis.

Proper functioning of the coagulation cascade requires the factors discussed earlier, along with adequate concentrations of calcium and vitamin K. Calcium is a cofactor that is required for the activation of various factors; its deficiency is associated with coagulopathy [72]. Vitamin K is required for the synthesis of factors II, VII, IX, and X, and proteins C and S. A third protein, protein Z, is also regulated by vitamin K; this protein appears to play a role in degradation of factors Xa and XI [73]. Defects in protein Z have been associated with hypercoagulable disorders [74].

20.3.6 Regulation

Regulation of the coagulation cascade relies on a variety of mediators. Protein C and S inhibit the production of factor Va, leading to cessation of further thrombin production. Protein C and S production are upregulated by thrombin, leading to a feedback inhibition reaction at the level of the final common pathway. Tissue factor pathway inhibitor inhibits tissue factor, temporizing clot formation at the extrinsic pathway level. Prostacyclin (PGI2) leads to the production of adenylyl cyclase and cAMP production by platelets, leading to sequestration of calcium and general inhibition of coagulation.

20.3.7 Thrombolytics

Two other complex systems help to control coagulation: the first is the thrombolytic system, which involves plasmin and tissue plasminogen activator (tPA), and the second involves a group of inhibitors of the coagulation factors, including antithrombin III, protein C, and protein S.

The thrombolytic system dissolves fibrin clots using the serine protease plasmin. Plasmin is formed from its inactive precursor, plasminogen. Interestingly, plasmin is also activated by thrombin, which thereby limits its own clot-forming ability.

The second anticoagulant system is made up of antithrombin III and proteins C and S. Antithrombin breaks down factors IXa, Xa, Xia, and XIIa and thrombin, leading to inhibition of coagulation at both the intrinsic and final common pathways, and its activity is enhanced up to 2,000-fold by heparin.

20.4 Monitoring

There are several general tests of clotting factors commonly used to measure overall function of the coagulation cascade. The activated partial thromboplastin time test (PTT) measures the intrinsic pathway and will be increased in deficiencies of factors VII, IX, XI, XII, von Willebrand fibrinogen. PTT testing is used to monitor heparin efficacy in patients on heparin drips. The prothrombin time test (PT) measures the extrinsic pathway and will be abnormal in deficiencies of factors II, V, VII, and X and fibrinogen. Because of variations in PT level reporting, the international normalized ratio (INR) was developed to allow comparison of levels across laboratories. PT/INR testing is used to monitor vitamin K and warfarin efficacy.

The coagulation cascade is a complex interplay between dozens of proteins and cells. Its seamless function is required to avoid coagulopathies and hypercoagulable states. The division into an intrinsic and extrinsic pathway plays unique roles in coagulation and offers scientists numerous targets to deal with disorders in coagulation.

20.5 Anatomic Considerations

Superficial venous thrombophlebitis (STP) refers to thrombosis occurring in the superficial veins. Patients with STP usually present with a painful, red, tender superficial vein. Ultrasound should be performed to delineate the extent of thrombosis and rule out concomitant DVT. Concomitant PE is also not uncommon and should be ruled out. Extensive STP above the knee, especially in the great saphenous vein, or STP near saphenofemoral or saphenopopliteal junctions, merits anticoagulation along with compression or even surgical saphenofemoral disconnection. Less extensive STP can be treated with nonsteroidal anti-inflammatory medicines and compression therapy. Close follow-up is important, since STP can progress to DVT or PE.

External venous obstruction in the pelvis and the thoracic outlet lead to acute and chronic venous thrombosis. In the pelvis, May-Thurner syndrome occurs due to sustained compression of the left iliac vein by the right iliac artery. Treatment mandates removal of the external forces through iliac stenting, and several series have shown improvements in intermediate quality of life following this type of intervention. In the thoracic outlet, Paget-Schroetter syndrome occurs when the subclavian vein becomes obstructed due to repeated trauma from adjacent bony, muscular and ligamentous attachments. While management of this entity is controversial, most practitioners agree that thrombolysis of subclavian clot and either selective or routine surgical decompression of the thoracic outlet is necessary for the optimal outcomes.

20.6 Presentation

Patients with DVT usually present with acute, unilateral extremity swelling or pain. Tenderness is common on examination, but Homan's sign (passive dorsiflexion of the foot produces calf pain) is unreliable. Redness and localized warmth are sometimes found. Differential diagnoses include cellulitis, Baker's cyst, lymphangitis, lymphedema, and local injuries.

Patients with pulmonary embolism usually present with shortness of breath or chest pain. The chest pain can be pleuritic or unilateral. The diagnosis less commonly presents, but should be considered, in patients with syncope, shock, or cardiopulmonary arrest. Other symptoms include cough, hemoptysis, anxiety, and sweats. Signs include tachypnea (respiratory rate over 16 breaths per minute) and tachycardia (heart rate over 100 beats per minute). Unexplained hypoxia should prompt aggressive investigation for PE.

The differential diagnosis for each of these symptoms is large, but common alternative diagnoses are acute myocardial infarction, aortic dissection, acute pericarditis, chronic obstructive pulmonary disease, asthma, congestive heart failure, and pneumonia.

20.7 Diagnosis

Many episodes of DVT and PE present with occult symptoms. Clinical scores have been developed to assist in diagnosis of both DVT and PE. A variety of risk assessment models exist for calibrating the risk of DVT formation and subsequent PE [43–50]. Among these various models, the Wells score stands out for its simplicity and applicability as a risk evaluation model for DVT and PE (Table 20.1). A score of two or higher indicates a significant risk for DVT, while a score less than two indicates that the risk of DVT is low. Patients with a risk of DVT should be evaluated with noninvasive imaging [51]. In the PE score, a total of 4 or less points means the risk for PE is low. When considering the diagnosis of PE, most patients receive an EKG and chest X-ray, tests useful mostly to exclude other diagnoses. However, EKG findings often consistent with PE include right heart strain and right heart block. Unexplained hypoxia also suggests PE.

Table 20.1 Clinical model for predicting the pretest probability of deep-vein thrombosis

Clinical characteristic	Score
Active cancer (patient receiving treatment for cancer within the previous 6 months or currently receiving palliative treatment)	1
Paralysis, paresis, or recent plaster immobilization of the lower extremities	1
Recently bedridden for 3 days or more, or major surgery within the previous 12 weeks requiring general or regional anesthesia	1
Localized tenderness along the distribution of the deep venous system	1
Entire leg swollen	1
Calf swelling at least 3 cm larger than that on the asymptomatic side (measured 10 cm below tibial tuberosity)	1
Pitting edema confined to the symptomatic leg	1
Collateral superficial veins (nonvaricose)	1
Previously documented deep-vein thrombosis	1
Alternative diagnosis at least as likely as deep-vein thrombosis	−2

A score of two or higher indicates that the probability of deep-vein thrombosis is likely; a score of less than two indicates that the probability of deep-vein thrombosis is unlikely. In patients with symptoms in both legs, the more symptomatic leg is used

Table 20.2 Pulmonary embolism score

Variable	Score
Clinical signs and symptoms of DVT (minimum of leg swelling and pain with palpation of deep veins)	3.0
Alternative diagnoses less likely than PE	3.0
Heart rate >100 beats per minute	1.5
Immobilization >3 days or surgery in the previous 4 weeks	1.5
Previous PE or DVT	1.5
Hemoptysis	1.0
Malignancy and receiving treatment, treated in the last 6 months, or palliative	1.0

D-dimers are a product of fibrinolysis that are often elevated in acute VTE. The D-dimer test is sensitive (85–95 %) but nonspecific (40–65 %) for acute VTE. Enzyme-linked immunosorbent assays and some immunoturbidimetric D-dimer tests are more sensitive than other methods, such as whole-blood and quantitative latex agglutination assays. Patients with a low risk DVT score and a negative D-dimer have less than a 1 % chance of having DVT [15]. Similarly, a low risk PE score and a negative D-dimer carries a less than 1 % risk of nonfatal PE [16]. These DVT and PE patients rarely need further testing (Table 20.2).

Duplex ultrasonography is the accepted standard for noninvasive venous imaging in suspected DVT. Ultrasound for thigh DVT has sensitivity of 97 %, specificity of 86 %, positive predictive value of 87 %, and negative predictive value of 97 % for evaluation of the femoropopliteal system. Accuracy from ultrasound is operator dependent. Small calf vein thrombi can be missed on ultrasound. For this reason, patients with continued suspicion of DVT and an initially negative ultrasound study should be rescanned in around a week to rule out a significant thrombus extension from an initially missed calf vein thrombus. Magnetic resonance venography (MRV) is an alternative to ultrasound useful for evaluation of pelvic and caval thrombi. Wide adoption of MRV is limited by rare but devastating cases of nephrogenic systemic fibrosis (NSF). In the future, additional contrast agents and technical refinements will permit increased use of magnetic resonance (MR) in the evaluation of VTE, particularly in cases of suspected central stenoses.

Computed tomographic angiography (CTA) diagnoses PE with a high sensitivity and specificity, enabling rapid diagnosis with minimal morbidity. The test is contraindicated in the setting of renal insufficiency due to the relative nephrotoxicity of the more than 100 mL of contrast required for the study [75]. Since the 1960s, pulmonary angiography has been the invasive gold standard for diagnosing emboli to the pulmonary vasculature. The procedure carries morbidity of approximately 6 %, related primarily to access complications, and mortality of less than 0.5 %, related to ventricular dysrhythmias due to right heart catheterization. Ventilation perfusion (V/Q) scans are another alternative but are insensitive and nonspecific and useful only if pretest clinical probability matches V/Q scan result.

20.8 Treatment

Now in its eighth edition, the American College of Chest Physicians (ACCP) has produced comprehensive clinical practice guidelines for VTE [76]. In patients with DVT, elastic compression stockings reduce the long-term risk of postthrombotic symptoms (such as chronic pain, swelling, or ulceration). Unfractionated heparin (UFH) or low molecular weight heparin (LMWH) is injected to prevent thrombus extension. The primary management of venous thromboembolism is medical anticoagulation and is discussed at length in Chap. 21. The following paragraphs discuss procedural management of acute VTE in the subgroups of patients who may benefit. Pulmonary emboli without hemodynamic derangement are treated like DVT patients with LMWH or UFH along with warfarin. In patients where the clinical suspicion is high and the risk of hemorrhagic complications is tolerable, anticoagulation can be initiated prior to confirmatory imaging. In the case of a hemodynamically significant PE, thrombolytic therapy (e.g., streptokinase or urokinase) is recommended. Catheter pulmonary thromboembolectomy is considered in cases of significant PE where thrombolysis fails or is contraindicated.

There is emerging data regarding the utility of a percutaneous approach to iliofemoral DVT. In the case of acute iliofemoral DVT, an interventional strategy may include mechanical thrombectomy, thrombolytic therapy, and/or stenting. Some groups advocate an interventional approach in the setting of chronic pathology. While longer-term data is needed, intermediate results demonstrate that an interventional approach to iliofemoral DVT improves venous valve function, symptoms, and quality of life. A recent large experience with an interventional approach to the iliofemoral venous segment demonstrates improved quality of life and primary patency at 3 years of greater than 50 %.

Approved and proposed indications for vena cava filter placement include, among others, a contraindication to anticoagulation in a patient with known DVT and new PE or DVT while anticoagulated. Based on the only randomized controlled data available regarding vena caval filters, these devices are proven to decrease the incidence of PE in patients with documented lower extremity DVT and a contraindication to anticoagulation. The introduction of retrievable filters has increased filter usage in high-risk patients who cannot be anticoagulated, despite a lack of randomized data on the utility of this technology in this ever-broadening patient population. The nationwide retrieval rate for removable filters is less than 50 %, and several groups advocate lifelong anticoagulation in the setting of a permanent IVC filter.

20.9 Natural History

Even patients properly treated have a significant risk of complications, which include recurrence, chronic venous insufficiency, or pulmonary hypertension. Chronic venous insufficiency

(CVI) results from chronic thrombus or venous valves damaged by thrombus, resulting in deep, superficial, or perforator reflux, and producing chronic venous disease symptoms like pain, swelling, varicose veins, and skin changes. Compression stockings, early anticoagulation to reduce clot extension, and thrombolysis when indicated are treatments that can reduce the risk for CVI. Massive or recurrent PE is a significant cause of pulmonary hypertension since the pulmonary arterial endothelium is somewhat ineffective at thrombolysis. A large enough chronic clot burden can result in chronic cor pulmonale. Duration of anticoagulation is increased past 3 months to decrease VTE recurrence risk (see Chap. 21).

Venous thromboembolic disease is a significant source of patient morbidity and mortality. Short- and long-term outcomes in patients with VTE will be improved by advances in the understanding of VTE biology, pharmacotherapy, and interventional strategies, combined with targeted risk factor reduction and appropriate prophylaxis.

References

1. Ludwig Christian Stern. Ebers G. ed (in German). PapyrosEbers: Das hermetischeBuchüber die Arzeneimittel der altenÄgypter in hieratischerSchrift, herausgegebenmitInhaltsangabe und Einleitungversehen von Georg Ebers, mitHieroglyphisch-LateinischemGlossar von Ludwig Stern, mitUnterstützung des KöniglichSächsischenCultusministerium. 2 (1st ed.). Leipzig: W. Englemann; 1875.
2. ANNING ST. The historical aspects of venous thrombosis. Med Hist. 1957;1(1):28–37.
3. Kempf EJ. From Hippocrates to Galen. Med Libr Hist J. 1904;2(4):282–307.
4. Dexter L, Folch-Pi W. Venous thrombosis. An account of the first documented case. JAMA. 1974;228(2): 195–6.
5. Hunter J. Observations on the inflammation of the internal coasts of veins. Trans Soc Improv Med Chir Knowl. 1793;1:18–25.
6. Virchow RLK. Ueber die akuteEntzuendung der Arterien. Archiv fur pathologische Anatomie und Physiologie und fur klinischeMedizin Berlin. 1847;1: 272–4.
7. Dickson BC. Venous thrombosis: on the history of Virchow's triad. Univ Toronto Med J. 2004;81:166–71.
8. Murray G. Anticoagulant therapy with heparin. Am J Med. 1947;3(4):468–71.
9. Hirsch DR, Ingenito EP, Goldhaber SZ. Prevalence of deep venous thrombosis among patients in medical intensive care. JAMA. 1995;274(4):335–7.
10. http://www.surgeongeneral.gov/topics/deepvein/calltoaction/call-to-action-on-dvt-2008.pdf
11. Douketis JD, Kearon C, Bates S, Duku EK, Ginsberg JS. Risk of fatal pulmonary embolism in patients with treated venous thromboembolism. JAMA. 1998;279(6):458–62.
12. Anderson FA, Wheeler HB, Goldberg RJ, et al. A population-based perspective of the hospital incidence and case-fatality rates of deep vein thrombosis and pulmonary embolism: the Worcester DVT study. Arch Intern Med. 1991;151:933–8.
13. Dalen JE, Alpert JS. Natural history of pulmonary embolism. Prog Cardiovasc Dis. 1975;17:257–70.
14. Alpert JS, Smith R, Carlson J, Ockene IS, Dexter L, Dalen JE. Mortality in patients treated for pulmonary embolism. JAMA. 1976;236:1477–80.
15. Salzman EW, Hirsh J. The epidemiology, pathogenesis, and natural history of venous thrombosis. In: Colman RW, Hirsh J, Salzman EW, editors. Hemostasis and thrombosis: basic principles and clinical practice. Philadelphia: JB Lippincott & Co; 1994. p. 1275–96.
16. Prandoni P, Lensing AWA, Cogo A, et al. The long-term clinical course of acute deep vein thrombosis. Ann Intern Med. 1996;125:1–7.
17. Ruggeri M, Tosetto A, Castaman G, Rodeghiero F. Congenital absence of the inferior vena cava: a rare risk factor for idiopathic deep-vein thrombosis. Lancet. 2001;357(9254):441.
18. Hamoud S, Nitecky S, Engel A, Goldsher D, Hayek T. Hypoplasia of the inferior vena cava with azygous continuation presenting as recurrent leg deep vein thrombosis. Am J Med Sci. 2000;319(6):414–6.
19. Greenfield LJ, Proctor MC. The percutaneous greenfield filter: outcomes and practice patterns. J Vasc Surg. 2000;32(5):888–93.
20. Tsuji Y, Goto A, Hara I, Ataka K, Yamashita C, Okita Y, et al. Renal cell carcinoma with extension of tumor thrombus into the vena cava: surgical strategy and prognosis. J Vasc Surg. 2001;33(4):789–96.
21. Stamatakis JD, Kakkar VV, Sagar S, Lawrence D, Nairn D, Bentley PG. Femoral vein thrombosis and total hip replacement. Br Med J. 1977;2(6081):223–5. [Full Text].
22. Alikhan R, Cohen AT, Combe S, Samama MM, Desjardins L, Eldor A, et al. Risk factors for venous thromboembolism in hospitalized patients with acute medical illness: analysis of the MEDENOX Study. Arch Intern Med. 2004;164(9):963–8.
23. Heit JA, Elliott CG, Trowbridge AA, Morrey BF, Gent M, Hirsh J. Ardeparin sodium for extended out-of-hospital prophylaxis against venous thromboembolism after total hip or knee replacement. A randomized, double-blind, placebo-controlled trial. Ann Intern Med. 2000;132(11):853–61.

24. Nordström M, Lindblad B, Bergqvist D, Kjellström T. A prospective study of the incidence of deep-vein thrombosis within a defined urban population. J Intern Med. 1992;232(2):155–60.
25. Dahlbäck B. Inherited thrombophilia: resistance to activated protein C as a pathogenic factor of venous thromboembolism. Blood. 1995;85(3):607–14.
26. Anderson Jr FA, Wheeler HB, Goldberg RJ, Hosmer DW, Forcier A. The prevalence of risk factors for venous thromboembolism among hospital patients. Arch Intern Med. 1992;152(8):1660–4.
27. Warlow C, Ogston D, Douglas AS. Deep venous thrombosis of the legs after strokes. Part I–incidence and predisposing factors. Br Med J. 1976;1(6019): 1178–81. [Full Text].
28. Monreal M, Lafoz E, Casals A, Inaraja L, Montserrat E, Callejas JM, et al. Occult cancer in patients with deep venous thrombosis. A systematic approach. Cancer. 1991;67(2):541–5.
29. Rickles FR, Levine M, Edwards RL. Hemostatic alterations in cancer patients. Cancer Metastasis Rev. 1992;11(3–4):237–48.
30. Levine MN, Gent M, Hirsh J, Arnold A, Goodyear MD, Hryniuk W, et al. The thrombogenic effect of anticancer drug therapy in women with stage II breast cancer. N Engl J Med. 1988;318(7):404–7.
31. Schroeder R. Massive thromboembolism captured by real-time echocardiography. J Surg Radiol. 2010;1:1(1).
32. Clagett GP, Reisch JS. Prevention of venous thromboembolism in general surgical patients. Results of meta-analysis. Ann Surg. 1988;208(2):227–40. [Full Text].
33. Clagett GP, Anderson Jr FA, Heit J, Levine MN, Wheeler HB. Prevention of venous thromboembolism. Chest. 1995;108(4 Suppl):312S–34.
34. Beaty JH, editor. Orthopaedic knowledge. Rosemont: AAOS; 1999. p. 63–72.
35. Rialon KL, Ceppa EP, Mureebe L. Case study: a 53-year-old female with lower abdominal pain. J Surg Radiol. 2011;1:2(3).
36. Kakkar VV, Howe CT, Nicolaides AN, Renney JT, Clarke MB. Deep vein thrombosis of the leg. Is there a "high risk" group? Am J Surg. 1970;120(4):527–30.
37. Motykie GD, Caprini JA, Arcelus JI, Zebala LP, Lee CE, Finke NM, et al. Risk factor assessment in the management of patients with suspected deep venous thrombosis. Int Angiol. 2000;19(1):47–51.
38. Motykie GD, Zebala LP, Caprini JA, Lee CE, Arcelus JI, Reyna JJ, et al. A guide to venous thromboembolism risk factor assessment. J Thromb Thrombolysis. 2000;9(3):253–62.
39. Schafer AI. Hypercoagulable states: molecular genetics to clinical practice. Lancet. 1994;344(8939–8940): 1739–42.
40. Meissner MH, Strandness E. Pathophysiology and natural history of acute deep venous thrombosis. In: Rutherford's vascular surgery. 2005. p. 2124–42.
41. Ho CH, Chau WK, Hsu HC, Gau JP, Yu TJ. Causes of venous thrombosis in fifty Chinese patients. Am J Hematol. 2000;63(2):74–8.
42. Vandenbrouke JP, Bloemenkamp KW, Rosendaal FR, Helmerhorst FM. Incidence of venous thromboembolism in users of combined oral contraceptives. Risk is particularly high with first use of oral contraceptives. BMJ. 2000;320(7226):57–8.
43. Neff MJ, ACEP. ACEP releases clinical policy on evaluation and management of pulmonary embolism. Am Fam Physician. 2003;68(4):759–60.
44. Wells P, Anderson D, Rodger M, Ginsberg J, Kearon C, Gent M, Turpie A, Bormanis J, Weitz J, Chamberlain M, Bowie D, Barnes D, Hirsh J. Derivation of a simple clinical model to categorize patients probability of pulmonary embolism: increasing the models utility with the SimpliRED D-dimer. Thromb Haemost. 2000;83(3):416–20.
45. Woller SC, Stevens SM, Jones JP, Lloyd JF, Evans RS, Aston VT, Elliott CG. Derivation and validation of a simple model to identify venous thromboembolism risk in medical patients. Am J Med. 2011;124(10): 947–954.e2.
46. Khorana AA. Risk assessment and prophylaxis for VTE in cancer patients. J Natl Compr Canc Netw. 2011;9(7):789–97.
47. Pannucci CJ, Bailey SH, Dreszer G, Fisher Wachtman C, Zumsteg JW, Jaber RM, Hamill JB, Hume KM, Rubin JP, Neligan PC, Kalliainen LK, Hoxworth RE, Pusic AL, Wilkins EG. Validation of the Caprini risk assessment model in plastic and reconstructive surgery patients. J Am Coll Surg. 2011;212(1):105–12. Epub 2010 Nov 18.
48. Barbar S, Noventa F, Rossetto V, Ferrari A, Brandolin B, Perlati M, De Bon E, Tormene D, Pagnan A, Prandoni P. A risk assessment model for the identification of hospitalized medical patients at risk for venous thromboembolism: the Padua Prediction Score. J Thromb Haemost. 2010;8(11):2450–7.
49. Eichinger S, Heinze G, Jandeck LM, Kyrle PA. Risk assessment of recurrence in patients with unprovoked deep vein thrombosis or pulmonary embolism: the Vienna prediction model. Circulation. 2010;121(14): 1630–6.
50. Mitchell L, Lambers M, Flege S, Kenet G, Li-Thiao-Te V, Holzhauer S, Bidlingmaier C, Frühwald MC, Heller C, Schmidt W, Pautard B, Nowak-Göttl U. Validation of a predictive model for identifying an increased risk for thromboembolism in children with acute lymphoblastic leukemia: results of a multicenter cohort study. Blood. 2010;115(24):4999–5004.
51. Wells PS, Anderson DR, Rodger M, et al. Evaluation of D-dimer in the diagnosis of suspected deep-vein thrombosis. N Engl J Med. 2003;349(13):1227–35.
52. Desai SS, Shortell CK, editors. Clinical review of vascular surgery. 1st ed. New York: Catalyst Publishers; 2010.
53. Mackman N, Tilley RE, Key NS. Role of the extrinsic pathway of blood coagulation in hemostasis and thrombosis. Arterioscler Thromb Vasc Biol. 2007; 27(8):1687–93.
54. Drake TA, Morrissey JH, Edgington TS. Selective cellular expression of tissue factor in human tissues.

Implications for disorders of hemostasis and thrombosis. Am J Pathol. 1989;134:1087–97.
55. Fleck RA, Rao LVM, Rapaport SI, Varki N. Localization of human tissue factor antigen by immunostaining with monospecific, polyclonal anti-human tissue factor antibody. Thromb Res. 1990;57:765–81.
56. Flössel C, Luther T, Müller M, Albrecht S, Kasper M. Immunohistochemical detection of tissue factor (TF) on paraffin sections of routinely fixed human tissue. Histochemistry. 1994;101:449–53.
57. Bouchard BA, Shatos MA, Tracy PB. Human brain pericytes differentially regulate expression of procoagulant enzyme complexes comprising the extrinsic pathway of blood coagulation. Arterioscler Thromb Vasc Biol. 1997;17:1–9.
58. Schecter AD, Spirn B, Rossikhina M, Giesen PL, Bogdanov V, Fallon JT, Fisher EA, Schnapp LM, Nemerson Y, Taubman MB. Release of active tissue factor by human arterial smooth muscle cells. Circ Res. 2000;87:126–32.
59. Mackman N, Sawdey MS, Keeton MR, Loskutoff DJ. Murine tissue factor gene expression in vivo: tissue and cell specificity and regulation by lipopolysaccharide. Am J Pathol. 1993;143:76–84.
60. Erlich JH, Parry GCN, Fearns C, Muller M, Carmeliet P, Luther T, Mackman N. Tissue factor is required for uterine hemostasis and maintenance of the placental labyrinth during gestation. Proc Natl Acad Sci U S A. 1999;96:8138–43.
61. Hartzell S, Ryder K, Lanahan A, Lau LF, Nathans D. A growth factor-responsive gene of murine BALB/c 3T3 cells encodes a protein homologous to human tissue factor. Mol Cell Biol. 1989;9:2567–73.
62. Toomey JR, Kratzer KE, Lasky NM, Stanton JJ, Broze Jr GJ. Targeted disruption of the murine tissue factor gene results in embryonic lethality. Blood. 1996;88:1583–7.
63. Taylor Jr FB, Chang A, Ruf W, Morrissey JH, Hinshaw L, Catlett R, Blick K, Edgington TS. Lethal E. coli septic shock is prevented by blocking tissue factor with monoclonal antibody. Circ Shock. 1991;33:127–34.
64. Gregory SA, Morrissey JH, Edgington TS. Regulation of tissue factor gene expression in the monocyte procoagulant response to endotoxin. Mol Cell Biol. 1989;9:2752–5.
65. Ritis K, Doumas M, Mastellos D, Micheli A, Giaglis S, Magotti P, Rafail S, Kartalis G, Sideras P, Lambris JD. A novel C5a receptor-tissue factor cross-talk in neutrophils links innate immunity to coagulation pathways. J Immunol. 2006;177:4794–802.
66. Hemker HC, Siepel T, Altman R, Loeliger EA. Kinetic aspects of the interaction of blood-clotting enzymes. II. The relation between clotting time and plasma concentration in prothrombin-time estimations. Thromb Diath Haemorrh. 1967;17(3–4): 349–57.
67. Salomon O, Steinberg D, Dardik R, Rosenberg N, Zivelin A, Tamarin I, Ravid B, Berliner S, Seligsohn U. Inherited factor XI deficiency confers no protection against acute myocardial infarction. J Thromb Haemost. 2003;1:658–61.
68. Doggen CJ, Rosendaal FR, Meijers JC. Levels of intrinsic coagulation factors and the risk of myocardial infarction among men: opposite and synergistic effects of factors XI and XII. Blood. 2006;108: 4045–51.
69. Gailani D, Renné T. The intrinsic pathway of coagulation: a target for treating thromboembolic disease? J Thromb Haemost. 2007;5:1106–12.
70. Naito K, Fujikawa K. Activation of human blood coagulation factor XI independent of factor XII. Factor XI is activated by thrombin and factor XIa in the presence of negatively charged surfaces. J Biol Chem. 1991;266:7353–8.
71. McGehee WG, Klotz TA, Epstein DJ, Rapaport SI. Coumarin necrosis associated with hereditary protein C deficiency. Ann Intern Med. 1984;101(1):59–60.
72. Gallop PM, Lian JB, Hauschka PV. Carboxylated calcium-binding proteins and vitamin K. N Engl J Med. 1980;302(26):1460–6.
73. Atoda H, Morita T. A novel blood coagulation factor IX/factor X-binding protein with anticoagulant activity from the venom of Trimeresurusflavoviridis (Habu snake): isolation and characterization. J Biochem. 1989;106(5):808–13.
74. Santacroce R, Sarno M, Cappucci F, Sessa F, Colaizzo D, Brancaccio V, Grandone E, Margaglione M. Low protein Z levels and risk of occurrence of deep vein thrombosis. J Thromb Haemost. 2006; 4(11):2417–22.
75. Stein PD, Fowler SE, Goodman LR, Gottschalk A, Hales CA, Hull RD, Leeper Jr KV, Popovich Jr J, Quinn DA, Sos TA, Sostman HD, Tapson VF, Wakefield TW, Weg JG, Woodard PK, PIOPED II Investigators. Multidectectorcomputed tomography for acute pulmonary embolism. N Engl J Med. 2006; 354(22):2317–27.
76. Kearon C, Kahn S, Agnelli G. Antithrombotic therapy for venous thromboembolic disease. Chest. 2008;133: 454S–545.

Anticoagulation for Venous Thromboembolism

21

Thomas L. Ortel

Contents

T.L. Ortel, MD, PhD
Departments of Medicine and Pathology,
Duke University Medical Center, Durham, NC, USA
e-mail: ortel001@mc.duke.edu

Abstract

Anticoagulation is a fundamental of management in venous disease. This chapter discusses anticoagulant therapy and a variety of agents. The current treatment for a new venous thromboembolic event in a patient is anticoagulant therapy, beginning with either unfractionated heparin (UFH) or low-molecular-weight heparin (LMWH), while warfarin is concomitantly initiated for chronic therapy.

21.1 Anticoagulant Therapy

The current treatment for a new venous thromboembolic event in a patient is anticoagulant therapy, beginning with either unfractionated heparin (UFH) or low-molecular-weight heparin (LMWH), while warfarin is concomitantly initiated for chronic therapy. Heparin is a polysulfated glycosaminoglycan prepared from porcine intestinal mucosa and bovine lung that exerts an anticoagulant effect by enhancing the inhibitory effect of antithrombin on thrombin, factor Xa, and other serine proteinases in the coagulation cascade (Fig. 21.1). LMWH is prepared from UFH by either chromatographic fractionation or enzymatic digestions to obtain smaller glycosaminoglycan chains that preferentially exert inhibitory activity against factor Xa instead of thrombin (Fig. 21.1). Enoxaparin, dalteparin, and tinzaparin are all LMWH that differ slightly in their relative anti-factor Xa/antithrombin activity, molecular weight, and

E. Mowatt-Larssen et al. (eds.), *Phlebology, Vein Surgery and Ultrasonography*,
DOI 10.1007/978-3-319-01812-6_21, © Springer International Publishing Switzerland 2014

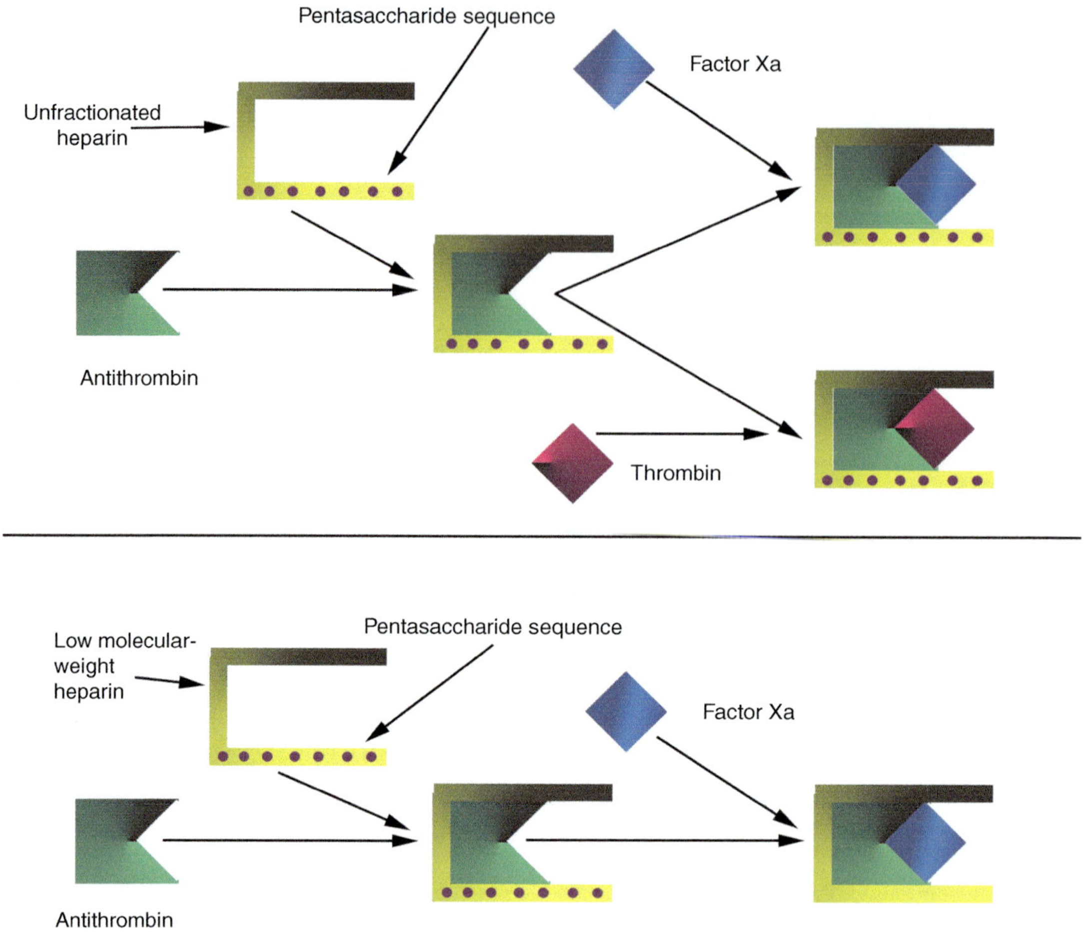

Fig. 21.1 Mechanism of action of unfractionated versus low-molecular-weight heparins (see text)

degree of clearance by the kidney. Fondaparinux is a synthetic pentasaccharide that exhibits inhibitory activity against factor Xa with only minimal effect on thrombin. Because of the mechanism whereby antithrombin inhibits factor Xa and thrombin, shorter glycosaminoglycan chains preferentially inhibit factor Xa rather than thrombin.

Warfarin exerts an anticoagulant effect by interfering with an essential posttranslational, vitamin K-dependent step that results in the gamma-carboxylation of specific glutamic acid residues in coagulation factors II, VII, IX, and X [1]. The resulting proteins exhibit dysfunctional calcium-dependent binding onto anionic phospholipid surfaces, interfering with rapid generation of thrombin. Warfarin and other vitamin K antagonists (e.g., dicoumarol, phenprocoumon, acenocoumarol) cause this effect by interfering with the cyclic conversion of vitamin K and its 2,3-epoxide, which blocks the regeneration of the reduced form of vitamin K1. Since the anticoagulant effect of warfarin is dependent on the synthesis of new, dysfunctional coagulation proteins, the antithrombotic efficacy of the drug is determined by the circulating half-life of the functional hemostatic proteins. The half-life of factor X is approximately 48 h and that of factor II is approximately 72 h; consequently, UFH or LMWH is used initially in the treatment of a patient with a new venous thromboembolism (VTE), generally for about 5 days, or until the anticoagulant effect of warfarin has sufficiently impacted the hemostatic proteins to manifest an antithrombotic effect.

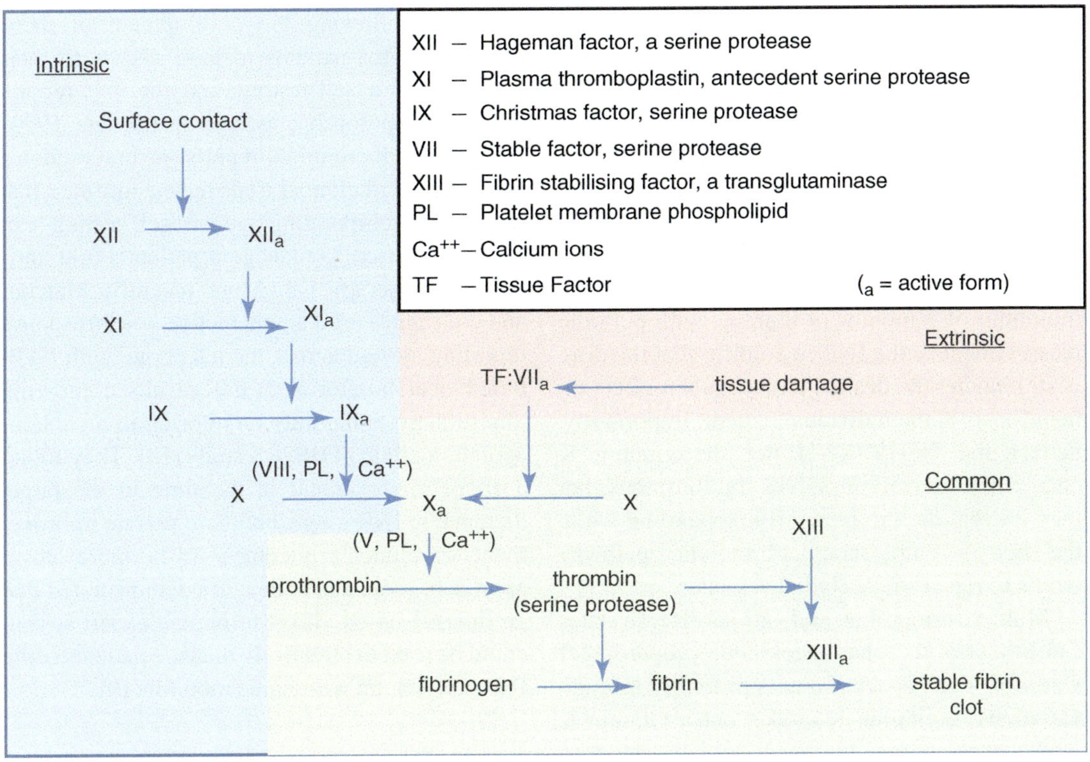

Fig. 21.2 Coagulation pathways (© Graham Colm, used with permission under the Creative Commons Atribution license)

21.2 Laboratory Monitoring of Anticoagulant Agents

For both UFH and the vitamin K antagonists, the therapeutic efficacy of the different agents has been shown to be optimal when a specific degree of anticoagulation, as measured by routine coagulation assays, has been achieved. For therapeutic UFH, the degree of anticoagulation is monitored by the activated partial thromboplastin time (aPTT), an assay that measures the intrinsic pathway of coagulation (Fig. 21.2). A subtherapeutic aPTT is associated with an increased risk of recurrent or progressive venous thromboembolism, whereas a supratherapeutic aPTT is associated with an increased risk of hemorrhage. Similarly, warfarin and the other vitamin K antagonists are also monitored for therapeutic efficacy, but in this case the test used is the prothrombin time (PT), an assay that measures the extrinsic pathway of coagulation (Fig. 21.2). To correct for variations in assay results due to differences in thromboplastin reagents and coagulometers, the PT is first converted to a ratio (patient PT by the mean of a normal range of PT values) that is then corrected with an adjustment factor to the international normalized ratio, or "INR." A target INR of 2–3 is the typical target range for treatment of patients with venous thromboembolism. As with UFH, subtherapeutic warfarin is associated with an increased risk for venous thromboembolism, whereas supratherapeutic warfarin is associated with an increased risk for hemorrhage.

The LMWH, although prepared from UFH, and with a similar, antithrombin-dependent, mechanism of action, does not need to be monitored for antithrombotic efficacy. These agents, typically administered subcutaneously with a weight-based dosage, exhibit a reproducible anticoagulant effect that does not require laboratory monitoring. They are cleared by the kidney, however, and can accumulate in patients with renal insufficiency. In this setting, checking anticoagulant efficacy can be performed using an anti-factor Xa assay.

21.3 Management Strategies

Patients with a new venous thromboembolism will be started on anticoagulation with UFH or LMWH concomitantly with a vitamin K antagonist, and the parenteral agent will be continued until the vitamin K antagonist is therapeutic as determined by the INR, at which time it will be stopped. Warfarin will then be continued for a minimum of 3 months of therapy, with periodic reassessment of the INR to confirm that the drug is still having the desired anticoagulant effect on hemostasis in the individual patient. Importantly, neither the UFH/LMWH nor the vitamin K antagonists actively dissolves the thrombus, but they prevent the thrombus from extending while the body's endogenous fibrinolytic pathway works to repair the occluded vessels.

Multiple drugs, diet, and various disease states can influence the pharmacokinetic properties of warfarin. The impact of diet is primarily through variations in vitamin K intake, but a vitamin K intake that is too low can actually lead to increased variation in the INR [2]. INR monitoring typically needs to be more frequent with medication or diet changes, and with certain illnesses. In addition to various acquired conditions, allelic variants have been identified in the genes encoding vitamin K epoxide reductase (VKORC1) and in the cytochrome P450 2C9 hepatic microsomal enzyme (CYP2C9) that modify the dose of warfarin necessary to achieve and maintain a target therapeutic INR [3, 4]. Dosing algorithms have been developed that incorporate the results of polymorphisms at CYP2C9 and VKOR1, but implementation of these algorithms more widely is dependent on completion of prospective randomized clinical trials with clinical outcome data.

Multiple studies have demonstrated that the optimal approach to therapeutic monitoring of the INR is through a dedicated anticoagulation management service rather than through routine medical care. Frequently, these anticoagulation management services will use a point-of-care monitor to measure the PT from a finger-stick sample of capillary whole blood to provide rapid access to necessary data for assessing the anticoagulant effect of the vitamin K antagonist. A natural extension following the development of these meters was for patients to have access to their own meter for self-testing, and the first reports using this approach appeared in the late 1980s [5, 6]. Since these initial reports, several randomized controlled clinical trials have confirmed that strategies incorporating patient self-testing can be reliably used to manage a patient's oral anticoagulant therapy [7]. More recently, Matchar and colleagues used an interactive voice-response reporting system across the telephone with Web-based local monitoring of INR results, comparing this strategy to monthly monitoring in an anticoagulation clinic (THINRS study) [8]. They found a slight improvement in the time in the target therapeutic INR range, but there was no improvement in clinical outcomes. In a more novel approach, Ryan and colleagues demonstrated that an Internet-based, direct-to-patient expert system could be used to effectively manage patients using INR self-testing with home monitors [9].

21.4 Complications of Anticoagulant Therapy

Hemorrhagic complications are the most frequent adverse event associated with the use of vitamin K antagonist therapy. Variables associated with an increased risk for therapy-related bleeding include the intensity of the anticoagulant effect (i.e., the target INR), the amount of time within the target INR (time in therapeutic range [TTR]), patient comorbidities, the concomitant use of drugs that interfere with hemostasis (e.g., antiplatelet agents), and the duration of therapy [1, 10]. The management of patients with elevated INR results is determined by the extent of the elevation of the INR, as well as whether or not the patient is having major bleeding (Table 21.1) [1]. Recently, Majeed and colleagues described 160 patients treated with prothrombin complex concentrates for emergency reversal of warfarin either for bleeding or the need for emergent surgery, demonstrating good clinical efficacy in more than 90 % of patients treated [11]. Thromboembolic complications were observed, but the frequency was relatively low (six patients, 3.8 %) [11]. Recombinant factor VIIa can also be

Table 21.1 Inherited thrombophilic disorders

Disorder	Prevalence in normals (%)	Frequency in patients with VTE (%)	Relative risk of first episode of DVT
Factor V Leiden (heterozygote)	0.05–4.8[a]	18.8	7
Factor V Leiden (homozygote)	0.02	1.5	80
Prothrombin G20210A allele	0.06–2.7[a]	7.1	2.8
Protein C deficiency	0.2–0.4	3.7	6.5
Protein S deficiency	0.16–0.21	2.3	5.0
Antithrombin deficiency	0.02	1.9	20
Dysfibrinogenemia	<0.01	0.8	Unknown
Elevated homocysteine levels[b]	5–7	10	2.95
Elevated factor VIII level	11	25	4.8
Elevated factor IX level	10	20	2.8
Elevated factor XI level	10	19	2.2
Elevated lipoprotein(a) level	7	20	3.2
Elevated thrombin-activatable fibrinolysis inhibitor (TAFI)	9	14	1.7

[a]Percent lowest in individuals of Asian or African descent, highest in individuals of Caucasian descent
[b]Greater than 18.5 mmol/L

used in the treatment of patients with hemorrhagic complications related to anticoagulant therapy, but its use in non-approved indications has been associated with an increased risk for thromboembolic complications [12]. The use of these agents in this setting needs to be individualized and managed by a clinician experienced in their use.

21.5 The Future of Vitamin K Antagonists

During the past decade, multiple new oral anticoagulants have been developed that do not require frequent laboratory monitoring or dose adjustments. These agents are not without their limitations, however, which are discussed further below. In addition, warfarin is one of the least expensive drugs, particularly when compared to other anticoagulant therapies. Although its management does incur significant health costs, these frequently involve different sources of funding. Consequently, certain patient populations are likely to continue use of warfarin and other vitamin K antagonists for some time, including patients with very stable INRs, patients with mechanical heart valves, and patients with limited financial resources.

21.6 Thrombolytic Therapy

In contrast to the passive reduction of thrombus size allowed by anticoagulant therapy, thrombolytic agents actively promote lysis of fibrin clot [13]. Although this approach is associated with an increased risk for bleeding, thrombolytic therapy should be considered in selected subsets of patients with venous thromboembolic disease [14]. Patients with extensive proximal deep venous thrombosis (DVT) (e.g., iliofemoral DVT) are at highest risk for postthrombotic morbidity, with up to 75 % having chronic painful edema and 40 % having venous claudication when treated with anticoagulant therapy alone (refs). Pharmacomechanical thrombolysis or catheter-directed thrombolysis, without mechanical thrombus fragmentation, would be the optimal approach in patients at low risk for hemorrhagic complications [14]. The ATTRACT (Acute Venous Thrombosis: Thrombus Removal with Adjunctive Catheter-Directed Thrombolysis) trial is a National Heart, Lung and Blood Institute (NHLBI)-sponsored prospective randomized trial that is comparing the use of adjunctive pharmacomechanical catheter-directed thrombolysis to optimal standard DVT therapy alone in patients with acute, symptomatic DVT (clinicaltrials.gov #NCT00790335). Importantly, this study will determine the development of postthrombotic syndrome to assess the development of this complication in patients treated with a more aggressive approach. For programs that lack expertise in interventional vascular procedures, systemic thrombolysis may be used in selected patients with acute DVT15, or the patient can be transferred to a center with the appropriate level of expertise [14].

Patients with pulmonary embolism (PE) should undergo risk stratification to evaluate for the role of thrombolytic therapy. For patients with massive acute pulmonary embolism, defined as acute PE with sustained hypotension, thrombolytic therapy should be considered unless there are contraindications owing to hemorrhagic risk [14]. Fibrinolysis may also be considered for patients with submassive acute PE who have additional clinical evidence of adverse prognosis and a low risk for hemorrhagic complications [14]. In contrast, patients with a low-risk PE, or submassive acute PE with minor right ventricular dysfunction or minor myocardial necrosis, should be treated with anticoagulant therapy and not fibrinolysis [14, 15]. Intravenous therapy via a peripheral vein is indicated in most patients who will be treated with thrombolysis [15].

21.6.1 Inferior Vena Cava Filter

The placement of a filter in the inferior vena cava (IVC) represents a strategy whereby pulmonary emboli (initial or recurrent) can be prevented in a patient who either cannot tolerate anticoagulant therapy (e.g., due to concomitant bleeding) or would be clinically compromised if a pulmonary embolism was sustained. It is important to recognize that these intravascular devices are not intended to treat a venous thromboembolic event but are designed to prevent thromboemboli from traveling to the pulmonary vasculature. Consequently, these devices have been shown to decrease the incidence of pulmonary emboli in the acute setting, but they are associated with an increased risk for IVC thrombosis in patients who are not on anticoagulant therapy with an IVC filter in place [16]. Retrievable filters are currently available and provide the option of subsequently removing the filter when it is no longer needed [17].

21.6.2 Duration of Therapy

Following completion of a standard course of anticoagulation, the next decision that must be made is whether anticoagulant therapy can be safely discontinued in the individual patient. Current evidence would suggest that the risk of recurrent VTE after stopping anticoagulant therapy is largely determined by two factors: (1) whether the acute episode of VTE has been effectively treated and (2) the patient's intrinsic risk of sustaining a new VTE [15]. Several studies have demonstrated that durations of therapy less than 3 months are associated with an increased risk for recurrent VTE, supporting the current overall recommendation for a minimal duration of therapy for acute VTE of 3 months [15]. The decision to continue therapy beyond 3 months should be based on an assessment of the continued benefit of anticoagulant therapy compared to the risk for bleeding, in addition to patient preference for continued anticoagulation or stopping therapy.

21.7 Spontaneous vs. Provoked Event

For patients with a VTE occurring in the setting of orthopedic surgery or other high-risk procedures, the risk of recurrent thromboembolic events after cessation of anticoagulant therapy is extremely low [18]. Consequently, the American College of Chest Physicians (ACCP) recommends that these patients only need 3 months of anticoagulant therapy which can be stopped after completion [15]. Patients who sustain VTE in the setting of other transient risk factors, such as during pregnancy or after other surgical procedures, also have a relatively low risk for recurrent VTE [18]. Conversely, other acquired risk factors are associated with an ongoing increased risk for recurrent VTE, such as antiphospholipid syndrome or malignancy, and patients with VTE and these conditions generally require chronic anticoagulant therapy. Acquired

Table 21.2 Recommendations for management of elevated INR results or bleeding in patients receiving vitamin K antagonist therapy

Condition	Intervention
INR above therapeutic range but <5.0; no significant bleeding	Decrease of hold dose; increase frequency of monitoring; if only minimally elevated, no dose reduction may be required
INR ≥5.0 but <9.0; no significant bleeding	Hold 1–2 doses, increase frequency of monitoring, and resume at lower dose when INR is in the therapeutic range. In addition, can give vitamin K if the patient is at an increased risk of bleeding or if the patient requires urgent surgery (typically 1–5 mg orally, depending on the indication)
INR ≥9.0; no significant bleeding	Hold warfarin therapy and give vitamin K; increase frequency of monitoring; give additional vitamin K if necessary. Resume therapy at a lower dose with INR therapeutic
Serious bleeding at any elevation of INR	Hold warfarin therapy and give vitamin K (10 mg by slow IV infusion). Depending on the urgency of the situation, may supplement with prothrombin complex concentrates, fresh frozen plasma, or recombinant factor VIIa. Vitamin K can be repeated every 12 h
Life-threatening bleeding	Hold warfarin therapy and give prothrombin complex concentrate or recombinant factor VIIa supplemented with vitamin K (10 mg by slow IV infusion); repeat if necessary depending on INR

Modified from Ansell et al. [1]

risk factors associated with an increase in the risk for VTE are listed in Table 21.2.

Patients who sustain a VTE in the absence of any acquired risk factors, on the other hand (referred to as “spontaneous” or “unprovoked” VTE), exhibit an increased risk for recurrent VTE after the cessation of anticoagulation [19]. The risk for recurrence has been reported to be as high as 22.6 % by 5 years after completion of therapy [20]. Consequently, the ACCP guidelines recommend that patients with a first unprovoked

Table 21.3 Acquired prothrombotic disorders

Antiphospholipid antibodies
Malignancy
Myeloproliferative disorders
Paroxysmal nocturnal hemoglobinuria
Nephrotic syndrome
Inflammatory bowel disease
Pregnancy/postpartum
Therapy-related (oral contraceptives, hormone replacement therapy)
Trauma
Surgery and the postoperative state
Prolonged bed rest or immobilization
Presence of a central venous catheter
Elevated homocysteine levels

VTE should receive treatment with a vitamin K antagonist for at least 3 months [15]. After 3 months of therapy has been completed, it is recommended that all patients should be evaluated for the risk-benefit ratio of continued anticoagulant therapy, and for those patients with a first unprovoked VTE that was a proximal DVT or PE, in whom risk factors for hemorrhage are minimal and for whom good anticoagulant monitoring is available, “long-term” treatment is recommended [15]. The definition of long-term frequently represents an indefinite course of therapy (or until hemorrhagic risk exceeds antithrombotic benefit), since patients who are treated with anticoagulant therapy for longer than 3 months exhibit the same risk for recurrent VTE as individuals treated for 3 months only [21].

Given the cumulative hemorrhagic risk associated with long-term anticoagulant therapy, investigators have studied multiple strategies to try and identify which patients are at low risk for recurrent VTE and could therefore safely stop anticoagulant therapy. Various approaches that have been used in this regard are summarized herewith.

21.8 Inherited Thrombophilia

Individuals who sustain an unprovoked VTE will frequently have an underlying inherited thrombophilic risk factor (Table 21.3) [22]. Common thrombophilic states, such as factor V Leiden or prothrombin G20210A, which may occur in as many as 20 and 9 % of patients with a first-time VTE, confer a relatively mild risk for recurrent venous thrombosis [23]. Deficiency states of the natural anticoagulant proteins antithrombin, protein C, or protein S confer a higher risk for recurrent VTE [24], and certain investigators have recommended that patients with these disorders might merit a longer course of anticoagulant therapy after an initial thrombotic event [25]. Elevated levels of coagulation factors, particularly factor VIII, can also be associated with an increased risk for VTE. When considering whether or not an individual patient could discontinue anticoagulation after a course of therapy has been completed, however, it is important to recognize that the *absence* of one of these disorders has not been found to identify a subset of individuals who appear to have a lower risk for recurrent VTE [26]. Consequently, thrombophilia evaluations, while identifying a potential risk factor for the initial event, are generally not particularly helpful when determining an individual patient's risk for recurrent VTE.

21.9 Gender

Multiple studies have demonstrated that men have a higher risk for recurrent VTE after an initial event than women [27]. This increased risk remains after adjustment for previous hormonal therapy-related VTE in women [19]. This difference in risk is not observed in patients with a provoked VTE [19].

21.10 D-Dimer

The D-dimer reflects an ongoing natural hemostatic process, fibrinolysis, which is enhanced in individuals presenting with an acute VTE. Thrombin converts fibrinogen to soluble fibrin, which forms soluble dimers, trimers, and larger multimers that eventually form an insoluble plug at the site of vascular injury. The strength of the nascent clot is then enhanced by cross-linking of individual fibrin molecules to one another by the transglutaminase factor XIIIa. The clot is subsequently remodeled and broken down by plasmin, which cleaves the cross-linked mass of fibrin, releasing various fragments into the circulation. The D-dimer is one of these degradation products, consisting of two D-domains originating from two different fibrin molecules that were cross-linked to one another and then released from the fibrin clot by the process of fibrinolysis.

In patients with an acute VTE, the D-dimer is characteristically markedly elevated, reflecting ongoing thrombus formation and endogenous fibrinolysis. In fact, the presence of a normal D-dimer level in a patient with a low clinical suspicion for VTE can effectively rule out that diagnosis [28]. Several recent studies have shown that the presence of an elevated D-dimer level while on anticoagulant therapy, or the new development of an elevated D-dimer level after anticoagulation has been stopped, is associated with an increased risk for recurrent VTE [29]. Neither the timing of measurement of the D-dimer after stopping anticoagulation nor the age of the individual patient affected the ability of this test to detect patients at an increased risk for recurrent VTE [30]. Furthermore, patients with an elevated D-dimer level who continue (or resume) anticoagulant therapy exhibit a lower risk for recurrent thromboembolic events, in some cases even lower than the risk for recurrence observed in individuals with a normal D-dimer level after stopping anticoagulation [31]. Consequently, the D-dimer does appear to be a useful laboratory test in the assessment of risk for recurrent VTE after an initial event.

21.11 Residual Venous Thrombosis

Several investigators have studied the role of residual venous thrombosis as a predictor for patients at risk of recurrent VTE. Patients with no evidence for residual vein thrombosis identified at the completion of 3 months of anticoagulant therapy exhibited a very-low risk for recurrent VTE in the Duration of Anticoagulation based on Compression UltraSonography (DACUS) study [32]. In addition, those patients with residual vein obstruction detected exhibited a lower incidence of recurrent VTE if they continued anticoagulant therapy, supporting the concept of an extended course of therapy [32]. In contrast, the REVERSE investigators found that the presence of residual vein obstruction at the time of withdrawal of oral anticoagulant therapy was not associated with a statistically higher risk of recurrent VTE in a cohort study [33]. A systematic review and meta-analysis of 14 studies (five randomized controlled trials and nine cohort studies) found that residual vein obstruction was associated with a modestly increased risk for recurrent VTE in all patients (provoked and unprovoked), but not in unprovoked patients alone [34]. Limitations to this analysis included a lack of standardization of how residual vein obstruction should be assessed and prior reports of poor interobserver agreement [34]. Further prospective studies are necessary to assess the role of residual vein obstruction in patients with DVT.

21.12 Prediction Rules

In an effort to improve the predictive value of the above variables in identifying patients who are at low risk for recurrent VTE and may therefore safely stop anticoagulation, several investigators have explored the development of prediction "rules" based on the presence of one or more of these identified predictors. Rodger and colleagues [35] collected data on 646 participants with a first, unprovoked major VTE enrolled over a 4-year period in a multicenter prospective cohort study (the REVERSE study). Information collected included data about demographic characteristics, risk factors at the time of the initial event, post-thrombotic symptoms, concomitant medications, results of thrombophilia testing, and imaging reports confirming the initial event. After completion of a standard course of anticoagulant therapy (5–7 months), anticoagulation was stopped and the participants were followed for recurrent VTE. Women who had none or only one of the following characteristics exhibited a low risk for recurrent VTE (annual risk 1.6, 95 % confidence interval [CI] 0.3–4.6 %): hyperpigmentation, edema or redness of either leg, elevated D-dimer level while taking warfarin, body mass index ≥30 kg/m^2, or age ≥65 years. Women with two or more of these characteristics had an annual risk of recurrent VTE of 14.1 % (95 % CI, 10.9–17.3 %). Men had a high risk for recurrent VTE (annual risk 13.7, 95 % CI 10.8–17.0 %), and no combination of clinical predictors could identify a subset of males at low risk for recurrent VTE.

Eichinger and colleagues [36] took a similar approach, enrolling 929 participants with a first unprovoked VTE and following them after a standard course of anticoagulant therapy. This study differed from the REVERSE study in that patients with a "strong" thrombophilic defect, such as a deficiency of antithrombin, protein C, or protein S, a lupus anticoagulant, or homozygous or combined defects involving other thrombophilic disorders (e.g., factor V Leiden, prothrombin G20210A). A higher risk for recurrent VTE was associated with male sex (hazard ratio vs. female sex 1.90, 95 % CI 1.31–2.75), proximal DVT (hazard ratio vs. distal DVT 2.08, 95 % CI 1.16–3.74), pulmonary embolism (hazard ratio vs. distal DVT 2.60, 95 % CI 1.49–4.53), and elevated levels of D-dimer (hazard ratio per doubling of the result 1.27, 95 % CI 1.08–1.51). These variables were combined to develop a nomogram to predict risk for recurrent VTE, and cross-validation of the model demonstrated that recurrence rates corresponded with the different risk categories.

21.13 Intensity of Anticoagulation with Vitamin K Antagonists in Patients on Extended Therapy for VTE

For patients who are determined to be at higher risk for recurrent VTE, anticoagulant therapy with warfarin would be continued indefinitely until the risk for hemorrhage exceeds the benefit of continued anticoagulation, or the patient desires to stop therapy. The optimal intensity of the anticoagulant effect with vitamin K antagonists has been investigated through several randomized trials. The Extended Low-Intensity Anticoagulation for Thromboembolism (ELATE) study was a randomized blinded trial that compared conventional-intensity vitamin K antagonist therapy (target INR range: 2.0–3.0) to a low-intensity regimen (target INR range: 1.5–1.9) [37]. This study found that the low-intensity vitamin K antagonist therapy was significantly less effective than conventional-intensity therapy without providing a safety advantage with decreased bleeding [37]. In contrast, the Prevention of Recurrent Venous Thromboembolism (PREVENT) study compared low-intensity warfarin therapy (target INR range: 1.5–2.0) with placebo and found that low-intensity therapy did significantly decrease the risk for recurrent VTE, without increasing the risk for major hemorrhage [38]. One potential advantage of the low-intensity regimen in the PREVENT study was the decreased need for INR measurements, making therapeutic monitoring less burdensome to patients and healthcare providers [38]. Long-term anticoagulant therapy for patients with VTE may be simplified even further, however, with the arrival of the new oral anticoagulants.

21.14 New Anticoagulants

Warfarin and related vitamin K antagonists have been the only oral anticoagulants available for more than 50 years. Although these agents are effective in the prevention and treatment of venous thromboembolism, they have various limitations that can complicate their safe and effective use. In particular, as a narrow therapeutic index agent, the anticoagulant effect of the vitamin K antagonists needs to be regularly monitored with the prothrombin time (PT), a test of the extrinsic pathway of hemostasis. A subtherapeutic level is associated with an increased risk for recurrent thrombosis, whereas a supratherapeutic level is associated with an increased risk for hemorrhagic complications. To facilitate comparison of PT results obtained with different coagulation reagents and different coagulometers, the international normalized ratio (INR) was developed. Although the INR substantially improved the ability to use the PT to monitor warfarin therapy, there are limitations to its use, including in certain patients with lupus anticoagulants and in patients with liver disease. Other limitations associated with the vitamin K antagonists include the necessity to maintain a relatively consistent amount of vitamin K in the diet (to minimize fluctuations in the INR) and the need to reevaluate a patient's anticoagulant status whenever a new medication is initiated.

Because of these various limitations and the desire to have an oral anticoagulant that did not need to be monitored for therapeutic efficacy and safety, investigators have explored multiple therapeutic agents as alternatives to warfarin. One approach that was particularly attractive was to specifically target individual components of the hemostatic mechanism with small molecule inhibitors that could be administered orally. Direct inhibition of thrombin has been known to be an effective antithrombotic strategy since the initial characterization of hirudin, a 65 amino acid protein isolated from leech saliva that binds to and neutralizes thrombin by forming noncovalent, yet irreversible, 1:1 complexes [39].

Although three parenteral direct thrombin inhibitors have been available for more than a dozen years, lepirudin and argatroban are seldom used except in patients suspected of having heparin-induced thrombocytopenia (HIT), and bivalirudin is primarily limited to patients with HIT or patients undergoing percutaneous coronary interventions. An important limitation to all three of these therapies is the lack of a specific antidote for reversal of the anticoagulant effect, a limitation shared with the new oral factor-specific therapies described below.

21.14.1 Ximelagatran

Ximelagatran is an orally administered direct thrombin inhibitor that is rapidly absorbed and converted to its active form, melagatran. Ximelagatran, administered as a fixed dose without coagulation monitoring, was shown to be as effective as enoxaparin/warfarin for the treatment of deep vein thrombosis, with or without pulmonary embolism [40]. Bleeding rates were low, but increased levels of liver enzymes were noted in 9.6 % of ximelagatran-treated patients, a problem which ultimately contributed to the decision by the Food and Drug Administration (FDA) not to approve the drug in the United

States. In addition, a retrospective analysis of adverse events revealed a higher rate of serious coronary events with ximelagatran compared with enoxaparin/warfarin [40]. After a brief release in Europe for use as a thromboprophylactic agent following hip or knee surgery, ximelagatran was withdrawn from the market and has not been further studied.

21.14.2 Dabigatran

Dabigatran etexilate is an oral prodrug that is rapidly converted after hepatic processing to dabigatran, which directly inhibits both free and clot-bound thrombin (Table 21.3). Dabigatran has been extensively investigated in the prevention of thromboembolism after orthopedic surgery and in the prevention of stroke or peripheral embolism in patients with atrial fibrillation [41]. Dabigatran became the first of the new oral anticoagulants to be approved for use in the United States in October 2010, when it was approved for use in patients with atrial fibrillation. Since dabigatran is predominantly eliminated by the kidneys, patients with renal insufficiency (creatinine clearance <30 mL/min) should be treated with a lower dose of the drug.

Dabigatran has also been studied in the treatment of patients with acute venous thromboembolism [42]. In this randomized, double-blind, non-inferiority trial, patients with acute VTE were initially treated with a parenteral anticoagulant (heparin or low-molecular-weight heparin) followed by 6 months of therapy with either dabigatran (150 mg twice daily) or warfarin with a target INR range of 2.0–3.0. Dabigatran was as effective as warfarin in preventing recurrent VTE during the course of therapy, with a similar frequency of bleeding events [42]. The numbers of deaths, acute coronary syndromes, and abnormal liver function studies were similar in the two groups, but a slightly increased number of patients discontinued study drug in the dabigatran arm compared to the warfarin arm ($p=0.05$) [42]. Dabigatran has also been shown to be effective as an alternative to warfarin for extended maintenance anticoagulant therapy for patients with VTE [43].

Although routine monitoring of coagulation assays is not necessary for patients taking dabigatran, there are certain clinical settings in which it would be potentially useful to be able to assess the anticoagulant effect in a given patient (e.g., with recurrent VTE or bleeding, or prior to a surgical procedure). Since it inhibits thrombin, dabigatran does have an effect on all of the routine coagulation assays. At clinically relevant plasma concentrations, dabigatran has relatively little effect on the PT or INR [44]. There is considerable variation in sensitivities for different thromboplastin reagents, with Innovin® being one of the more sensitive reagents [45]. Prolongation of the aPTT occurs with increasing dabigatran concentration, but the concentration-response curve is curvilinear and flattens at higher concentrations [44]. The thrombin time is particularly sensitive to the presence of dabigatran, and a diluted form of the thrombin time has been developed as a sensitive assay that spans the therapeutic range of the drug [44]. The ecarin clotting time (ECT) also provides a linear relationship with dabigatran concentration, but this assay is not widely available. At peak concentrations, the fibrinogen concentration may be considerably underestimated with certain fibrinogen reagents using a Clauss-type clotting assay [45]. When interpreting a coagulation assay obtained from a patient on dabigatran therapy, it is important to note the time of blood sampling in relation to drug administration, given the relatively short half-life and the notable differences obtained at peak and trough levels of the drug.

One potential drawback to therapy with dabigatran is the lack of an antidote. Regardless of the relatively short half-life of the drug, immediate reversal of the anticoagulant effect may be needed in case of major bleeding or emergency surgery. Protamine sulfate and vitamin K are not expected to affect the anticoagulant activity of dabigatran. Similarly, there is neither expected benefit nor experience with other systemic hemostatic agents, such as desmopressin, aprotinin, aminocaproic acid, or tranexamic acid. Prothrombin complex concentrate, but not recombinant factor VIIa, was shown to be effective in preventing hematoma expansion in a murine

Table 21.4 Oral direct thrombin and factor Xa inhibitors

	Dabigatran	Apixaban	Rivaroxaban	Edoxaban
Target	Thrombin	Factor Xa	Factor Xa	Factor Xa
Time to maximum plasma concentration	1.25–3 h	1–3 h	2–4 h	1–4 h
Half-life	12–14 h	8–15 h	9–13 h	9–11 h
Renal excretion	80 %	~25 %	66 %	~35 %
Food effect	Delays absorption	No effect	Delays absorption	No effect
Effect on thrombin time	Prolonged	Normal	Normal	Normal
Effect on PT	Prolonged	Prolonged	Prolonged	Prolonged
Effect on aPTT	Prolonged	Prolonged	Prolonged	Prolonged
Anti-factor Xa activity	None	Present	Present	Present
Substrate of cytochrome P450 enzymes	No	Yes (CYP3A4, CYP2J2)	Yes (CYP3A4)	Yes (CYP3A4)
Substrate of P-glycoprotein drug transporter	Yes	Yes	Yes	Yes

model of intracerebral hemorrhage associated with dabigatran [46]. In contrast, administration of a four-component prothrombin complex concentrate (Cofact) had relatively little effect on the prolonged coagulation assays in healthy subjects taking dabigatran [47]. Dabigatran is dialyzable due to its relatively low (approximately 35 %) plasma protein binding and hemodialysis could be potentially effective in accelerating plasma clearance of dabigatran [44].

21.14.3 Rivaroxaban

Rivaroxaban is an oral agent that directly inhibits factor Xa, both in its free form, as well as in the prothrombinase complex (Table 21.4) [48]. As with dabigatran, it has been studied for the prevention of venous thromboembolism following orthopedic surgery, the prevention of stroke and peripheral arterial thromboembolism in patients with atrial fibrillation, and in the treatment of patients with venous thromboembolism. It is currently available in the USA for thromboprophylaxis following total hip or knee arthroplasty.

Rivaroxaban was studied in an open label, randomized, event-driven, non-inferiority study that compared oral rivaroxaban alone with subcutaneous enoxaparin followed by vitamin K antagonist therapy in patients with acute, symptomatic DVT [49]. A total of 3,449 patients were enrolled, and rivaroxaban was non-inferior in efficacy with respect to the primary outcome of recurrent VTE (36 events [2.1 %] vs. 51 events with enoxaparin/vitamin K antagonist [3.0 %]; hazard ratio, 0.68; 95 % CI, 0.44–1.04, $P<.001$). Major bleeding and clinically relevant nonmajor bleeding events were similar in both treatment groups. In a parallel study, rivaroxaban alone was compared to placebo for an additional 6–12 months of therapy after completion of an initial 6–12 months of anticoagulation. In this study, rivaroxaban had superior efficacy compared to placebo, although there was an increase in nonfatal major bleeding in the rivaroxaban group compared to the placebo group.

In contrast to dabigatran, rivaroxaban has no effect on the ecarin clotting time or the thrombin time, since its inhibitory effect is at the level of factor Xa. Rivaroxaban does prolong the PT, but the response varies markedly with different thromboplastin reagents [50]. Prolongation of the aPTT also varies with different reagents, although the effect on the aPTT is relatively weak at lower concentrations of rivaroxaban [50]. The fibrinogen content, measured with a Clauss-type fibrinogen assay, was almost unaffected by rivaroxaban in plasma [50]. One approach that may prove useful for evaluating patients on rivaroxaban therapy would be an anti-factor Xa assay, similar to the assay used for assessing low-molecular-weight heparins.

As with dabigatran, there is no antidote for the anticoagulant effect of rivaroxaban. The four-component prothrombin complex concentrate Cofact immediately and completely reversed the prolonged PT in healthy subjects on rivaroxaban therapy [47]. In contrast to dabigatran, rivaroxaban is highly protein-bound and therefore not removed by dialysis [51].

21.14.4 Apixaban

Apixaban is an orally available direct factor Xa inhibitor that inhibits free factor Xa, as well as factor Xa in the prothrombinase complex. It has been extensively studied in patients with atrial fibrillation and is a safe and effective alternative to warfarin for these patients [52]. The safety and efficacy of apixaban in the treatment of patients with an acute VTE is currently being studied (Clinicaltrials.gov #NCT00643201). Apixaban has also been studied in patients with an acute coronary syndrome, but the addition of apixaban with antiplatelet agents was associated with an increased risk for major bleeding without a significant reduction in recurrent ischemic events [53].

Apixaban prolongs the PT in a concentration-dependent manner which varied for the different reagents, but the sensitivity of the PT for apixaban is low [54]. In addition, converting the PT values to INR did not reduce the variability between different thromboplastin reagents, but actually produced a wider spread of values [54]. An anti-factor Xa assay provided linear results that correlated with apixaban plasma concentrations measured by liquid chromatography/mass spectrometry [54]. Similar results were obtained in a pharmacokinetic/pharmacodynamics substudy of the APPRAISE-1 study, with anti-factor Xa activity, determined by either an anti-factor Xa/LMWH or anti-factor Xa/apixaban method correlating strongly and linearly with apixaban plasma concentrations [55].

No data are available concerning the management of bleeding episodes in patients on apixaban therapy, although similar strategies as used for patients on rivaroxaban would appear to be reasonable.

21.14.5 Edoxaban

Edoxaban is an orally available, highly specific direct inhibitor of factor Xa. It has been studied in Phase 2 studies investigating safety and efficacy as a thromboprophylactic agent in patients undergoing total hip arthroplasty [56, 57]. It is currently being investigated in a prospective, randomized, double-blind trial in the treatment of patients with acute VTE (Clinicaltrials.gov #NCT00986154). The PT, aPTT, and anti-factor Xa assays are all prolonged with Edoxaban [58], although studies with multiple reagents have not been performed.

The new oral anticoagulant agents will open a new chapter in the treatment of patients with VTE, both in the acute setting and with chronic therapy. Warfarin is likely to be around for years to come, however, for a variety of reasons. Development of clinical laboratory strategies to quickly distinguish these therapeutic agents, as well as to assess anticoagulant effect, will be essential for managing hemorrhagic, as well as recurrent thromboembolic complications related to these drugs.

References

1. Ansell J, Hirsh J, Hylek E, Jacobson A, Crowther M, Palareti G. Pharmacology and management of the vitamin K antagonists: American College of Chest Physicians Evidence-Based Clinical Practice Guidelines (8th Edition). Chest. 2008;133(6 Suppl):160S–98S.
2. Kim KH, Choi WS, Lee JH, Lee H, Yang DH, Chae SC. Relationship between dietary vitamin K intake and the stability of anticoagulation effect in patients taking long-term warfarin. Thromb Haemost. 2010;104(4):755–9.
3. Sanderson S, Emery J, Higgins J. CYP2C9 gene variants, drug dose, and bleeding risk in warfarin-treated patients: a HuGEnet systematic review and meta-analysis. Genet Med. 2005;7(2):97–104.
4. Yang L, Ge W, Yu F, Zhu H. Impact of VKORC1 gene polymorphism on interindividual and interethnic warfarin dosage requirement – a systematic review and meta analysis. Thromb Res. 2010;125(4):e159–66.
5. White RH, McCurdy SA, von Marensdorff H, Woodruff Jr DE, Leftgoff L. Home prothrombin time monitoring after the initiation of warfarin therapy. A randomized, prospective study. Ann Intern Med. 1989;111(9):730–7.
6. Ansell J, Holden A, Knapic N. Patient self-management of oral anticoagulation guided by capillary (fingerstick) whole blood prothrombin times. Arch Intern Med. 1989;149(11):2509–11.

7. Heneghan C, Alonso-Coello P, Garcia-Alamino JM, Perera R, Meats E, Glasziou P. Self-monitoring of oral anticoagulation: a systematic review and meta-analysis. Lancet. 2006;367(9508):404–11.
8. Matchar DB, Jacobson A, Dolor R, Edson R, Uyeda L, Phibbs CS, et al. Effect of home testing of international normalized ratio on clinical events. N Engl J Med. 2010;363(17):1608–20.
9. Ryan F, Byrne S, O'Shea S. Randomized controlled trial of supervised patient self-testing of warfarin therapy using an internet-based expert system. J Thromb Haemost. 2009;7(8):1284–90.
10. Schulman S, Beyth RJ, Kearon C, Levine MN. Hemorrhagic complications of anticoagulant and thrombolytic treatment: American College of Chest Physicians Evidence-Based Clinical Practice Guidelines (8th Edition). Chest. 2008;133(6 Suppl): 257S–98S.
11. Majeed A, Eelde A, Agren A, Schulman S, Holmstrom M. Thromboembolic safety and efficacy of prothrombin complex concentrates in the emergency reversal of warfarin coagulopathy. Thromb Res. 2012;129: 146–51.
12. O'Connell KA, Wood JJ, Wise RP, Lozier JN, Braun MM. Thromboembolic adverse events after use of recombinant human coagulation factor VIIa. JAMA. 2006;295(3):293–8.
13. Bell WR. Present-day thrombolytic therapy: therapeutic agents – pharmacokinetics and pharmacodynamics. Rev Cardiovasc Med. 2002;3 Suppl 2:S34–44.
14. Jaff MR, McMurtry MS, Archer SL, Cushman M, Goldenberg N, Goldhaber SZ, et al. Management of massive and submassive pulmonary embolism, iliofemoral deep vein thrombosis, and chronic thromboembolic pulmonary hypertension: a scientific statement from the American Heart Association. Circulation. 2011;123(16):1788–830.
15. Kearon C, Kahn SR, Agnelli G, Goldhaber S, Raskob GE, Comerota AJ. Antithrombotic therapy for venous thromboembolic disease: American College of Chest Physicians Evidence-Based Clinical Practice Guidelines (8th Edition). Chest. 2008;133(6 Suppl): 454S–545S.
16. Decousus H, Leizorovicz A, Parent F, Page Y, Tardy B, Girard P, et al. A clinical trial of vena caval filters in the prevention of pulmonary embolism in patients with proximal deep-vein thrombosis. Prevention du Risqued'EmboliePulmonaire par Interruption Cave Study Group. N Engl J Med. 1998;338(7):409–15.
17. Mismetti P, Rivron-Guillot K, Quenet S, Decousus H, Laporte S, Epinat M, et al. A prospective long-term study of 220 patients with a retrievable vena cava filter for secondary prevention of venous thromboembolism. Chest. 2007;131(1):223–9.
18. Baglin T, Luddington R, Brown K, Baglin C. Incidence of recurrent venous thromboembolism in relation to clinical and thrombophilic risk factors: prospective cohort study. Lancet. 2003;362(9383):523–6.
19. Douketis J, Tosetto A, Marcucci M, Baglin T, Cosmi B, Cushman M, et al. Risk of recurrence after venous thromboembolism in men and women: patient level meta-analysis. BMJ. 2011;342:d813.
20. Baglin T, Douketis J, Tosetto A, Marcucci M, Cushman M, Kyrle P, et al. Does the clinical presentation and extent of venous thrombosis predict likelihood and type of recurrence? A patient-level meta-analysis. J Thromb Haemost. 2010;8(11):2436–42.
21. Boutitie F, Pinede L, Schulman S, Agnelli G, Raskob G, Julian J, et al. Influence of preceding length of anticoagulant treatment and initial presentation of venous thromboembolism on risk of recurrence after stopping treatment: analysis of individual participants' data from seven trials. BMJ. 2011;342:d3036.
22. Crowther MA, Kelton JG. Congenital thrombophilic states associated with venous thrombosis: a qualitative overview and proposed classification system. Ann Intern Med. 2003;138(2):128–34.
23. Ho WK, Hankey GJ, Quinlan DJ, Eikelboom JW. Risk of recurrent venous thromboembolism in patients with common thrombophilia: a systematic review. Arch Intern Med. 2006;166(7):729–36.
24. van den Belt AG, Sanson BJ, Simioni P, Prandoni P, Buller HR, Girolami A, et al. Recurrence of venous thromboembolism in patients with familial thrombophilia. Arch Intern Med. 1997;157(19):2227–32.
25. Brouwer JL, Lijfering WM, Ten Kate MK, Kluin-Nelemans HC, Veeger NJ, van der Meer J. High long-term absolute risk of recurrent venous thromboembolism in patients with hereditary deficiencies of protein S, protein C or antithrombin. Thromb Haemost. 2009; 101(1):93–9.
26. Christiansen SC, Cannegieter SC, Koster T, Vandenbroucke JP, Rosendaal FR. Thrombophilia, clinical factors, and recurrent venous thrombotic events. JAMA. 2005;293(19):2352–61.
27. McRae S, Tran H, Schulman S, Ginsberg J, Kearon C. Effect of patient's sex on risk of recurrent venous thromboembolism: a meta-analysis. Lancet. 2006; 368(9533):371–8.
28. Kearon C, Ginsberg JS, Douketis J, Turpie AG, Bates SM, Lee AY, et al. An evaluation of D-dimer in the diagnosis of pulmonary embolism: a randomized trial. Ann Intern Med. 2006;144(11):812–21.
29. Verhovsek M, Douketis JD, Yi Q, Shrivastava S, Tait RC, Baglin T, et al. Systematic review: D-dimer to predict recurrent disease after stopping anticoagulant therapy for unprovoked venous thromboembolism. Ann Intern Med. 2008;149(7):481–90, W94.
30. Douketis J, Tosetto A, Marcucci M, Baglin T, Cushman M, Eichinger S, et al. Patient-level meta-analysis: effect of measurement timing, threshold, and patient age on ability of D-dimer testing to assess recurrence risk after unprovoked venous thromboembolism. Ann Intern Med. 2010;153(8):523–31.
31. Palareti G, Cosmi B, Legnani C, Tosetto A, Brusi C, Iorio A, et al. D-dimer testing to determine the duration of anticoagulation therapy. N Engl J Med. 2006;355(17):1780–9.
32. Siragusa S, Malato A, Anastasio R, Cigna V, Milio G, Amato C, et al. Residual vein thrombosis to establish duration of anticoagulation after a first episode of deep vein thrombosis: the Duration of Anticoagulation based on Compression UltraSonography (DACUS) study. Blood. 2008;112(3):511–5.

33. Le Gal G, Carrier M, Kovacs MJ, Betancourt MT, Kahn SR, Wells PS, et al. Residual vein obstruction as a predictor for recurrent thromboembolic events after a first unprovoked episode: data from the REVERSE cohort study. J Thromb Haemost. 2011;9(6): 1126–32.
34. Carrier M, Rodger MA, Wells PS, Righini M, LEG G. Residual vein obstruction to predict the risk of recurrent venous thromboembolism in patients with deep vein thrombosis: a systematic review and meta-analysis. J Thromb Haemost. 2011;9(6):1119–25.
35. Rodger MA, Kahn SR, Wells PS, Anderson DA, Chagnon I, Le Gal G, et al. Identifying unprovoked thromboembolism patients at low risk for recurrence who can discontinue anticoagulant therapy. CMAJ. 2008;179(5):417–26.
36. Eichinger S, Heinze G, Jandeck LM, Kyrle PA. Risk assessment of recurrence in patients with unprovoked deep vein thrombosis or pulmonary embolism: the Vienna prediction model. Circulation. 2010;121(14): 1630–6.
37. Kearon C, Ginsberg JS, Kovacs MJ, Anderson DR, Wells P, Julian JA, et al. Comparison of low-intensity warfarin therapy with conventional-intensity warfarin therapy for long-term prevention of recurrent venous thromboembolism. N Engl J Med. 2003;349(7): 631–9.
38. Ridker PM, Goldhaber SZ, Danielson E, Rosenberg Y, Eby CS, Deitcher SR, et al. Long-term, low-intensity warfarin therapy for the prevention of recurrent venous thromboembolism. N Engl J Med. 2003;348(15):1425–34.
39. Greinacher A, Warkentin TE. The direct thrombin inhibitor hirudin. Thromb Haemost. 2008;99(5): 819–29.
40. Fiessinger JN, Huisman MV, Davidson BL, Bounameaux H, Francis CW, Eriksson H, et al. Ximelagatran vs low-molecular-weight heparin and warfarin for the treatment of deep vein thrombosis: a randomized trial. JAMA. 2005;293(6): 681–9.
41. Connolly SJ, Ezekowitz MD, Yusuf S, Eikelboom J, Oldgren J, Parekh A, et al. Dabigatran versus warfarin in patients with atrial fibrillation. N Engl J Med. 2009;361(12):1139–51.
42. Schulman S, Kearon C, Kakkar AK, Mismetti P, Schellong S, Eriksson H, et al. Dabigatran versus warfarin in the treatment of acute venous thromboembolism. N Engl J Med. 2009;361(24):2342–52.
43. Schulman S, Eriksson H, Goldhaber SZ, Kakkar AK, Kearon C, Kvamme AM, et al. Dabigatran or warfarin for extended maintenance therapy of venous thromboembolism. J ThrombHaemost. 2011:O-TH-033.
44. Van Ryn J, Stangier J, Haertter S, Liesenfeld KH, Wienen W, Feuring M, et al. Dabigatran etexilate – a novel, reversible, oral direct thrombin inhibitor: interpretation of coagulation assays and reversal of anticoagulant activity. Thromb Haemost. 2010;103(6):1116–27.
45. Lindahl TL, Baghaei F, Blixter IF, Gustafsson KM, Stigendal L, Sten-Linder M, et al. Effects of the oral, direct thrombin inhibitor dabigatran on five common coagulation assays. Thromb Haemost. 2011;105(2): 371–8.
46. Zhou W, Schwarting S, Illanes S, Liesz A, Middelhoff M, Zorn M, et al. Hemostatic therapy in experimental intracerebral hemorrhage associated with the direct thrombin inhibitor dabigatran. Stroke. 2011;42: 3594–9.
47. Eerenberg ES, Kamphuisen PW, Sijpkens MK, Meijers JC, Buller HR, Levi M. Reversal of rivaroxaban and dabigatran by prothrombin complex concentrate: a randomized, placebo-controlled, crossover study in healthy subjects. Circulation. 2011;124(14):1573–9.
48. Orfeo T, Butenas S, Brummel-Ziedins KE, Gissel M, Mann KG. Anticoagulation by factor Xa inhibitors. J Thromb Haemost. 2010;8(8):1745–53.
49. Bauersachs R, Berkowitz SD, Brenner B, Buller HR, Decousus H, Gallus AS, et al. Oral rivaroxaban for symptomatic venous thromboembolism. N Engl J Med. 2010;363(26):2499–510.
50. Hillarp A, Baghaei F, FagerbergBlixter I, Gustafsson KM, Stigendal L, Sten-Linder M, et al. Effects of the oral, direct factor Xa inhibitor rivaroxaban on commonly used coagulation assays. J Thromb Haemost. 2011;9(1):133–9.
51. Romualdi E, Rancan E, Siragusa S, Ageno W. Managing bleeding complications in patients treated with the old and the new anticoagulants. Curr Pharm Des. 2010;16(31):3478–82.
52. Granger CB, Alexander JH, McMurray JJ, Lopes RD, Hylek EM, Hanna M, et al. Apixaban versus warfarin in patients with atrial fibrillation. N Engl J Med. 2011;365(11):981–92.
53. Alexander JH, Lopes RD, James S, Kilaru R, He Y, Mohan P, et al. Apixaban with antiplatelet therapy after acute coronary syndrome. N Engl J Med. 2011;365(8):699–708.
54. Barrett YC, Wang Z, Frost C, Shenker A. Clinical laboratory measurement of direct factor Xa inhibitors: anti-Xa assay is preferable to prothrombin time assay. Thromb Haemost. 2010;104(6):1263–71.
55. Becker RC, Yang H, Barrett Y, Mohan P, Wang J, Wallentin L, et al. Chromogenic laboratory assays to measure the factor Xa-inhibiting properties of apixaban – an oral, direct and selective factor Xa inhibitor. J Thromb Thrombolysis. 2011;32(2):183–7.
56. Weitz JI, Connolly SJ, Patel I, Salazar D, Rohatagi S, Mendell J, et al. Randomised, parallel-group, multicentre, multinational phase 2 study comparing edoxaban, an oral factor Xa inhibitor, with warfarin for stroke prevention in patients with atrial fibrillation. Thromb Haemost. 2010;104(3):633–41.
57. Raskob G, Cohen AT, Eriksson BI, Puskas D, Shi M, Bocanegra T, et al. Oral direct factor Xa inhibition with edoxaban for thromboprophylaxis after elective total hip replacement. A randomised double-blind dose–response study. Thromb Haemost. 2010;104(3):642–9.
58. Ogata K, Mendell-Harary J, Tachibana M, Masumoto H, Oguma T, Kojima M, et al. Clinical safety, tolerability, pharmacokinetics, and pharmacodynamics of the novel factor Xa inhibitor edoxaban in healthy volunteers. J Clin Pharmacol. 2010;50(7):743–53.

Thrombophilias

22

Stephanie M. Dentoni

Contents

S.M. Dentoni, MD, FSVM
California Vein & Vascular Institute,
Stockton, CA, USA
e-mail: dentonimd@veinandvascularinstitute.com

Abstract

The precise mechanism of hemostasis maintains constant regulation of fluidity and thrombosis. Many factors can disrupt this delicate balance and shift the paradigm to a hypercoagulable or hemophilic state. A high clinical suspicion is required for adequate diagnosis, prophylaxis, and treatment of thrombophilia. If left concealed, potentially, a life-threatening thromboembolic event may occur. With the advances in vein treatment and the evolving area of thrombophilia, a clear understanding of lurking hypercoagulable states is imperative when providing the best possible care and treatment for a patient. Both inherited and acquired thrombophilic states are identified when the appropriate level of clinical suspicion is used. Disease states and illnesses not often recognized as risk factors for venous thromboembolism (VTE) are defined. The appropriate diagnosis, prophylaxis, and treatment will improve the patient's outcome and prevent long-term consequences that carry high morbidity. Genetic testing is controversial in many instances and may be

E. Mowatt-Larssen et al. (eds.), *Phlebology, Vein Surgery and Ultrasonography*,
DOI 10.1007/978-3-319-01812-6_22, © Springer International Publishing Switzerland 2014

recommended if the result will have a significant impact on the patient. This chapter focuses on different disease processes that result in thrombophilia.

22.1 Introduction

The body's intricate compilation of microenvironments function cohesively to maintain a constant state that allows blood to flow without coagulating and bleeding inhibited by clotting. The precise mechanism of hemostasis maintains constant regulation of fluidity and thrombosis. Many factors can disrupt this delicate balance and shift the paradigm to a hypercoagulable or hemophilic state. A high clinical suspicion is required for adequate diagnosis, prophylaxis, and treatment of thrombophilia. If left concealed, potentially, a life-threatening thromboembolic event may occur.

Patients are often unaware of the possibility of an underlying hypercoagulable tendency. However, the astute clinician will identify subtle clues that would suggest the likelihood. As clues are uncovered, more questions and testing lead to the appropriate intervention. Even overt clues such as an unprovoked deep venous thrombosis or recurrent superficial thrombophlebitis episodes often go overlooked and ignored. Having an underlying hypercoagulable tendency does not necessarily lead to an event in an otherwise healthy individual. In combination with a reversible risk factor, however, the patient may be at a substantial risk. A firm understanding of the mechanisms that regulate hemostasis, risk factors, and disease states demystifies the daunting term "thrombophilia."

22.2 History and Physical Examination

Many styles of history taking are effective. Although open-ended questions are the standard for medical history taking, asking specific questions have an imperative role in determining the patient's hypercoagulable risk. Such questions should become part of a routine history with every patient, especially those undergoing treatment with an inherent risk of deep venous thrombosis.

22.3 Medical History

Chronic illnesses, obstetrical history, recent and current medication history, and the general overall health, including age-appropriate cancer screening, are useful in determining thrombophilic risk (Tables 22.1 and 22.2). Different mechanisms are involved in a myriad of chronic illnesses that predispose the patient to a hypercoagulable state. Inflammatory bowel disease, paroxysmal nocturnal hemoglobinuria, collagen vascular disorders, myeloproliferative disorders, hyperviscosity syndromes, nephrotic syndrome, infectious diseases (cytomegalovirus, HIV, mycobacterium, Q fever, syphilis, malaria, pneumocystis), and malignancies, especially mucin-secreting adenocarcinomas of the gastrointestinal tract, should alert the practitioner to a potential underlying clotting disorder given the correct circumstance [1, 2].

A complete obstetrical history is important to assess a patient's risk for thrombophilia. Recurrent first trimester spontaneous abortions,

Table 22.1 Age-appropriate cancer screening recommended by the National Cancer Institute

Sufficient evidence for a benefit in mortality	Insufficient evidence for a benefit in mortality but may be considered in specific patient populations
Breast cancer	Prostate cancer
Cervical cancer	Lung cancer
Colon and rectal cancers	Other cancers (ovarian, endometrial, testicular, bladder, esophageal, gastric, liver, neuroblastoma, oral, skin)

Table 22.2 Vitamin K-dependent proteins

Factor II – thrombin
Factor VII – stable factor or proconvertin
Factor IX – Christmas factor
Factor X – Stuart-Prower factor
Protein C
Protein S

preeclampsia, low birth weight babies, placental abruption, and unexplained fetal demise are seen in women who have a factor V Leiden mutation, prothrombin gene mutation, or antiphospholipid antibody syndrome. The highest risk of a thrombosis during pregnancy is in the postpartum period. Clotting factors are at a relative imbalance during pregnancy and into the postpartum period. It may take several months for the balance to stabilize after delivery [3].

22.4 Physical Examination

Physical findings are sparse when looking for evidence of an underlying hypercoagulable state. Subtle findings may be noted on a routine physical examination. Particular attention to detail is rewarding and can offer direction to the appropriate differential diagnosis. Evidence of recurrent superficial thrombophlebitis in different vein segments is found in Trousseau syndrome and a work-up for an occult malignancy is indicated [4]. Livedo reticularis, a fine lacey rash, may accompany antiphospholipid antibody syndrome [1, 2]. Necrotic lesions in the presence of warfarin (warfarin skin necrosis) imply a deficiency in protein C or protein S. The diagnosis of a deep venous thrombosis (DVT) is the most common clinical manifestation of thrombophilia. Clinical findings of DVT are pain or edema, but DVT can be clinically silent. Diagnostic venous duplex ultrasound or contrast venography is necessary to confirm the presence of a deep venous thrombosis.

22.5 Hemostasis

Maintaining hemostasis is a pathophysiological process regulated by primary and secondary hemostasis. The two exist in an almost simultaneous fashion. As this mechanism ensues, the common end point, thrombosis, is inevitable. Primary hemostasis consists of platelet aggregation, adhesion, and activation [5]. Disruption of the subendothelial layer exposes collagen and von Willebrand factor to circulating factors that would otherwise remain concealed. As platelets become activated, they adhere to the site of vessel injury. Subsequently, they release alpha and dense granules, which perpetuate the cycle. Glycoprotein IIb/IIIa mediates cross-linking of platelets and fibrin to produce a barricade to prevent further damage.

The coagulation cascade constitutes secondary hemostasis. It is a self-perpetuating series of reactions that lead to the production of cross-linked fibrin and thrombin through the activation of the extrinsic and intrinsic pathways. Inactive protein zymogens are converted to active serine proteases in the cascade with multiple feedback mechanisms which accelerate the cycle and form a fibrin rich venous clot. The exposure of tissue factor on the damaged subendothelium initiates the extrinsic pathway. Tissue factor (TF) activates and forms a complex with factor VII which in turn leads to the production of thrombin through the activation of factor X. The extrinsic pathway is inhibited and regulated by tissue factor pathway inhibitor (TFPI). However, due to the powerful factor already activated, factor II, thrombin, the cycle continues and becomes more difficult to regulate by the inherent inhibitors. Generated thrombin now activates numerous zymogens and proteins. The intrinsic pathway becomes involved through the production of thrombin and to a lesser extent the interaction of TF-VII complex with factor IX. Thrombin controls the cascade with both positive and negative feedback mechanisms. Factor XI is activated which activates factor IX and further causes the activation of factor X, and thrombin is produced. Fibrin is converted to cross-linked fibrin polymer by factor XIII which is triggered by thrombin. Factor V and factor VIII are positively affected by thrombin. They function as cofactors to enhance the intrinsic pathway. Production of activated factor X, thrombin, and fibrin is the same mechanism of thrombus formation in both the intrinsic and extrinsic pathways, the final common pathway.

Regulators of the coagulation cascade minimize thrombus formation. Natural anticoagulants limit thrombus formation and inhibit its development. Antithrombin, protein C, and the fibrinolytic pathway are the main contributors of this regulatory process. Thrombomodulin binds thrombin and with the aid of its cofactor, protein S, protein C is activated and inhibits activated factors V and VIII. Antithrombin is a potent anticoagulant and cleaves thrombin and activated factor X which renders them ineffective. In fact, heparin and low-molecular-weight heparin (LMWH) potentiate antithrombin and halt the coagulation cascade. At the time of initial vessel injury, fibrinolysis begins. Plasminogen is cleaved to plasmin by the activation of tissue plasminogen activator (tPA) derived from the endothelial cells. Plasmin degrades fibrin and fibrinogen which lyses clot. This is the essence of fibrinolysis for the treatment of an extensive acute deep venous thrombosis.

22.6 Hypercoagulable Disorders

Certain risk factors predispose one to developing a venous thromboembolism. A combination of risk factors may substantially increase the risk. Congenital or acquired abnormalities of hemostasis are the underlying mechanism. Classification of acquired and inherited disorders may overlap as with hyperhomocysteinemia and protein C and S deficiencies. Insight into the formation of a platelet plug, procoagulant factors and cofactors, and circulating inhibitors is fundamental in understanding thrombophilia. Overproduction or underproduction of coagulation factors are at the basis of thrombophilia. Only 15 % of hypercoagulable states are due to deficiencies of natural anticoagulants. Thrombosis may occur in any vein. One in an unusual location warrants an investigation into a hypercoagulable state. Only a few congenital and acquired abnormities have the ability to predispose to both arterial and venous thrombosis (Table 22.3). An appreciation of the coagulation cascade and the intricate interaction of disease processes allow one to formulate the appropriate differential diagnosis.

Table 22.3 Disorders with arterial and venous thrombotic consequences

1. Heparin-induced thrombocytopenia (with or without thrombosis)
2. Cancer/malignancy
3. Antiphospholipid antibody syndrome (lupus anticoagulant or anticardiolipin antibody)
4. Hyperhomocysteinemia
5. Prothrombin gene mutation

22.7 Exclusive Congenital Hypercoagulable Disorders

Congenital hypercoagulable disorders vary in epidemiology, inheritance patterns, associated gestational complications, and potential risk for a thromboembolic event. Genetic causes of a thromboembolic event account for approximately one-fourth of all events and up to 63 % with a familial predisposition [6]. Of the inherited hypercoagulable disorders, only factor V Leiden and prothrombin gene mutation are exclusively familial. Protein C and S deficiencies, antithrombin deficiency, hyperhomocysteinemia, and dysfibrogenemia may be congenitally transmitted but also acquired later in life (Fig. 22.1).

22.7.1 Factor V Leiden

Of all the possible inherited hypercoagulable disorders, factor V R506Q Leiden is the most common. Its inheritance pattern is autosomal dominant and has a single point mutation with the replacement of guanine by adenine thereby changing arginine to glutamine [7]. Activated protein C (APC) resistance and factor V Leiden mutation is often referred to synonymously even though it is an incorrect reference. The mutation causes incomplete resistance of activated protein C, an inherent anticoagulant [8]. Therefore, the action of activated protein C is decreased, there is ineffective degradation of factor Va, and consequently, the coagulation cascade is upregulated. Only 92 % of APC resistance is due to factor V Leiden. The remaining etiologies for APC resistance include

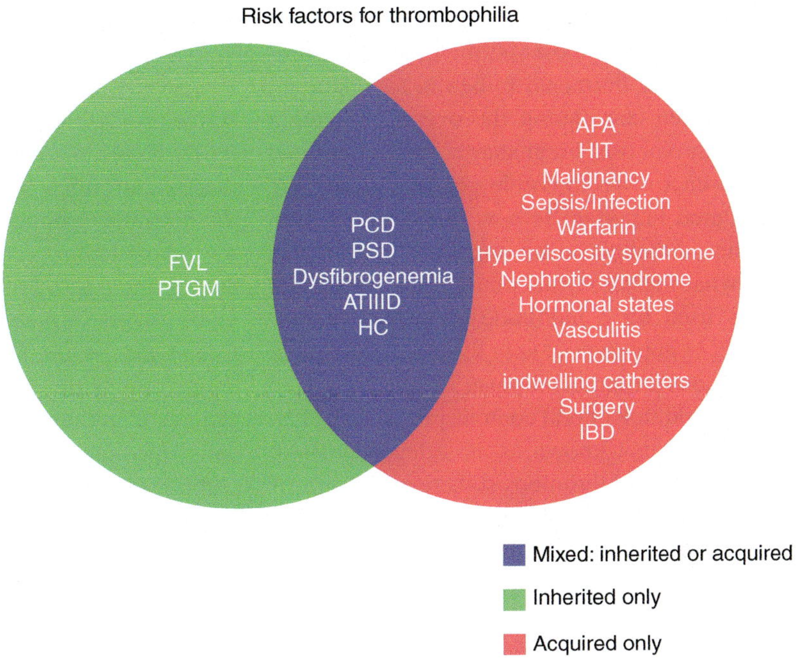

Fig. 22.1 Risk factors for thrombophilia (see text). *FVL* factor V Leiden mutation, *PTGM* prothrombin gene mutation, *PCD* protein C deficiency, *PCD* protein S deficiency, *ATIIID* antithrombin III deficiency, *HC* hyperhomocysteinemia, *APA* antiphospholipid antibody syndrome, *HIT* heparin-induced thrombocytopenia, *IBD* inflammatory bowel disease

pregnancy, oral contraceptive use, malignancy, antiphospholipid antibodies, and other factor V mutations [5]. Factor V Leiden affects 5 % of white northern European descent and is rare in Asian and African descent. It is accountable for 20 % of first idiopathic deep venous thrombotic events [6]. Heterozygosity imparts a five- to sevenfold increase relative risk over the general population for a thromboembolic event whereas a homozygote has an 80-fold increased risk. Unfortunately, there are no warning signs for early detection of the condition. The initial presentation is generally a deep venous thrombosis in the lower extremities. However, less frequently, other deep and superficial veins may be involved at the time of diagnosis.

Up to 60 % of venous thromboembolic events in pregnant women are caused by factor V Leiden. The highest risk for having a thromboembolic event during pregnancy is in the immediate postpartum state [9]. Pregnancy complications may alert the astute physician to a possible underlying thrombophilic tendency. Recurrent spontaneous abortions, low birth weight babies or slow fetal intrauterine growth, preeclampsia, and placental abruption are associated with factor V Leiden. When oral contraceptives are added to a patient with factor V Leiden heterozygosity, the relative risk for a venous thromboembolic event is 30–35 [10]. When a clinical suspicion for factor V Leiden mutation is present, APC resistance is determined by laboratory testing and confirmation is made with polymerase chain reaction (PCR).

22.7.2 Prothrombin Gene Mutation

Prothrombin gene mutation, second to factor V Leiden, is the next most commonly inherited defect affecting hemostasis with the predilection for venous thrombosis. It is inherited in an autosomal dominant manner and the relative risk per lifetime for developing a deep venous thrombosis is 2–6 [11]. Prevalent in southern Europe with a presence in the Middle East and Indian territories, it is almost nonexistent in Asian and African descent. Prothrombin, factor II, is vitamin K dependent, hence, its depletion with warfarin. The mechanism of action is poorly identified. It is postulated that an overproduction of prothrombin floods the available pool of zymogen precursors which increases its availability for activation.

Prothrombin gene mutation and factor V Leiden are similar not only in its mode of inheritance but also in the clinical presentation. Deep venous thrombosis is often the initial presentation. The hormonal milieu is an important aspect when considering the overall risk for a venous thrombosis. Pregnancy complications and the presence of prothrombin gene mutation once considered important is now disputed. Its relationship is thought to be important but remains somewhat unclear. Oral contraceptives are commonly used for a multitude of medical conditions. It is important to note that the relative risk of a venous thromboembolism in a heterozygote with the addition of oral contraceptives is 16 [12].

Although not known as an independent risk factor for arterial thrombosis, there are reports of a possible association between prothrombin gene mutation and arterial thrombosis including stroke and myocardial infarction. Currently, it is unknown if a homozygous state increases the risk for an arterial event. It has been suggested that risk factor modification contributes more to the prevention of arterial thrombosis. Diagnosis of the presence of prothrombin gene mutation is by PCR.

22.7.3 Mixed Congenital and Acquired Hypercoagulable Disorders

Protein S, protein C, antithrombin deficiencies, and hyperhomocysteinemia are known causes of thrombophilias but are less prevalent than factor V Leiden and prothrombin gene mutation. Dysfibrogenemia is even less recognized as a potential risk factor for a thrombotic event and is rarely implicated. These disorders may be acquired or inherited through genetic transmission.

In general, deficiencies are categorized as type I or type II. Type I is identified by a quantitative reduction in the amount of protein produced. However, if there are adequate amounts produced that are qualitatively dysfunctional, then type II is identified. Occasionally, there will be type III. This is seen in the presence of a cofactor and is distinguished by adequate amounts of total protein with reduced amounts of free, active protein, such as the case with protein S [13].

22.7.4 Protein C Deficiency

Protein C is a vitamin K-dependent, trypsin-like serine protease that utilizes protein S as a cofactor for activation. After posttranscriptional modification, thrombin cleaves protein C and removes the activation peptide, and in combination with thrombomodulin, activated protein C is generated. Protein S, a cofactor which enhances activated protein C, potentiates the effects of protein C and inactivates factors Va and VIIIa, hence decreasing fibrin clot formation. The activation process is initiated on the surface of endothelial cells mediated by thrombomodulin-thrombin complex (Fig. 22.2). Protein C has potent anti-inflammatory and cytoprotective effects as well. This is important in patients with overwhelming infection or sepsis. In fact, recombinant-activated protein C is used in the treatment of sepsis to halt the coagulation cascade and inflammatory pathways. Multiple acquired etiologies of protein C deficiency are listed in Table 22.4. It is reported that 0.2 % of the general population has protein C deficiency with a sevenfold increased risk of thrombosis [14].

Complications of protein C deficiency mirror those seen with protein S deficiency. In the homozygous state, purpura fulminans, a detrimental systemic thrombosis, ensues. Heterozygotes generally present with a lower extremity deep venous thrombosis. It is well recognized that other sites may be involved with thrombosis including the inferior vena cava and cerebral, retinal, and mesenteric veins [5]. Therefore, clinical presentation depends on the site of involvement. Protein C levels less than 50 % of normal are clinically relevant. Treatment is based on the presence of thrombosis which requires anticoagulation.

22.7.5 Protein S Deficiency

Of the congenital and acquired thrombophilias, protein S deficiency is unique. Protein S attaches to protein C and serves as a cofactor to potentiate the anticoagulant effect of activated protein C (Fig. 22.2). Protein S also acts independently to directly inhibit thrombin [15] as well as two

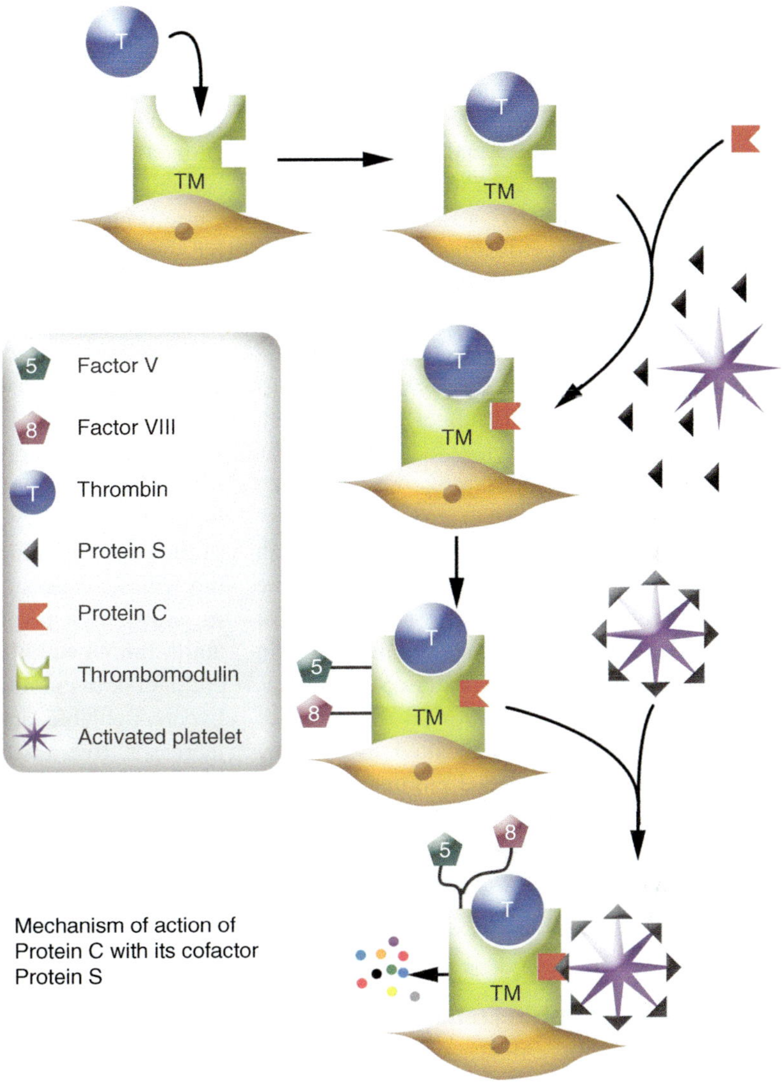

Fig. 22.2 Mechanism of action of protein C with its cofactor protein S

Table 22.4 Acquired protein C deficiency

Thrombosis
Acute DIC
Malignancy
Pregnancy, oral contraceptives, HRT
Antiphospholipid antibody syndrome
Hemolytic uremic syndrome
Acute respiratory distress syndrome
Infection
Severe liver disease
Postoperative state
Vitamin K deficiency, vitamin K antagonists

procoagulant complexes, factor X clotting factor-activating complex and prothrombin-activating complex. Protein S exists in two forms, free and bound, with 50–70 % of protein S representing the bound state [16, 17]. Therefore, protein S deficiency is classified into type I, type II, and type III because of its collaboration with protein C and other proteins. It is an autosomal dominant trait and thrombosis is found in both the heterozygous and homozygous states. Like homozygous protein C and antithrombin deficiencies, the homozygous state is lethal, resulting in purpura fulminans [18].

There are two genes identified on chromosome 3 for human protein S: the active gene, PROS-b and a pseudogene (named for its multiple coding errors), PROS-b. Deletions and point mutations alter the protein and allow for phenotypic variation. Deficiencies in protein S are not only congenital but also acquired in disease states. Liver disease or dysfunction and vitamin K deficiency are most common [19, 20].

Of patients with a diagnosed venous thromboembolic event, 2 % will be positive for protein S deficiency. American and European Caucasians historically are the highest affected group [20]. Japanese populations are now identified conferring the highest prevalence of protein S deficiency which is approximately five to ten times more frequent than seen in Caucasians. Presentation with an initial thrombosis usually occurs prior to the age of 45 with protein S levels less than 50 % of normal. There is no purified recombinant protein available in cases of severe protein S deficiency. Treatment with anticoagulation in the presence of an acute thrombosis is warranted, as with any thrombosis, except in special circumstances. In a case of a confirmed protein S deficiency and a life-threatening thromboembolic event, consideration may be given to the use of fresh frozen plasma.

22.7.6 Antithrombin Deficiency

Historically, antithrombin deficiency was the first described genetic abnormality linked to thrombophilia [21]. Congenital acquisition is rare compared to the presence of the acquired state. Its name is somewhat of a misnomer since it affects not only thrombin but many factors in the coagulation cascade. It primarily affects activated factors II, IX, and X and to a lesser extent factors VIIa, XIa, and XIIa. Antithrombin irreversibly binds to thrombin. With the addition of heparin to the thrombin-antithrombin complex, a conformational change enhances the ability of antithrombin to bind thrombin. Through its interaction with heparin, anticoagulant properties are accelerated up to 2,000 times. Other mechanisms of action are with thrombomodulin on endothelial cells. Antithrombin adheres to thrombomodulin and in turn accelerates neutralization of the coagulation cascade. Therefore, it is a potent natural anticoagulant that helps maintain hemostasis. It is thought that a type I homozygote develops deleterious clotting abnormalities and is incompatible with life. Heterozygotes, compatible with life, have a fivefold increase risk of developing a venous thrombosis [22].

Congenitally acquired antithrombin deficiency is considered more ominous than inherited deficiencies of protein C or S due to the variability of thrombotic manifestations. The type of mutation in the antithrombin gene determines the severity of thrombophilia. Replacement of threonine by nonpolar methionine, antithrombin wibble, causes a mild hypercoagulable state in adults; if a polar lysine replaces threonine, antithrombin wobble, thrombosis occurs in early childhood. In combination with another inherited hypercoagulable state, the risk of thrombosis increases five times. Antithrombin deficiency combined with an acquired risk factor escalates the risk to 20-fold [23].

Whether acquired or congenital, the initial presentation is venous thrombosis. Onset may be in childhood to adolescent or adulthood depending on the genetic defect and co-inheritance of other thrombophilias. Testing to confirm the diagnosis involves measuring the antithrombin level. An antithrombin level of 30–60 % of normal is significant with the exception of neonates which normally have 60 % of adult levels without having a hypercoagulable state. Monitoring blood levels in a patient with a family history of antithrombin deficiency is prudent. If the familial mutation is known, genetic analysis confirms the diagnosis.

22.7.7 Hyperhomocysteinemia

Hyperhomocysteinemia is a well-known risk factor for a thrombotic event. The mechanism of vascular injury is mediated through vascular endothelial disruption, platelet activation, and subsequent thrombosis. Both arterial and venous involvement (Table 22.3) is a consequence of increased plasma homocysteine levels. Homocysteine metabolism utilizes vitamins B_6, B_9 (folate), and B_{12} with enzymatic conversion of homocysteine to methionine or cysteine [24]. Increases in homocysteine are due to vitamin B deficiencies or mutations in specific enzymes methylenetetrahydrofolate reductase (MTHFR and thermolabile variant MTHFR) and cystathionine beta-synthase (CBS). Both heterozygous and homozygous states are found to be associated with hyperhomocysteinemia. Profound hyperhomocysteinemia is identified in patients homozygous for CBS deficiency or MTHFR deficiency. These patients are severely affected and have mental retardation or severe developmental delay, ectopia lentis and extreme myopia, excessive height, and hypercoagulability [25]. Heterozygotes for CBS and MTHFR deficiency or homozygous for thermolabile variant MTHFR mildly increases plasma homocysteine levels and increases the risk for arterial or venous thrombosis.

Hyperhomocysteinemia may be acquired through vitamin B deficiencies or renal disease. In theory, malabsorptive states or malnutrition may play a role in elevating homocysteine levels; however, this is not proven [26]. Nonetheless, regardless of the underlying cause of elevated homocysteine levels, diagnosis depends on the value of a fasting plasma homocysteine level. Further testing with a methionine load test to assess a possible heterozygous CBS abnormality may be indicated if the plasma homocysteine levels are normal or mildly increased and there is a high clinical suspicion for the disorder.

Treatment depends on the presence or absence of a thrombotic event. Elevated homocysteine levels are treated with folic acid, B6, and B12 supplements. If hyperhomocysteinemia is accompanied by an arterial or venous thrombosis, anticoagulation is immediately initiated. It is unclear if normalization of plasma homocysteine levels removes the underlying hypercoagulable tendency. Individual assessments for future risk should be evaluated.

22.7.8 Dysfibrogenemia

Of all the inherited and acquired thrombophilias, dysfibrogenemia has the most variable effects on the hemostatic system. Congenitally transmitted, it is exceedingly rare. In the face of an acute illness with severe liver dysfunction, it is common. There are also reports of an association between renal cell carcinoma or liver tumors and dysfibrogenemia. When inherited, 40 % of the patients are asymptomatic. Of the remaining patients, 50 % will present with a bleeding diathesis and 10 % will have a venous thromboembolic event with or without an associated bleeding tendency [27]. The inheritance pattern is usually autosomal dominant or codominant with the main defect in polymerization of the fibrin monomer [28]. When thrombosis is present, it is mild and associated with plasmin resistance. This is the fibrinogen Oslo I variant.

Clinically, the patient presents with bleeding after a procedure or surgery. There may be a history of easy bruisability, menorrhagia, epistaxis, poor wound healing, miscarriage, or venous thrombosis. A combination of bleeding and clotting are only associated with the congenital form. Baseline prolongations of the prothrombin time (PT), activated partial thromboplastin time (aPTT), thrombin time (TT), and reptilase time are present. Treatment depends on symptoms and complications. If bleeding is present, fresh frozen plasma or cryoprecipitate may be indicated. An acute thrombosis requires anticoagulation if there are no concurrent bleeding complications.

22.8 Acquired Thrombophilia

As we develop and age, we are susceptible to many extrinsic and intrinsic factors that influence our internal milieu. Fortunately, the majority of these changes are beneficial but some may trigger disease and health risk. Hypercoagulable states that are purely acquired may affect anyone and predispose them to a possible life-threatening event. Venous thromboembolism is a consequence and in certain circumstances, arterial thrombosis may be equally as devastating. There are many acquired thrombophilic risk factors that we encounter throughout our lifetime.

22.8.1 Antiphospholipid Antibody Syndrome/Hughes Syndrome

First described in 1952, antiphospholipid antibody syndrome (APS) was initially associated with systemic lupus erythematosus (SLE) with hypercoagulability. Historically, patients with syphilis test positive for the antibody. The term "Hughes syndrome" was later coined in recognition of Dr. Graham Hughes, who described the association of thrombosis with antiphospholipids. APS is the general term that describes the presence of antiphospholipids and a clinical event. It is further categorized into three classes depending on the antibody type: anticardiolipin antibodies, antiphospholipid antibodies, and antibodies against beta-2 glycoprotein 1. Lupus anticoagulant (LAC) describes the presence of antiphospholipid antibodies, whereas anticardiolipin antibody syndrome denotes the presence of anticardiolipin antibodies or antibodies to beta-2 glycoprotein 1. The term "LAC" is confusing due to the implications of its name. "Anticoagulant" represents vitro findings, but in vivo, a hypercoagulable state is produced. Frequently, systemic lupus erythematosus is not associated with APS. However, the association between an identifiable underlying disease process, such as SLE or another autoimmune disorder, is referred to as "secondary APS," whereas "primary APS" signifies that it is independent of a chronic illness [29, 30].

Pathophysiology of APS is not clearly defined. There are multiple postulated theories of interaction of antibodies with the coagulation cascade. Despite a mysterious mechanism of hypercoagulability, antibodies are readily identified in plasma. The frequency of APS is unknown. The prevalence of antiphospholipid antibodies in the general population is 1–5 % [31, 32]. Thirty-four to forty-two percent of patients with SLE will develop APS [32, 33]. Healthy individuals with positive antibody titers are not uncommon. The presence of anticardiolipin antibodies increases with age and are more common than the presence of antiphospholipid antibodies.

Both arterial and venous thromboses are observed in APS. Patients present with cerebral vascular accidents, myocardial infarction, deep venous thrombosis or pulmonary embolism, endocarditis associated with SLE, and pregnancy complications such as preterm labor, preeclampsia or low birth weight, recurrent miscarriages, or fetal demise [32]. Even though APS is a hypercoagulable disorder, an association between thrombocytopenia and APS is well documented in 20–40 % of patients. Despite the presence of a low platelet count, thrombosis can occur in any vessel and in any organ system. Adrenal infarction or hemorrhage, retinal thrombosis, cerebral venous sinus thrombosis, and avascular necrosis are possible complications. Therefore, APS should be considered in any patient with a thrombosis in an unusual site. It is suggested that recurrent thrombosis has a higher likelihood of occurring in the same vessel type (venous or arterial). In the most severe form and often fatal, catastrophic APS is rare and manifests as multiorgan involvement with infarction.

The diagnosis of APS is based on clinical criteria with supporting laboratory findings [34]. Arterial or venous thrombosis and pregnancy mortality establish the syndrome. Specifically, one of the following pregnancy complications must be present: fetal demise more than 10 weeks gestation, prematurity of less than 34 weeks, and three or more consecutive spontaneous abortions at less than 10 weeks gestation. The presence of antiphospholipid antibodies, anticardiolipin antibodies, beta-2 glycoprotein I, prolonged aPTT at baseline and without normalization with mixing studies, and dilute Russell's viper venom time confirms the clinical suspicion. Treatment consists of anticoagulation, which may be indefinite depending on the clinical situation. There remains controversy over the level of anticoagulation. In general, the international ratio is kept between two and three, but there are some who believe the range should be increased to between three and four. It is crucial to assess the patient and the clinical circumstances surrounding thrombotic events prior to determining the length and intensity of treatment.

22.8.2 Heparin-Induced Thrombocytopenia

Heparin-induced thrombocytopenia carries significant morbidity and mortality when clinically unnoticed. Heparin or heparin products are commonly used for thromboprophylaxis and patients are often exposed to it when hospitalized or with procedures or surgeries. Thrombocytopenia, the initial presentation, is often disregarded because of its commonality among these patients.

Classically, there are two types of heparin-induced thrombocytopenia described. Type I is nonimmune, benign, and associated with a milder decrease in the platelet count. The platelet count, which will rebound without withdraw of heparin, will rarely fall below 100,000 platelets/μl. In contrast, type II is associated with a significant reduction in the platelet count and considerable morbidity and mortality. Type II heparin-induced thrombocytopenia will be considered here due to its clinical significance and referred to as "HIT."

HIT is found in up to 5 % [35, 36] of hospitalized patients and 33 % of those patients go on to develop an arterial or venous thrombosis [37, 38]. Antibodies to platelet factor 4 found in alpha granules in platelets complex with heparin to form the antigen. These IgG antibodies form through exposure to unfractionated heparin may cross-react with low-molecular-weight heparin [37]. These complexes are removed by the reticuloendothelial system, resulting in thrombocytopenia. Thrombocytopenia may be evident at different times after heparin exposure. In a heparin-naïve patient, the platelet count will be at 50 % of the baseline value or fall below 100,000 μl after the fifth day of treatment. A patient who is re-exposed to heparin may experience thrombocytopenia within the first 3 days of heparin initiation. Moreover, delayed-onset HIT is found at 5 or more days after the elimination of heparin therapy [39]. Antibody detection is present up to 3 months after heparin discontinuation [40] and, hence, the need for anticoagulation therapy with vitamin K antagonist for at least 3 months. Even low-dose, subcutaneous heparin prophylaxis has been associated with HIT in 1 % of this patient population [41].

Special consideration should be given to patients with a cardiac history. Heparin exposure is common as is thrombocytopenia. These patients invariably have repeated exposures to heparin and glycoprotein IIb/IIIa inhibitors with a history of thrombocytopenia. The incorrect diagnosis leaves the patient at a substantially increased risk of hemorrhage. However, on the contrary, a missed diagnosis of HIT may have life-threatening thrombotic consequences. Pursuit of the correct diagnosis in a timely manner is of the essence.

Thrombotic complications may be present with HIT. Arterial or venous manifestations occur in up to 30 % of the patients. The site and type of vessel involved may be associated with the thrombotic risk factor profile of the patient [35]. Indwelling catheters, orthopedic patients, and neurological surgical patients are at risk for venous thrombosis whereas cardiac patients present with arterial thrombosis. A severe form of generalized thrombosis similar to disseminated intravascular coagulation has been reported and often fatal [42].

Other clinical clues not to be overlooked when considering the diagnosis of HIT are skin necrosis at the site of subcutaneous administration of heparin and heparin resistance [37]. To confirm the diagnosis after the identification of thrombocytopenia with the predicted platelet rebound on removal of heparin, heparin-induced platelet aggregation (HIPA) and serotonin release assay (SRA) are performed. HIPA is less sensitive when compared to SRA. Enzyme-linked immunosorbent assay (ELISA) recognizes platelet factor 4/heparin complex antibodies and are sensitive like SRA, but less specific [35]. Treatment consists of urgent withdraw of heparin products and immediate initiation of a direct thrombin inhibitor (DTI). Anticoagulation with warfarin is initiated and overlapped with a DTI after the platelet count recovers. Warfarin is continued for at least 3 months or longer depending on the clinical circumstance.

22.8.3 Malignancy

Venous thromboembolism may complicate a patient's course with a history of malignancy. The presence of cancer increases the risk for a thromboembolic event by four- to sevenfold [43, 44]. In fact, an idiopathic venous thrombosis may be the initial presentation in a patient with an occult malignancy. Other factors including the patient profile, those inherent to malignancy, and chemotherapy increase the incidence of thrombosis.

Obesity, immobility, older age, and other medical comorbidities are independent risk factors for an acquired hypercoagulable state in cancer patients. The two most commonly inherited thrombophilic disorders, factor V Leiden and prothrombin gene mutation, do not seem to increase the overall risk of a venous thrombosis in a patient with an underlying malignancy [43]. Specific histological characteristic as well as a particular location of the tumor impart a higher risk than others. Generally, patients with adenocarcinomas, especially mucin-secreting, and brain tumors, have a high risk of going on to develop a thrombosis [45]. Both solid tumors and hematological malignancies are associated with a hypercoagulable state. Increased risks for VTE in pancreatic, ovarian, uterine, testicular, gastric, lung, and renal malignancies are reported [46, 47]. Non-Hodgkin's lymphoma may cause a mass effect on a deep vein, resulting in outflow obstruction and thrombosis. Acute promyelocytic leukemia and high-grade lymphoma confer a higher risk than other hematologic cancers [48]. Factors such as hyperviscosity, treatment with thalidomide or its derivatives, and the presence of cancer itself are associated with an elevated risk of developing a thrombotic event in patients with multiple myeloma [49]. Cytotoxic chemotherapeutic agents, hormonal therapy, and antiangiogenic agents are often used in conjunction with other treatment modalities in cancer patients. These agents are situational risk factors and carry an increased VTE risk.

Inflammation is a key feature in the pathophysiology of thrombosis in a patient with an underlying malignancy. Tumor cells activate a cascade of inflammatory products, cytokines, and procoagulants. The increase of circulating factors and exposure of prothrombotic proteins, such as cancer procoagulant (directly activates factor X), factor VIII, von Willebrand factor, fibrinogen, thrombin, and tissue factor, trigger the coagulation cascade. Platelets are activated and both primary and secondary hemostasis act in concert with positive feedback mechanisms that shift the balance toward thrombosis.

Malignancies are often under-recognized as a significant risk factor for both arterial and venous thrombotic events. Symptoms of a deep or superficial venous thrombosis, recurrent thrombophlebitis or Trousseau syndrome, or arterial occlusion are classical presentations. An idiopathic deep venous thrombosis in a person less than 45 years of age or recurrent thrombotic events requires a thrombophilia workup including a search for occult malignancy. Patients with a history of a malignancy who develop a thrombotic event require treatment with anticoagulation and an oncological reevaluation. The CLOT (randomized comparison of low-molecular-weight heparin versus oral anticoagulant therapy for the prevention of recurrent VTE in patients with cancer) trial shows a significant risk reduction in recurrent VTE with malignancy-related thrombosis when low-molecular-weight heparin (LMW) is used instead of vitamin K antagonists. A minimum of a 6-month treatment course with LMWH is recommended for patients with active malignancy and VTE. Continuation of treatment beyond 6 months is individualized after assessing the patient's clinical situation and risk factor profile.

22.8.4 Increased Estrogen States

Pregnancy, hormone replacement therapy, and oral contraceptives (OCPs) are well-known risk factors for thrombophilia. Oral contraceptive use is a common drug regimen for the treatment of many gynecological disorders. By using OCPs alone, without other risk factors identified, the relative risk of a venous thromboembolic event is seven. A dramatic increase in the risk of a venous thrombosis with a combination of an increased estrogen state and an inherited thrombophilia is reported. In fact, the combination of OCPs with factor V Leiden heterozygosity increases the risk of VTE 35-fold [50]. Heterozygous prothrombin gene mutation is less affected but still significant at 16-fold [12]. Shockingly, the risk of cerebral venous thrombosis with prothrombin gene mutation and OCP use is increased by a factor of approximately 150 [51].

Thrombophilia may present as maternal or fetal complications during pregnancy. In developed countries, the leading cause of maternal death is due to pulmonary embolism (PE) and morbidity caused from PE is as high as 20 % [51]. Thirty to fifty percent of pregnancy-associated VTE have an identifiable inherited hypercoagulable state. Even though factor V Leiden and prothrombin gene mutation are most commonly found, these patients are at low risk for VTE with pregnancy. Genetic thrombophilias that are associated with a high risk of venous thrombosis are protein C or S deficiency, antithrombin deficiency, homozygous states, and compound heterozygosity for prothrombin gene mutation and factor V Leiden [52]. Fetal complications that should increase the suspicion for a possible underlying thrombophilia are preeclampsia and fetal demise. Like the antepartum state, the risk of venous thrombosis continues into the postpartum state and is higher than that of the antepartum state [53]. This risk is present for 6 weeks to 2 months after delivery. No official guideline for thromboprophylaxis during pregnancy is established to date. The risk is individualized and unfractionated heparin, as well as LMWH, has been used for treatment and prophylaxis in the appropriate clinical situation.

Hormone replacement therapy (HRT) has been a subject of controversy and debate. It is clear that oral HRT is risk factor for venous thrombosis. There is a two- to threefold increased risk of VTE in the presence of oral HRT. The risk is highest within the first year of initiation. This risk is not equivalent when comparing oral estrogens to transdermal estrogen formulations. Hepatic metabolism of oral estrogens through the first-pass effect shifts the hemostatic balance in favor of thrombosis. There is also a decrease in antithrombin production when oral estrogens are used. Due to the difference in metabolism, these changes are not as readily observed with a transdermal preparation. With the addition of an inherited thrombophilia, the risk of VTE increases appreciably [10].

Table 22.5 Chronic illnesses with an increased risk for thromboembolism

Chronic illnesses	Infectious diseases
Malignancy	HIV
Crohn's disease	CMV
Ulcerative colitis	Q fever
Collagen vascular disorders	Syphilis
Paroxysmal nocturiahemoglobinuria (PNH)	Malaria
Hyperviscosity syndromes	Pneumocystis
Myeloproliferative disorders	
Nephrotic syndrome	

22.8.5 Chronic Illnesses or Diseases

Many chronic illnesses, controlled or uncontrolled, may increase the incidence of developing a thrombosis (Table 22.5). Some illnesses may have an underlying genetic susceptibility that becomes activated later in life which initiates a reaction that further triggers the onset of the disease. A patient may have a genetic predisposition for the illness but it is acquired until later in life. The exact circumstance that induces the expression of the disease is often not identified. Inflammatory bowel disease is a disorder that is well known to have an association with an increased risk of venous thromboembolism. However, other illnesses, such as rheumatoid arthritis, are reported to have possible associations. A thorough patient history may uncover a potential hypercoagulable state.

22.9 Genetic Testing for Family Members

When compared to the vast list of acquired hypercoagulable risk factors, there are few inherited abnormalities of coagulation that should be considered for familial testing. Siblings and children of the affected person are candidates for evaluation. However, genetic testing is not routine and consequences of a positive test must be considered prior to evaluation. When determining who is a candidate for testing, the underlying familial abnormality impacts who is tested. Some genetic disorders are regarded as more powerful based on their VTE risk profile. Homozygous factor V Leiden, homozygous prothrombin gene mutation, double heterozygous factor V Leiden and prothrombin gene mutation, protein C and S deficiencies, and antithrombin deficiencies are established as a high risk group and fit into this category. An argument can be made for familial testing depending on clinical risk factors of the individual such as a the possible acquisition of a reversible risk factor which may have an impact on long-term morbidity and mortality (i.e., immobilization, long travel, medications, or pregnancy). The presence of heterozygous factor V Leiden or heterozygous prothrombin gene mutation without other risk factors generally has no impact on current management [54, 55].

22.10 Anticoagulation Prophylaxis During Lower Extremity Venous Procedures in Thrombophilic Patients

Currently, there are no guidelines available for the indication of prophylactic intensity anticoagulation during lower extremity venous procedures. To make matters more confusing, there is no consensus among phlebologists for the use of prophylactic anticoagulation during these procedures.

Understanding thrombophilia, identifying potential hypercoagulable patients, and evaluating situational risk factors will help guide decision in the use prophylactic intensity anticoagulation. The risk/benefit profile of low-dose anticoagulation is favorable in most situations and should be considered in any patient who may be predisposed to having a periprocedural venous thromboembolism. In fact, at the time of a minimally invasive venous procedure, if a patient is on anticoagulation for reasons other than a venous thromboembolic event, some phlebologists feel that it is not necessary to interrupt anticoagulation and the procedure can be accomplished on full anticoagulation. This author believes that in most circumstances, a patient with a congenital, acquired, or situational hypercoagulable state should be on prophylactic intensity anticoagulation (if not already on therapeutic intensity anticoagulation) starting the morning of the procedure and continued for 7–10 days. At the completion of anticoagulation, the absence of thrombus extension at or near the junction of the deep venous system should be documented by ultrasound evaluation. It is my practice to again evaluate the treated lower extremity by ultrasound 1 week after discontinuation of anticoagulation to ensure the absence of thrombus in the deep venous system and document the stability of any superficial thrombus previously identified. It is important to realize that recommendations regarding anticoagulation prophylaxis for venous procedures are variable within the phlebologic community. All risks and benefits of the proposed procedures and the patient's thrombophilic profile must be well thought-out prior to determining the most appropriate treatment course. Patients must have a clear understanding of all the options and possible outcomes. If uncomfortable with the clinical situation, reevaluate the treatment plan. Not every patient with varicose vein disease is an appropriate candidate for invasive or minimally invasive treatment. Conservative treatment with the daily use of medical strength compression stockings may be the best option.

Conclusion

With the advances in vein treatment and the evolving area of thrombophilia, a clear understanding of lurking hypercoagulable states is imperative when providing the best possible care and treatment for a patient. Both inherited and acquired thrombophilic states are identified when the appropriate level of clinical suspicion is used. Disease states and illnesses not often recognized as risk factors for VTE are defined. The appropriate diagnosis, prophylaxis, and treatment will improve the patient's outcome and prevent long-term consequences that carry high morbidity. Genetic testing is controversial in many instances and may be recommended if the result will have a significant impact on the patient.

References

1. Levine JS, Branch DW, Rauch J. The antiphospholipid syndrome. N Engl J Med. 2002;346:752–63.
2. Shapiro SS. The Lupus anticoagulant/antiphospholipid syndrome. Annu Rev Med. 1996;47:533–53.
3. Kupferminc MJ. Thrombophilia and pregnancy. Reprod Biol Endocrinol. 2003;1:111.
4. Varki A. Trousseau's syndrome: multiple definitions and multiple mechanisms. Blood. 2007;110(6):1723–9.
5. Deitcher S. Hypercoagulable states. Cleveland Clinic Center for Continuing Education. 2010. www.clevelandclinicmeded.com.
6. Grody WW, Griffin JH, Taylor AK, Korf BR, Heit JA, ACMG Factor V Leiden Working Group. American College of Medial Genetics consensus statement on factor V Leiden mutation testing. Genet Med. 2001;3:139–48.
7. Lane DA, Mannucci PM, Bauer KA, et al. Inherited thrombophilia: part 1. Thromb Haemost. 2001;85:584–95.
8. Gandrille S, Greengard JS, Alhenc-Gelas M, et al. Incidence of activated protein c resistance caused by the ARG 506GLN mutation in factor V in 113 unrelated symptomatic protein C-deficienct patients. The French Network on the behalf of INSERM. Blood. 1995;86:219–22.
9. Vandenbrouche JP, Koster T, Briet E, et al. Increased risk of venous thrombosis in oral-contraceptive users who are carriers of factor V Leiden mutation. Lancet. 1994;344:1453–7.
10. Bank I, Libourel EJ, Middeldorp S, Van Pampuse C, Koopman MM, Hamulyak K, et al. Prothrombin 20210A mutation: a mild risk factor for venous thromboembolism but not for arterial thrombotic disease and pregnancy-related complications in a family study. Arch Intern Med. 2004;164:1932–7.
11. Deitcher SR, Caiola E, Jaffer A. Demystifying two common genetic predispositions to venous thrombosis. Cleve Clin J Med. 2000;67:825–6, 833–6.
12. Martinelli I, Taioli E, Bucciarelli P, et al. Interaction between the G20210A mutation of the prothrombin gene and oral contraceptive use in deep vein thrombosis. Arterioscler Thromb Vasc Biol. 1999;19:700–3.
13. Johnson CM, Mureebe L, Silver D. Hypercoagulable states: a review. Vasc Endovascular Surg. 2005;39:123–33.
14. Goldenberg NA, Manco-Johnson MJ. Protein C deficiency. Haemophilia. 2008;14:1214–21.
15. Heeb MJ, Prashun D, Griffin JH, Bouma BN. Plasma protein S contains zinc essential for efficient activated protein C-independent anticoagulant activity and binding to factor Xa, but not for efficient binding to tissue factor pathway inhibitor. FASEB J. 2009;23(7):2244–53.
16. Leroy-Matheron C, Gouault-Heilmann M, Aiach M, Gandrille S. A mutation of the active protein S gene leading to an EGF1-lacking protein in a family with qualitative (type II) deficiency. Blood. 1998;91:4608.
17. Rezende SM, Simmonds RE, Lane DA. Coagulation, inflammation, and apoptosis: different roles for protein S and the protein S-C4b binding protein complex. Blood. 2004;103:1192.
18. Edlich RF, Cross CL, Dahlstrom JJ, Long 3rd WB. Modern concepts of the diagnosis and treatment of purpura fulminans. J Environ Pathol Toxicol Oncol. 2008;27(3):191–6.
19. Lijfering WM, Brouwer JL, Veeger NJ, Bank I, Coppens M, Middeldorp S, et al. Selective testing for thrombophilia in patients with first venous thrombosis: results from a retrospective family cohort study on absolute thrombotic risk for currently known thrombophilic defects in 2479 relatives. Blood. 2009;113(21):5314–22.
20. Kate MK, van der Meer J. Protein S deficiency: a clinical perspective. Haemophilia. 2008;14:1222–8.
21. Egeberg O. Inherited antithrombin deficiency causing thrombophilia. Thromb Diath Haemorrh. 1965;13:516–30.
22. Maclean P, Tait RC. Hereditary and acquired antithrombin deficiency; epidemiology, pathogenesis and treatment options. Drugs. 2007;67(10):1429–40.
23. Van Boven HH, Vandenbroucke JP, Briët E, Rosendaal FR. Gene-gene and gene-environment interactions determine risk of thrombosis in families with inherited antithrombin deficiency. Blood. 1999;94(8):2590–4.
24. GN W, Loscalzo J. Homocysteine and atherothrombosis. N Engl J Med. 1998;338:1042–50.
25. Picker JD, Levy HL. Homocystinuria caused by cystathionine beta-synthase deficiency. NCBI Bookshelf. 2011. www.ncbinm.nih.gov.
26. Casella G, Bassoti G, Villanacci V, Di Bella C, et al. Is hyperhomocysteinemia relevant in patients with celiac disease? World J Gastroenterol. 2011;17(24):2941–4.
27. Acharya SS, Dimichele DM. Rare inherited disorders of fibrinogen. Haemophilia. 2008;14(6):1151–8.
28. Kotlin R, Reicheltova Z, Maly M, et al. Two cases of congenital dysfibrinogenemia associated with thrombosis – Fibrinogen Praha III and Fibrinogen Pizen. Thromb Haemost. 2009;102(3):479–86.
29. Amigo MC, Khamashta MA. Antiphospholipid (Hughes) syndrome in systemic lupus erythematosus. Rheum Dis Clin North Am. 2000;26(2):331–48.
30. Love PE, Santoro SA. Antiphospholipid antibodies: anticardiolipin and the lupus anticoagulant in systemic lupus erythematosus (SLE) and in non-SLE disorders. Prevalence and clinical significance. Ann Intern Med. 1990;112:682–98.

31. Manoussakis MN, Tzioufas AG, Silis MP, et al. High prevalence of anticardiolipin and other autoantibodies in healthy elderly population. Clin Exp Immunol. 1987;68:557–65.
32. Tektonidou M. Orphanet encyclopedia. 2004. http://www.orpha.net/data/patho/Pro/en/Antiphospholipid-FRenPro5517.pdf
33. Tektonidou MG, Ioannidis JPA, Boki KA, Vlachoyiannopoulos PG, Moutsopoulos HM. Prognostic factors and clustering of serious clinical outcomes in antiphospholipid antibody syndrome. QJM. 2000;93:523–30.
34. Aserson RA, Cervera R, de Groot PG, et al. Catastrophic antiphospholipid syndrome: international consensus statement on classification criteria and treatment guidelines. Lupus. 2003;12(7):530–4 [Guideline].
35. Franchini M. Heparin-induced thrombocytopenia: an update. Clin Lab. 2006;52(1–2):11–7.
36. Baglin TP. Heparin-induced thrombocytopenia/thrombosis syndrome (HIT): diagnosis and treatment. Platelets. 1997;8:72–82.
37. Comunale ME, van Cott IM. Heparin-induced thrombocytopenia. Int Anesthesiol Clin. 2004;42:27–43.
38. Nand S, Wong W, Yuen B, Yetter A, Schmulbach E, Gross Fisher S. Heparin-induced thrombocytopenia with thrombosis: incidence, analysis if risk factors, and clinical outcomes in 108 consecutive patients treated at a single institution. Am J Hematol. 1997;56: 12–6.
39. Warkentin TE, Kelton JG. Delayed-onset heparin-induced thrombocytopenia and thrombosis. Ann Intern Med. 2001;135:502–6.
40. Kelton JG. Heparin-induced thrombocytopenia: an overview. Blood Rev. 2002;16:77–80.
41. Girolami B, Prandoni P, Stefani PM, et al. The incidence of heparin-induced thrombocytopenia in hospitalized medical patients treated with subcutaneous unfractionated heparin: a prospective cohort study. Blood. 2003;101:2955–9.
42. Klein HG, Bell WR. Disseminated intravascular coagulation during heparin therapy. Ann Intern Med. 1974;80:477–81.
43. Blom JW, Doggen CJM, Osanto S, Rosendaal FR. Malignancies, prethrombotic mutations, and the risk of venous thrombosis. JAMA. 2005;293:715–22.
44. Heit JA, Silverstein MD, Mohr DN, et al. Risk factors for deep vein thrombosis and pulmonary embolism: a population-based case–control study. Arch Intern Med. 2000;160:809–15.
45. Gerber DE, Grossman SA, Streiff MB. Management of venous thromboembolism in patients with primary and metastatic brain tumors. J Clin Oncol. 2003;24: 1310–8.
46. Khorana AA, Francis CW, Culakova E, et al. Thromboembolism in hospitalized neutropenic cancer patients. J Clin Oncol. 2006;24:484–90.
47. Connolly GC, Khorana AA. Emerging risk stratification approaches to cancer-associated thrombosis: risk factors, biomarkers and a risk score. Thromb Res. 2010;125 Suppl 2:1–7.
48. Ottinger H, Belka C, Kozole G, et al. Deep venous thrombosis and pulmonary artery embolism in high-grade non Hodgkin's lymphoma: incidence causes and prognostic relevance. Eur J Haematol. 1995;54: 186–94.
49. Palumbo A, Rajkumar SV, Dimopoulos MA, et al. Prevention of thalidomide- and lenalidomide-associated thrombosis in myeloma. Leukemia. 2008; 22:414–23.
50. Vandernbrouche JP, Koster T, Briet E, et al. Increased risk of venous thrombosis in oral-contraceptive users who are carriers of factor V Leiden mutation. Lancet. 1994;344:1453–7.
51. Martinelli I, Sacchi E, Landi G, et al. High risk of cerebral-vein thrombosis in carriers of a prothrombin-gene mutation and in users of oral contraceptives. N Engl J Med. 1998;338:1793–7.
52. Ronsmans C, Graham WJ. Maternal mortality: who, when, where, and why. Lancet. 2006;368: 1189–200.
53. Martinelli I, Legnani C, Bucciarelli P, Grandone E, De Stefano V, Mannucci PM. Risk of pregnancy-related venous thrombosis in carriers of severe inherited thrombophilia. Thromb Haemost. 2001;86:800–3.
54. Canonica M, Plu-Bureau G, Lowe G, Scarabin PY. Hormone replacement therapy and risk of venous thromboembolism in postmenopausal women: systematic review and meta-analysis. BMJ. 2008;336:1227.
55. Moll S. Who should be tested for thrombophilia? Genet Med. 2011;13:19–20.

Part VI

Special Topics

Lymphedema

23

James Laredo and Byung Boong Lee

Contents

J. Laredo, MD, PhD, FACS, RVT, RPVI (✉)
Department of Surgery, Division of Vascular Surgery, George Washington University Medical Center, 22nd and I Street, NW, 6th Floor, Washington, DC, USA
e-mail: jlaredo@mfa.gwu.edu

B.B. Lee, MD, PhD, FACS
George Washington University Medical Center, Washington, DC, USA
e-mail: bblee38@comcast.net

Abstract

Lymphedema is the result of impaired lymphatic function. Lymphedema is characterized by swelling of tissues, most commonly involving the lower extremities in 80 % of cases. It can also occur in the arms, face, trunk, and external genitalia. Leg edema is a common condition that is seen by all practicing clinicians. The differential diagnosis of lower extremity edema is extensive and includes systemic causes such as congestive heart failure, renal insufficiency, hepatic insufficiency, hypoalbuminemia, and medications and local causes such as deep vein thrombosis, venous insufficiency, lymphedema, lipedema, and cellulitis. A detailed understanding of the anatomy and physiology of the lymphatic system and the pathophysiology of lymphedema will contribute to the proper diagnosis and treatment of this complex and important clinical condition.

23.1 Introduction

Lymphedema is the result of impaired lymphatic function. The lymphatic system is an essential component of the human circulatory system. It is comprised of a complex network of vessels. The major function of the lymphatic system is the maintenance of interstitial fluid homeostasis and prevention of edema [1, 2]. Other important functions include transportation of white blood cells and antigen-presenting cells to the lymphoid

E. Mowatt-Larssen et al. (eds.), *Phlebology, Vein Surgery and Ultrasonography*,
DOI 10.1007/978-3-319-01812-6_23, © Springer International Publishing Switzerland 2014

organs and lipid absorption from the gastrointestinal tract [1, 2].

Lymphedema is characterized by swelling of tissues, most commonly involving the lower extremities in 80 % of cases [3, 4]. It can also occur in the arms, face, trunk, and external genitalia. Leg edema is a common condition that is seen by all practicing clinicians. The differential diagnosis of lower extremity edema is extensive and includes systemic causes such as congestive heart failure, renal insufficiency, hepatic insufficiency, hypoalbuminemia, and medications and local causes such as deep vein thrombosis, venous insufficiency, lymphedema, lipedema, and cellulitis [2–5].

A detailed understanding of the anatomy and physiology of the lymphatic system and the pathophysiology of lymphedema will contribute to the proper diagnosis and treatment of this complex and important clinical condition.

23.2 Anatomy and Physiology

The lymphatic system is found throughout the body and is composed of four components: lymphatic vessels, lymph fluid, lymph nodes, and lymphocytes [1, 2]. Lymphatic vessels generally accompany the venous system throughout the body except in the central nervous system, hepatic sinusoids, and cortical bony skeleton, where these perivascular spaces serve the function of the lymphatic vessels [1–3]. Lymphatic fluid from the lower extremities, pelvis, abdominal viscera, thorax, left arm, and left head and neck drains into the central venous system via the thoracic duct. Lymphatic fluid from the right arm, right head and neck, and parts of the thorax drains into the central venous system via the right lymphatic duct [1–3]. Numerous interconnections exist as well as significant variants [1]. In addition, an extensive system of superficial lymphatic vessels extends over the surface of the entire body draining into communication watersheds, regional lymph nodes, and ultimately the deep lymphatic system.

Analogous to the venous system, the lymphatic system has both a superficial and deep system in the extremities that is separated by the muscle fascia (Fig. 23.1). The superficial lymphatic system collects lymph from the skin and subcutaneous tissue, and the deep lymphatic system collects lymph from subfascial structures, such as the muscle, bone, and deep blood vessels. The superficial and deep systems of the lower extremities merge within the pelvis and those of the upper extremity merge in the axilla. The two drainage systems function in an interdependent fashion such that the deep lymphatic system participates in lymph transport for the skin during lymphatic obstruction [1–3].

The lymphatic vasculature is composed of a hierarchal network of initial and collecting lymphatic vessels that exhibit molecular, cellular, and functional differences. Initial lymphatic vessels consist of a single layer of endothelial cells with end-to-end or overlapping junctions [1, 2, 6]. The basement membrane is scant or absent around the initial lymphatic vessels, which are connected to the extracellular matrix by fibrillin-containing anchoring filaments. These anchoring filaments may modulate the uptake of interstitial fluid through molecular signaling in addition to pulling apart endothelial cells. The initial lymphatic vessels drain into the collecting lymphatics (Fig. 23.2) [1, 6].

Collecting lymphatic vessels are composed of endothelial cells that are surrounded by a well-defined basement membrane. Intraluminal bicuspid valves are present within the collecting lymphatic vessels. Valves partition collecting lymphatic vessels into discrete contractile segments, termed "lymphangions," which are surrounded by the smooth muscle and contract to actively transport lymphatic fluid through lymph nodes and throughout the lymphatic system (Fig. 23.2) [1, 2, 6].

Since the lymphatics lack a central pump, lymphatic fluid is propelled through the lymphatics through the concerted effects of respiratory motions, skeletal muscle contractions, and the autocontractility of the mural smooth muscle of the vasculature itself. In the skeletal muscle, lymphatics are usually paired with arterioles, so that arterial pulsations can also contribute to the periodic expansion and compression of the initial lymphatic vessels to enhance fluid uptake [1–3, 7].

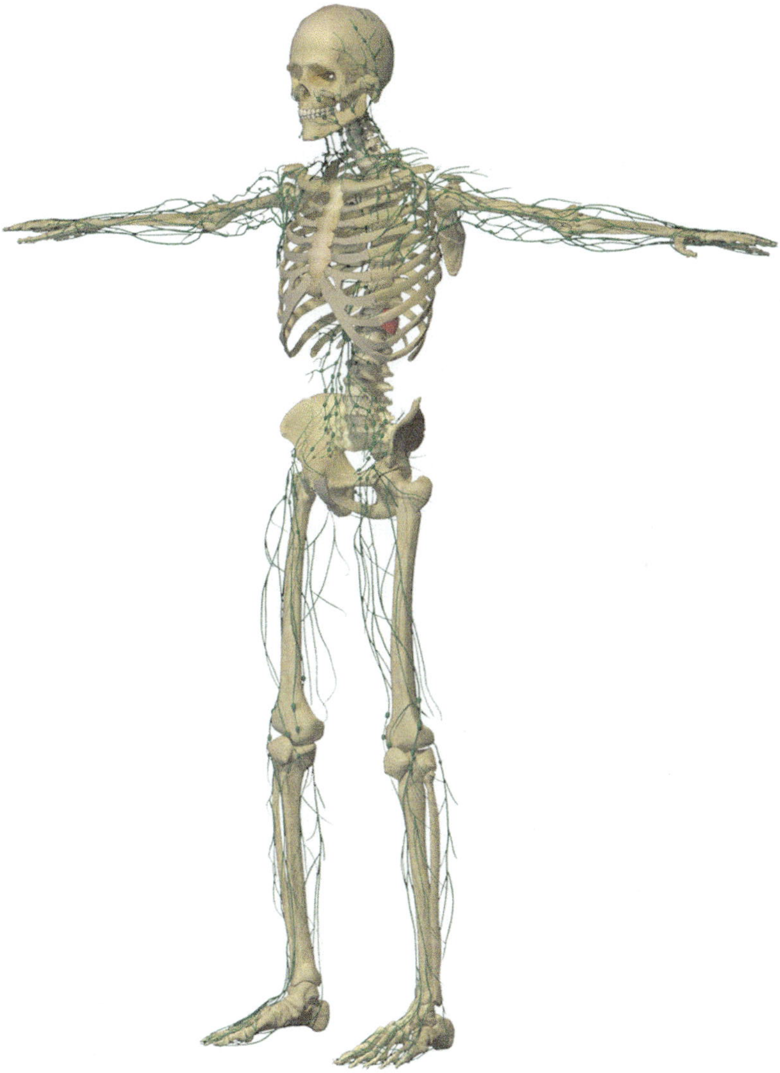

Fig. 23.1 Schematic diagram of the lymphatic system demonstrating the superficial and deep lymphatics and lymph nodes

23.3 Pathophysiology

Lymphedema is an imbalance between lymphatic fluid formation and lymphatic fluid absorption, representing a high-output or low-output failure of the lymphatic system or a combination of both. The increase of interstitial fluid leads to a cascade of remodeling that leads to permanent changes in the tissues of the affected limb [1–3, 7].

High-output failure (also known as dynamic insufficiency) occurs when excessive lymphatic fluid formation exceeds the transport capacity of the intact lymphatic system. Increases in lymphatic fluid production may arise when Starling forces shift net pressure to favor the flow of fluid into the interstitium. Increases in venous pressure result in increased hydrostatic pressure within the venules, and capillaries increase the driving force for ultrafiltration [1–3]. The loss of oncotic pressure, as seen in hypoproteinemic states such as malnutrition, has a similar effect. Elevated venous pressure occurs in patients with right heart failure, deep vein thrombosis, and venous insufficiency. Local inflammation increases capillary permeability, accelerating the loss of fluid and plasma proteins into the interstitium [1–3].

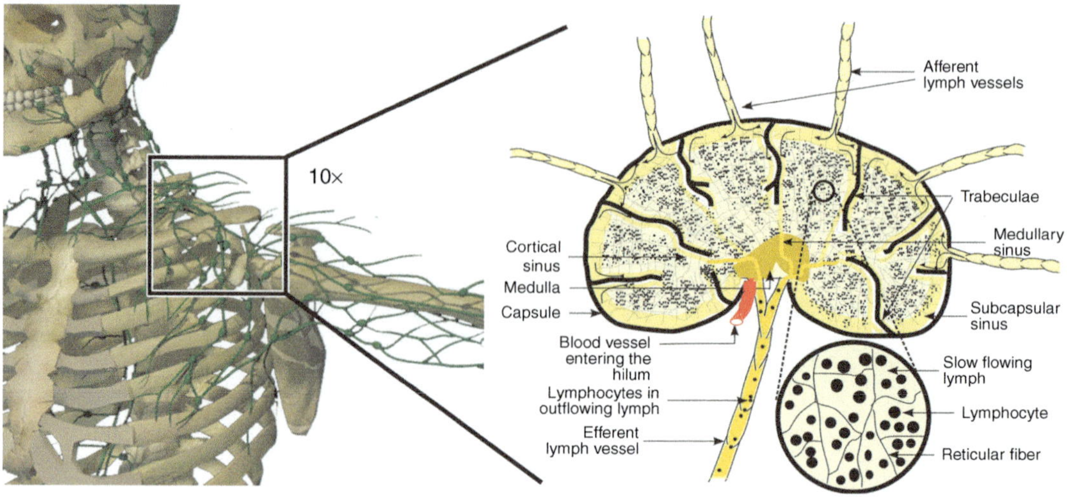

Fig. 23.2 Schematic diagram of the lymphatic vessels. Note the initial lymphatic vessels that are represented as solid green, smaller-diameter vessels that drain into the larger-diameter collecting lymphatic vessels. Note the smooth muscle cells around the collecting lymphatics and the presence of valves. Segments of collecting lymphatic vessels located between two valves are known as "lymphangions"

In contrast, low-output failure (also known as mechanical insufficiency) occurs when there is injury or impairment of the lymphatic system due to paralysis, obstruction, or inadequacy of the lymphatics (e.g., lymphedema from filarial lymphatic obstruction or congenital hypoplasia) [1–3]. As lymphatic obstruction progresses, tortuosity, dilatation, and pooling of lymphatic fluid give way to massive ectasia, valvular destruction, retrograde lymph flow, and lymph coagulation. Intrinsic truncal contractions fail; intraluminal valves give way, and hydrostatic pressure increases in the superficial valveless lymphatic watersheds. Chronic inflammation results in mast cell infiltration, disruption of the interstitial elastin fiber network, intense lymphangiogenesis and hemangiogenesis, fibrosis, progressive fat deposits, and skin thickening [1–3].

Dermal edema is the hallmark of lymphedema and represents the earliest clinical manifestation of lymphatic impairment [1, 2]. The presence of dilated lymphatic vessels may also be evident. With prolonged lymphatic impairment, tissue changes include fibroplasia, hyperkeratosis, and increases in stromal cells. In addition, elastic tissue fragmentation, clumping, and loss of mature elastic fibers also occur. Abundant subcutaneous fat becomes a predominant component of the swelling seen in the affected limb [3, 7].

The inflammatory cells present in the edematous tissue contribute to the ongoing fibrosis. It is believed that the inflammatory cells fail to migrate to the lymph nodes due to impaired lymphatic transport and dysfunctional lymphangiogenesis, leading to worsening edema and further inflammation. This ultimately results in impaired immune trafficking and decreased clearance of pathogens [1, 2].

Lymphedema is a progressive and usually painless swelling of the limbs or genitals that is the result of decreased transport capacity of the lymphatic system. Lymphedema can be primary or secondary. Primary lymphedema is due to a defect in the lymph conducting pathways. Secondary lymphedema is due to an acquired cause (such as filariasis, previous surgery, radiation therapy, malignancy, infection, and inflammation) that results in injury and impairment of the lymphatic system (Fig. 23.3) [2–4, 7, 8].

23.4 Stages of Lymphedema

Regardless of the etiology, lymphedema is clinically staged by the extent of visible tissue degradation (Table 23.1) [9–12]. In the early stages of lymphedema (stage I), the associated limb swelling resembles other types of edema such as that

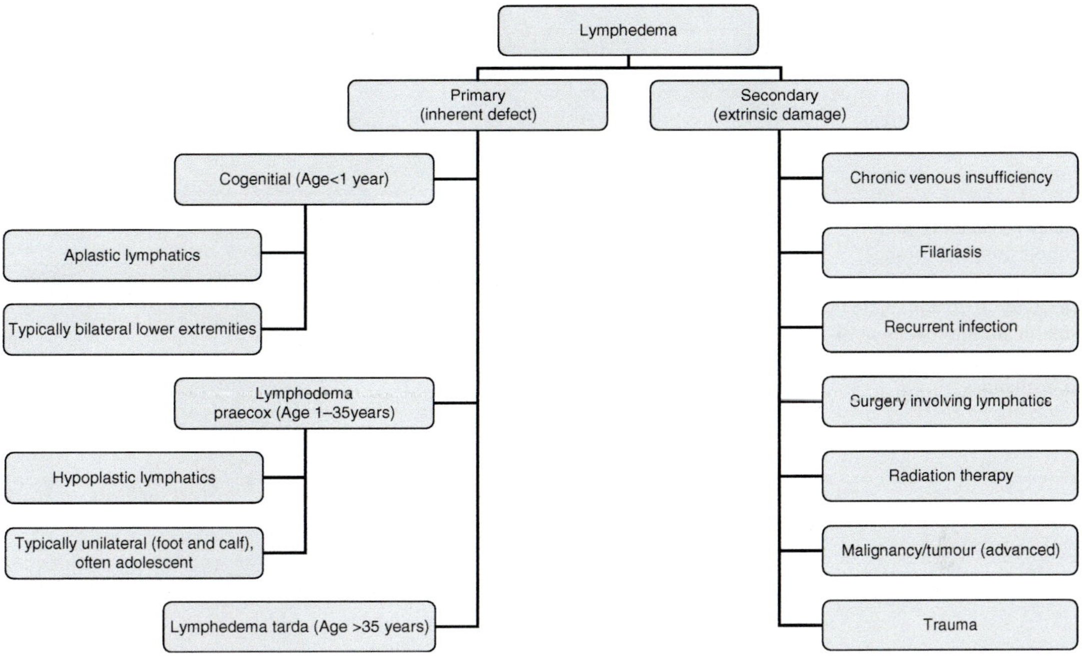

Fig. 23.3 Primary and secondary lymphedema. Lymphedema is the result of decreased transport capacity of the lymphatic system. Lymphedema can be primary or secondary. Primary lymphedema is due to a defect in the lymph conducting pathways. Secondary lymphedema is due to an acquired cause

Table 23.1 Stages of lymphedema

Latency	Risk for lymphedema present. No clinical change evident
Stage I	Pitting, reduces overnight with simple measures (elevation). No fibrosis
Stage II	No longer pitting, no full reduction with elevation, evident fibrosis
Stage III	Nonreversible, hardened fibrosis and sclerosis of cutaneous and subcutaneous tissues

seen with congestive heart failure, renal insufficiency, and venous disease. At this stage, the swelling is completely relieved with elevation and/or overnight rest. The tissues are soft and usually pitting with no evidence of fibrosis. As the condition progresses (stage II), the edema is no longer relieved with elevation or rest, and skin changes begin to appear such as induration of the skin and progressive hardening. The edema also becomes nonpitting. In the late, chronic stage of lymphedema (stage III), the edema is severe, and the skin is fibrotic with numerous skin changes that include hyperkeratosis, warty projections, cobblestoning, and lichenification (Fig. 23.4). Stage III lymphedema is also known as "elephantiasis" because the affected limb begins to resemble the leg of an elephant [9, 10, 13].

23.5 Primary Lymphedema

In patients with primary lymphedema, the cause of decreased lymphatic transport can be an intrinsic "defect" or a malfunction of the lymph conducting elements, which is believed to be a genetically determined abnormality of lymph drainage [2]. The majority of lymphedemas classified as primary lymphedema have inborn abnormalities of the lymphatic system that manifest mostly with irregular or abnormal structural development caused by abnormal (mutant) genes [2, 11]. These abnormalities result in lymphatic hypoplasia, aplasia, numerical hyperplasia, or dilation (lymphangiectasia) with valvular incompetence [2, 11].

Primary lymphedemas have been classified into three groups, depending on the age of onset: congenital (before age 2), praecox (onset between ages 2 and 35), and tarda (after age 35). Lymphedema praecox is the most common form of primary

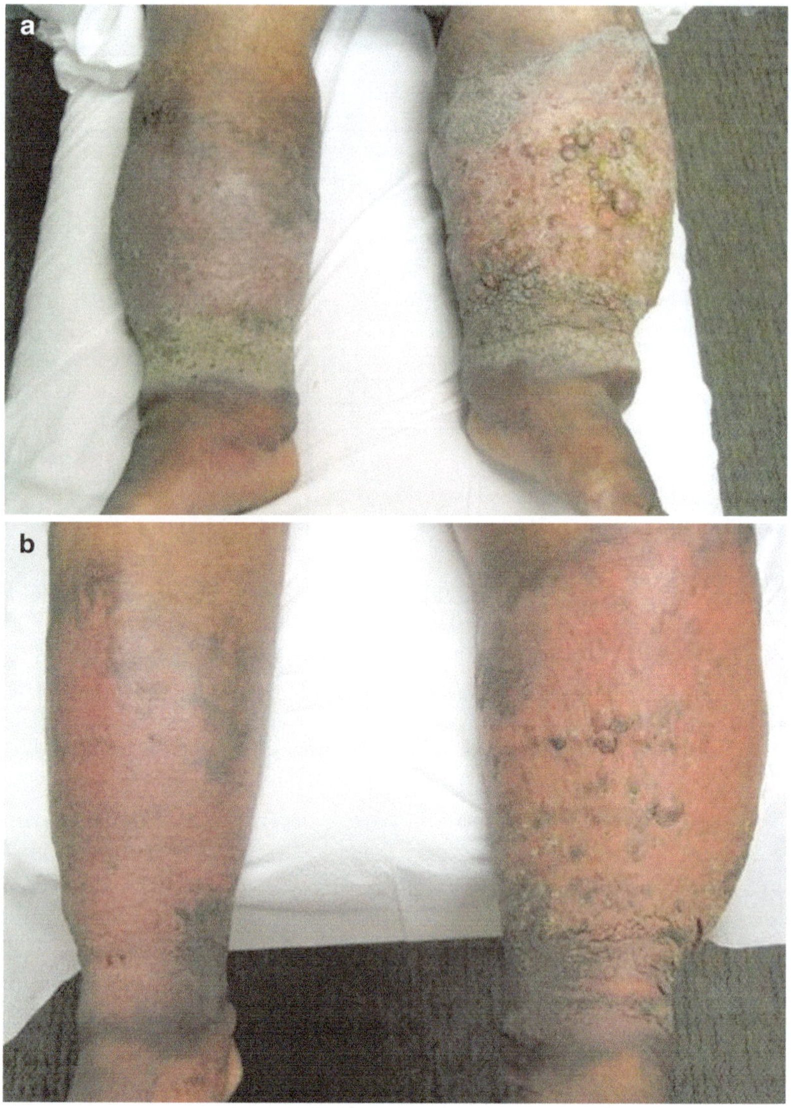

Fig. 23.4 Bilateral lower extremity lymphedema in a 56-year-old man before and after complex decongestive therapy. (**a**) Before treatment. Note the significant limb swelling and chronic skin changes (lichenification, warty projections, and cobblestone appearance) associated with lymphedema. (**b**) After treatment. Note the significant improvement in limb swelling and chronic skin changes

lymphedema with a female to male ratio of 10:1. It is usually unilateral and often limited to the foot and calf in most patients (Fig. 23.3) [2, 8, 11].

23.6 Secondary Lymphedema

Secondary lymphedema is far more common than primary lymphedema and represents 90 % of cases of lymphedema. The most common causes of lower extremity lymphedema are tumor (e.g., lymphoma, prostate cancer, ovarian cancer), surgery involving the lymphatics, radiation therapy, obesity, trauma, and infection. Worldwide, infection with the parasitic nematode Wuchereria bancrofti (also known as filariasis) is the most common cause of lymphedema (Fig. 23.3) [2, 4, 8].

23.7 Diagnosis

23.7.1 Clinical Evaluation

Evaluation of patients with lymphedema must include a detailed, careful history and thorough physical examination [3, 4, 7, 11, 12]. The history should include age at onset, travel to tropical countries, and history of all causes that could

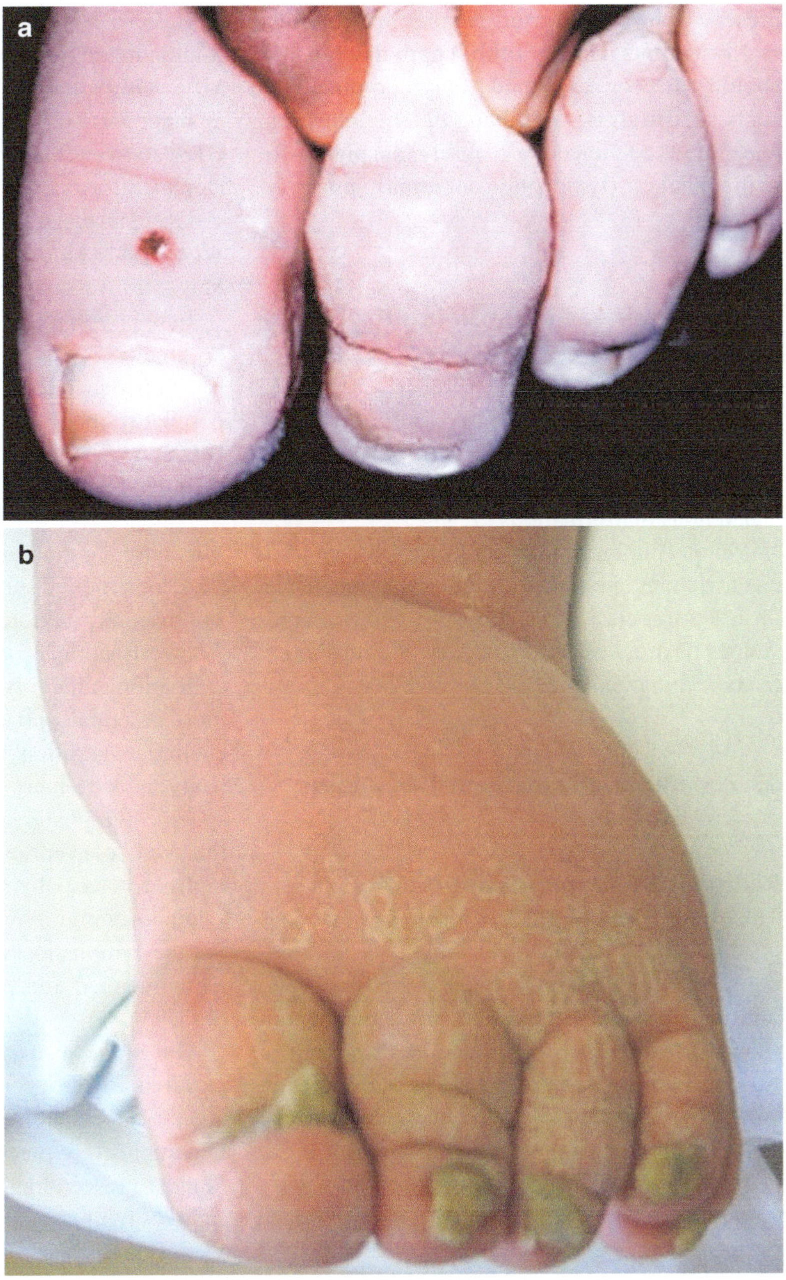

Fig. 23.5 Clinical signs of lymphedema. (**a**) Positive Stemmer's sign (a failure by the examiner to pick up or pinch a fold of skin at the base of the second toe). (**b**) Buffalo hump on the dorsum of the left foot in a patient with lymphedema

result in secondary lymphedema such as surgery, malignancy, venous insufficiency, trauma, and cellulitis. A history of temporary edema of the affected limb or other areas must be noted, and a detailed family history of limb swelling should also be recorded.

Signs and symptoms of lymphedema should be documented. These include nonpitting edema, skin changes such as "peau d'orange," pinkish-red skin discoloration, hyperkeratosis, dermatitis, eczema, ulceration, varicosity, lymph vesicles, warty projections, drainage of fluid (clear or milky), or yellow discoloration or other abnormalities of the nails (Fig. 23.4). The presence of Stemmer's sign (inability to pinch a fold of skin at the base of the second toe) or puffiness of the forefoot (buffalo hump) should be noted (Fig. 23.5) [3, 7, 11, 12]. The presence of venous, arteriovenous, or capillary malformations and any limb length discrepancy should be recorded. Finally, any complications such as cellulitis, lymphangitis, malnutrition, and immunodeficiency or, rarely, suspicion for malignancies (lymphangiosarcoma) must be documented [3, 7, 11].

23.7.2 Noninvasive Radiologic Studies

Plain film X-rays will identify limb length discrepancies, bone abnormalities, or phleboliths in patients with combined lymphatic malformations and venous malformations [7, 11].

Venous duplex studies will confirm any associated venous anomalies (valvular incompetence, obstruction, ectasia, or aneurysms) and assess for venous obstruction as an etiology or contributing factor to lymphedema [7, 11].

23.7.3 Minimally Invasive Radiologic Studies

Radionuclide Lymphoscintigraphy

This study is performed with a subcutaneous injection of 99mTc-labeled human serum albumin (HAS) or 99mTc-labeled sulfur colloid (SC) into the first and second web space of the toes (fingers), followed by radionuclide scanning at various time intervals [7, 11]. It is the test of choice to confirm or exclude lymphedema as the cause of chronic limb swelling. Removal of the colloid from the injection site; appearance time of activity at the knee, groins, or axilla; absence or presence of major lymphatic collectors; number and size of vessels and nodes; the presence of collaterals and reflux; and symmetric activity with the opposite side are recorded and used for interpretation.

An appropriate combination of non- to minimally invasive tests normally should provide all the information necessary to insure an adequate diagnosis and lead to the correct multidisciplinary, specifically targeted and sequenced treatment strategy. The tests and the information they provide are indicated here [11].

Basic/essential tests:

Radionuclide lymphoscintigraphy

MRI with/without contrast for the differential diagnosis

CT scan to exclude underlying pathology

Duplex ultrasonography

Optional tests:

Whole body blood pool scintigraphy (WBBPS)

Magnetic resonance (MR) and/or ultrasound lymphography

Volumetry

Bio-impedance spectrometry

Air plethysmography

Ultrasonographic lymphangiography: investigational for the reconstructive surgery candidate patient

MR lymphangiography: investigational for the reconstructive surgery candidate patient

Microscopic fluorescent lymphangiography: investigational for phlebolymphedema

Radionuclide lymphoscintigraphy is the most essential part of the diagnosis of lymphedema in addition to clinical evaluation. This study is extremely useful for delineating the specific lymphatic abnormality and has largely replaced conventional oil contrast lymphography for visualizing the lymphatic network. Lymphoscintigraphy remains the gold standard for the lymphatic function evaluation, which is recommended for proper clinical management [3, 7, 11].

On some occasions an invasive study is required for an accurate diagnosis. These tests and the information they provide are listed below:

Direct puncture percutaneous lymphangiography

Standard (ascending) lymphangiography

Indirect lymphography using water-soluble contrast media

Fine needle aspiration biopsy of lymph node

Skin biopsy in cases of suspected sarcoma and skin cancer or differential diagnosis of warty lesions

Invasive tests are seldom required for diagnosis but are occasionally needed for confirming the diagnosis or planning surgical therapy.

Conventional oil contrast lymphangiography, especially if coupled with computed tomography (CT) scanning, is still advantageous in selected patients with chylous dysplasia and gravitational reflux disorders in order to define more clearly the extension of the pathologic alterations and sites of lymphatic and chylous leakage [11]. It is the only diagnostic study that can clearly demonstrate pathologies of chylous vessels, chylous cyst, and thoracic duct in cases of chylothorax, chylous ascites, protein-losing enteropathy, etc.

As a part of the diagnostic procedure, the systemic causes of edema (e.g., heart failure, hypoproteinemia, pulmonary hypertension, hypothyroidism, cyclic edema) should be ruled out. Duplex ultrasonography should be performed initially in all forms of lymphedema to assess for concomitant venous disease.

Diagnostic evaluation should also include appropriate assessment of the patient's understanding of the disease process and ability to be compliant with the treatment regimen, since the outcome of successful management is totally dependent on the patient's active participation in the care of his or her lymphedema.

23.8 Treatment of Lymphedema

23.8.1 General Considerations

The importance of patient education and compliance cannot be overemphasized when treating patients with both primary and secondary lymphedema. The patient must first understand that lymphedema is a chronic condition and will never be completely cured. In addition they must also understand that there is no "quick fix" operation, medication, or therapy that will completely reverse the clinical condition. Treatment of lymphedema is essentially management of the medical condition and prevention of progression of the disease process. Lymphedema can be successfully managed.

The goals of lymphedema therapy are to arrest progression, reduce swelling, maintain that reduction, prevent infection, restore mobility and range of motion, and train patients for self-management [4, 10, 14].

The treatment of lymphedema requires diligence and motivation on the part of the patient. The patient must be an active, compliant participant for successful management. The mainstay of lymphedema treatment is through physical therapeutic measures occurring in the setting of a specific lymphedema therapy program, performed by specially trained lymphedema therapists [3, 10, 14, 15].

23.8.2 Physical Treatments

Physical treatment to reduce swelling is aimed at controlling lymph formation and improving lymph drainage through existing lymphatic vessels and collateral routes by applying normal physical processes which stimulate lymph flow (Table 23.2) [3, 10, 12, 14–16]. Manual therapies in multiple forms remain the most widely used interventions for the therapeutic management of lymphedema, regardless of etiology.

Table 23.2 Physical treatments for lymphedema

Treatment	Effect
Exercise	Dynamic muscle contractions encourage movement of lymph along tissue planes and noncontractile, initial lymph vessels (passive drainage) and increased contractility of collecting lymph vessels (active drainage)
Compression garments	Opposes capillary filtration Acts as a counterforce to muscle contractions generating greater interstitial pressure changes
Manual lymphatic drainage	Form of massage therapy that stimulates lymph flow in more proximal, normally draining lymphatics to "siphon" lymph from congested areas
Compression bandaging	Used as an intensive treatment in combination with exercise to reduce large, misshapen lower limbs and permit subsequent maintenance treatment with compression stockings
Pneumatic compression	Softens and reduces limb volume but can forcibly displace fluid into the trunk and genitalia. Compression garments must be worn after treatment
Elevation	Does not stimulate lymph drainage, but lowers venous pressure and therefore capillary filtration, allowing lymph drainage to catch up

Table 23.3 Complex decongestive therapy

Phase I: intensive reduction therapy
Manual lymphatic drainage massage
Multilayered low-stretch wrapping techniques
Specific exercise regimen
Skin care education and techniques
Phase II: maintenance therapy
Daily wear of pressure garment
Continued nightly multilayered wrapping
Self-manual lymphatic drainage massage
Exercise
Continued meticulous skin management

Manual lymphatic drainage (MLD) is a highly specialized form of massage therapy that employs very light and gentle cutaneous distension to enhance lymph transport. MLD is believed to stimulate and increase the intrinsic contractility of lymph collecting vessels and encourage increased protein molecule sequestration and subsequent transport [10, 14–16]. MLD is often combined with other manual therapies including compression bandaging, exercise regimens, skin care techniques, pressure gradient garments, and pneumatic compression devices [15–20].

Complex decongestive therapy (CDT) is a combined approach to lymphedema therapy that has been standardized by multiple international lymphatic treatment organizations and specialized lymphedema treatment programs [10, 14–16]. The treatment regimen is composed of two phases: intensive reduction therapy followed by maintenance therapy (Table 23.3). This treatment regimen utilizes MLD, compression wrapping, exercise therapy, and skin care. This highly successful treatment regimen has become the standard of care for lymphedema management [10, 14–16]. Significant improvement and reduction of swelling is often readily apparent after treatment (Fig. 23.4).

Compression wrapping in various forms has been a long-standing treatment of both venous and lymphatic edema [10, 17–20]. Lymphatic wrapping techniques are complex and utilize low-stretch bandages instead of the more traditional high-stretch elastic bandages. High-stretch wrapping produces high pressures at rest that decrease with limb muscle contraction and movement. This decreases the ability of the wrap to raise the tissue pressure during exercise, reducing the hydrostatic pressure gradient and resulting in a reduction in stimulation of lymphatic flow [10, 17–20].

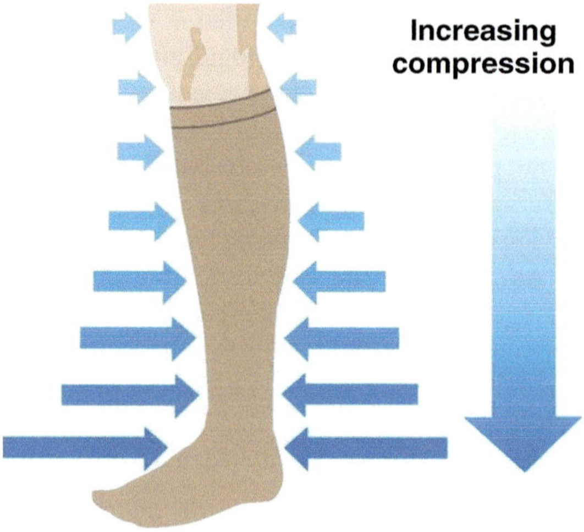

Fig. 23.6 Graduated compression stockings. Graduated compression stockings have the highest pressure at the ankle level. The pressure decreases up the leg where the pressure is the lowest at the highest level. The ideal compression for lymphedema treatment is 30–40 mmHg

In contrast, low-stretch wrapping provides resistance during muscle pump action that results in an increase in pressure gradient and stimulates increased fluid flow [10, 17–20]. Patients with significant obesity, pain problems, or advanced disease may not be able to comply with the complexities of wrapping. For these patients, static gradient compression devices are available.

The use of elastic compression garments is the mainstay of the maintenance portion of any lymphedema management program [10, 17–21]. Compliance with daily use of compression stockings or sleeves is critical for maintenance of limb size and volume. Compression garments should have graduated compression where pressure is highest distally and decreases proximally where the pressure is lowest at the highest level (Fig. 23.6). For an upper extremity graduated compression sleeve, pressure is highest at the hand/wrist and is lowest at the shoulder. For a lower extremity graduated compression stocking, pressure is highest at the ankle and is lowest at the

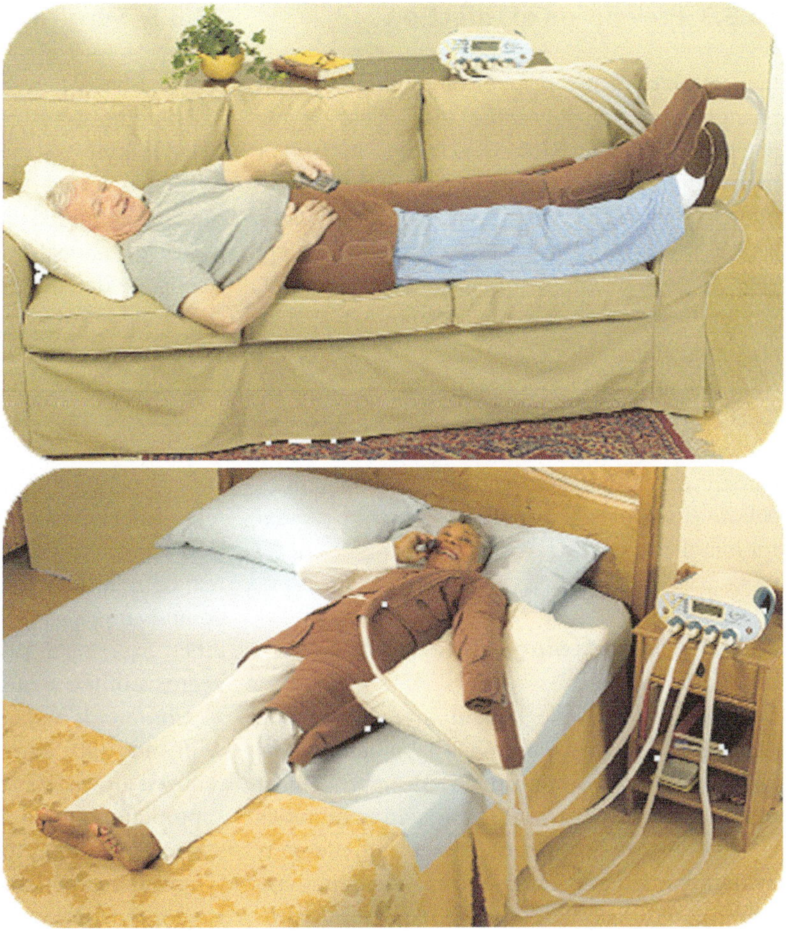

Fig. 23.7 The Flexitouch system pneumatic compression device. This pneumatic compression device closely mimics manual lymphatic drainage with the use of multiple small compression chambers. Compression sleeves for the lower extremity (*top*) and upper extremities and trunk (*bottom*) are available

knee, thigh, or waist, depending on the length of the stocking. Recommended graduated compression is 30–40 mmHg for the lower extremity [10, 18]. Upper extremity lymphedema sleeves are available with a graduated compression of 20–30 mmHg, which is usually adequate [10, 18].

In addition to providing graduated compression, compression stockings and sleeves also assist with venous return, help preserve skin integrity, and protect the skin from trauma [10]. Currently, there are many manufacturers who produce graduated compression stockings and sleeves with different pressure strengths, different fabrics, and multiple color options. The ability to independently don the compression garment is critical. Numerous devices are available to assist with stocking and sleeve donning.

For decades prior to the introduction of CDT, pneumatic compression pumps were the mainstay of lymphedema therapy. Since the mid-1990s, when CDT became more widely available, the use of pneumatic compression pump therapy has largely become an adjunct to CDT in both the reductive and maintenance phases [3, 10, 14, 22]. The majority of pneumatic compression pumps perform sequential pumping of the affected lymphedematous limb from distal to proximal. These devices augment the beneficial effects of the standard modalities of CDT. There is a new class of sequential pneumatic compression device, known as the Flexitouch system. This pneumatic compression device closely mimics MLD with the use of multiple small compression chambers (Fig. 23.7).

23.8.3 Prevention of Infection

Prevention of acute episodes of cellulitis or lymphangitis is critical because they cause severe deterioration in swelling and result in further injury to the lymphatic system [12, 21, 22]. Care of the skin, good hygiene, control of skin diseases such as tinea pedis, and careful antiseptic dressing application after minor wounds are all important. Antibiotics must be administered promptly when an acute inflammatory episode occurs. There are no definitive studies addressing antibiotic prophylaxis for patients at risk for lymphedema, but evidence has shown the relationship between chronic fungal infection and the development of cellulitis, which is known to increase the potential for lymphatic failure [12, 22].

23.8.4 Pharmacologic Treatment

Diuretics are of little benefit in patients with lymphedema because the pharmacologic effects only limit capillary filtration [2, 3]. Improvement in lymphedema patients who are taking diuretics suggests that the predominant cause of edema is not lymphatic and is likely due to another undiagnosed etiology. In cases where increased hydrostatic pressure is also elevated, such as the postphlebitic syndrome with secondary hypertension, low-dose thiazide-induced diuresis may play a beneficial complementary role to compression therapy [12].

Coumarin, a benzopyrone medication, has been reported to be of benefit to patients with lymphedema [23]. However, the poor study design of most of the coumarin trials limits interpretability. The therapeutic benefit, if present, has been theoretically ascribed to its effects on cutaneous macrophages and, thereby, on local proteolysis. The medication also stimulates other cellular elements of the immune system and may promote protein reabsorption. Despite some encouraging early trials, coumarin must still be considered experimental [23–25]. In addition, its associated risk of hepatotoxicity makes this medication an even much less attractive treatment option [3, 23].

23.8.5 Surgical Therapy

In situations where CDT fails to improve the size and weight of a lymphedematous limb that is so large, it inhibits its use and interferes with mobility and function, and surgery may be of value. Surgery is aimed at either removing excessive tissue (excisional procedures) or bypassing local lymphatic defects (lymphatic reconstruction procedures) [4, 26]. CDT is still required after surgical excision and reconstruction.

Excisional procedures usually involve staged removal of the lymphedematous subcutaneous tissue of the leg [26–29]. The most radical excisional operation, the Charles procedure, involves total skin and subcutaneous tissue excision of the lower extremity from the tibial tuberosity to the malleoli, followed by skin grafting. The main complications associated with this procedure and other excisional procedures are infection and necrosis of the skin graft [26].

Chronic lymphedematous tissue transforms with time into adipose tissue, which cannot be reduced by massage or compression treatment. Liposuction aimed at removing this adipose tissue has been reported to be beneficial in treating lymphedematous limbs [28, 29]. This procedure is not routinely performed for treatment of lymphedema.

Developments in microvascular techniques have allowed surgical attempts at direct lymphatic reconstructions, performance of lymphatic-venous anastomoses, or lymphatic grafting [26, 30, 31]. These reconstructions are usually indicated in only a small subset of patients who have proximal obstruction with preserved lymphatic vessels distally.

The best outcomes are seen in patients with secondary lymphedema, with well-defined trauma to the lymphatics, seen on lymphatic imaging, who underwent lymphatic to venous anastomoses [30, 31].

Lymphatic bypass procedures are only performed in a few selected cases and in only a few specialized medical centers. This is reflected in the literature by small patient numbers in most series reported [26]. Results are variable, and lymphatic bypass procedures are generally not routinely performed except at these few specialized medical centers.

References

1. Dellinger MT, Bernas MJ, Witte MH. Lymphatic biology and pathobiology. In: Dieter RS, Dieter Jr RA, Dieter RA, editors. Venous and lymphatic diseases. New York: McGraw Hill; 2011. p. 17–36.
2. Thanaporn PK, Rockson SG. Disease of the lymphatic vasculature. In: Dieter RS, Dieter Jr RA, Dieter RA, editors. Venous and lymphatic diseases. New York: McGraw Hill; 2011. p. 569–94.
3. Rockson SG. Diagnosis and management of lymphatic vascular disease. J Am Coll Cardiol. 2008; 52(10):799–806.
4. Tiwari A, Cheng KS, Button M, Myint F, Hamilton G. Differential diagnosis, investigation, and current treatment of lower limb lymphedema. Arch Surg. 2003;138(2):152–61.
5. Ely JW, Osheroff JA, Chambliss ML, Ebell MH. Approach to leg edema of unclear etiology. J Am Board Fam Med. 2006;19(2):148–60.
6. Alitalo K, Tammela T, Petrova TV. Lymphangiogenesis in development and human disease. Nature. 2005; 438:946–53.
7. Rooke TW, Felty C. Lymphedema: pathophysiology, classification, and clinical evaluation. In: Gloviczki P, editor. Handbook of venous disorders. 3rd ed. London: Hodder Arnold; 2009. p. 629–34.
8. Kerchner K, Fleischer A, Yosipovitch G. Lower extremity lymphedema update: pathophysiology, diagnosis, and treatment guidelines. J Am Acad Dermatol. 2008;59(2):324–31.
9. International Society of Lymphology. The diagnosis and treatment of peripheral lymphedema. 2009 Concensus Document of the International Society of Lymphology. Lymphology. 2009;42(2):51–60.
10. Gamble GL, Cheville A, Strick D. Lymphedema: medical and physical therapy. In: Gloviczki P, editor. Handbook of venous disorders. 3rd ed. London: Hodder Arnold; 2009. p. 649–57.
11. Lee B, Andrade M, Bergan J, Boccardo F, Campisi C, Damstra R, et al. Diagnosis and treatment of primary lymphedema. Consensus document of the International Union of Phlebology (IUP)-2009. Int Angiol. 2010;29(5):454–70.
12. Mortimer PS. ABC of arterial and venous disease swollen lower limb – 2: Lymphoedema. BMJ. 2000; 320:1527–9.
13. Dean SM, Zirwas MJ, Horst AV. Elephantiasis nostras verrucosa: an institutional analysis of 21 cases. J Am Acad Dermatol. 2011;64(6):1104–10.
14. Cheville AL, McGarvey CL, Petrek JA, Russo SA, Taylor ME, Thiadens SR. Lymphedema management. Semin Radiat Oncol. 2003;13(3):290–301.
15. Mayrovitz HN. The standard of care for lymphedema: current concepts and physiological considerations. Lymphat Res Biol. 2009;7(2):101–8.
16. Badger C, Preston N, Seers K, Mortimer P. Physical therapies for reducing and controlling lymphoedema of the limbs. Cochrane Database Syst Rev. 2004;4, CD003141.
17. Partsch H, Mosti G. Thigh compression. Phlebology. 2008;23(6):252–8.
18. Partsch H, Flour M, Smith PC, International Compression Club. Indications for compression therapy in venous and lymphatic disease consensus based on experimental data and scientific evidence. Under the auspices of the IUP. Int Angiol. 2008;27(3): 193–219.
19. Pappas CJ, O'Donnell Jr TF. Long-term results of compression treatment for lymphedema. J Vasc Surg. 1992;16(4):555–62.
20. Damstra RJ, Brouwer ER, Partsch H. Controlled, comparative study of relation between volume changes and interface pressure under short-stretch bandages in leg lymphedema patients. Dermatol Surg. 2008;34(6):773–8.
21. Mortimer PS. Therapy approaches for lymphedema. Angiology. 1997;48(1):87–91.
22. Keeley VL. Lymphoedema and cellulitis: chicken or egg? Br J Dermatol. 2008;158(6):1175–6.
23. Badger C, Preston N, Seers K, Mortimer P. Benzo-pyrones for reducing and controlling lymphoedema of the limbs. Cochrane Database Syst Rev. 2004;2, CD003140.
24. Casley-Smith JR. Benzo-pyrones in the treatment of lymphoedema. Int Angiol. 1999;18(1):31–41.
25. Loprinzi CL, Kugler JW, Sloan JA, Rooke TW, Quella SK, Novotny P, et al. Lack of effect of coumarin in women with lymphedema after treatment for breast cancer. N Engl J Med. 1999;340(5):346–50.
26. Gloviczki P. Principles of surgical treatment of chronic lymphedema. In: Gloviczki P, editor. Handbook of venous disorders. 3rd ed. London: Hodder Arnold; 2009. p. 658–64.
27. Miller TA, Wyatt LE, Rudkin GH. Staged skin and subcutaneous excision for lymphedema: a favorable report of long-term results. Plast Reconstr Surg. 1998;102(5):1486–98.
28. Brorson H. From lymph to fat: complete reduction of lymphoedema. Phlebology. 2010;25 Suppl 1:52–63.
29. Brorson H, Ohlin K, Olsson G, Svensson B, Svensson H. Controlled compression and liposuction treatment for lower extremity lymphedema. Lymphology. 2008;41(2):52–63.
30. Campisi C, Bellini C, Campisi C, Accogli S, Bonioli E, Boccardo F. Microsurgery for lymphedema: clinical research and long-term results. Microsurgery. 2010;30(4):256–60.
31. Campisi C, Eretta C, Pertile D, Da Rin E, Campisi C, Macciò A, et al. Microsurgery for treatment of peripheral lymphedema: long-term outcome and future perspectives. Microsurgery. 2007;27(4):333–8.

Venous Leg Ulcers

24

Robert B. McLafferty

Contents

Abstract

Venous leg ulcers are the most common form of leg ulcer. While there are many rare causes of ulcerations that can occur from knee to the toes, the overview provided herein gives the practitioner guidance on how to evaluate a patient presenting with a leg ulcer and care for and heal the venous ulcer and information about other more common types of ulcers that are in the differential diagnosis. Fortunately, history and physical examination can help determine, with some confirmatory tests, the type of ulcer. Nevertheless, the essentials of wound healing remain the same for the large majority of ulcers on the lower extremities. Healing will hasten if treatment of all leg ulcers includes assuring adequate perfusion; removing nonviable tissue; reducing inflammation and eliminating infection, relieving edema; optimizing tissue growth; off-loading or providing pressure relief; controlling pain; and treating host systemic disease or conditions such as diabetes and nutrition.

24.1 Introduction

Chronic ulceration of the lower leg and foot continues to be one of the more formidable clinical problems in medicine. Conditions leading to ulceration of this susceptible region of the body frequently cause pain, disability, social stigma, and considerable costs. Burden on family

R.B. McLafferty, MD, FACS, RVT
Division of Vascular Surgery, Department of Surgery, Southern Illinois University, School of Medicine, Springfield, IL, USA
e-mail: robert.mclafferty@va.gov

E. Mowatt-Larssen et al. (eds.), *Phlebology, Vein Surgery and Ultrasonography*,
DOI 10.1007/978-3-319-01812-6_24, © Springer International Publishing Switzerland 2014

members, caretakers, and medical facilities as well as the economic strain from inability to work can be high, further complicating the pathway to healing. A staggering 1 % of the population will suffer from chronic ulceration of the leg during some time over a lifetime [1, 2]. The prevalence of leg ulcerations increases with age and ranges from 3 to 5 % in the adult population over the age of 65 years [1–4]. In one study from the UK, the prevalence of venous ulcers alone in individuals over the age of 65 was estimated to be 1–2 % [5].

Although there are varying definitions of the term ulcer, the two prerequisites include full thickness obliteration of the epidermis and dermis with no sources of epithelialization in the center of the ulcer combined with the tendency of slow healing. Generally, as compared to an acute wound, a slow-healing ulcer is defined as being present for more than 4 weeks. Reasons for chronic ulcers are not necessarily related to depth and size but often associated with an underlying disease manifestation (systemic, local, or both) that requires specialized treatment in order to induce healing.

Dividing the causes of ulcers into common and rare etiologies helps in the construction of an accurate differential diagnosis. The most common causes of leg ulcers are chronic venous disease (45–90 %), diabetes mellitus (15–25 %), arterial ischemia (10–20 %), or a combination of two or more of these etiologies (10–15 %) [6–9]. Less common causes of ulcers, but not necessarily rare, include infections, decubitus (pressure), and vasculitis. This chapter will primarily focus on the diagnosis and care for venous leg ulcers and also briefly outline evaluation and treatment options of other causes of leg ulcers in the differential diagnosis. The importance of correct diagnosis cannot be over emphasized as diagnostic tests and treatments can vary dramatically. Alternatively stated, incorrect diagnosis can lead to incorrect treatment and hence result in further harm to the patient with a leg ulcer.

24.2 Basic Principles

24.2.1 History and Physical Examination

When performing a first-time evaluation on a new patient with a chronic leg ulcer, several basic principles should be followed in addition to a complete history and physical examination. The patient's story of how the ulceration began is important and may give rise to clues as to the type of ulcer. Did the ulcer occur spontaneously from seemingly normal-appearing skin or were there preceding symptoms or signs such as pain, tenderness, itching, swelling, skin discoloration, inflammatory changes, or blisters? Other important aspects of the ulcer include location, size, duration, and symptoms. Do the symptoms vary with time of day or position?

Further clues in the history regarding the patient's overall medical condition include whether or not the patient has had deep venous thrombosis or pulmonary embolism; whether the patient has diabetes mellitus; and whether the patient has risk factors for atherosclerotic disease such as smoking, hypertension, hyperlipidemia, or chronic renal insufficiency. Past history of other events related to atherosclerosis such as stroke, coronary artery disease, or claudication should be elicited. Inflammatory conditions such as rheumatoid arthritis, lupus erythematosus, or inflammatory bowel disease are also important. Other pertinent information include whether the patient has had fever or rigors, recent trauma or surgery, a change in types of shoes being worn, or a history of whether there are any sensory deficits, particularly in the forefoot.

The physical exam from below the knees to the toes requires close methodical inspection and palpation. Vitally important areas to be assessed include the skin on the posterior heel and ankle as well as the web spaces between the toes. Nails deserve close scrutiny and should be described in detail. Bony deformities such as partial foot amputation, bunion, hammertoes, metatarsal head prominence, valgus toe deformity, and/or midfoot collapse (Charcot deformity/joint) should be documented. Edema, varicose veins, inflammatory changes, skin lesions, hypo- or hyperpigmentation, erythema, dependent rubor, cyanosis, and bullae should be noted in addition to a detailed description of the ulcer. Inspection of edema should include whether the foot and/or toes are involved. Characterization of the ulcer should include location, nature of wound edges, depth, moisture content, exposed muscle tendon and/or bone, presence of granulation tissue, and characteristics of necrotic tissue. Palpation includes assessing for pitting edema, tenderness, crepitus, fluctuance, bogginess, and sensation. The presence of neuropathy can be established utilizing a 5.0 monofilament that delivers a standard 10 g of force. The femoral, popliteal, posterior tibial, and dorsal pedal arteries should also be palpated. Vital signs should be performed with particular attention to fever, tachycardia, and hypotension.

24.2.2 Laboratory Assessment

All patients with leg ulcers undergoing initial evaluation deserve the same general blood chemistry testing in order to understand the underlying cause of the ulcer or other contributing factors to nonhealing. Further breadth of laboratory testing can vary depending on the history, examination, and initial results of general blood chemistry testing. All patients should have a complete blood count and a complete metabolic panel. For patients with ulcers that seem to be caused by venous disease, diabetes mellitus, arterial disease, or a combination thereof, additional testing should include hemoglobin A1 C, serum B-12 (cyanocobalamin), thyroid-stimulating hormone (TSH) level, T4 level, fasting lipid panel with attention to high-density lipoprotein cholesterol (HDL-C) and subfractions HDL2-C and HDL3-C, lipoprotein level, and homocysteine level. If a systemic inflammatory condition or immunologic problem is suspected, other blood chemistries should include C-reactive protein, sedimentation rate, rheumatoid factor, antinuclear antibodies, quantitative immunoglobulins, protein electrophoresis, immune complexes, complement (CH50, C3, C4), a-ANCA, and p-ANCA. Patients who have had multiple occurrences of arterial or venous thromboses, thrombosis at a young age (<30), or a strong family history of thrombophilia may benefit from a hypercoagulable evaluation. These laboratory tests include antithrombin III, proteins C and S, factor V Leiden, prothrombin gene mutation, IgG or IgM anticardiolipin antibodies, lupus anticoagulants, hemoglobin electrophoresis for sickle cell disease, and cryoglobulins. Nutritional assessment remains paramount in those patients showing signs of depletion or having coexisting diseases that may hinder wound healing. These include total protein, albumin, prealbumin, transferrin, and absolute lymphocyte count.

24.2.3 Microbial Culture Evaluation

All leg wounds require microbial evaluation whether or not they appear clinically infected. Often, increased bioburden of bacteria, without other signs or symptoms of infection, can be a major detriment to healing. Bacterial cultures can be quantitative, semiquantitative, or qualitative. The most accurate method of qualitative analysis comes from taking a punch biopsy of viable tissue at the margin of the ulcer and having the laboratory immediately determine the number of organisms per gram. If the specimen has greater than 105 organisms, this is sufficient evidence for a clinically infected wound, even when other signs of infection may be lacking. A swab can also be used for a quantitative technique by generously swabbing over a 1 cm^2 area. Using serial dilution techniques, the laboratory can determine the number of organisms per milliliter. Semiquantitative swab technique involves swabbing over the "clean" wound surface which is then streaked onto a Petri dish. Growth is then graded as none, light, moderate, or heavy. Heavy growth represents active infection. Qualitative analysis allows for determination of types of bacteria present as well as fungus, if suspected. Gram stain and aerobic and anaerobic cultures should be routinely obtained. Depending on the results, empiric followed by definitive antibiotic therapy should start immediately.

24.2.4 Skin/Ulcer Biopsy

Tissue biopsy of the skin and ulcer assists in the differential diagnosis of vasculitis syndromes, microthrombotic disorders, inflammatory conditions, and malignancy. A biopsy should be considered if the leg ulcer has an atypical appearance or has shown minimal signs of healing after 2–4 weeks. Typically, a 3–4 mm punch biopsy is used to obtain the tissue, and care should be taken to avoid crushing the specimen. The biopsy should be obtained along the newest or most recent edge of the ulcer and include a rim of "normal" tissue/skin. When examining under light microscopy for inflammatory changes, microthrombi, or necrosis of vessels, specimens should be placed in formaldehyde. Evaluation of autoantibodies, compliment, and fibrin require immunofluorescence and the use of a special transport media for the specimen. Contraindications to tissue biopsy can include bleeding disorders or anticoagulant therapy, moderate to severe immunosuppression, and severe peripheral arterial disease.

24.2.5 Wound Assessment

When assessing a lower extremity ulcer, there are certain features that should be commented upon in order to track changes and improvements. This is particularly important when more than one physician may be involved in the patient's care. Important aspects of the examination and documentation include wound size, length, width, and depth; the quality and quantity of exudate; the wound bed appearance including the presence of granulation tissue, necrotic tissue, and friability; presence of deep tissue structures such as tendon or bone; presence of undermining; and quality of the skin surrounding the ulcer such as eczema, maceration, erythema, or induration. The level of pain and tenderness should be noted with the use of a validated pain scale.

24.2.6 Noninvasive Vascular Testing

Noninvasive vascular testing remains one of the most important parts of assessing patients with a chronic ulcer of the lower extremities. These tests can identify what components of the vascular tree are involved, what pathologic process may be, and what level is involved. Different aspects of venous disease are primarily diagnosed by duplex ultrasound imaging. Acute and chronic deep venous thrombosis or abnormal venous wall pathology is diagnosed by the use of duplex ultrasound. Additionally, venous valve reflux can be performed by using duplex ultrasound and measuring venous valve closure times [10]. All patients should undergo ankle and toe blood pressures to assess for arterial insufficiency as the primary cause or a contributing factor to a nonhealing leg ulcer. Further adjunctive testing for arterial insufficiency may include transcutaneous oxygen measurement, pulse volume recordings, and Doppler waveform studies. These tests may be helpful if patients have heavily calcified tibial arteries or are those with toe amputations (Table 24.1).

24.2.7 X-Ray Evaluation

Evaluation with x-ray helps determine if there is underlying pathology contributing to the severity or cause of the leg ulcer. Patients with clear infection of the foot should undergo plain x-rays of the foot to screen for changes in the bone consistent with osteomyelitis. Computed tomography or magnetic resonance imaging can help determine the presence of deep infection, the presence of soft tissue mass, or the presence of an arteriovenous malformation. Radionucleotide scans can sometimes be helpful in also determining the presence of occult or deeper infected tissue or abscess.

Table 24.1 Noninvasive vascular testing options showing different levels of arterial insufficiency

Ankle-brachial index	
≥0.9–1.3	Normal range
≥0.6–0.8	Borderline perfusion
≤0.5	Severe ischemia
Ankle pressure ≤40 mmHg	Critical limb ischemia
Toe pressure ≤30 mmHg	Critical limb ischemia
Transcutaneous oxygen pressure measurement ($TcPO_2$)	
>40 mmHg	Sufficient to support ulcer healing
20–40 mmHg	Equivocal wound ulcer healing
<20 mmHg	Inability to support ulcer healing
Pulse volume recordings or Doppler waveforms	
Triphasic	Normal
Biphasic	Mild to moderate arterial obstruction
Monophasic	Severe arterial obstruction

24.3 Venous Ulcers

24.3.1 Epidemiology

Venous ulcers are the most common cause of leg ulcers, representing 45–90 % of all leg ulcers [6–9]. Although the exact prevalence of venous ulcers is unknown, the range is estimated to be between 1 and 3 % of the general population in developed countries [11–14]. Of the six to seven million people in the United States with chronic venous disease, about one million individuals have venous ulcers. Contracting these ulcers leads to major economic implications with the lifetime average cost exceeding $40,000 and total cost of care in the United States exceeding one billion dollars per year [7, 14, 15]. These costs are further exacerbated at all levels due to the high recurrence rates of venous ulcers which can be as high as 57–97 % [12].

24.3.2 Pathophysiology

Venous ulcers are a direct result of venous ambulatory hypertension from chronic venous disease. The causes of chronic venous disease include venous insufficiency from valve reflux, venous obstruction, calf muscle pump dysfunction, or a combination of two or more of these causes. The end result is venous hypertension in the upright position which leads to congestion of the deep and superficial venous system. This increase in pressure is ultimately transmitted to the capillaries which in turn leads to leaking of protein-rich serum and erythrocytes into the subcutaneous space. This leads to migration of neutrophils and a pronounced inflammatory response. The physical signs of this process are edema, dermatitis, hyperpigmentation, lipodermatosclerosis, and ulceration. The large majority of venous ulcers occur in the gaiter area of the leg around the medial or lateral malleolus. These ulcers can occur spontaneously or begin after a minor trauma.

24.3.3 History and Physical Examination

Past history of deep venous thrombosis remains a vital part of determining whether chronic venous disease may play a role in a chronic leg ulcer. Location and when the DVT occurred should be noted. History should also include probing questions as to whether the patient may have had an occult deep venous thrombosis. This would include past trauma or surgery to the leg, particularly orthopedic surgery. Historical features unique to deciphering whether venous disease plays a role in a leg ulcer include a past or present history of deep venous thrombosis, pregnancy, obesity, arthritis or other conditions affecting calf muscle pump, varicose veins, trauma to the leg, sedentary lifestyle with chronic dependency of the leg, or a known hypercoagulable state.

Many of the findings on physical examination of leg ulcer are unique only to chronic venous disease. Edema in the early stages can be pitting and then over a longer time becomes "brawny," or nonpitting. The location of edema in chronic venous disease is in the lower leg below the knee and down to the ankle. Edema from chronic venous disease does not involve the foot.

Hyperpigmentation occurs primarily in the ankle area from chronic deposition of erythrocytes that are broken down and deposit hemosiderin [16, 17]. Telangiectasias, reticular veins, and varicose veins are often present. Stasis or venous dermatitis results from the pronounced inflammatory response in the dermis and epidermis. The skin can appear with erythema, scaling, crusting, weeping, and erosions. These areas can incite extreme pruritus, and subsequent scratching can cause mild breaks in the skin which can become a nidus for venous ulceration formation and/or cellulitis. Lipodermatosclerosis can be noted to form in the gaiter area of the leg. This fibrosis and hardening of the subcutaneous space can begin to limit how much edema can occur and subsequently cause the lower leg to appear like an upside-down champagne bottle. These fibrotic changes are thought to be a combination of chronic inflammation and deposition of fibrin and collagen. In some areas within the ankle, smooth white plaques on the skin can occur which are called atrophie blanche. These lesions can be a precursor to venous ulceration.

The venous ulcer is classically located around or on the medial or lateral malleolus (Fig. 24.1). These ulcers can vary in size depending on the chronicity. They are typically exudative and shallow with a dark-red base or possess yellow necrotic slough. The skin borders are generally irregular and maceration and intense skin inflammatory changes are also present. Intensity of pain and tenderness varies from patient to patient.

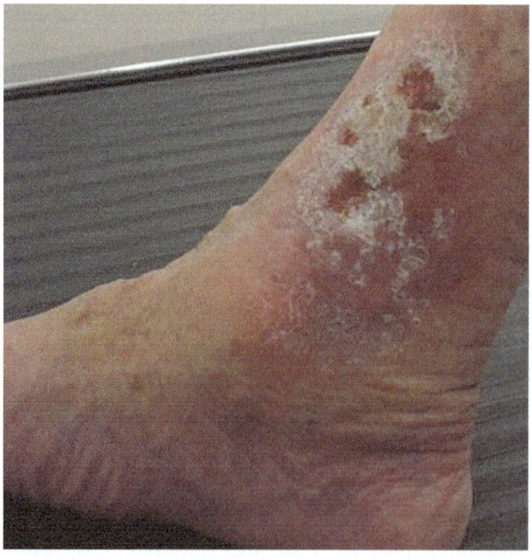

Fig. 24.1 Classical location for a venous ulcer near the medial or lateral malleolus

24.3.4 Management

The mainstay of therapy for the treatment of chronic venous disease and healing venous ulcers is compression therapy [18, 19]. Used as early as the seventeenth century, the application of externally applied pressure or static support helps to return the venous system back to a "normal physiologic state." There are multiple types of compression therapy and all have certain advantages and disadvantages. The basic mechanism of action provides graduated pressure from the ankle to the knee and augments the dysfunctional calf muscle pump during ambulation. With every dorsiflexion, venous return is augmented. Compression also increases the interstitial pressure in the subcutaneous space and muscular compartments while partially collapsing superficial veins. This action promotes normal function of the venous valves, increases velocity of blood flow, and reduces aggregation and extravasation of neutrophils [20, 21].

Compression devices can be categorized as either sustained/static or intermittent/dynamic. Sustained or static compression includes different types of compression wraps, stockings, or orthoses. Intermittent or dynamic compression includes pneumatic pump devices. Table 24.2 lists the breakdown of types of compression with advantages and considerations. Generally, when a patient presents with a venous ulcer, the leg is edematous, weeping, and macerated. Multilayered compression wraps such as Profore (Smith and Nephew, London, England) with multiple layers of elastic and nonelastic components including a thick layer of gauze are the early choice of treatment. Advantages include the ability to absorb exudate, adapt to a changing leg diameter while maintaining compression, and provide continuous compression either with ambulation or at rest. Once the edema is reduced considerably, skin integrity is improved, and the

Table 24.2 Classification of types of leg compression that can be used for chronic venous disease and the venous leg ulcer

Sustained (static)		
Subtypes	Advantages	Considerations
Elastic		
Multilayered compression wraps	For early treatment to control exudates and edema, for sedentary or ambulating patients	Requires skilled personnel to apply
Single-layer elastic wraps	Early treatment or maintenance therapy	Applied by trained caregiver, reusable
Compression stockings	Later treatment or maintenance therapy	Needs fitting, requires patient skill and strength to apply
Inelastic		
Unna boot	Early treatment for edema and exudate, good for ambulating patient	Applied by trained caregiver
Short-stretch wrap	Early treatment or maintenance therapy, good for ambulating patient, permissible for patients with ABIs of 0.5–0.8	Applied by trained caregiver, reusable
Orthoses	Maintenance treatment, used when edema is controlled, easier to apply	Requires fitting, bulky
Intermittent (dynamic)		
Pneumatic compression	Applicable to patients with arterial or venous disease	Avoid in patients with heart disease

ulcer has decreased in size, maintenance compression can be started. For elderly individuals, patients with weakened upper extremity strength, or the morbidly obese, an orthosis such as CircAid (Coloplast Corp, Marietta, Georgia) may be the best option to continue ulcer healing while maintaining control of edema. Younger patients may do better with transition to elastic compression stockings for maintenance therapy. In the United States, elastic compression stockings come in four classes, depending on their strength of support (Table 24.3). In the large majority of patients, below-knee compression suffices for treatment of a venous ulcer when in a maintenance stage.

Table 24.3 Levels of compression for elastic stockings

Class	Strength (mm Hg)
I	20–30 (light)
II	30–40 (moderate)
III	40–50 (strong)
IV	50–60

Not every patient should have compression therapy instituted as there are two primary contraindications. Patients with uncompensated heart failure can be put into acute pulmonary edema with mobilization of interstitial fluid into the intravascular space. Patients with ankle-brachial indices less than 0.5 can have further tissue compromise if high-level elastic compression (30–40 mmHg) is applied. Application of this strength of compression stocking can also incite ischemic rest pain. This type of therapy should only be used on patients with an ankle-brachial index greater than 0.8. For patients between 0.5 and 0.8, moderate compression therapy may suffice. It is also important that arterial perfusion be corrected if the ABI is less than 0.8. This will improve healing potential of the venous ulcer as well as allow the use of a higher level of compression therapy.

The medication pentoxifylline has been shown to increase healing of venous ulcers. One meta-analysis of nine prospective trials comparing the drug to placebo showed significantly better healing with a relative risk of 1.30 ($p < 0.05$) [22]. The mechanism of healing action of this rheologic is thought to be through the inhibition of cytokine-mediated neutrophil activation. Micronized purified flavonoid fraction (MPFF; trade name Daflon, Servier Company, Neuilly-sur-Seine, France) is thought to increase venous tone. A meta-analysis of randomized placebo-controlled trials showed a relative risk reduction in ulcer healing by 32 % with a shorter time to healing of 16 versus 21 weeks ($p < 0.05$) [23]. Pale sulfonated shale oil (PSSO) applied topically has been shown to enhance proliferation of growth factor expression and stimulate wound healing. A multicenter, randomized, observer-blinded, placebo-controlled study demonstrated a significant reduction in ulcer size in treatment group versus control group [24]. One hundred and nineteen class 6 patients received 20 weeks of treatment. Results showed the treatment arm went from a mean ulcer size of 15–6.2 cm^2 and placebo arm from a mean of 11.4–10.8 cm^2. While MPFF and PSSO are not available in the United States, patients with venous ulcers should be started on pentoxifylline 400 mg by mouth three times a day. The most common side effect is generalized stomach upset.

The human skin equivalent Apligraf (Organogenesis, Canton, Massachusetts) has been shown in a prospective randomized trial to have greater healing of venous ulcers compared to a placebo arm at 6 months (63 % versus 49 %, $p = 0.02$) [25]. Additionally, the median time to complete ulcer closure was significantly shorter at 61 days versus 181 days ($p = 0.003$). Apligraf is manufactured from cultured human fibroblasts and keratinocytes derived from donated foreskin with each sheet derived from a single donor. Apligraf can only be applied to the venous ulcer when bioburden has been dramatically decreased and the ulcer bed is free of necrotic tissue or fibrinous debris. Apligraf is believed to have three mechanisms of possible action. First, the skin graft may "take" with persistence of graft cells in the wound which stimulate increased healing. Second, cells within Apligraf detect a wound and begin to secret growth factors that stimulate healing. Third, the graft serves as a semipermanent bio-occlusive cover to the wound bed [26]. Apligraf is indicated after a venous ulcer has failed to show any remarkable healing after 1 month of conventional (compression) therapy. Apligraf is applied to the wound with the appropriate bolster dressing in addition to conventional multilayer compression bandage. Compression should be changed weekly and more frequently if the wound is exudative. Up to five applications can be used for the treatment of venous ulcer.

For ulcers that are large, recurrent, or recalcitrant to healing from standard compression and other previously cited adjuvant therapies, treatment of venous reflux and/or obstruction should be seriously considered. How to proceed depends on the history. For patients with no previous history of venous thromboembolism and presumed primary chronic venous disease, treatment of venous reflux can be helpful in reducing static pressure at the ankle. If venous reflux testing shows only superficial venous reflux in the great and/or small saphenous veins, then surgical removal or venous ablation of these segments should have a significant positive impact on healing the ulcer [27, 28]. Additionally, if there is concomitant superficial and deep reflux present, surgical removal or ablation of the superficial great and/or small saphenous veins has been shown to improve valvular function of the deep axial venous system [29].

In patients with a history of venous thromboembolism or who continue to show recalcitrance in venous ulcer healing after ablation or surgical removal of the refluxing superficial venous segments, an evaluation of obstruction may be indicated [30, 31]. Magnetic resonance venography can demonstrate iliac venous stenosis from either chronic venous changes within the vein from previous deep venous thrombosis or external compression such as May-Thurner syndrome [32]. This syndrome is characterized by iliac artery compression points on the iliac veins – most commonly the right common iliac artery compressing the left common iliac vein between the sacral promontories. Treatment involves an endovascular antegrade approach in a deep venous segment, most commonly the popliteal vein, and then crossing the obstruction in order to stent open the obstruction. It is important to note that in performing endovascular procedures on the iliac veins for obstruction, intravascular ultrasound remains the criterion standard for determining the presence of obstruction and success of treatment with stenting [33].

Some patients may also have evidence of perforator vein incompetence. While treatment of these veins remains somewhat controversial, evaluation involves ultrasound examination of the veins that connect the deep tibial veins through the muscular fascia to the posterior arch vein along the medial calf. The American Venous Forum consensus opinion is to treat perforator veins near a healed or active leg ulcer if the perforator vein is greater than 3.5 mm in diameter and if the reversal of flow from the deep compartment to the superficial venous system with augmentation is greater than 0.5 s [34]. Treatment of incompetent perforator veins can be accomplished by sub-endoscopic perforator surgery (SEPS) or percutaneous ablation of perforators (PAPs) using radio frequency or laser ablation [35].

Open surgical techniques for the correction of venous reflux to treat recalcitrant venous ulcers have had mixed results in the success of healing [36–38]. While performed more routinely at some specialty centers, valve correction, creation, or transfer often is not necessary in virtually all patients with venous ulcer who have undergone the recommended progression of the aforementioned treatments. Nevertheless, in highly selective cases, it may be an option to help some patients in healing a venous ulcer.

24.4 Leg Ulcer Differential Diagnosis

24.4.1 Arterial Ulcers

Arterial ulcers occur due to decreased tissue perfusion from obstruction of arteries supplying the lower extremities. Atherosclerotic occlusive disease causes the large majority of arterial obstruction leading to ulcer. Common risk factors for atherosclerosis such as smoking, hypertension, hyperlipidemia, and diabetes mellitus are most often part of the history. The prevalence of these ulcers is more common in men and increases with age. These ulcers are extremely painful and if not treated can progress to gangrene which could lead to the need for amputation. Examination reveals diminished and/or absent lower extremity pulses and decreased ankle-brachial index (Table 24.1). In addition to these ulcers presenting most often on the tips of the toes, inspection reveals trophic changes on the foot including dry cracking and thinning of the skin, hair loss, and dystrophic nails. Arterial ulcers tend to be small, dry, non-exudative, pale, and necrotic (Fig. 24.2). Improving arterial perfusion represents the mainstay of treatment. Primary treatments include endovascular or open surgery in order to deliver enough oxygenated blood to begin the healing process. Other adjuvant treatments include lifestyle changes, atherosclerotic risk factor reduction, pharmacologic treatment, intermittent pneumatic compression, and hyperbaric oxygen treatment. Rarely, amputation is necessary if all other treatment options fail and the ulcer continues to worsen.

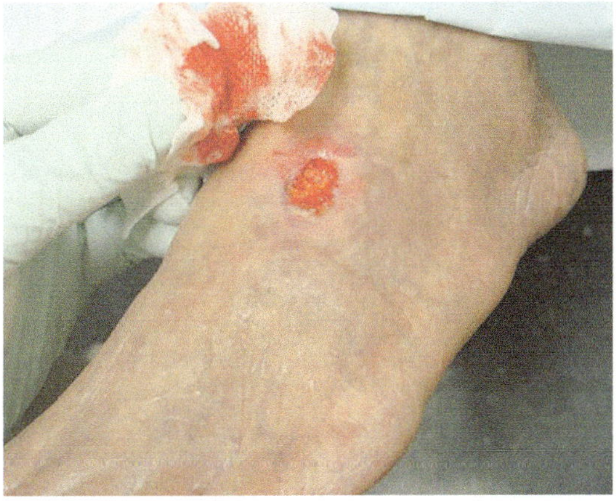

Fig. 24.2 Arterial ulcers typically present as small, dry, non-exudative, pale, and necrotic breakdowns

24.4.2 Diabetic Ulcers

Ulcers in the lower extremity from diabetes occur almost universally on the foot and are also referred to as neurotrophic, perforating, or mal perforans ulcers. Approximately 2–3 % of patients with diabetes will develop a foot ulcer per year with a cumulative lifetime incidence of 15 % [39, 40]. In the large majority of diabetic foot ulcers, distal sensorimotor and autonomic neuropathies play a major role in the pathophysiology. With these neuropathic changes come

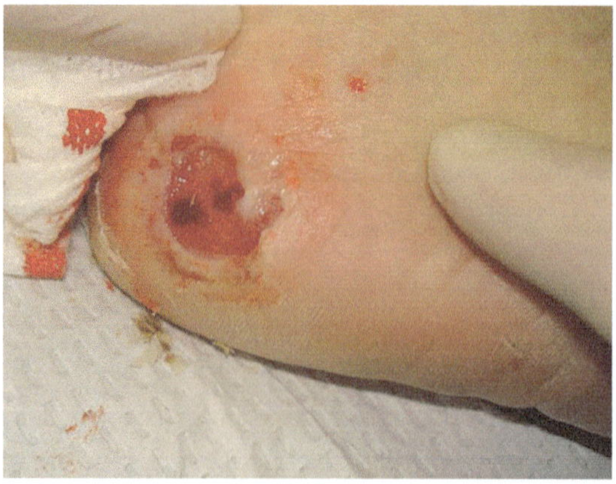

Fig. 24.3 Tissue necrosis from focal pressure compounded by a sensorimotor deficit from diabetes

foot deformities including hammertoes, prominent metatarsal heads with thinning of the foot fat pad, ankle joint equinus, and Charcot arthropathy. All of these deformities, in combination with neuropathy, lead to pressure points whereby repetitive focal pressure can lead to tissue necrosis (Fig. 24.3). Patients with sensorimotor deficit have no protective response to the repetitive pressure injury, thus leading to potentially limb-threatening ulceration and infection. On examination, the sensory deficit takes on a stocking distribution. Patients may have callus which fully covers an ulcer, thus necessitating trimming to assure no deeper tissue necrosis. Some patients may have such profound sensory deficit that sepsis may be the presenting symptom with an undiagnosed diabetic foot ulcer and deep foot abscess. Other causes of diabetic foot ulcers include the presence of peripheral arterial disease in combination with increased risk of infection from impairment of granulocyte function and chemotaxis. Often mild trauma will create a break in the skin, thus leading to a nonhealing ulcer. These typically occur on the toes or within their web spaces. Treatment includes aggressive surgical debridement, treatment of infection, relief of pressure at the wound site, arterial reconstruction if necessary, and strict control of glucose levels. If these standard measures fail, then other adjuvant therapies can be used to help stimulate healing. These include the use of recombinant human growth factors, bioengineered skin substitutes, and hyperbaric oxygen therapy [41, 42].

24.4.3 Pressure Ulcers

Tissue breakdown can occur on the lower extremity when constant focal pressure is applied between a bony prominence and an external surface. For the lower leg, these occur on the heel and malleoli. Often patients have other comorbidities such as diabetes, obesity, or peripheral artery disease which further increases susceptibility. Most often pressure ulcers occur when a patient has an illness whereby spontaneous movement of the lower extremities becomes severely limited. Examples include prolonged general anesthesia, critical illness with sedation, coma, paralysis, or lower extremity orthopedic surgery. Pressure ulcers can be divided into four stages including stage I, nonblanchable erythema; stage II, partial thickness loss of skin such as blistering; stage III, full thickness skin loss exposing the subcutaneous fatty tissue; and stage IV, full thickness skin loss with exposure of the muscle and/or bone. While prevention of pressure ulcers remains a more critical issue, treatment of pressure ulcers includes aggressive changes in position, special foam padding, and/or orthotics to relieve pressure completely. Surgical debridement of necrotic tissue and providing a moist dressing will facilitate healing. Other contributing factors to healing such as peripheral arterial disease, edema, infection, diabetes, and nutrition should all be corrected.

24.4.4 Infectious Ulcers

While all leg ulcers have bacterial contamination, some are the direct result of bacterial infection of the skin which then can cause varying degrees of skin necrosis. Alpha hemolytic Streptococcus pyogenes can cause a wide range of serious infections including erysipelas, punched-out leg ulcers called ecthyma, fasciitis necroticans, and sepsis with multiorgan failure. Other direct infections that can cause skin necrosis with or without ulceration include ulcerating pyoderma from Staphylococcus aureus, ecthyma gangrenosum from pseudomonas, and gas gangrene from clostridium. These types of infections require immediate high-dose and potent antibiotics because of the tendency for rapid spread with further skin involvement and the increased risk of systemic involvement [43].

24.4.5 Vasculitic Ulcers

Vasculitis results from inflammation of the blood vessels of which any size or site can be affected. Most often, vasculitis comes from a systemic immunologic or inflammatory disorder. Examples include rheumatoid arthritis, systemic lupus erythematosus, polyarteritis nodosa, hypersensitivity vasculitis, Wegener's granulomatosis, Sjőgren's syndrome, cryoglobulinemia, scleroderma, and dermatomyositis [44, 45]. Inflammation of small vessels in the skin and subcutaneous fatty tissue of the lower extremity can lead to petechiae, erythematous nonblanching macules or nodules, purpura, necrosis, and subsequent ulceration. Patients may also harbor systemic features of fever, myalgias, arthralgias, and malaise. Skin biopsy and blood chemistry testing, which checks for systemic inflammation, are critical to the diagnosis. Treatment focuses on control of the systemic disease and often involves antihistamines, corticosteroids, and immunosuppressive agents. Ulcer treatment should include debridement of necrotic tissue, control of infection, absorption of excess exudate, protection against further trauma, and providing a moist wound healing environment.

24.4.6 Pyoderma Gangrenosum

The etiology of pyoderma gangrenosum stems from a noninfectious neutrophilic dermatosis that often occurs in association with an underlying systemic disease such inflammatory bowel disease, rheumatoid arthritis, hematologic disease, or malignancy. Lesions develop from sterile pustules which can rapidly progress to a painful ulcer with undermining. The base of pyoderma gangrenosum often appears purulent, and the surrounding skin borders appear with erythematous violaceous borders. Histopathology from skin biopsy appears as general inflammation with no specific features to the ulcer. The correct diagnosis relates to exclusion of other ulcer etiologies, presence of a possible systemic condition, presentation and ulcer appearance, and a high index of suspicion. The hallmark of treatment is high-dose corticosteroids in combination with cytotoxic drugs. Combination therapy with sulfa-based drugs such as dapsone, clofazimine, minocycline, or thalidomide can also be given. Ulcer treatment is supportive with debridement of necrotic tissue, control of infection, providing moist bandage for an optimal healing environment, and pain control [45].

24.5 Summary

Venous leg ulcers are the most common form of leg ulcer. While there are many rare causes of ulcerations that can occur from the knee to the toes, the overview provided herein gives the practitioner guidance on how to evaluate a patient presenting with a leg ulcer and care for and heal the venous ulcer and information about other more common types of ulcers that are in the differential diagnosis. Fortunately, history and physical examination can help determine, with some confirmatory tests, the type of ulcer. Nevertheless, the essentials of wound healing remain the same for the large majority of ulcers on the lower extremities. Healing will hasten if treatment of all leg ulcers includes assuring adequate perfusion; removing nonviable tissue; reducing inflammation and eliminating infection, relieving edema; optimizing tissue growth; off-loading or providing pressure relief; controlling pain; and treating host systemic disease or conditions such as diabetes and nutrition.

References

1. Ryan TJ. The epidemiology of leg ulcers. In: Westerhof W, editor. Leg ulcers: diagnosis and treatment. Amsterdam: Elsevier Science Publishers BV; 1993. p. 19–27.
2. Baker SR, Stacey MC, Jopp-McKay AB, et al. Epidemiology of chronic venous ulcers. Br J Surg. 1991;78:864–7.
3. Callam MJ, Harper DR, Dale JJ, Ruckley CV. Chronic ulcer of the leg: clinical history. Br Med J (Clin Res Ed). 1987;294(6584):1389–91.
4. Nelzen O, Berqvist D, Lindhagen A, Hallbook T. Chronic leg ulcers: an underestimated problem in primary health care among elderly patients. J Epidemiol Community Health. 1991;45:184–7.
5. Margolis DJ, Bilker W, Santanna J, Baumgarten M. Venous leg ulcer: incidence and prevalence in the elderly. J Am Acad Dermatol. 2002;46:381–6.
6. Bello YM, Phillips TJ. Management of venous ulcers. J Cutan Med Surg. 1998;3:6–12.
7. Valencia IC, Falabella A, Kirsner RS, Eaglstein WH. Chronic venous insufficiency and venous leg ulceration. J Am Acad Dermatol. 2001;44:401–21.
8. Mekkes JR, Loots MAM, Van Der Wal AC, Bos JD. Causes, investigation and treatment of leg ulceration. Br J Dermatol. 2003;148:388–401.
9. Van Bemmelen PS, Bedford G, Beach K, Strandness DE. Qualitative segmental evaluation of venous valvular reflux with duplex ultrasound scanning. J Vasc Surg. 1989;10:425–31.
10. de Araujo T, Valencia I, Federman DG, Kirsner RS. Managing the patient with venous ulcers. Ann Intern Med. 2003;138:326.
11. Paquette D, Falanga V. Leg ulcers. Geriatr Dermatol. 2002;18:77–88.
12. Phillips T. Current approaches to venous ulcers and compression. Dermatol Surg. 2001;27:611–21.
13. Weingarten MS. State-of-the-art treatment of chronic venous disease. Clin Infect Dis. 2001;32:949.
14. Simka M, Majewski E. The social and economic burden of venous leg ulcers: focus on the role of micronized purified flavonoid fraction adjuvant therapy. Am J Clin Dermatol. 2003;4:573–81.
15. Lopez A, Phillips T. Venous ulcers. Wounds. 1998;10:149.
16. Reichhardt L. Venous ulceration: compression as the mainstay of therapy. J Wound Ostomy Continence Nurs. 1999;26:39.
17. O'Meara S, Cullum NA, Nelson EA. Compression for venous leg ulcers. Cochrane Database Syst Rev. 2009;(21):CD000265.
18. Kantor J, Margolis D. Management of leg ulcers. Semi Cutan Med Surg. 2003;22:212.
19. Choucair M, Phillips T. Compression therapy. Dermatol Surg. 1998;24:141.
20. Kunimoto B. Management and prevention of venous leg ulcers: a literature-guided approach. Ostomy Wound Manage. 2001;47:36.
21. Jull AB, Waters J, Arroll BI. Pentoxifylline for treating venous leg ulcers. Cochrane Database Syst Rev. 2002;(1):CD001733.
22. Smith PC. Daflon 500 mg and venous leg ulcer: new results from a meta-analysis. Angiology. 2005;l56:S33–9.
23. Beckert S, Warnecke J, Zelenkova H, Kovnerystyy O, Stege H, Cholcha W, Konigsrainer A, Coerper S. Efficacy of topical pale sulfonated shale oil in the treatment of venous leg ulcers: a randomized, controlled multicenter study. J Vasc Surg. 2006;43:94–100.
24. Falanga V, Margolis D, Alvarez O, Auletta M, Maggiacomo F, Altman M, Jensen J, Sabolinski M, Hardin-Young J. Rapid healing of venous ulcers and lack of clinical rejection with an allogeneic cultured human skin equivalent. Human Skin Equivalent Investigators group. Arch Dermatol. 1998;134:293–300.
25. Alvarez OM, Fahey CB, Auletta MJ, Fernandez-Obregon A. A novel treatment for venous leg ulcers. J Foot Ankle Surg. 1998;37:319–24.
26. Barwell JR, Davies CE, Deacon J, et al. Comparison of surgery and compression with compression alone in chronic venous ulceration (ESCHAR study): randomised controlled trial. Lancet. 2004;363:1854–9.
27. Marrocco CJ, Atkins MD, Bohannon WT, Warren TR, Buckley CJ, Bush RL. Endovenous ablation for the treatment of chronic venous insufficiency and venous ulcerations. World J Surg. 2010;34:2299–304.
28. Harlander-Locke M, Lawrence PF, Alktaifi A, Jimenez JC, Rigberg D, Derubertis B. The impact of ablation of incompetent superficial and perforator veins on ulcer healing rates. J Vasc Surg. 2012;55(2):458–64.
29. Neglen P, Hollis KC, Olivier J, Raju S. Stenting of venous outflow in chronic venous disease: long-term stent-related outcome, clinical, and hemodynamic result. J Vasc Surg. 2007;46:979–90.
30. Raju S, Darcey R, Neglen P. Unexpected major role for venous stenting in deep reflux disease. J Vasc Surg. 2010;51:401–8.
31. Wolpert LM, Rahmani O, Stein B, Gallagher JJ, Drezner AD. Magnetic resonance venography in the diagnosis and management of May-Thurner syndrome. Vasc Endovascular Surg. 2002;36:51–7.
32. Alhalbouni S, Hingorani A, Shiferson A, Gopal K, Jung D, Novak D, Marks N, Ascher E. Iliac-femoral venous stenting for lower extremity venous stasis symptoms. Ann Vasc Surg. 2012;26(2):185–9.
33. Gloviczki P, Comerota A, Dalsing M, Eklof B, Gillespie D, Gloviczki M, Lohr J, McLafferty R, Meissner M, Murad M, Padberg F, Pappas P, Passman M, Raffetto J, Vasquez M, Wakefield T. The care of patients with varicose veins and associated chronic venous diseases: clinical practice guidelines of the Society for Vascular Surgery and the American Venous Forum. J Vasc Surg. 2011;53:2S–48.
34. O'Donnell TF. The role of perforators in chronic venous insufficiency. Phlebology. 2010;25:3–10.

35. Raju S, Fredericks RK, Neglen PN, Bass JD. Durability of venous valve reconstruction techniques for "primary" and postthrombotic reflux. J Vasc Surg. 1996;23:357–66.
36. Masuda EM, Kistner RL. Long-term results of venous valve reconstruction: a four – to twenty-one-year follow-up. J Vasc Surg. 1994;19:391–403.
37. Tripathi R, Sieunarine K, Abbas M, Durrani N. Deep venous valve reconstruction for non-healing ulcers: techniques and results. ANZ J Surg. 2004;74: 34–9.
38. Frykberg RG. Epidemiology of the diabetic foot: ulcerations and amputations. Adv Wound Care. 1999;12:139–41.
39. Reiber GE, Lipsky BA, Gibbons GW. The burden of diabetic foot ulcers. Am J Surg. 1998;176(Suppl 2A):5–10.
40. American Diabetes Association. Consensus development conference on diabetic foot wound care. Diabetes Care. 1999;22:1354–60.
41. Kranke P, Bennett M, Roeckl-Wiedmann I, Debus S. Cochrane Database Syst Rev. 2004;(2):CD004123.
42. Phillips TJ. Chronic cutaneous ulcers: etiology and epidemiology. J Invest Dermatol. 1994;102:38–41.
43. Roenigk H, Young J. Leg ulcers. In: Young J, Olin J, Bartholomew J, editors. Peripheral vascular diseases. 2nd ed. St. Louis: Mosby; 1996.
44. Rubano J, Kerstein M. Arterial insufficiency and vasculitides. J Wound Ostomy Continence Nurs. 1996;28:147–52.
45. Shah JB. Approach to commonly misdiagnosed wounds and unusual leg ulcers. In: Sheffield PJ, Fife CE, editors. Wound care practice. 2nd ed. Flagstaff: Best Publishing; 2006. p. 590–1.

Biostatistics

25

Elaheh Rahbar, Sapan S. Desai, Eric Mowatt-Larssen, and Mohammad Hossein Rahbar

Contents

E. Rahbar, PhD (✉)
Department of Surgery, Center for Translational Injury Research, University of Texas Medical School at Houston, Houston, TX, USA
e-mail: elaheh.rahbar@uth.tmc.edu

S.S. Desai, MD, PhD, MBA
Department of Surgery, Duke University Medical Center, Durham, NC, USA

Department of Cardiothoracic and Vascular Surgery, University of Texas at Houston Medical School, Houston, TX, USA
e-mail: sapan.desai@surgisphere.com

E. Mowatt-Larssen, MD, FACPh, RPhS
Vein Specialists of Monterey, Pacific Street 757, Monterey, CA 93940, USA
e-mail: eric.mowatt.larssen@gmail.com

M.H. Rahbar, PhD
Department of Epidemiology and Biostatistics, Human Genetic and Environmental Sciences, University of Texas School of Public Health at Houston, Houston, TX, USA
e-mail: mohammad.h.rahbar@uth.tmc.edu

E. Mowatt-Larssen et al. (eds.), *Phlebology, Vein Surgery and Ultrasonography* ,
DOI 10.1007/978-3-319-01812-6_25, © Springer International Publishing Switzerland 2014

Abstract
Biostatistics is a branch of statistics that applies statistical methods to medical and biological problems. It is of essential importance in the successful conduct of clinical and translational studies. An understanding of biostatistics enables the critical analysis of scholarly articles and their proper assimilation into one's own practice. In this section, we provide an introduction to biostatistics and cover the essentials of descriptive and inferential statistics including estimation and hypothesis testing. In addition, we discuss major types of study designs and the importance of sensitivity and specificity, measures of absolute and relative risk, common errors, and sources of bias in scientific studies.

25.1 Introduction

Biostatistics is a branch of statistics that applies statistical methods to medical and biological problems. It is of essential importance in the successful conduct of clinical and translational studies. An understanding of biostatistics enables the critical analysis of scholarly articles and their proper assimilation into one's own practice. In recent years, as a result of extraordinary advancement in computational capabilities, there have been significant improvements in statistical techniques and research design methodologies, including adaptive designs, randomization, and Bayesian methods in clinical trials. However, clinical and translational investigators are often unaware of these new statistical methods. The lack of awareness is compounded by the tendency for individual clinical and translational studies to have either too few study subjects, too much random noise in the study data, or too much potential for bias. In this section, we provide an introduction to biostatistics and cover the essentials of descriptive and inferential statistics including estimation and hypothesis testing. In addition, we discuss major types of study designs and the importance of sensitivity and specificity, measures of absolute and relative risk, common errors, and sources of bias in scientific studies [1–4].

25.2 Descriptive Statistics

Before we can discuss the steps in developing a good clinical study and the appropriate statistical testing methods, we must go over the basics of descriptive statistics. The basic statistical problem is that we are trying to infer the properties of the underlying population from a limited number of measurements from the population. In order to successfully do this, we must understand how to describe the sample data and define the relationships between the sample and population.

25.2.1 Measures of Central Tendency: Mean, Median, and Mode

The mean, median, and mode are statistics used to describe a distribution. The mean is the average of all measurements. It is important to distinguish the difference between the mean of a measurement in a population and the mean of a measurement in a sample; the population mean is often denoted by μ. The sample mean, denoted by $\bar{x}$, is simply a point estimate for the population mean. This will be further discussed in the following section. The median is the middle measurement when all of the measurements are sorted in ascending or descending order, which can be a better measure of central tendency in skewed distributions. In normal (bell-shaped) distributions, the average and median values are the same. The mode is the measurement with the highest frequency. Based on these three measures of central tendency, one can understand the shape of the distribution. Furthermore, depending on the type of measurements and shape of the distribution, one may choose one or more of these measures of central tendency to describe their data set.

25.2.2 Measures of Spread: Range, Variance, and Standard Deviation

Sample range is the difference between the highest and the lowest measurements. Therefore, it is a very sensitive measure of variability because it is influenced by the extreme observations. For situations in which there are extreme observations, some researchers use the interquartile range (IQR) which represents the difference between the 25th percentile and 75th percentile. Sample variance (s^2) is another important measure of variability, which is calculated by the following formula (Eq. 25.1), where x_i are the individual measurements, $\bar{x}$ is the sample mean and n is the sample size:

$$s^2 = \frac{\sum_{i=1}^{n}(x_i - \bar{x})^2}{n-1} \quad (25.1)$$

Since the unit of variance is squared of the original unit of measure, the sample standard deviation (s) is often used as another measure of spread, which is simply the square root of the sample variance (Eq. 25.2):

$$s = \sqrt{s^2} = \sqrt{\frac{\sum_{i=1}^{n}(x_i - \bar{x})^2}{n-1}} \quad (25.2)$$

It is important to distinguish the difference between population and sample measures of spread. For example, population standard deviation (σ) is a measure of spread over the entire population of size N with a mean of μ (Eq. 25.3); similarly, population variance is denoted by σ^2. The reason for using "$n-1$" in calculating sample variance (s^2) and standard deviation (s) is to ensure that the estimates for variability remain unbiased. This concept is discussed in standard statistical textbooks, and we refer the reader to *Fundamentals of Biostatistics* by Bernard Rosner for additional information.

$$\sigma = \sqrt{\frac{\sum_{i=1}^{N}(x_i - \mu)^2}{N}} \quad (25.3)$$

25.2.3 Normal Distributions

In practice, many measurements including weight and height have a bell-shaped distribution.

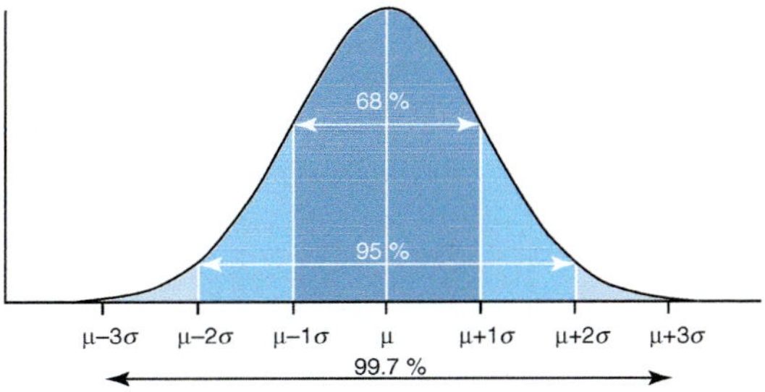

Fig. 25.1 A normal distribution of the population with mean μ and standard deviation (sigma)

Mathematically these distributions can be characterized by a normal (Gaussian) distribution with mean μ and standard deviation σ. The normal distribution is symmetrical and has the property that about 68 % of the observations lie within one standard deviation from the mean, 95 % within 2 standard deviations, and 99.7 % within 3 standard deviations (Fig. 25.1).

25.2.4 Skewed Distributions

Not all distributions are normal in nature. In fact, skewed distributions are common in clinical data. In a negatively skewed distribution (i.e., skewed towards the left), the mean is less than the median. In a positively skewed distribution (i.e., skewed towards the right), the median is less than the mean. In a bimodal distribution, there are two modes, one mean, and one median. For irregular distributions, one may be interested in describing the data in terms of the median and interquartile range (Fig. 25.2).

25.2.5 Estimation and Bias

As stated earlier, one of the objectives of statistics is to infer the properties of the underlying population from a sample (i.e., subset of the population). Statistical inference can be subdivided into two main areas: estimation and hypothesis testing. Estimation is concerned with estimating the values of specific population parameters. It is therefore, very important to understand the

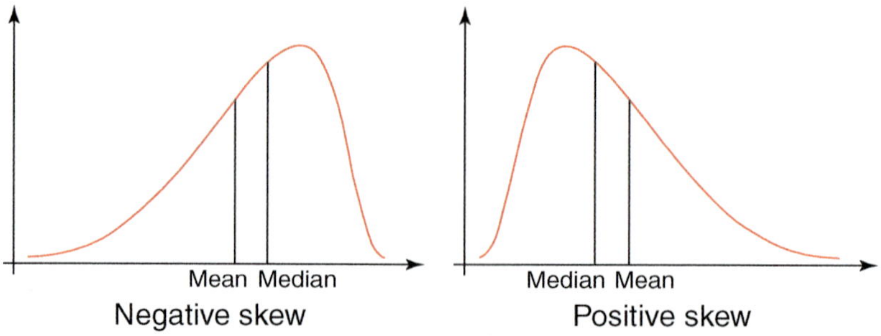

Fig. 25.2 A negatively skewed curve has a mode that is greater than the median, which is greater than the mean (left-skewed). A positively skewed curve has the opposite finding (right-skewed)

relationships between the sample characteristics and population parameters [5–10].

25.2.6 Point and Interval Estimators for the Population Mean

A natural estimator for μ is the sample mean $\bar{x}$, which is referred to as a point estimate. Suppose we want to determine the appropriate sample size for estimating the mean of a population (μ) which is unknown. We can start by taking a random sample to determine the sample mean and sample variance. However, the sample mean values can change from sample to sample. Therefore, it is necessary for us to determine the variation in the point estimate (e.g., sample mean). Assuming that the sample size is large ($n>30$), we can determine an interval estimate (e.g., 95 % confidence interval) for the population parameters. For example, if the population parameter is μ, a 95 % confidence interval can be calculated by the following formula (Eq. 25.4). The value 1.96 is the exact value determined from the normal distribution, which is based on the fact that 95 % of the measurements are within 1.96 (approximately 2) standard deviations of the mean.

$$\bar{x} \pm 1.96\sqrt{\frac{s^2}{n}} \quad (25.4)$$

The quantity to the right of the mean in Eq. 25.4 is known as the margin of error or the bound on the error of estimation (B). In general, as sample size increases, B decreases. However, this inverse relationship is not linear. In order to decrease B by half, one must increase the sample size by a factor of 4. This relationship between margin of error, B, and sample size allows researchers to calculate the appropriate sample size to achieve the desired bound on the error with 95 % confidence and will be further elaborated in the sample size determination section.

25.2.7 Standard Error of the Mean

The standard error of the mean (SEM) or standard error (SE) is the standard deviation of sample mean. There is a mathematical relationship between the standard deviation of the measurements in the population and the SEM. This mathematical relationship helps to calculated SEM based on one random sample of size n. SEM is equal to the standard deviation divided by the square root of the sample size n. The SEM is affected by the sample size; as the sample size increases, the SEM decreases (Eq. 25.5):

$$\text{SEM} = \frac{s}{\sqrt{n}} \quad (25.5)$$

25.2.8 Point and Interval Estimators for the Population Proportion

In clinical studies, one is often interested in assessing the prevalence of a certain characteristic of the population. In this case, it is important to determine the point and interval estimators for the population proportion (p). The point estimator for the population proportion $\hat{p}$ is defined as the proportion of the observed characteristic of interest in the sample (Eq. 25.6):

$$\hat{p} = \frac{x}{n} \tag{25.6}$$

For large samples with a 95 % confidence interval, the population proportion p is calculated as follows:

$$\hat{p} \pm 1.96\sqrt{\frac{\hat{p}(1-\hat{p})}{n}} \tag{25.7}$$

The quantity to the right of the sample proportion in Eq. 25.7 is known as the margin of error or the bound on the error of estimation (B). As shown before in the case of point estimates for the population mean, this relationship can be used to estimate the appropriate sample size, which will be explained later.

25.2.9 Bias

Generally, bias is defined as "a partiality that prevents objective consideration of an issue." In statistics, bias means "a tendency of an estimate to deviate in one direction from a true value." In terms of the population means and proportion estimates described in the previous sections, bias can be defined as:

$$\begin{aligned} \text{Bias} &= (\bar{x} - \mu) \\ \text{Bias} &= (\hat{p} - p) \end{aligned} \tag{25.8}$$

From a statistical perspective, an estimator is considered unbiased if the average bias based on repeated sampling is zero. For example, $\bar{x}$ is an unbiased estimator of μ and $\hat{p}$ is an unbiased estimator for p. However, there are multiple sources of bias inherent in any study that may occur during the course of the study, from allocation of participants and delivery of interventions to measurement of outcomes. Bias can also occur before the study begins or after the study during analysis. Late-look bias occurs with re-examination and re-interpretation of the collected data after the study has been unblinded. Lead-time bias occurs when earlier examination of patients with a particular disease leads to earlier diagnosis, giving the false impression that the patient will live longer. Measurement bias occurs when an investigator familiar with the study does the measurement and makes a series of errors towards the conclusion they expect. Recall bias occurs when patients informed about their disease are more likely to recall risk factors than uninformed patients. Sampling bias occurs when the sample used in the study is not representative of the population and so conclusions may not be generalizable to the whole population. Finally, selection bias occurs when the lack of randomization leads to patients choosing their experimental group which could introduce confounding [11–14].

25.3 Hypothesis Testing

25.3.1 Developing a Hypothesis

A research question can be formulated into null and alternative hypotheses for statistical testing. The null hypothesis states that there is no difference between the parameter of interest and the hypothesized value of the parameter. Whereas the alternative hypothesis is that there is some kind of difference. The alternative hypothesis cannot be tested directly; it is accepted by default if the test of statistical significance rejects the null hypothesis. In the case of comparing two population parameters, the null hypothesis is that there is no difference between groups (A or B) on the measured outcome, whereas the alternative hypothesis is that there is a difference between the measured outcome and the group (A or B). Alternatively, the null hypothesis can be written as no association between group (A or B) and measured outcome vs. alternative hypothesis that there is an association between group (A or B) and the measured outcome. In later sections, you will see that some researchers prefer to write the hypotheses in terms of the ratio of the two population parameters [e.g., relative risk (RR) or odds ratio (OR)]. In this case the null hypothesis can be written as RR = 1 (OR = 1) vs. RR ≠ 1 (OR ≠ 1).

25.3.2 Other Elements of Testing Hypothesis

In addition to the null and alternative hypotheses, we must have a test statistic, a rejection region, and p-value to conduct a formal testing hypothesis. A test statistic calculates the difference between the observed data and the hypothesized values of the parameters assuming the null hypothesis is true. For example, for comparing means of two normal distributions, we can use a test statistic, which has a t-distribution under the null hypothesis. Rejection region is the range of values of the distribution of the test statistic for which the null hypothesis is rejected, in favor of the alternative hypothesis. Traditionally, for each testing hypothesis one must determine a cutoff value for the rejection region, based on a probability of type I error ($\alpha = 0.05$).

25.3.3 Types of Error

Type I error occurs when the null hypothesis is rejected despite being true. The probability of type I error (α) is usually considered acceptable at 5 %. P-value is the probability of observing more extreme values than what has been already observed in the sample assuming the null hypothesis is true. If p-value $< \alpha$, then the null hypothesis can be rejected. On the other hand, type II error occurs when the null hypothesis is not rejected when it should be. The probability of type II error (β) is more difficult to calculate because we usually do not know the true value of the parameter of interest under the alternative hypothesis. Additionally, it is important to note that as alpha increases, beta decreases and the power of the study increases.

25.3.4 Power

The power of a test is the probability of rejecting the null hypothesis when it is false. Mathematically, power is defined as $1-\beta$. The power of a test is directly related to its sample size; increasing sample size results in a higher power. However, the power is also directly dependent upon the variance of the measurement. In fact, it is inversely related to the variance of the measurement. If the variance is higher then the power will be lower. Using more sensitive and specific instruments that can measure a finer gradient (such as reliably estimating high-density lipoproteins to three decimal places) can also improve the power of a study. An insufficiently powered study can lead to false acceptance of the null hypothesis and thereby lead to a higher likelihood of type II error. In other words, a study may incorrectly conclude that there is no difference between two groups (e.g., two treatments) when one really existed. To avoid these errors, the power of a study must be determined by an estimate of the expected differences between two groups.

25.3.5 Sample Size Determination

The sample size (n) is the total number of patients enrolled in a particular study. This number plays a critical role in the statistical power and relevance of the findings from the study. The sample size can be determined through two inferential techniques. First, for determining the minimum sample size required to estimate a certain parameter of interest within a certain margin of error, we need the variance of the measurement, level of confidence, and the margin of error. Referring back to the definition of margin of error, we can calculate the sample size for estimating the difference between two means ($\mu_1 - \mu_2$) based on two independent samples of equal size with the following formula:

$$n_1 = n_2 \geq \left(\frac{1.96}{B}\right)^2 \cdot \left(\sigma_1^2 + \sigma_2^2\right) \tag{25.9}$$

For estimating the mean of one population, the sample size formula is slightly different, and we refer the reader to Rosner's textbook, *Fundamentals of Biostatistics*.

Example #1: Suppose we are interested in estimating the effect of a new cholesterol-fighting medication in a two arm clinical trial with a known standard deviation of 15 mg/dL in serum cholesterol levels. Note that you do not know what the exact effect of this new drug. In order to determine the required sample size for estimating the treatment effect of the new cholesterol-fighting medication, within a pre-specified bound on the error of estimation (for example, 10 mg/dL) with 95 % confidence, we will use Equation 25.9 to calculate the sample size in each arm of the study, assuming equal number of subjects are enrolled per arm. This is done as follows, where B=10 and σ=15.

$$n_1 = n_2 \geq \left(\frac{1.96}{10}\right)^2 .\left(15^2 + 15^2\right)$$
$$n_1 = n_2 \geq 17.29$$

Therefore, at least 18 subjects must be enrolled in each arm of this study to estimate a difference in effect between the treatment and control groups with 95 % confidence.

Another method of determining sample size is based on the power of a hypothesis test. For the testing hypothesis, sample size is determined from variance of the measurement, level of confidence, and effect size. For comparing two population means, the effect size is defined as the absolute difference between the means of the two populations divided by the standard deviation of the measurement of the control group. Together, the formula for sample size for a two-population study with an $\alpha = 0.05$ and $\beta = 0.2$ (i.e., 80 % power) is as follows (Equation 25.10):

$$n_1 = n_2 \geq \frac{(1.96 + 0.84)^2 \left[\sigma_1^2 + \sigma_2^2\right]}{\Delta^2} \qquad (25.10)$$

This method is only appropriate when the sample size between the two groups is the equal. For unequal groups we refer you to Rosner's textbook, *Fundamentals of Biostatistics*.

Example #2: Recall example 1 regarding the cholesterol-fighting medication. Let's assume now that we are interested in testing whether the new cholesterol-fighting medication is effective in reducing cholesterol levels compared to the control group. Based on previous information, we know that a reduction of cholesterol levels by 5 mg/dL, on average, is considered clinically significant. In order to determine the sample size in each study arm that will allow a detection of at least 5 mg/dL in the mean cholesterol levels between the two groups with at least 80% power at 5% level of significance, we will use Equation 25.10, where σ=15 (as indicated in Example 1) and Δ=5 mg/dL.

$$n_1 = n_2 \geq \frac{(1.96 + 0.84)^2 .\left(15^2 + 15^2\right)}{5^2}$$
$$n_1 = n_2 \geq 141.12$$

Therefore, at least 142 subjects must be enrolled in each arm of this study to test the difference in mean cholesterol levels between the treatment and control groups with power of at least 80% at 5% level of significance

To determine the sample size for estimating a population proportion (p) within a certain margin of error (B) with 95 % confidence, we need to have an initial estimate for the population proportion of interest. If no such estimate is available, the most conservative sample size can be determined by replacing $p = 0.5$ in the following formula (Equation 25.11):

$$n \geq \left(\frac{1.96}{B}\right)^2 (p)(1 - p) \qquad (25.11)$$

Example #3: Let's assume now that we are interested in estimating the proportion of subjects in the population who have cholesterol levels >200 mg/dL within 4 % of its actual proportion in the population, and with 95 % confidence. This means that B = 0.04, and p can be extracted from the literature. If it is entirely unknown, then use p = 0.5 for the most conservative estimate of sample size (i.e. largest sample size). Using equation 25.11, we calculate:

$$n \geq \left(\frac{1.96}{0.04}\right)^2 . (0.5)(1 - 0.5)$$
$$n \geq 600.25$$

Therefore, you will need at least 601 subjects to be able to estimate the proportion of subjects with elevated cholesterol levels (i.e. >200 mg/dL). Please note that since we use p=0.5, in the formula, this is the most conservative estimate for required sample size.

Furthermore, to determine the required sample size for comparing two population proportions assuming an absolute difference of delta (p_1-p_2) and equal sample sizes in both groups, we will use the following formula. This formula is specifically for having at least 80 % power ($\beta=0.2$) with $\alpha=0.05$, where:

$$n_1 = n_2 \geq \frac{(1.96+0.84)^2\left[p_1(1-p_1)+p_2(1-p_2)\right]}{\Delta^2} \quad (25.12)$$

Similar to before, if p_1 and p_2 are unknown, the most conservative estimate of n_1 and n_2 can be obtained by assuming a value of 0.5 for p_1 and p_2 in the above formula. This method is only appropriate when the sample size between the two groups is equal. For unequal groups we refer you to Rosner's textbook, *Fundamentals of Biostatistics*.

25.4 Tests of Significance

25.4.1 T-Test

Student's t-test was developed in 1908 by William S. Gosset using the pen name Student. He created this statistical test as a method of monitoring the quality of Guinness stout, comparing one batch to another and ensuring that production was of consistent quality. The t-test assumes that the groups being compared come from a normally distributed population. There are three different types of t-tests: one-sample t-test, two-sample t-test, and paired-sample t-test. The one-sample t-test compares the mean of a population to a specified (hypothesized) value. In the two-sample t-test, two independent samples are compared for differences between the population means. However, if the two samples being compared are dependent or matched, a paired t-test must be used. The limitation of the t-test is that it can only compare two groups at any given time. For comparing more than two group means, we will introduce one-way analysis of variance (ANOVA) in the next section.

25.4.2 ANOVA

The analysis of variance (ANOVA) is a statistical procedure based on the F-test that can be used to simultaneously compare means from more than two groups. Similar to the t-test, ANOVA assumes that the populations being compared have normal distributions. It is particularly useful when comparing dose–response curves of a medication given at differing doses to a group of patients. ANOVA helps to avoid inflation of type I error potentially caused by conducting multiple t-tests between groups when there are more than two groups. For additional information about the ANOVA and the F-test, please see Rosner's book on *Fundamentals of Biostatistics*.

25.4.3 Chi-Square Test of Independence

The chi-square test of independence allows testing for association or lack of it between two categorical variables. For example, in testing associations between disease status (D+/D–) and ethnicity (Caucasian, African American, Hispanic, other), we can form a contingency table that provides the count for the frequency of observations in each combination of the rows and columns. The chi-square test of independence has $(r-1)(c-1)$ degrees of freedom where r is the number of rows and c is the number of columns in the contingency table. The rejection region for the chi-square test will be on the right tail of the chi-square distribution. Any major statistical software can be used for computation of test statistics and p-values.

25.4.4 Regressions and Correlations

Up to this point we have discussed hypothesis and statistical testing methods; the next step is to evaluate if there are any correlations between the outcome variable and group (class) variables.

Linear-regression methods allow one to study how an outcome variable (y) is related to one or more predictor variables ($x_1, x_2, \ldots. x_k$).

25.4.5 Simple Linear Regression

Simple linear regressions are often fitted to the data using the least squares method where the best-fit line is determined by minimizing the sum of squared distances of the data points from the regression line. The simple linear regression equation often takes the following form, where α is the y-intercept and β is the slope of the regression line in the population (Eq. 25.13):

$$E(y) = \alpha + \beta x \quad (25.13)$$

The slope of the regression line (β coefficient) represents the estimated average increase in y per one-unit increase in x. It is used to make predictions between the two variables, x and y. However, predictions are not always easy to make with clinical data, and often we are interested in describing the relationship between x and y. In this case, the sample correlation coefficient (r) is a useful tool for quantifying the relationship between variables and is better suited than the estimated regression coefficient. The population correlation coefficient is denoted by ρ. In other words, r is a natural point estimator for ρ.

25.4.6 Correlation

Correlation coefficients help to describe linear relationships between two variables. It is of vital importance to understand that correlation does not imply causation. In correlation analysis, it is important to look at the scatter plot which is a graphical presentation of pairs of (X, Y) coordinates plotted on the X-Y axis. The X is the independent variable and the Y is the dependent variable. The correlation coefficient must lie between −1 and 1. A correlation coefficient of 0 means that there is no linear relationship between the two variables (or X and Y are uncorrelated). However, the two variables might still be otherwise related (e.g., U-shaped relationship). A correlation coefficient between 0 and 1 means a positive correlation exists: as X goes up, the Y variable generally goes up. A negative correlation implies an inverse relationship: as X increases, the Y variable generally decreases. Thus, the correlation coefficient provides a quantitative measure of dependence between the two variables. Please note that dependence of Y on X does not imply that there is a causal relationship between X and Y.

25.5 Study Designs and Measures of Association

As mentioned in the previous section, it is important to determine correlations and associations between the dependent and independent variables. In this section we discuss the concepts of associations in relation to the study designs implemented.

25.5.1 Study Design

It is important to design a study that will answer the proposed research question in an unbiased and efficient manner. As stated earlier, it is important to clearly define the "disease" and "treatment" variables so that one can effectively assess a disease-treatment relationship. Randomization, blinding, minimizing bias, using placebos, controls, and a sufficient sample size should be used whenever possible. However, not all scientific questions are practically answered by high-quality, multi-institutional, randomized controlled trials. As a result, a variety of study designs are available for various types of epidemiologic, clinical, and translational research.

25.5.2 Case Study

Case studies examine the outcome of a single patient with a disease who received a particular treatment. Case studies are useful to note interesting or odd effects of treatment or to note an off-label use of a medication, and they may spur more rigorous clinical investigations.

25.5.3 Case-Control Study

Case-control studies are retrospective studies that identify two groups of patients; one group with the known disease (cases) and another group without the disease (controls). The goal is to compare the proportion of a certain exposure between case and control groups. These studies are often susceptible to recall bias as patients with knowledge of their disease are likely to recall being subjected to a particular exposure (e.g., high-tension power lines). However, case-control studies are very useful for identifying risk factors of a rare disease. Additionally, confounding factors (i.e., factors that are associated with both the disease and exposure) may also introduce bias. In this case, matched case-control studies are used to minimize confounding. For example, when attempting to identify risk factors for type II diabetes through a case-control study, it is important to control for age because age is associated with both type II diabetes and various exposures.

25.5.4 Cohort Study

Cohort studies are prospective studies that follow a predetermined disease-free group of patients over a period of time. As the study progresses, some individuals develop the disease and others do not. The development of the disease is then related to the exposure variables observed over the time period of the study. These studies sometimes require a long span of time, during which loss of patients is likely to occur. Cohort studies are useful when examining the effect of various risk factors on the development of disease.

25.5.5 Cross-Sectional Study

In cross-sectional studies, the patient population is asked about their current disease status and current and/or past exposure status to various risk factors. Cross-sectional studies compare the prevalence of disease at one point in time between exposed and unexposed individuals. This is different than the prospective (cohort) study where the incidence of disease rather than prevalence of disease is investigated.

25.5.6 Clinical Trials

Clinical trials are distinguished by several traits that help make their findings more valid and reliable. Good clinical trials are randomized, which helps to minimize selection bias. They could be double-blinded, which minimizes measurement bias by reducing confounding by investigators and patients who may be aware of the therapy they are giving or receiving. Multi-centered trials reduce confounding due to local or regional differences and limited sample sizes. Placebo controls help to ensure that the trial is double-blind and helps to reduce measurement bias. A crossover design ensures that a patient receives a therapy for at least half of the trial and a placebo for the remainder – it helps to serve as an internal control and reduces measurement bias. The best clinical trials incorporate as many of these traits as possible. They are designed in such a way that their outcomes can typically be trusted if all tenets of the study design are faithfully followed. The major determent to clinical trials is their high cost. One note regarding clinical trials: in order for a randomized study to be properly evaluated, the sample size must be carefully predetermined.

25.6 Measures of Associations Between Two Binary Variables

Depending on the study design, different measures of association can be used to display relationships between variables. As mentioned earlier, the chi-square test of independence can be used to test the null hypothesis that the exposure and disease are not associated with each other against the alternative that there is an association. However, there are several methods to measure associations between two binary variables including odds ratio and relative risk. In a case-control study, where a

		Disease	
		+	−
Exposure	+	*a*	*b*
	−	*c*	*d*

Fig. 25.3 Illustration of the four possible scenarios from a "disease-exposure" relationship

group of patients who have the disease are compared to a group of patients who do not have the disease with respect to their exposure, the data can be organized in the form of a 2×2 contingency table, as shown in Fig. 25.3.

25.6.1 Odds Ratio

The odds ratio is a descriptive statistic that can be thought of as determining the strength of an association between two binary variables. The odds ratio is defined as the ratio of odds of exposure among patients who have the disease relative to the odds of exposure among patients who do not have the disease. The odds of an event refers to the probability of the event occurring over the probability of the event not occurring. Simply, the odds ratio is calculated by the formula given in Eq. 25.14. It is often used in retrospective, case-control and cross-sectional studies to evaluate the particular effect of a risk factor on disease.

$$\text{Odds Ratio} = \frac{d}{b} \tag{25.14}$$

Standard statistical packages provide 95 % confidence intervals for odds ratios. If the 95 % confidence intervals for odds ratios do not include 1, then one can conclude that there is an association between the disease and exposure. Also there is a formula for calculating the 95 % confidence intervals for odds ratios based on the information in the contingency table. For additional information we refer the reader to Rosner's textbook, *Fundamentals of Biostatistics*.

25.6.2 Relative Risk

Relative risk is used to compare the chance of a particular disease between the exposed and non-exposed groups. For example, in a cohort study, the risk of a smoker developing lung cancer would be compared to the group of nonsmokers and the result given in terms of the relative risk of lung cancer. Relative risk is calculated as follows:

$$\text{Relative Risk} = \frac{\mathrm{a}/(a+b)}{c/(c+d)} \tag{25.15}$$

Standard statistical packages also provide 95 % confidence intervals for relative risk. If the 95 % confidence intervals for relative risks do not include 1, then one can conclude that there is an association between the disease and exposure. The formula for calculating the 95 % confidence intervals for relative risks can be found in Rosner's textbook, *Fundamentals of Biostatistics*. The relative risk must be used with care as minor differences in risks between the two groups can result in a large ratio. In these cases, you must also report the absolute risk for the disease, which is simply the probability of the disease.

25.6.3 Attributable Risk

To compare risks of disease between exposed and non-exposed groups in a cohort study, one can calculate the attributable risk. It is calculated as the difference between the incidence of disease in exposed group and incidence of disease in non-exposed group (Eq. 25.16). Therefore, it represents the additional incidence of disease related to exposures and often called the risk difference.

$$\text{Attributable Risk} = \frac{a}{a+b} - \frac{c}{c+d} \tag{25.16}$$

25.6.4 Associations vs. Causal Relationships

It is important to note that associations do not imply causal relationships. In fact, in clinical research it is very difficult to establish causal relationships. Depending on the study design, one can build evidence for or against a causal relationship. For example, in randomized control trials it is easier to establish causal relationships than in retrospective studies. Randomized controlled trials with adequate sample size and blinding are usually the best evidence for a cause and effect relationship.

When investigating whether an exposure has a causal relationship with a disease, it is important to evaluate if the association is an artifact of measurement bias or random variation (chance). If the association is not due to bias and seems unlikely, then one must consider if the association is occurring indirectly, potentially through confounding factors. If one does not find confounding and the study is well designed, a causal relationship is likely. For more detailed discussion on causality, we refer the reader to Fletcher's book, *Clinical Epidemiology*, and Rothman's book, *Modern Epidemiology*.

25.7 Diagnostic Tests

So far the focus of this chapter has been on the use of statistics in the development of various clinical studies to investigate the associations between exposures and disease. However, clinicians are also interested in assessing the predictive power of diagnostic tests. In order to assess the accuracy of a diagnostic test result, one must know the person's true status of the disease. Results from a diagnostic test can be classified as true positives, true negatives, false positives, and false negatives, as illustrated in Fig. 25.4. A true positive occurs when a test designed to determine the presence of a disease reports a correct answer. A true negative occurs when a test correctly reports that a disease is not present. False positives can be psychologically detrimental to a patient, such as when a test reports positive HIV status when the patient actually does not have this disease. They can also result in increased cost of care for unnecessary treatments since the patient has been falsely identified as diseased. False negatives can prevent a patient from receiving therapy when a test incorrectly reports that a patient does not have a disease.

		Disease		Total
		+	−	
Test	+	TP	FP	TP + FP
	−	FN	TN	FN + TN
Total		TP + FN	FP + TN	

Fig. 25.4 The four results that can be obtained from a test for a particular disease, along with the calculations for sensitivity, specificity, positive predictive value, and negative predictive value

25.7.1 Sensitivity

Sensitivity is a measure of the proportion of true positives, calculated as the number of people who tested positive among all who have the disease (Eq. 25.17). A highly sensitive test will have a low rate of false negatives. Further, if the sensitivity is high enough and the test results negative, one can trust that the patient does not have a disease. Sensitive tests are often valuable as screening tests for a population.

$$\text{Sensitivity} = \frac{\text{TP}}{\text{TP} + \text{FN}} \tag{25.17}$$

25.7.2 Specificity

Specificity is a measure of the proportion of true negatives, calculated as the number of people who tested negative among all who do not have the disease (Eq. 25.18). Specific tests have very low rates of false positives, so a true-positive result is considered to be trustworthy. If a patient obtains a positive result on a specific test, they are effectively ruled in for a particular disease.

$$\text{Specificity} = \frac{\text{TN}}{\text{TN} + \text{FP}} \quad (25.18)$$

25.7.3 Positive Predictive Value

Positive predictive values are used to determine the chance of having a disease given a positive test result. It is calculated as the number of true positives divided by the total of positive test results (Eq. 25.19). The positive predictive value is used in conjunction with the pretest probability to determine the chance the patient truly has a disease. For example, doing a test for the Ebola virus is unlikely to be meaningful, even with a positive result, on a healthy American in Nebraska who has never traveled to Africa.

$$\text{Positive Predictive Value} = \frac{\text{TP}}{\text{TP} + \text{FP}} \quad (25.19)$$

25.7.4 Negative Predictive Value

The negative predictive value determines the chance of not having a particular disease given a negative test result. It is calculated as the number of true negatives divided by the total number of negative test results (Eq. 25.20). The negative predictive value is also used in conjunction with pretest probability and clinical suspicion to determine whether a patient is likely to have a particular disease.

$$\text{Negative Predictive Value} = \frac{\text{TN}}{\text{TN} + \text{FN}} \quad (25.20)$$

25.8 Summary and Conclusions

In this chapter we discussed the steps towards developing a successful clinical study beginning with identifying one's target population. Once the population is identified, a research question is formulated into a testing hypothesis, when possible, and an appropriate study design is implemented. Accordingly, data is collected in a randomized non-bias fashion to improve data quality and is analyzed using various significance tests. Additionally, associations can be assessed using odds ratio, relative risk, and attributable risk. We hope that this chapter has provided a basic understanding of clinical study design and testing hypotheses and illustrated the importance of biostatistics in clinical and translational research. However, we acknowledge that the material provided here may not be sufficient to independently design a clinical study. Therefore, we strongly recommend that you consult biostatisticians and epidemiologists when designing complex clinical and translational studies.

References

1. Guyatt G, Jaeschke R, Heddle N, Cook D, Shannon H, Walter S. Basic statistics for clinicians: 1. Hypothesis testing. CMAJ. 1995;152(1):27–32. Review.
2. Guyatt G, Jaeschke R, Heddle N, Cook D, Shannon H, Walter S. Basic statistics for clinicians: 2. Interpreting study results: confidence intervals. CMAJ. 1995;152(2):169–73.
3. Jaeschke R, Guyatt G, Shannon H, Walter S, Cook D, Heddle N. Basic statistics for clinicians: 3. Assessing the effects of treatment: measures of association. CMAJ. 1995;152(3):351–7.
4. Guyatt G, Walter S, Shannon H, Cook D, Jaeschke R, Heddle N. Basic statistics for clinicians: 4. Correlation and regression. CMAJ. 1995;152(4): 497–504.
5. Hayward RS, Wilson MC, Tunis SR, Bass EB, Guyatt G. Users' Guides to the medical literature. VIII. How to use clinical practice guidelines. A. Are the recommendations valid? The Evidence-Based Medicine Working Group. JAMA. 1995;274(7): 570–4.
6. Wilson MC, Hayward RS, Tunis SR, Bass EB, Guyatt G. Users' guides to the Medical Literature. VIII. How to use clinical practice guidelines. B. what are the recommendations and will they help you in caring for your patients? The Evidence-Based Medicine Working Group. JAMA. 1995;274(20): 1630–2.
7. Guyatt GH, Sackett DL, Sinclair JC, Hayward R, Cook DJ, Cook RJ. Users' guides to the medical literature. IX. A method for grading health care recommendations. Evidence-Based Medicine Working Group. JAMA. 1995;274(22):1800–4.
8. Levin LA, Danesh-Meyer HV. Lost in translation: bumps in the road between bench and bedside. JAMA. 2010;303:1533–4.

9. Baggerly KA, Morris JS, Edmonson SR, Coombes KR. Signal in Noise: Evaluating Reported Reproducibility of Serum Proteomic Tests for Ovarian Cancer. J Natl Cancer Inst. 2005;97:307–9.
10. Ransohoff DF, Gourlay ML. Sources of bias in specimens for research about molecular markers for cancer. J Clin Oncol. 2010;28:698–704.
11. Ioannidis JP. Why most published research findings are false. PLoS Med. 2005;2:e124.
12. Rosner B. Fundamentals of biostatistics. 6th ed. Stamford: Thomson Learning; 2006.
13. Fletcher R, Fletcher S. Clinical epidemiology: the essentials. 4th ed. New York: Lippincott Williams and Wilkins; 2005.
14. Rothman KJ, Greenland S, editors. Modern epidemiology. 2nd ed. Philadelphia: Lippincott Williams & Wilkins; 1998.

Vein Anesthesia

26

David O. Joseph, Jessica L. Myers, and Eugene W. Moretti

Contents

Abstract

Local anesthesia and tumescent anesthesia play a key role in the success of phlebology procedures. This chapter reviews key principles of these procedures. Local anesthetics have been used for decades by physicians to provide pain relief during simple surgical procedures. The utility of this is twofold: first, they provide a degree of anesthesia at the operative site that decreases or even eliminates the need for general anesthesia; second, they can provide several hours of analgesia that decreases the amount of narcotic given both intra- and postoperatively.

26.1 Introduction

Local anesthesia and tumescent anesthesia play a key role in the success of phlebology procedures. This chapter reviews key principles of these procedures.

26.2 Local Anesthesia

26.2.1 Discovery and Development

Local anesthetics have been used for decades by physicians to provide pain relief during simple surgical procedures. The utility of this is twofold: first, they provide a degree of anesthesia at the operative site that decreases or even eliminates the need for general anesthesia; second, they can

D.O. Joseph, MD, MS
Department of Anesthesia, University of Texas at Houston Medical School, Houston, TX, USA
e-mail: david.o.joseph@uth.tmc.edu

J.L. Myers, MD • E.W. Moretti, MD, MHsc (✉)
Department of Anesthesiology, Duke University Medical Center, Durham, NC, USA
e-mail: jmeyers728@yahoo.com
eugene.moretti@dm.duke.edu

E. Mowatt-Larssen et al. (eds.), *Phlebology, Vein Surgery and Ultrasonography*,
DOI 10.1007/978-3-319-01812-6_26, © Springer International Publishing Switzerland 2014

provide several hours of analgesia that decreases the amount of narcotic given both intra- and postoperatively.

Cocaine was the first local anesthetic discovered. South American Indians would chew the leaves of the plant *Erythroxylum coca* to increase their physical endurance when working. They also found that chewing coca leaves would make their mouths and tongues numb. This finding prompted a German graduate student by the name of Niemann to isolate cocaine from the leaves of the coca plant in 1860. Eventually, due to its ability to anesthetize the cornea, it was used as a local anesthetic for glaucoma surgery [1, 2]. Subsequent to this, cocaine use for regional and local anesthesia became widespread in Europe and the USA. However, the toxic effects of the drug were soon elucidated after deaths were reported of both patients and medical staff whom had become addicted. It was not until advances in organic chemistry in 1891 that newer local anesthetics could be synthesized, specifically the amino esters (e.g., tropocaine, eucaine, holocaine, orthoform, benzocaine, and tetracaine). The amino amides were developed between 1898 and 1972 (e.g., nirvaquine, procaine, chloroprocaine, cinchocaine, lidocaine, mepivacaine, prilocaine, efocaine, bupivacaine, etidocaine, and articaine). Both the amino esters and amino amides demonstrated significantly less toxicity than cocaine, and many are still in mainstream use today (Table 26.1).

Bupivacaine was first synthesized in 1957 and was of particular interest because of its long duration of action. Major side effects of bupivacaine include central nervous system and cardiovascular toxicity [3–6]. Ropivacaine is an alternative local anesthetic with fewer toxicities and is derived from the optically active isomers of mepivacaine [3, 7].

Table 26.1 Commonly used local anesthetics

Esters	Amides
Procaine (Novocain®)	Lidocaine (Xylocaine®)
Chloroprocaine (Nesacaine®)	Mepivacaine (Polocaine® or Carbocaine®)
	Bupivacaine (Marcaine®)
	Prilocaine (Citanest®)
	Ropivacaine (Naropin®)

26.2.2 Pharmacology

The mechanism of action for local anesthetics is an alteration of sodium conduction across the neuronal cell membrane. The resting membrane potential is established across a neuronal membrane by the sodium/potassium ATPase pump. This results in a cell membrane with a negative electrical potential of about −70 mV. When a stimulus is applied to a neuron, there is an initial opening of the sodium channels and a positive change in membrane potential. When a certain threshold is met (approximately −55 mV), a larger opening of voltage-gated sodium channels produces an action potential which is propagated as an impulse along the neuronal cell (Fig. 26.1). This impulse also conducts pain signals from a peripheral nerve to the spinal cord and subsequently to the brain. Local anesthetics exert their effect mainly by blocking the sodium conduction necessary for the initiation and propagation of the action potential. Sodium channels are membrane proteins that consist of a large alpha subunit and one or two smaller beta subunits. The alpha subunit allows the passage of sodium ions [8, 9]. Local anesthetics bind to a specific site on the alpha subunit from inside the cell. The voltage-gated sodium channels exist in three states: the resting, activated, and inactivated states. Local anesthetics have a greater affinity for the sodium channel when in the inactivated and activated states as compared to the resting state; therefore, local anesthetics exert their greatest effect on nerves that are firing rapidly [10].

Local anesthetics are compounds that exist in solution. The pKa of a compound in solution is the pH at which 50 % of the compound exists in ionic form and 50 % exists in nonionic form. The tendency to release hydrogen ion determines a compound's strength as an acid, and the tendency to bind hydrogen ion determines its strength as a base. As the pH decreases, there are more hydrogen ions in solution and therefore a greater tendency for the compound to hold on to hydrogen. As the pH increases, there are fewer hydrogen ions in solution, and therefore it increases the tendency of the compound to release hydrogen into solution. Local anesthetics are weak bases. Structurally they exist

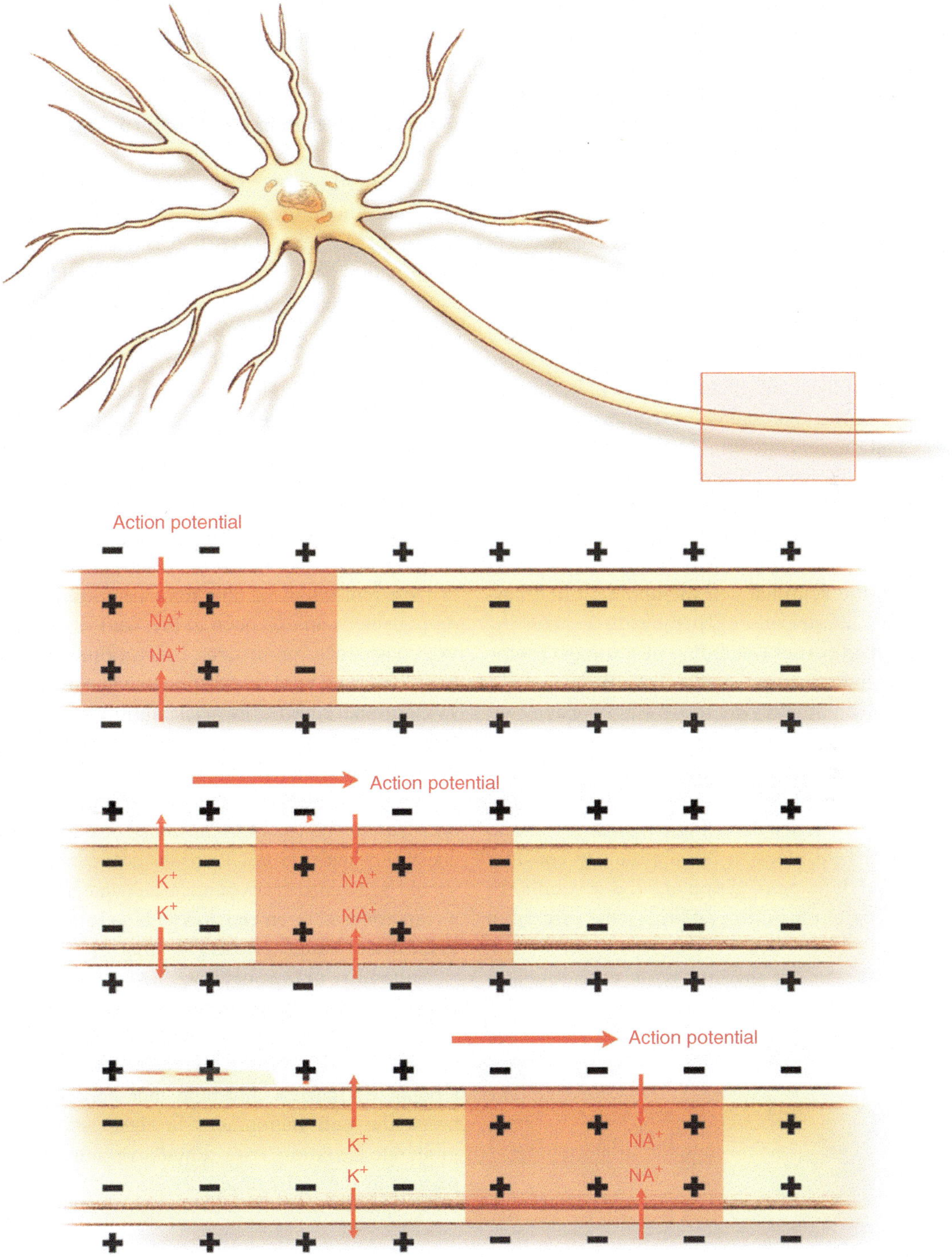

Fig. 26.1 Propagation of an action potential

as amino esters or amino amides. The amino group when bound to a hydrogen ion forms a charged species. It should be noted also that the amino group on local anesthetics has a pKa that is higher than physiological pH.

Therefore, if a local anesthetic has a low pKa or one that is close to physiological pH, it has a higher proportion of non-ionized species and can gain access to a neuronal cell better compared to a compound that has a high pKa; this is the case as non-ionized compounds tend to be more lipophilic and thereby penetrate the cell membrane more readily. An alternative explanation for the function of local anesthetics involves altering the fluidity of the neuronal cell membrane in such a way that the conformation of the sodium channel changes, thereby changing its conductance [2, 11]. When a local anesthetic has a pKa close to physiological pH, it has a higher concentration of its non-ionized, lipophilic form that can pass through the neuronal cell membrane; this translates into a faster onset [7]. Table 26.2 shows the physical properties (including pKa values) for the more commonly used local anesthetics [10–13].

Local anesthetics in the form of esters are eliminated via plasma esterases, while the amides are absorbed into the circulation and eventually metabolized by the liver and excreted by the kidneys [1, 14]. When choosing which anesthetic to use for a field block, it is important to consider onset and duration of action and the suitability of tissue for a block. In addition, the use of a vasoconstrictor and the maximum dose of local anesthetic are of equal importance.

Table 26.2 Physical properties of the commonly used local anesthetics

	Concentration (%)	pKa	pH	Onset
Esters				
Procaine	0.25–0.5	8.9	3.5–5	Fast
Chloroprocaine	1–2	9	4.5	Fast
Amides				
Lidocaine	1–2	7.7	5.0–7.0	Fast
Prilocaine	1	7.7	4.5	Fast
Mepivacaine	1	7.6	4.5–6.8	Fast
Bupivacaine	0.25	8.1	4–6.5	Fast
Ropivacaine[a]	0.5	8.2	5.5–6.0	Fast

[a]Onset is listed with regard to local infiltration. Ropivacaine has a slower onset time when used for peripheral nerve blocks

26.2.3 Onset and Duration of Action

Lipid solubility can affect onset of action for a local anesthetic (Table 26.2). Increased concentration of the drug (even if it is known to be a drug of slow onset) can speed up the initiation of the block; such is the case with chloroprocaine (pKa 9 and ionized proportion of 97 %). The onset and duration of action are also affected by the target tissue: highly vascular tissues may take the drug away from the site and limit its maximum effect. Uptake is slower for highly lipid-soluble drugs and those that avidly bind to protein. Generally, amides tend to have a longer duration of action than esters (Table 26.3).

Most local anesthetics are vasodilators which increase removal of the drug from the operative site; ropivacaine is an exception to this with its intrinsic vasoconstrictive properties. Epinephrine can be added to most local anesthetics to cause vasoconstriction and improve its availability to the tissue. Epinephrine also significantly increases duration of action for infiltration anesthesia and peripheral nerve blocks when used with the shorter-duration local anesthetics. The use of a vasoconstrictor and local anesthetics with intrinsic vasoconstrictive properties should be avoided in an operative field that has either a compromised or an end arterial blood supply due to the risk of tissue necrosis [14, 15].

Suitability of the operative site is an important consideration; infected tissue is a poor target site for an infiltrative local anesthetic block. Infection causes a lowering of the pH, leading to a greater amount of ionized molecule that poorly penetrates the cell membrane. In these situations, moderate sedation with adjunctive intravenous pain control may be necessary.

26.2.4 Calculating Dosage and Drug Administration

When administering local anesthetics, the maximum dosage of the drug that can be safely given

Table 26.3 Maximum dosages allowable for the administration of infiltrative local anesthesia

Esters	Maximum dose (plain) (mg/kg)	Duration of action (plain)	Maximum dose (with epinephrine)	Duration of action (with epinephrine)
Procaine	5	20–30 min	7 mg/kg	30 min
Chloroprocaine	11	15–30 min	14 mg/kg	30 min
Lidocaine	4	30 min to 2 h	7 mg/kg	Up to 3 h
Mepivacaine[a]	4	1.5–3 h	7 mg/kg	Approximately 20–30 % longer
Prilocaine	7	30 min to 1.5 h	8 mg/kg	Up to 2 h
Bupivacaine[b]	2	2–4 h	3 mg/kg	3–4 h
Ropivacaine	5	2–6 h	N/A	N/A

[a]Avoid in pregnancy
[b]Avoid in pregnancy until term

is of great importance. Due to its vasoconstrictive properties, epinephrine often allows greater amounts of local anesthesia to be used as it limits systemic toxicity by decreasing absorption from the operative site. The maximum dose is expressed in milligrams per kilogram of the patient's body weight. Concentration of local anesthetics is expressed as a percentage (e.g., 0.25 % bupivacaine or 1 % lidocaine). The conversion is as follows: 1 % = 10 mg/mL. The relative contraindication for the use of epinephrine is in patients at risk of myocardial ischemia, as accidental intravenous injection can lead to tachyarrhythmias and myocardial ischemia. Other patients at increased risk are those with hyperthyroidism or on medications that alter the effects of catecholamines (e.g., monoamine oxidase inhibitors and tricyclic antidepressants) [1].

26.2.5 Toxicity and Treatment of Toxicity

Toxicity to local anesthetics can be either local or systemic; local adverse effects can manifest as paresthesias, while systemic toxicity manifests as cardiovascular (CV) or central nervous system (CNS) problems such as hypotension, tinnitus, confusion, and respiratory depression. Toxic reactions such as anaphylaxis or methemoglobinemia can also occasionally occur, especially with benzocaine, lidocaine, and prilocaine. Higher levels of methemoglobin (20–45 %) may cause headache, lethargy, tachycardia, or dizziness. Shortness of breath, arrhythmias, cardiac failure, and seizures occur at levels >45 %. Above 70 %, there is a high risk of mortality. Methylene blue 1 % can be given at a dose of 1–2 mL/kg for treatment. If methemoglobinemia persists, this dose can be repeated 30–60 min later [2, 12].

Comorbidities like renal or hepatic failure, respiratory acidosis, heart block, or other cardiac problems can worsen the severity of these reactions. Pregnancy and extremes of age are also conditions that warrant caution with the use of local anesthetics [7]. In fact, mepivacaine is contraindicated in pregnancy because of poor fetal metabolism (hepatic immaturity). Bupivacaine is also contraindicated in the parturient due to the physiological changes associated with pregnancy as well as direct effects of progesterone [12]. It is important to remember, however, that the primary cause for systemic toxicity is an unintentional intravascular injection of local anesthetic [7].

Allergies to local anesthetics can manifest as rash or urticaria. Anaphylaxis is extremely uncommon, but it should never be overlooked. Acute allergic reactions associated with the amino esters are usually caused by a hypersensitivity reaction to para-aminobenzoic acid (PABA). Some preparations of amino amides contain methylparaben, a compound chemically similar to PABA, and this may be a source of allergic reactions that occur in this group [7, 15].

The American Society of Regional Anesthesia and the Association of Anaesthetists of Great Britain and Ireland suggest a management strategy for systemic local anesthetic toxicity [16, 17]. The first step is to stop the injection of local anesthetic and call for help. Next, an airway should be established and maintained, providing the patient with 100 % oxygen. IV access should be quickly established if not already present. Seizures should be controlled with a benzodiazepine or propofol given in small boluses. The cardiovascular status of the patient should be continuously monitored, and in the event of collapse, cardiopulmonary resuscitation (CPR) should be performed and arrhythmias should be identified and treated appropriately.

Another option is treatment with a lipid emulsion, commercially known as Intralipid®. This should be a 20 % solution given as a bolus of 1.5 mL/kg over 1 min with an infusion started at 0.25 mL/kg/min. The boluses may be repeated every 5 min if needed. Recovery from local anesthetic-induced cardiac arrest can take up to an hour; success in these cases is noted to occur with lipid emulsion treatment after local anesthetic toxicity was recognized [18–21]. Animal studies have also shown recovery from local anesthetic-induced cardiac toxicity with the same treatment [22–25].

Small needle size and slow injection are very important. Subcutaneous infiltration can cause a lot of pain. Also, remember to always draw back on the syringe after advancing the needle to avoid an inadvertent intravascular injection of local anesthetic.

26.3 Tumescent Anesthesia

First described by Klein for liposuction in 1987, tumescent anesthesia (TA) is now used during thermal ablation and ambulatory phlebectomy. During TA, dilute lidocaine is infiltrated around a target vein that will be ablated or removed. In thermal ablation, the surrounding fluid acts as a heat sink for the laser or radiofrequency energy to prevent perivenous structure damage, provides local anesthesia, and compresses the vein to improve the thermal effect. In ambulatory phlebectomy, TA provides local anesthesia, hypodissects targeted veins to make their removal easier, and reduces postoperative hematoma and ecchymosis risk due to the compression of surrounding tissues.

Table 26.4 A common formula to produce 500 mL of tumescent anesthesia

445 mL of saline 0.9 %
50 mL of lidocaine 1 % with epinephrine 1:100,000
5 mL of sodium bicarbonate 8.4 %

A common TA dilution of lidocaine is 0.1 %. Epinephrine is often used to assist in vasoconstriction. Epinephrine can be withheld in patients who may be at risk for adverse events, such as patients with a history of tachydysrhythmias or myocardial ischemia. Sodium bicarbonate can also be added to decrease injection pain.

One common formula to produce 500 mL of TA is shown in Table 26.4. This formula provides a total of 500 mg of lidocaine, close to the 7 mg/kg dose if used with epinephrine for a 70 kg patient. This recommended dose has not been verified in the medical literature, although it is still commonly respected. Still, doses of 35 mg/kg and even 55 mg/kg have been found safe in separate studies.

There are pumps which can assist in delivery of TA. Chapters 7, 10, and 12 provide further details of ultrasound guidance and TA use in thermal and surgical ablations.

References

1. Ahlstrom KK, Frodel JL. Local anesthetics for facial plastic procedures. Otolaryngol Clin North Am. 2002;35:29–53.
2. Culp Jr WC, Culp Sr WC. Practical application of local anesthetics. J Vasc Interv Radiol. 2010;22:111–8.
3. Ruetsch YA, Boni T, Borgeat A. From cocaine to ropivacaine: the history of local anesthetic drugs. Curr Top Med Chem. 2001;1(3):175–82.
4. Mather LE, Long GJ, Thomas J. The intravenous toxicity and clearance of bupivacaine in man. Clin Pharmacol Ther. 1971;12(6):935–43.
5. Scott DB. Evaluation of the local toxicity of anaesthetics in man. Br J Anaesth. 1975;47(1):56–61.
6. Scott DB, Jebson PJ, Boyes RN. Pharmacokinetic study of the local anaesthetics bupivacaine (Marcain) and etidocaine (Duranest) in man. Br J Anaesth. 1973;45(10):1010–2.

7. Kapitanyan R, Su M. Toxicity, local anesthetics. eMedicine. Available at http://emedicine.medscape.com. 2010. Accessed on 24 Feb 2011.
8. Bray JJ, Cragg PA, Macknight AD, Mills RG, Taylor DW. Lecture notes on human physiology. 3rd ed. Oxford/Boston: Blackwell Science; 1994.
9. Marban E, Yamagishi T, Tomaselli GF. Structure and function of voltage-gated sodium channels. J Physiol. 1998;308(5):647–57.
10. Morgan GE, Mikhail MS, Murray ML. Clinical anesthesiology. 4th ed. New York: McGraw Hill; 2006.
11. Barash PG, Cullen BF, Stoelting RK. Clinical anesthesia. 5th ed. Philadelphia: Lippincott Williams & Wilkins; 2006.
12. Tetzlaff JE. The pharmacology of local anesthetics. Anesthesiol Clin North America. 2000;18: 217–31.
13. Windle ML. Local anesthetic agents, infiltrative administration. eMedicine. http://emedicine.medscape.com. 2009. Accessed on 25 Feb 2011.
14. Miller RD. Miller's anesthesia. 6th ed. New York: Elsevier Churchill Livingstone; 2005.
15. Achar S, Kundu S. Principles of office anesthesia: part I. Infiltrative anesthesia. Am Fam Physician. 2002;66(1):91–4.
16. Neal JM, Bernards CM, Butterworth JF, DiGregorio G, Drasner K, Hejtmanek MR, Mulroy MF, Rosenquist RW, Weinberg GL. ASRA practice advisory on local anesthetic systemic toxicity. Reg Anesth Pain Med. 2010;35(2):152–61.
17. Guidelines for the management of severe local anaesthetic toxicity. The Association of Anaesthetists of Great Britain and Ireland. Available at http://www.aagbi.org/news.htm#115. 2007. Accessed on 25 Feb 2011.
18. Dix SK, Rosner GF, Nayar M, Harris JJ, Guglin ME, Winterfield JR, Xiong Z, Mudge Jr GH. Intractable cardiac arrest due to lidocaine toxicity successfully resuscitated with lipid emulsion. Crit Care Med. 2011;39(4):872–4.
19. Litz RJ, Popp M, Stehr SN, Koch T. Successful resuscitation of a patient with ropivacaine-induced asystole after axillary plexus block using lipid infusion. Anaesthesia. 2006;61(8):800–1.
20. Litz RJ, Roessel T, Heller AR, Stehr SN. Reversal of central nervous system and cardiac toxicity after local anesthetic intoxication by lipid emulsion injection. Anesth Analg. 2008;106(5):1575–7.
21. Ludot H, Tharin JY, Belouadah M, Mazoit JX, Malinovsky JM. Successful resuscitation after ropivacaine and lidocaine-induced ventricular arrhythmia following posterior lumbar plexus block in a child. Anesth Analg. 2008;106(5):1572–4.
22. Cave G, Harvey MG, Winterbottom T. Evaluation of the Association of Anaesthetists of Great Britain and Ireland lipid infusion protocol in bupivacaine-induced cardiac arrest in rabbits. Anaesthesia. 2009;64(7): 732–7.
23. Weinberg G, Ripper R, Feinstein DL, Hoffman W. Lipid emulsion infusion rescues dogs from bupivacaine-induced cardiac toxicity. Reg Anesth Pain Med. 2003;28(3):198–202.
24. Weinberg G, VadeBoncouer T, Ramaraju GA, Garcia-Amaro MF, Cwik MJ. Pretreatment or resuscitation with a lipid infusion shifts the dose–response to bupivacaine-induced asystole in rats. Anesthesiology. 1998;88:1071–5.
25. Corman S, Skledar S. Use of lipid emulsion to reverse local anesthetic-induced toxicity. Ann Pharmacother. 2007;41:1873–7.

Index

E. Mowatt-Larssen et al. (eds.), *Phlebology, Vein Surgery and Ultrasonography*,
DOI 10.1007/978-3-319-01812-6, © Springer International Publishing Switzerland 2014

D

M

W

GPSR Compliance

The European Union's (EU) General Product Safety Regulation (GPSR) is a set of rules that requires consumer products to be safe and our obligations to ensure this.

If you have any concerns about our products, you can contact us on ProductSafety@springernature.com

In case Publisher is established outside the EU, the EU authorized representative is:

Springer Nature Customer Service Center GmbH
Europaplatz 3
69115 Heidelberg, Germany

Batch number: 10632888

Printed by Printforce, the Netherlands